Pain Management in Vulnerable Populations

Pain Management in Vulnerable Populations

Edited by

PAUL J. CHRISTO, ROLLIN M. GALLAGHER,
JOANNA G. KATZMAN, AND KAYODE A. WILLIAMS

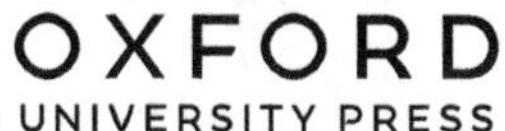

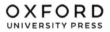

OXFORD
UNIVERSITY PRESS

Oxford University Press is a department of the University of Oxford. It furthers the University's objective of excellence in research, scholarship, and education by publishing worldwide. Oxford is a registered trade mark of Oxford University Press in the UK and certain other countries.

Published in the United States of America by Oxford University Press
198 Madison Avenue, New York, NY 10016, United States of America.

Library of Congress Cataloging-in-Publication Data
Names: Christo, Paul J., editor. | Gallagher, Rollin M., editor | Katzman, Joanna G., editor.
Title: Pain management in vulnerable populations /
edited by Paul J. Christo, Rollin M. Gallagher, Joanna G. Katzman, and Kayode A. Williams
Description: New York, NY : Oxford University Press, [2024] |
Includes bibliographical references and index.
Identifiers: LCCN 2023040834 (print) | LCCN 2023040835 (ebook) |
ISBN 9780197649176 (paperback) | ISBN 9780197649190 (epub) |
ISBN 9780197649206 (online)
Subjects: MESH: Chronic Pain | Pain Management | Vulnerable Populations |
Social Determinants of Health | Health Status Disparities
Classification: LCC RB127.5.C48 (print) | LCC RB127.5.C48 (ebook) |
NLM WL 704 | DDC 616/.0472—dc23/eng/20231117
LC record available at https://lccn.loc.gov/2023040834
LC ebook record available at https://lccn.loc.gov/2023040835

DOI: 10.1093/med/9780197649176.001.0001

Printed by Marquis Book Printing, Canada

Contents

Contributors

Steven Amaefuna, MD
Department of Anesthesiology and Critical Care Medicine
Johns Hopkins School of Medicine
Baltimore, MD, USA

Marcus Anthony, MD
Department of Medicine
New York University Grossman School of Medicine
New York, NY, USA

Maya Armstrong, MD
Attending Physician, Turquoise Lodge Hospital
Albuquerque, NM, USA
Volunteer Faculty, Family and Community Medicine
University of New Mexico
Albuquerque, NM, USA

Ramin Asgary, MD, MPH, FASTMH
Professor of Global Health and International Affairs
Department of Global Health, Milken Institute School of Public Health
George Washington University
Washington, DC, USA
and
Associate Clinical Professor of Medicine
Department of Medicine
Icahn School of Medicine at Mount Sinai
New York, USA

Antje M. Barreveld, MD
Tufts University School of Medicine
Boston, Massachusetts
Commonwealth Anesthesia Associates
Newton-Wellesley Hospital
Newton, MA, USA

Austin G. Bell, MD, MAJ, MC, USA
Department of Anesthesiology
Dwight D. Eisenhower Army Medical Center
Fort Gordon, Georgia

Allison M. Berken, MD, MPH
Tufts University School of Medicine
Boston, MA, USA
Commonwealth Anesthesia Associates
Newton-Wellesley Hospital
Newton, MA, USA

Lauren E. Berninger, DO, MBE
Assistant Professor, Department of Medicine
Division of General Internal Medicine, Johns Hopkins University School of Medicine
Section of Palliative Medicine
Baltimore, MD, USA

Snehal Bhatt, MD
Department of Psychiatry and Behavioral Sciences
University of New Mexico School of Medicine
Albuquerque, NM, USA

Donna Boruchov, MD
Department of Pediatric Hematology/Oncology at Connecticut Children's Medical Center
Associate Professor, University of Connecticut School of Medicine
Farmington, CT, USA

Nitin Budhwar, MD
Associate Professor, Department of Internal Medicine/Section of Geriatric Medicine
Health Sciences Center
University of New Mexico
Albuquerque, New Mexico

Mariana Bueno, RN, PhD
Child Health Evaluative Sciences
The Hospital for Sick Children
Toronto, Ontario, Canada

Captain Taylor J. Byrne, DO
CPT Taylor Byrne, DO
Department of Anesthesiology
Walter Reed Army Medical Center
Washington, DC, USA

Karen E. Cardon, MD, FASAM
VA New Mexico Healthcare System
Albuquerque, NM, USA
University of New Mexico School of Medicine
Albuquerque, NM, USA

Sydnee Chavis, DMD, MS
Special Care and Geriatrics
Department of Oral Surgery
University of Maryland School of Dentistry
Baltimore, MD, USA

Martin D. Cheatle, PhD
Department of Psychiatry and Anesthesiology and Critical Care
Perelman School of Medicine
University of Pennsylvania
Philadelphia, PA, USA

Sandy Christiansen, MD
Associate Professor
Department of Anesthesiology and Perioperative Medicine
Oregon Health and Science University
Portland, OR, USA

Paul J. Christo, MD, MBA
Departments of Anesthesiology and Critical Care Medicine, Physical Medicine and Rehabilitation
Interim Chief, Division of Pain Medicine
Associate Professor
Johns Hopkins University School of Medicine
Baltimore, MD, USA

Megan Coco, PhD, APRN, CPNP
Connecticut Children's Hospital
Center for Cancer and Blood Disorders
Chennai, India

Steven P. Cohen, MD
Departments of Anesthesiology and Critical Care Medicine, Neurology, Physical Medicine and Rehabilitation, and Psychiatry and Behavioral Sciences
Johns Hopkins School of Medicine
Baltimore, MD, USA
Departments of Physical Medicine and Rehabilitation, Anesthesiology, and Neurology
Walter Reed National Military Medical Center
Uniformed Services University of the Health Sciences
Bethesda, MD, USA

Kaitlyn Coyle, BS, MPH
Icahn School of Medicine at Mount Sinai
New York, NY, USA

Shae Datta, MD
Department of Neurology
NYU Long Island School of Medicine
Mineola, NY, USA
Concussion Center
NYU Langone Health
New York, NY, USA

Barbara DeLateur, MD, MS
Department of Physical Medicine and Rehabilitation
Johns Hopkins University School of Medicine
Baltimore, MD, USA

Anilla Del Fabbro, MD
Department of Psychiatry and Behavioral Medicine
Virginia Tech Carilion School of Medicine
Roanoke, VA, USA

Keisha G. Dodman, MD
Tufts University School of Medicine
Boston, Massachusetts
Commonwealth Anesthesia Associates
Newton-Wellesley Hospital
Newton, MA, USA

Tina Doshi, MD
Assistant Professor
Department of Anesthesiology and Critical Care Medicine | Division of Pain Medicine
Department of Neurosurgery
Johns Hopkins University School of Medicine
Baltimore, MD, USA

Sotonye Douglas, MS
The Frank H. Netter School of Medicine
Quinnipiac University

North Haven, CT, USA
Volunteer
Icahn School of Medicine at Mount Sinai
New York, NY, USA

David A. Edwards, MD, PhD
Departments of Anesthesiology and Neurological Surgery
Division of Pain Medicine
Vanderbilt University Medical Center
Nashville, TN, USA

Fola Faponle, MCBhB
Obafemi Awolowo University
Banjul City Council, The Gambia

Helen M. Fernandez, MD, MPH
Brookdale Department of Geriatrics and Palliative Medicine
Icahn School of Medicine at Mount Sinai
New York, NY, USA

Allen Finley, MD, FRCPC, FAAP
Department of Anesthesia
Dalhousie University
Halifax, Nova Scotia, Canada

Rebecca Freeland, MD
Department of Anesthesiology and Critical Care Medicine
Division of Pain Medicine
Johns Hopkins University School of Medicine
Baltimore, MD, USA

Rollin M. Gallagher, MD, MPH
Founding Editor-in-Chief, *Pain Medicine*
Retired: Clinical Professor of Psychiatry and Anesthesiology
Director for Pain Policy Research and Primary Care
Penn Pain Medicine, University of Pennsylvania (2004–18)
Philadelphia, PA, USA

Harold J. Gelfand, MD, FASA, CAPT, MC, USN
Defense and Veterans Center for Integrative Pain Management
Uniformed Services University of the Health Sciences
Bethesda, MD, USA

Mary Catherine George, MM, PhD
Icahn School of Medicine at Mount Sinai
New York, NY, USA

Cynthia M. A. Geppert, MD, PhD, DPS, MA, MPH, MSB, MSJ, FACLP, DFAPA, FASAM, HEC
Western Region VA National Center for Ethics in Health Care
Departments of Psychiatry and Internal Medicine
University of New Mexico School of Medicine
Albuquerque, NM, USA
Alden March Bioethics Institute
Albany Medical College
Albany, NY, USA

Suzanne Goldhirsch, MA, MSEd
Brookdale Department of Geriatrics and Palliative Medicine
Icahn School of Medicine at Mount Sinai
New York, NY, USA

Shanna-Kay Christa Griffiths, BA
Icahn School of Medicine at Mount Sinai
New York, NY, USA

Frey Gugsa, MD, MSc
Department of Anesthesiology & Critical Care Medicine
The Johns Hopkins University School of Medicine
Baltimore, MD, USA

Andrew Han, BS
Medical student
Georgetown University School of Medicine
Washington, DC, USA

Emily A. Haozous, PhD, RN, FAAN
Pacific Institute for Research and Evaluation
Albuquerque, NM, USA

Denise Harrison, RN, RM, BScN, PhD
Department of Nursing
The University of Melbourne
Melbourne, Victoria, Australia
School of Nursing
University of Ottawa
Ottawa, Ontario, Canada
Murdoch Children's Research Institute
Melbourne, Victoria, Australia
Royal Children's Hospital
Melbourne, Victoria, Australia

Vanessa Jacobsohn, MD
Department of Psychiatry and Behavioral Sciences
School of Medicine University of New Mexico
Albuquerque, NM, USA

Mary R. Janevic, PhD, MPH
Research Associate Professor
Department of Health Behavior and Health Education
University of Michigan School of Public Health
Washington, MI, USA

Kellie Jaremko, MD, PhD
Department of Anesthesiology and Critical Care Medicine
Johns Hopkins School of Medicine
Baltimore, MD, USA

Noelle Marie Javier, MD
Brookdale Department of Geriatrics and Palliative Medicine
Icahn School of Medicine at Mount Sinai
New York, NY, USA

Taranjeet S. Jolly, MD
Departments of Anesthesiology and Critical Care Medicine and Psychiatry and Behavioral Sciences
Johns Hopkins School of Medicine
Baltimore, MD, USA

Donna Kalauokalani, MD, MPH
Deputy Medical Executive
California Correctional Healthcare Services
California Department of Corrections and Rehabilitation
Elk Grove, CA, USA

William G. Katzman, MA
Clinical Psychology Program
Long Island University
Brooklyn, NY, USA

Lauren A. Kelly, MD, MPH, MS
Brookdale Department of Geriatrics and Palliative Medicine
Icahn School of Medicine at Mount Sinai
New York, NY, USA

Brinda Krish, MD
Department of Anesthesiology and Critical Care Medicine
Johns Hopkins School of Medicine
Baltimore, MD, USA

Caitlyn Kuwata, MD
Brookdale Department of Geriatrics and Palliative Medicine
Icahn School of Medicine at Mount Sinai
New York, NY, USA

Jeffrey M. Lackner, PhD
Department of Medicine
Division of Behavioral Medicine
University of Buffalo, The State University of New York
Buffalo, NY, USA

Michael Lynch, MD, FACMT
PA Department of Drug and Alcohol Programs
UPMC Health Plan Quality and Substance Use Disorder Services
UPMC Medical Toxicology Telemedicine Bridge Clinic
Pittsburgh, PA, USA
University of Pittsburgh School of Medicine
Pittsburgh, PA, USA

Shuran Ma, MD
Pain Medicine Fellow
Department of Anesthesiology and Perioperative Medicine
Oregon Health and Science University
Portland, OR, USA

Salvador L. Manrriquez, DDS
Department of Diagnostic Sciences, Anesthesia, and Emergency Medicine
Orofacial Pain and Oral Medicine Center
Herman Ostrow School of Dentistry of USC
Los Angeles, CA, USA

Salimah H. Meghani, PhD, MBE, RN, FAAN
Department of Biobehavioral Health Sciences
University of Pennsylvania
Philadelphia, PA, USA

Juan Andres Moncayo, MD
Pontificia Universidad Católica del Ecuador
School of Medicine
Quito, Pichincha, Ecuador

Jana M. Mossey, PhD, MPH, MSN
Department of Epidemiology
Dornsife School of Public Health
Drexel University
Philadelphia, PA, USA

Siddika S. Mulchan, PsyD
Assistant Professor, Department of Pediatrics
University of Connecticut School of Medicine
Farmington, CT, USA

Katarina Nikolic, MD
Department of Anesthesiology and Critical Care Medicine
Johns Hopkins School of Medicine
Baltimore, MD, USA

Gaston Nyirigira, MMed
King Faisal Hospital
Kigali, Rwanda
University of Rwanda
Kigali, Rwanda

Ashli A. Owen-Smith, PhD, SM
Associate Professor and MPH Program Director
Department of Health Policy and Behavioral Sciences
Georgia State University
School of Public Health
Atlanta, GA, USA

Tejas Ozarkar, MD
Department of Anesthesiology
Burnett School of Medicine at TCU
Fort Worth, TX, USA
Riordan Medical Institute
Southlake, TX, USA

Nicole Marie Pope, BN, RN, MPhil
The Royal Children's Hospital
Melbourne, Victoria, Australia
The University of Melbourne
Melbourne, Victoria, Australia

Hassan Rayaz, MD
Department of Anesthesiology and Critical Care Medicine
Johns Hopkins School of Medicine
Baltimore, MD, USA

Marcela Romero Reyes, DDS, PhD
Brotman Facial Pain Clinic
Department of Neural and Pain Sciences
University of Maryland School of Dentistry
Baltimore, MD, USA

Jessica Robinson-Papp, MD, MS, FAAN
Icahn School of Medicine at
Mount Sinai
New York, NY, USA

John Sampson, MD
Department of Anesthesiology and Critical Care Medicine
Johns Hopkins School of Medicine
Baltimore, MD, USA

Friedhelm Sandbrink, MD
Department of Neurology
Washington DC VA Medical Center
Washington, DC, USA
Uniformed Services University of the Health Sciences
Bethesda, MD, USA
George Washington University School of Medicine and Health Sciences
Washington, DC, USA

Jeffrey F. Scherrer
Vice Chair for Research, Department of Family and Community Medicine
Professor Department of Family and Community Medicine and
Professor in the Department of Psychiatry and Behavioral Neuroscience
Executive Director of Research, AHEAD Institute
Saint Louis University School of Medicine
St. Louis, MO, USA

Thomas J. Smith, MD, FACP, FASCO, FAAHPM
Director of Palliative Medicine, Johns Hopkins Medical Institutions
Division of General Internal Medicine, Section of Palliative Medicine, JHUSOM
Professor of Oncology, Sidney Kimmel Comprehensive Cancer Center
Harry J. Duffey Family Professor of Palliative Medicine
Baltimore, MD, USA

Olivia Sutton, MD
Department of Anesthesiology and Critical Care Medicine
Johns Hopkins School of Medicine
Baltimore, MD, USA

Raymond C. Tait, PhD
Department of Psychiatry and Behavioral Neuroscience
Saint Louis University School of Medicine
St. Louis, MO, USA

Oluwakemi Tomobi, MD, MEHP
Global Alliance of Perioperative Professionals
Department of Anesthesiology and Critical Care Medicine
Johns Hopkins University School of Medicine
Baltimore, MD, USA

Arissa Torrie, MD, MHS
Research Associate
Department of Orthopaedics
University of Maryland School of Medicine
Baltimore, MD, USA

Erin A. Tracy, MD, MAJ, MC, USAF
Department of Anesthesiology
Uniformed Services University of the Health Sciences
Bethesda, MD, USA

Annie T. Wang, MD
Department of Anesthesiology and Critical Care Medicine
Johns Hopkins University School of Medicine
Baltimore, MD, USA

Eric J. Wang, MD
Assistant Professor
Division of Pain Medicine
Department of Anesthesiology and Critical Care Medicine
Johns Hopkins University School of Medicine
Baltimore, MD, USA

Amanda C. de C. Williams, PhD, CPsychol
Professor of Clinical Health Psychology UCL
Research Department of Clinical, Educational & Health Psychology
University College London
London, UK

Major Sara M. Wilson, MD
Anesthesiology and Pain Management
Uniformed Services University of the Health Sciences
Bethesda, MD, USA

Rediet Shimeles Workneh, M.B.B.S
Addis Ababa University
College of Health Science
Black Lion Hospital
Addis Ababa, Ethiopia

1

Model of Pain in Vulnerable Populations and the Role of Social Determinants of Health

Salimah H. Meghani and Mary R. Janevic

Introduction

More than 50 million Americans report chronic pain most days or every day during the previous 3 months (Figure 1.1).[1–3] In addition, approximately 8–14% adult Americans report high-impact chronic pain (HICP), which incorporates both a persistent pain duration of 3–6 months[1,3,4] and measures of disability to identify a more severely impacted chronic pain population for whom pain frequently limits daily function.[5,6] People comprising population are more likely to suffer mental and cognitive health impairments,[5] have lower quality of life,[6] and use health care services more frequently.[5,6] More than 80% of people in this group are unable to work, and one-third report difficulty with basic self-care activities.[5]

Defining Vulnerability

Healthy People 2030[7] defines social determinants of health (SDOH) as "the conditions in the environments where people are born, live, learn, work, play, worship, and age that affect a wide range of health, functioning, and quality-of-life outcomes and risks." The five domains of SDOH broadly include measures of health care access and quality, economic stability, education quality and access, social and community context, and neighborhood built environment.[7]

Although the term vulnerability and related terms (e.g., vulnerable, marginalized, disadvantaged, disenfranchised, and high risk) are frequently employed in pain literature, especially in pain care disparities literature, it has not been consistently defined. Lack of deliberate use of the language around SDOH can be disempowering and create gaps in equity through perpetuating and maintaining social norms that cause inequities in the first place.[8] Conceptually, references to vulnerability can include contexts that are both intrinsic to an individual (e.g., referring to persons having limited capacity, are too sick, or impoverished) or external (e.g., explicitly or implicitly assigning a subordinate position, such as those rendered by established social power norms).[9] Using the term in these contexts may underemphasize the multidimensional antecedents and processes that result in unequal distributions of a wide range of material, cultural, and sociopolitical resources.[10]

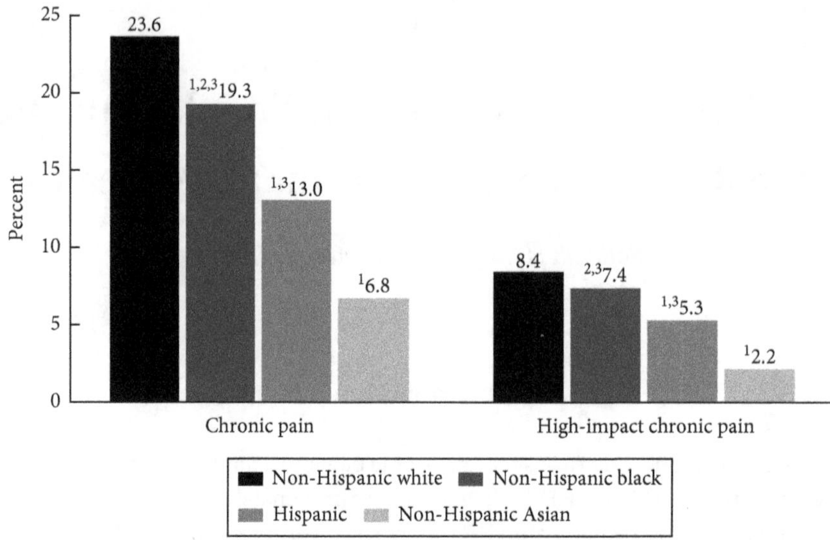

Figure 1.1 Percentage of adults aged 18 years or older with chronic pain and high-impact chronic pain in the past 3 months, by race and Hispanic origin: United States, 2019.[1] Chronic pain is based on responses of "most days" or "every day" to the survey question, "In the past 3 months. how often did you have pain? Would you say never, some days, most days, or every day?" High-impact chronic pain is defined as adults who have chronic pain and who responded "most days" or "every day" to the survey question, "Over the past 3 months, how often did your pain limit your life or work activities? Would you say never, some days, most days, or every day?" Estimates are based on household interviews of a sample of the civilian non-institutionalized population.

[1] Significantly different from non-Hispanic White adults ($p < .05$).

[2] Significantly different from Hispanic adults ($p < .05$).

[3] Significantly different from non-Hispanic Asian adults ($p < .05$).

Source: National Center for Health Statistics, National Health Interview Survey, 2019.

An additional application of the term occurs when groups are categorized as vulnerable because of their health care experiences and outcomes *due to* SDOH. In this context, the concept of vulnerability may be used to compare and benchmark improvements in access to resources as well as to apply moral and ethical codes to justify commitments and obligations (e.g., clinical, system, or policy interventions) to improve relevant outcomes. To avoid stigmatization of subgroups, the term vulnerability and related terms should be carefully employed.

Thus, we use the term vulnerability in this chapter to imply groups based on differential pain care and outcomes and to identify areas of opportunities to close pain care disparities. Box 1.1 highlights other terms that are used in this chapter, drawing from recent published work on diversity, equity, inclusion, and anti-racism in pain research.[8,11–15]

Box 1.1 Definitions of Key Terms

Social determinants of health (SDOH): "Social determinants of health (SDOH) are the conditions in the environments where people are born, live, learn, work, play, worship, and age that affect a wide range of health, functioning, and quality-of-life outcomes and risks."[7]

Social vulnerability: Refers to "potential harm to people . . . and . . . involves a combination of factors that determine the degree to which someone's life and livelihood are put at risk by a discrete and identifiable event in nature or in society."[109]

Anti-racism: Active process of eliminating racism by changing systems, structures, policies, and practices.[8]

Inequities: Unjust and avoidable differences related to health outcomes or health care; has a moral and ethical dimension.[90,110]

Disparities: Denotes difference, although often used interchangeably with *inequities* to mean unjust differences;[91,111] "Health disparities are the metric we use to measure progress toward achieving health equity."[112]

Racialized: Used in the context of people of color; Black, Indigenous, and people of color; and non-White persons. Refers to a dynamic sociopolitical process of "othering" certain individuals/groups based on physical characteristics; acknowledges that race is a social rather than biological construct.[8]

Minoritized: Replaces the term "minority" to recognize that "minority" status is socially constructed and is a result of systemic marginalization.[113]

Note: To further explore the concepts and definitions of vulnerability, health equity, and social determinants of health, see references 7, 114, and 115.

Chronic Pain and Pain Care: Who Is Vulnerable?

Racialized and Ethnic Identities

According to recent estimates based on a national survey of U.S. adults by the National Center for Health Statistics, non-Hispanic Whites report the highest prevalence (24%) of chronic pain in the past 3 months, followed by non-Hispanic Black (19%), Hispanic (13%), and non-Hispanic Asian (7%) adults.[1] For the more consequential HICP, both non-Hispanic White and non-Hispanic Black adults have the highest prevalence (8%), followed by Hispanics (5%) and non-Hispanic Asians (2%).[1]

Race and ethnicity are highly heterogeneous social constructs warranting careful extrapolation of findings from broad racial and ethnic categories to individuals and subgroups. For example, a study using longitudinal National Health Interview Survey (NHIS) data (2010–2017) demonstrated that whereas many Hispanic subgroups (e.g., White Central/South Americans and White Cubans) showed lower pain prevalence than did non-Hispanics Whites, the pain prevalence for other Hispanic subpopulations (e.g., White Puerto Ricans) was comparable or greater than that for non-Hispanics Whites, depending on the specific pain measure used.[16] Similarly, within Whites, any-Hispanic Whites reported a chronic pain prevalence of 14% compared to 23% for non-Hispanic Whites.[16] However, consistent with the findings of the recent National Center for Health Statistics national survey mentioned previously, only small, nonsignificant differences emerged when comparing non-Hispanic Whites and non-Hispanic Blacks on reports of HICP.[16,17]

Race, Ethnicity, and Pain: Structural Influences

Sizable disparities in prevalence of chronic pain have been reported by socioeconomic status (SES), including education, income, and wealth.[17–19] The 2016 NHIS found a higher prevalence of both chronic pain and HICP in adults living in poverty, those with public health insurance, rural residents, and persons who were previously but not currently employed. In addition, prevalence is lower among adults covered by private health insurance (14%) and almost double in adults covered by Medicaid or other public programs (30%). The disparity in prevalence of HICP was approximately five times greater (3.8% vs. 17.8%) between adults with private and public health insurance, respectively.[3]

The significant influence of psychosocial factors on the pain experience has long been recognized in the field of pain science, and the dominant framework guiding chronic pain research and treatment is the biopsychosocial model.[20] However, until recently, far less attention has been paid to the underlying structural factors that "sit outside" this model and influence each of its components. Structural racism and an economic and political context that does not provide an adequate safety net result in an inequitable societal distribution of resources, power, and risk or protective factors for health. In order to understand causes, mechanisms, and potential ways to address pain in vulnerable populations, it is necessary to consider how higher order factors—at the level of neighborhoods, communities, institutions, and societal structures—impact the biological, psychological, and social determinants of pain and pain-related disability.

Consequences of past and present structural racism include residential, economic, and educational segregation; health-damaging physical environments: mass incarceration; and severe, protracted psychosocial stress. These are root causes of the strikingly disproportionate morbidity and mortality experienced by African Americans, which includes a heavy burden of disabling pain.[12,19,21–26] Using a nationally representative sample of midlife and older adults, Janevic and colleagues[4] found that African American adults with chronic pain experienced more pain-related disability in most activity domains compared with White non-Hispanic adults. Overall, the largest predictor of having disabling pain was household wealth, its likelihood being three times greater in the lowest compared to the highest wealth quartile. The authors suggest several mechanisms that explain how personal financial resources might protect against disabling pain. For example, people with more resources are less likely to be exposed to occupational hazards that are risks for disabling pain; they have greater ability to modify their physical environment to minimize disability; and they are more able to pay for safe, health-promoting nonpharmacological pain treatments such as yoga or massage.

Interpreting Models of Vulnerability by Race and Ethnicity and Socioeconomic Status

A key consideration in understanding models of vulnerability is to recognize that minoritized race and disadvantageous SES factors overlap systematically and substantially in the United States to maintain structures of power and privilege.[27,28] SES variables such as education, income, wealth, and health insurance coverage have been found to be associated with general health, prevalence of specific health conditions, as well as patients' access to health services and treatments.[27,28]

Meghani and Chittams[29] have cautioned about interpreting race disparities findings in studies when authors control for SES variables and the race significance either attenuates or disappears. This is because SES is not only a confounder of racial disparities in health but is in the causal pathway by which race affects health.[27]

According to the U.S. Census Bureau's federally defined poverty thresholds, one in five Blacks (20%) have income below the federally established poverty threshold compared with 8% of Whites.[30] In the United States, there are startling wealth differentials by racialized group, such that White non-Latinx/o/e American households have 10 times the accumulated wealth of Black households, making wealth one of the most "prominent features of U.S. racial inequality."[31] Thus, racialized wealth disparities are likely a major contributor to the burden of pain-related disability among African Americans and Hispanics.

Blacks fare poorly compared with Whites on all measures of economic opportunities, health, and access to health care. Structural factors such as labor market discrimination and persistent real estate practices such as redlining and racial residential segregation continue to sustain structural racial inequities.[28,32,33]

Racialized Clinical Disparities in Pain Care

The majority of the prevalence studies presented above have been conducted with general populations in the United States. Disparities in pain care are expected to be more prominent in clinical settings, in which additional factors such as provider bias and stereotypes,[34–38] clinical uncertainty,[39] and differential application of empathy[34] operate and intersect with SDOH variables, compounding disparities through pathways of differential pain care.[16]

In 2012, Meghani et al.[40] performed a meta-analysis of 20 years of published evidence and found that Black patients were 34% less likely than Whites to be prescribed opioids for similar pain conditions (mostly acute pain conditions) when a source of pain was not readily identifiable, such as backaches and abdominal pain. They were also 14% less likely to receive opioids for verifiable causes such as injuries or surgery.[40] These findings have remained consistent in a more recent meta-analysis that demonstrates the continued presence of racial disparities in analgesia use for the management of acute pain in the United States.[41] Disparities in analgesic treatment for pain are observed for Hispanic patients, although the magnitude of the effect has been consistently less sizable than that for Blacks in independently completed accumulated systematic studies.[40,41]

In chronic pain management settings also, Blacks are likely to receive lower opioid morphine milligram equivalent doses, despite higher average pain and less injection drug use.[35] Blacks are at a greater risk of being mislabeled as drug-seeking or showing signs of aberrant behaviors, and they are subject to a greater burden of opioid risk assessment than their White counterparts.[42] Black claimants of workers' compensation for low back pain are also more likely to experience disparities in workers' compensation, including receipt of diagnosis, surgery, and long-term adjustment outcomes.[43–46]

In persons with cancer pain, Black and other minoritized patients consistently report more severe pain intensity than Whites,[47–61] are less likely to receive long-acting opioids to manage background cancer pain,[50] are more likely to receive types of opioids that cause clinical risks,[48] and are more likely to have inadequate cancer pain treatment relative to their reported pain severity.[50,52]

Health literacy is another SDOH factor linked to poor clinician–patient communication outcomes. Health literacy, in theory, is associated with a better understanding of chronic pain and of how it can be optimally self-managed and negotiated with providers.[53] Moreover, individuals with low levels of literacy and/or health literacy are at risk for poor perceived control over pain and needs in specific self-management domains (medication adherence and pain knowledge), as well as pain intensity.[54]

Minoritized Sex and Gender Identity

Research on pain-related disability and other aspects of the pain experience among minoritized sex and gender groups is still limited but is anticipated to grow rapidly as issues related to LGBTQ2S (lesbian, gay, bisexual, transgender, queer, two-spirit) individuals have come to the forefront in recent years.

Reasons for the vulnerability of LGBTQ2S groups to poor pain outcomes are explicated in "minority stress theory,"[55] which was developed to explain the added risk of mental health disorders among lesbian, gay, and bisexual people. This theory posits that the stress engendered by a stigmatized social position, including stigmatized sexual orientation, leads to psychological distress and adverse mental health outcomes. Distress, trauma, and chronic stress all have strong and consistent associations with pain and pain disability, which could explain higher rates of pain in these groups.

Moreover, due to bias, discrimination, and lack of awareness on the part of providers, in many instances LGBTQ2S individuals do not receive culturally safe, appropriate health care.[56,57] There is guidance elsewhere on how to make medical care more LGBTQ2S+ friendly[56]; to our knowledge, this has not yet been tailored to the specific context of pain care. Craig and colleagues[57] note that culturally safe care for LGBTQ2S individuals includes not assuming by default that patients are heterosexual and cisgender. Fuller guidance specific to pain treatment that encompasses the diversity of LGBTQ2S identities and experiences is eagerly awaited.

In a national study of older adults, lesbian, gay, and bisexual older adults had higher rates of back and neck pain, disability, and mental distress compared with their heterosexual counterparts.[58] Given the lessening of stigma in many segments of U.S. society related to diverse sexual orientations, it is possible that sexual orientation could interact with age cohort (e.g., older individuals are more likely to have been exposed to stigmatizing attitudes and behaviors) to differentially affect pain outcomes; however, this has yet to be explored.

Transgender and gender-diverse individuals experience "minority stress" along with other unique stressors related to their identity, including gender dysphoria, or the disconnect between sex assigned at birth and lived gender experience, and societal transphobia.[59,60] These conditions likely lead to higher pain burden in gender-diverse and nonconforming groups, but the pain experience of transgender individuals is just beginning to receive research attention.[61–64] In one study using national Medicare service claims data, transgender compared to cisgender individuals had higher rates of fibromyalgia (37.2% vs. 20.7%) and migraine (14.8% vs. 4.4%).[65]

There remains much yet to learn about gender-affirming care for transgender and gender-diverse people and its effect on pain. For example, given evidence that gender-affirming care is associated with better mental health outcomes,[66] it is possible that such treatment may also have a positive impact on experiences of pain and pain-related disability. Furthermore, although sex hormones are posited to play a role in pain processing, it is not known whether and how gender-affirming hormone treatment impacts pain processing[67] or specific pain conditions such as headache[68] that are linked to hormones in cisgender individuals.

The proportion of Americans who identify as transgender or otherwise gender nonconforming is markedly higher in younger compared to older cohorts[69]; hence, understanding how these still-marginalized identities can impact pain, and how to provide optimal pain care to these groups, must be a high priority going forward.

Older Adults

Older adults are more likely to suffer from painful conditions, including osteoarthritis, diabetic neuropathy, and post-stroke pain, and have less ability to recover from injury. Chronic pain also increases the risk of falls, a significant risk factor for disability and loss of independence. At a time when social networks tend to become smaller, older adults with persistent pain are more likely to experience negative impacts of pain on social functioning (see Chapter 6 for a more detailed discussion).[70]

Neonates and Children

Pain is frequently underdiagnosed and undertreated in children of all ages. Compared to adults, assessment and management of pain are different in children.[71,72] Population-based evidence on the prevalence of pain in children remains limited. For example, the NHIS does not collect data on chronic pain or HICP in children.[3] However, condition-specific prevalence and clinical data on pain prevalence point to a high prevalence of chronic pain and associated comorbidities in children. For example, conditions characterized as neurodivergence, such as autism, can predispose children with pain to additional risks characterized by social communication difficulties. Also, due to differences in sensory processing, autistic children and individuals may experience and express pain differently. Comorbid mental health disorders that are associated with chronic pain—including anxiety, substance-related and addictive disorders, depression, and others—are much more common in autistic people than in the general population.[73] One study using nationally representative data from the National Survey of Children's Health confirmed that children with autism spectrum disorder had elevated pain prevalence.[74] Autistic individuals experience the stressors of being in a marginalized group, per minority stress theory, and autism acceptance is associated with decreased depression.[75]

Similarly, a systematic review based on 57 studies of children and young adults with cerebral palsy found that pain prevalence ranged from 14% to 76% across studies.[76] Pain prevalence was higher in females, older age groups, and those with more severe gross motor function impairment.[76] A meta-analysis of low back pain in children and adolescents found a high mean 12-month period prevalence of 33% obtained from 13 studies.[77] It also found that the most recent studies report higher prevalence rates of low back pain than the oldest ones, possibly indicating a rising prevalence among children.

A nationally representative U.S. survey of ambulatory physician office visits for chronic musculoskeletal pain condition (2007–2015) found more than 28.6 million ambulatory visits over a 9-year period among persons younger than age 25 years (an average of 3 million visits per year).[78] The numbers of visits were higher among older age groups, females, non-Hispanic White ethnicity/race, and those with greater health care use and medical visits in the past year.[78]

Consistent with the findings in adults, findings of racialized status and SES extend to children and are linked with both differential pain assessment and pain treatment in acute care settings.[79–84] For example, minoritized and low-income children have lower rates of imaging for appendicitis, including computed tomography scans.[80] Similarly, studies evaluating unique contributions of SDOH factors found that Black children have significantly lower odds of receiving opioid medications in the emergency department compared to White children. Specially, Black girls were found to have the lowest odds of receiving rehabilitation referrals compared with both Black male children and White children overall.[79] Although some studies have reported mixed findings around racialized disparities, especially regarding long-bone fracture, these studies also identify consistent racialized disparities in type of analgesic received and optimal treatment of pain among Black children.[85]

How Is Vulnerability Expressed?

Pain-Related Disability

Pain-related disability is both a cause and a consequence of vulnerability. Pain-related disability, pain-related functioning, and pain interference are overlapping concepts referring to chronic pain's impact on multiple domains of functioning, including sleep and activities of daily living.[86] These closely related phenomena are distinct from pain intensity, and because functioning is potentially modified through behavioral changes, it is commonly a treatment target of psychosocial interventions for pain (e.g., through behavioral activation and increasing moderate physical activity). Because the degree of disability experienced by a person depends on their social and physical environment as well as on their own health and functional ability,[87] it is particularly necessary to consider multilevel factors when examining who is vulnerable to pain-related disability.

Being able to engage in personally meaningful activities is a key component of well-being and, in later life, is considered a core part of successful aging.[88] In contrast, not being able to carry out daily activities and/or decreased mobility due to pain are significant stressors.[54] This bidirectionality may result in a negative feedback loop, in which stress exacerbates pain intensity, ultimately leading to greater disability. Vulnerable groups, including marginalized and minoritized populations, are particularly at risk for experiencing high levels of pain-related disability, as described previously.

Clinician/Provider–Patient Communication

Certain groups, such as people living with cognitive impairment or those with autism spectrum disorder, can be considered vulnerable to poor pain care and outcomes due, in part, to communication difficulties. Henry and Matthias[89] write that almost every aspect of pain management relies on communication between patients and provider. This communication includes pain assessment, arriving at mutually agreed decisions about a pain management plan, and evaluating how well the plan is working.[89] Communication poses particular challenges in the context of pain, given its subjective nature, its frequently unclear etiology, and challenges related to the current effort to reduce the use of opioids as a chronic pain treatment. All these have the potential to lead to a lack of certainty and mutual mistrust—posing communication challenges and leaving room for inequities to occur.[90] On the other hand, high-quality communication, when it can be achieved, is associated with satisfaction, adherence, and better outcomes, including reduced pain intensity.[89]

Some studies have examined whether the quality of patient–provider communication affects treatment outcomes for pain; as has also been reported for studies of other chronic conditions (e.g., asthma),[91 92] it was found that more positive, patient-centered communication between patients with pain and providers predicted better pain outcomes (intensity and interference)—an association that was mediated by pain self-efficacy. With regard to pain treatment, there is evidence that a strong therapeutic alliance—that is, a relationship characterized by rapport, trust, and mutual goals—is linked to better outcomes in physical therapy.[93]

Notably, communication occurs in a cultural context, which determines how pain is socially constructed and experienced.[90] Henry and Matthias[89] present a comprehensive model of patient–provider communication for pain, which serves to highlight where vulnerabilities can occur. These potential areas include the interaction (e.g., "relational communication," which includes the extent to which communication is reassuring and fosters autonomy, respect, support, and collaboration) and the patient level—for example, the patient pain experience and understanding of pain. Henry and Matthias call for additional studies that consider key factors such as gender and racialized group/ethnicity and the role these play in interactions between patients with pain and providers;

as well as the extent to which quality of communication plays a role in producing inequities in pain treatment.

Resilience—The "Flip Side" of Vulnerability

When considering factors that contribute to the vulnerability of certain groups, it is also important to consider the other side of the coin—that is, resilience and protective factors. For instance, a strong sense of purpose in life can promote maintenance of function and quality of life, regardless of pain,[94] and positive emotions and experiences are associated with less pain.[95] Robinson-Lane and colleagues[96] describe a variety of culturally mediated resources and self-care practices for pain management among African American older adults, particularly application of spiritual coping strategies such as prayer and meditation, and maintaining a positive mindset. A note of caution is that although it is important to recognize and leverage strength and resilience in vulnerable groups, Meyer[55] describes a "tension between the view of the minority person as a victim versus a resilient actor. . . . The peril lies in that the weight of responsibility for social oppression can shift from society to the individual." In other words, an over-focus on resilience can detract from attention to the oppressive forces that keep marginalized groups living under chronically stressful and health-damaging conditions, including those that produce and perpetuate pain.

Remediation

In recent years, awareness of the existence of health disparities by SDOH factors has grown, in part as a result of the COVID-19 pandemic and the stark inequities it exposed. Yet less talked about is that these disparities spring from the "same systemic and structural sources of racism that poison so many other areas of life for people of color in the United States."[24] Causes of vulnerability of the other populations discussed in this chapter are similarly deep-rooted and entrenched.

Therefore, multiple levels of sustained interventions (individual, family, community, health care system, and policy) are needed to adequately address the conditions that contribute to pain vulnerability.[97] Arguably, policy-level changes are the most important, given their potential for sustained effects on populations.

As discussed above, structural racism is a root cause of pain inequities.[8] In their seminal *Lancet* series on structural racism in the United States, Bailey and colleagues[21] describe possible interventions to combat this deeply entrenched discriminatory system. According to them, multi-sector, place-based partnerships with a focus on equity can effectively apply pressure to the systems of structural racism at play within a particular geographical region. Place-based initiatives establish the necessary structures for reinvesting in neighborhoods that have long been marginalized. Bailey et al. also note that improvements in housing inevitably lead to improvements in health. Finally, Black reparations for slavery and centuries of economic exclusion have been described as a powerful, multigenerational intervention for health equity, by decreasing chronic stress and providing Black Americans with health-promoting resources such as better neighborhoods and higher quality schools.[98]

A recent and prominent example of how a major policy change promoting access to health care can have a positive downstream impact on health is seen in the expansion of the Medicaid program (i.e., federally provided health insurance for low-income Americans) that was a key component of the 2010 Affordable Care Act. Medicaid expansion was offered as an option for states, and some states chose it, whereas others did not. Research on the health impacts of Medicaid expansion, although somewhat equivocal, suggests that it has been generally associated with improved health, including chronic disease outcomes, and reductions in mortality.[99] Even stronger evidence demonstrates that Medicaid expansion improves financial well-being and health care access.[99] Given the known links between economic variables and the presence of pain and pain disability, we can speculate that this policy change will, over the long term, inevitably serve to improve pain outcomes, and the undeniably improved access to health care may result in higher quality pain treatment that ameliorates the disproportionate burden of pain in vulnerable groups. To date, no analyses have examined the impact of Medicaid expansion on pain specifically, although expansion appears to have a beneficial effect on certain chronic conditions that are associated with pain (e.g., improved diabetes management), as well as on receiving regular care for chronic conditions.[100]

Although not related to Medicaid expansion per se, a 2016 Oregon policy to expand benefits for evidence-based complementary and alternative medicine (CAM) services for Medicaid enrollees resulted in increased use of services such as chiropractic, acupuncture, and massage among Medicaid enrollees with back pain. Notably, there were still disparities by racialized groups such that Black, Indigenous, and Latino/x/e enrollees were less likely to use complementary services compared to other groups. Rural adults, males, and younger enrollees were also less likely to use these treatments. The study authors concluded that overall, "Oregon's back pain policy appears successful at boosting use of CAM therapies in this patient population."[101]

Although changes related to economic and health policies are likely to have the most profound impact on the pain experience of vulnerable groups by mitigating the conditions that make them vulnerable, there is still a role for individual-level interventions for pain tailored to address specific vulnerabilities. An example of such interventions is the efficacious LAMP (Learning About My Pain) cognitive–behavioral intervention for people living with pain who have low health literacy.[102]

Conclusion

Chronic pain and HICP create a sequela of vulnerability, and there are subgroups that are at particular risk due to social disadvantages that exist where people live and grow and where they seek care. These disadvantages seep into clinical settings in the forms of power differentials, clinician stereotypes and biases, and differential access to care, which are reflected in poor pain outcomes. In this chapter, we set the tone for care and deliberate use of terminologies that are consistent with the mechanisms that occasion inequities in pain prevalence, experience, and outcomes in that certain groups discussed are rendered vulnerable due to social risks, including being members of minoritized, racialized, or certain age groups; gender identities; cognitive impairment; and disability status.

We also acknowledge that most of the extant literature on disparities in pain care relates to racialized disparities as reflected in this chapter. These disparities continue to be prevalent based on accumulating literature. To this end, we refer readers to important recent work calling to confront racism in pain care in all forms[8,12,14,97] that can be applied to clinical practice and research, including preclinical research, to correctly attribute mechanisms to address pain care disparities using an anti-racism framework.[8,103] The anti-racism framework aims to identifying, challenging, and eliminating racism"[8] in pain research and supports cultural humility and critical self-reflection as the foundational tenets in ameliorating disparities.

In addition, many policy interventions based on previous national calls to action—including legislative actions, expanding insurance access, increasing public and health provider education, primary care and pain specialist training, improving workforce diversity, achieving uniformity in SDOH-related data collection, and emphasizing patient-centered outcomes in pain research—still create opportunities for action toward equitable pain care.[104] Consistent with recent federal reports, there is also a need for more equitable access to multimodal and non-opioid and nonpharmacological chronic pain interventions,[105,106] access to which, unfortunately, remains limited in general and especially by SDOH characteristics.[107,108]

Finally, we note that our exploration of vulnerable populations is selective rather than exhaustive. For example, Craig et al.[57] discuss how social marginalization affects the pain experience of other groups not discussed here, including people experiencing homelessness, torture survivors, Indigenous populations, refugees, and people living with HIV, who are also at similar risks of pain and pain undertreatment due to intersectionality of many social risk factors that can compound to create degrees of disadvantages.

In examining disparities in different subgroups, we urge readers to interrogate these disparities carefully rather than make biological or behavioral attributions and invoke easy misconceptions about mechanism of differences, which based on recent reports are still prevalent among health care providers and clinicians.[38] Also, as described in this chapter, because most disparities are due to social risks, we do not consider SDOH variables to be fixed but, rather, addressable to change through appropriate interventions that address these social risks or even epigenetic risks in the long term. Some of these interventions will require continued structural and policy reforms, and others will involve increasing clinician education and accountability. We acknowledge that interventions to ameliorate vulnerabilities in pain care remain limited, and much work lies ahead for the pain community to create equitable models of pain care to ultimately reduce the burden of pain and enhance the well-being of all persons and communities.

References

1. Zelaya CE, Dahlhamer JM, Lucas JW, Connor EM. Chronic pain and high-impact chronic pain among U.S. adults, 2019. *NCHS Data Brief*. 2020;(390):1–8.
2. Yong RJ, Mullins PM, Bhattacharyya N. Prevalence of chronic pain among adults in the United States. *Pain*. 2022;163:e328–e332.

3. Dahlhamer J, Lucas J, Zelaya C, et al. Prevalence of chronic pain and high-impact chronic pain among adults—United States, 2016. *MMWR Morb Mortal Wkly Rep.* 2018;67(36):1001–1006.
4. Janevic MR, McLaughlin SJ, Heapy AA, et al. Racial and socioeconomic disparities in disabling chronic pain: Findings from the Health and Retirement Study. *J Pain.* 2017;18:1459–1467.
5. Pitcher MH, Von Korff M, Bushnell MC, et al. Prevalence and profile of high-impact chronic pain in the United States. *J Pain.* 2019;20:146–160.
6. Von Korff M, Scher AI, Helmick C, et al. United States National Pain Strategy for population research: Concepts, definitions, and pilot data. *J Pain.* 2016;17:1068–1080.
7. U.S. Department of Health and Human Services, Office of Disease Prevention and Health Promotion. Healthy People 2030. n.d. Accessed August 6, 2022. https://health.gov/healthypeople/objectives-and-data/social-determinants-health
8. Morais CA, Aroke EN, Letzen JE, et al. Confronting racism in pain research: A call to action. *J Pain.* 2022;23(6):878–892.
9. Clark B, Preto N. Exploring the concept of vulnerability in health care. CMAJ 2018;190:E308–E309.
10. National Collaborating Centre for Determinants of Health. *Let's Talk: Populations and the Power of Language.* National Collaborating Centre for Determinants of Health, St. Francis Xavier University; 2013.
11. Strand NH, Mariano ER, Goree JH, et al. Racism in pain medicine: We can and should do more. *Mayo Clin Proc.* 2021;96:1394–400.
12. Letzen JE, Mathur VA, Janevic MR, et al. Confronting racism in all forms of pain research: Reframing study designs. *J Pain.* 2022;23:893–912.
13. Jean-Pierre J, James CE. Beyond pain and outrage: Understanding and addressing anti-Black racism in Canada. *Can Rev Sociol.* 2020;57:708–712.
14. Hood AM, Booker SQ, Morais CA, et al. Confronting racism in all forms of pain research: A shared commitment for engagement, diversity, and dissemination. *J Pain.* 2022;23:913–928.
15. Ghoshal M, Shapiro H, Todd K, Schatman ME. Chronic noncancer pain management and systemic racism: Time to move toward equal care standards. *J Pain Res.* 2020;13:2825–2836.
16. Nahin RL. Pain prevalence, chronicity and impact within subpopulations based on both Hispanic ancestry and race: United States, 2010–2017. *J Pain.* 2021;22:826–851.
17. Grol-Prokopczyk H. Sociodemographic disparities in chronic pain, based on 12-year longitudinal data. *Pain.* 2017;158:313–322.
18. Riskowski JL. Associations of socioeconomic position and pain prevalence in the United States: Findings from the National Health and Nutrition Examination Survey. *Pain Med.* 2014;15:1508–1521.
19. Portenoy RK, Ugarte C, Fuller I, Haas G. Population-based survey of pain in the United States: Differences among White, African American, and Hispanic subjects. *J Pain.* 2004;5:317–328.
20. Gatchel RJ, Peng YB, Peters ML, et al. The biopsychosocial approach to chronic pain: Scientific advances and future directions. *Psychol Bull.* 2007;133:581–624.
21. Bailey ZD, Krieger N, Agénor M, et al. Structural racism and health inequities in the USA: Evidence and interventions. *Lancet.* 2017;389:1453–1463.
22. Williams DR, Lawrence JA, Davis BA. Racism and health: Evidence and needed research. *Annu Rev Public Health.* 2019;40:105–125.
23. Morales ME, Yong RJ. Racial and ethnic disparities in the treatment of chronic pain. *Pain Med.* 2021;22:75–90.
24. Booker SQ, Bartley EJ, Powell-Roach K, et al. The imperative for racial equality in pain science: A way forward. *J Pain.* 2021;22(12):1578–1585.
25. Green CR, Anderson KO, Baker TA, et al. The unequal burden of pain: Confronting racial and ethnic disparities in pain. *Pain Med.* 2003;4:277–294.
26. Reyes-Gibby CC, Aday LA, Todd KH, Cleeland CS, et al. Pain in aging community-dwelling adults in the United States: Non-Hispanic whites, non-Hispanic blacks, and Hispanics. *J Pain.* 2007;8:75–84.

27. Williams DR. Race, socioeconomic status, and health: The added effects of racism and discrimination. *Ann N Y Acad Sci.* 1999;896:173–188.
28. Williams DR, Collins C. Racial residential segregation: A fundamental cause of racial disparities in health. *Public Health Rep.* 2001;116:404–416.
29. Meghani SH, Chittams J. Controlling for socioeconomic status in pain disparities research: All-else-equal analysis when "all else" is not equal. *Pain Med.* 2015;16:2222–2225.
30. KFF. Poverty rate by race/ethnicity (CPS). 2020. https://develop.kff.org/other/state-indicator/poverty-rate-by-race-ethnicity-cps/?currentTimeframe=0&sortModel=%7B%22colId%22:%22Location%22,%22sort%22:%22asc%22%7D
31. Levy BL. Wealth, race, and place: How neighborhood (dis)advantage from emerging to middle adulthood affects wealth inequality and the racial wealth gap. *Demography.* 2022;59:293–320.
32. Washington HA, Baker RB, Olakanmi O, et al. Segregation, civil rights, and health disparities: The legacy of African American physicians and organized medicine, 1910–1968. *J Natl Med Assoc.* 2009;101:513–527.
33. White K, Haas JS, Williams DR. Elucidating the role of place in health care disparities: The example of racial/ethnic residential segregation. *Health Serv Res.* 2012;47:1278–1299.
34. Forgiarini M, Gallucci M, Maravita A. Racism and the empathy for pain on our skin. *Front Psychol.* 2011;2: Article 108.
35. Haq N, McMahan VM, Torres A, et al. Race, pain, and opioids among patients with chronic pain in a safety-net health system. *Drug Alcohol Depend.* 2021;222:108671.
36. Hirsh AT, Miller MM, Hollingshead NA, et al. A randomized controlled trial testing a virtual perspective-taking intervention to reduce race and socioeconomic status disparities in pain care. *Pain.* 2019;160:2229–2240.
37. Mathur VA, Richeson JA, Paice JA, et al. Racial bias in pain perception and response: Experimental examination of automatic and deliberate processes. *J Pain.* 2014;15:476–484.
38. Hoffman KM, Trawalter S, Axt JR, et al. Racial bias in pain assessment and treatment recommendations, and false beliefs about biological differences between blacks and whites. *Proc Natl Acad Sci USA.* 2016;113:4296–4301.
39. Hirsh AT, Hollingshead NA, Ashburn-Nardo L, et al. The interaction of patient race, provider bias, and clinical ambiguity on pain management decisions. *J Pain.* 2015;16:558–568.
40. Meghani SH, Byun E, Gallagher RM. Time to take stock: A meta-analysis and systematic review of analgesic treatment disparities for pain in the United States. *Pain Med.* 2012;13:150–174.
41. Lee P, Le Saux M, Siegel R, et al. Racial and ethnic disparities in the management of acute pain in US emergency departments: Meta-analysis and systematic review. *Am J Emerg Med.* 2019;37:1770–1777.
42. Becker WC, Starrels JL, Heo M, et al. Racial differences in primary care opioid risk reduction strategies. *Ann Fam Med.* 2011;9:219–225.
43. Chibnall JT, Tait RC. Long-term adjustment to work-related low back pain: Associations with socio-demographics, claim processes, and post-settlement adjustment. *Pain Med.* 2009;10:1378–1388.
44. Chibnall JT, Tait RC, Andresen EM, et al. Race and socioeconomic differences in post-settlement outcomes for African American and Caucasian Workers' Compensation claimants with low back injuries. *Pain.* 2005;114:462–472.
45. Chibnall JT, Tait RC, Andresen EM, Hadler NM. Clinical and social predictors of application for social security disability insurance by workers' compensation claimants with low back pain. *J Occup Environ Med.* 2006;48:733–740.
46. Chibnall JT, Tait RC, Andresen EM, Hadler NM. Race differences in diagnosis and surgery for occupational low back injuries. *Spine.* 2006;31:1272–1275.
47. Vallerand AH, Hasenau S, Templin T, et al. Disparities between black and white patients with cancer pain: The effect of perception of control over pain. *Pain Med.* 2005;6:242–250.

48. Meghani SH, Kang Y, Chittams J, et al. African Americans with cancer pain are more likely to receive an analgesic with toxic metabolite despite clinical risks: A mediation analysis study. *J Clin Oncol*. 2014;32:2773–2779.
49. Meghani SH, Knafl GJ. Patterns of analgesic adherence predict health care utilization among outpatients with cancer pain. *Patient Prefer Adherence*. 2016;10:81–98.
50. Meghani SH, Thompson AM, Chittams J, et al. Adherence to analgesics for cancer pain: A comparative study of African Americans and Whites using an electronic monitoring device. *J Pain*. 2015;16:825–835.
51. Green CR, Montague L, Hart-Johnson TA. Consistent and breakthrough pain in diverse advanced cancer patients: A longitudinal examination. *J Pain Symptom Manage*. 2009;37:831–847.
52. Stephenson N, Dalton JA, Carlson J, et al. Racial and ethnic disparities in cancer pain management. *J Natl Black Nurses Assoc*. 2009;20:11–18.
53. Kim K, Yang Y, Wang Z, et al. *A Systematic Review of the Association Between Health Literacy and Pain Self-Management*. Patient Education and Counseling; 2021.
54. Vallerand AH, Crawley J, Pieper B, et al. The perceived control over pain construct and functional status. *Pain Med*. 2016;17:692–703.
55. Meyer IH. Prejudice, social stress, and mental health in lesbian, gay, and bisexual populations: Conceptual issues and research evidence. *Psychol Bull*. 2003;129:674.
56. Safer JD, Tangpricha V. Care of the transgender patient. *Ann intern Med*. 2019;171:ITC1–ITC16.
57. Craig KD, Holmes C, Hudspith M, et al. Pain in persons who are marginalized by social conditions. *Pain* 2020;161:261–265.
58. Fredriksen-Goldsen KI, Kim H-J, Shui C, et al. Chronic health conditions and key health indicators among lesbian, gay, and bisexual older US adults, 2013–2014. *Am J Public Health*. 2017;107:1332–1338.
59. Tan KK, Treharne GJ, Ellis SJ, et al. Gender minority stress: A critical review. *J Homosex*. 2020;67:1471–1489.
60. Lenning E, Buist CL. Social, psychological and economic challenges faced by transgender individuals and their significant others: Gaining insight through personal narratives. *Cult Health Sex*. 2013;15:44–57.
61. Abern L, Maguire K, Cook J; Carugno J. Prevalence of vulvar pain and dyspareunia in trans masculine individuals. *LGBT Health*. 2022;9:194–198.
62. Grimstad FW, Boskey E, Grey M. New-onset abdominopelvic pain after initiation of testosterone therapy among trans-masculine persons: A community-based exploratory survey. *LGBT Health*. 2020;7:248–253.
63. Moulder JK, Carrillo J, Carey ET. Pelvic pain in the transgender man. *Curr Obstet Gynecol Rep*. 2020;9:138–145.
64. Strath LJ, Sorge RE, Owens MA, et al. Sex and gender are not the same: Why identity is important for people living with HIV and chronic pain. *J Pain Res*. 2020;13:829–835.
65. Dragon CN, Guerino P, Ewald E, Laffan AM. Transgender Medicare beneficiaries and chronic conditions: Exploring fee-for-service claims data. *LGBT Health*. 2017;4:404–411.
66. Tordoff DM, Wanta JW, Collin A, et al. Mental health outcomes in transgender and nonbinary youths receiving gender-affirming care. *JAMA Netw Open*. 2022;5:e220978.
67. Aloisi AM, Bachiocco V, Costantino A, et al. Cross-sex hormone administration changes pain in transsexual women and men. *Pain*. 2007;132:S60–S67.
68. Hranilovich JA, Kaiser EA, Pace A, et al. Headache in transgender and gender-diverse patients: A narrative review. *Headache*. 2021;61:1040–1050.
69. Herman JL, Flores AR, O'Neill AK. How many adults and youth identify as transgender in the United States? Williams Institute; 2022.
70. Kelly L, Kuwata C, Goldhirsch S. *Pain in Older Adults Pain in Vulnerable Populations*. Oxford University Press; 2023.
71. Furyk J, Sumner M. Pain score documentation and analgesia: A comparison of children and adults with appendicitis. *Emerg Med Australas*. 2008;20:482–487.

72. Mathews L. Pain in children: Neglected, unaddressed and mismanaged. *Indian J Palliat Care.* 2011;17:S70–S73.
73. Lai M-C, Kassee C, Besney R, et al. Prevalence of co-occurring mental health diagnoses in the autism population: A systematic review and meta-analysis. *Lancet Psychiatry.* 2019;6:819–829.
74. Whitney DG, Shapiro DN. National prevalence of pain among children and adolescents with autism spectrum disorders. *JAMA Pediatr.* 2019;173:1203–1205.
75. Kalichman SC, Rompa D, Cage M, et al. Effectiveness of an intervention to reduce HIV transmission risks in HIV-positive people. *Am J Prev Med.* 2001;21:84–92.
76. McKinnon CT, Meehan EM, Harvey AR, et al. Prevalence and characteristics of pain in children and young adults with cerebral palsy: A systematic review. *Dev Med Child Neurol.* 2019;61:305–314.
77. Calvo-Munoz I, Gomez-Conesa A, Sanchez-Meca J. Prevalence of low back pain in children and adolescents: A meta-analysis. *BMC Pediatr.* 2013;13: Article 14.
78. Feldman DE, Nahin RL. National estimates of chronic musculoskeletal pain and its treatment in children, adolescents, and young adults in the United States: Data from the 2007–2015 National Ambulatory Medical Care Survey. *J Pediatr.* 2021;233:212–219.
79. Dickens H, Rao U, Sarver D, et al. Racial, gender, and neighborhood-level disparities in pediatric trauma care. *J Racial Ethn Health Disparities* 2023;10:1006–1017.
80. Wang L, Haberland C, Thurm C, et al. Health outcomes in US children with abdominal pain at major emergency departments associated with race and socioeconomic status. *PLoS One.* 2015;10:e0132758.
81. Wing E, Saadat S, Bhargava R, et al. Racial disparities in opioid prescriptions for fractures in the pediatric population. *Am J Emerg Med.* 2022;51:210–213.
82. Guedj R, Marini M, Kossowsky J, et al. Explicit and implicit bias based on race, ethnicity, and weight among pediatric emergency physicians. *Acad Emerg Med.* 2021;28:1073–1076.
83. Guedj R, Marini M, Kossowsky J, et al. Racial and ethnic disparities in pain management of children with limb fractures or suspected appendicitis: A retrospective cross-sectional study. *Front Pediatr.* 2021;9:652854.
84. Goyal MK, Kuppermann N, Cleary SD, et al. Racial disparities in pain management of children with appendicitis in emergency departments. *JAMA Pediatr.* 2015;169:996–1002.
85. Goyal MK, Johnson TJ, Chamberlain JM, et al. Racial and ethnic differences in emergency department pain management of children with fractures. *Pediatrics.* 2020;145:e20193370.
86. Dworkin RH, Turk DC, McDermott MP, et al. Interpreting the clinical importance of group differences in chronic pain clinical trials: IMMPACT recommendations. *Pain.* 2009;146:238–244.
87. Verbrugge LM, Jette AM. The disablement process. *Soc Sci Med.* 1994;38:1–14.
88. Regier NG, Parisi JM, Perrin N, et al. Engagement in favorite activity and implications for cognition, mental health, and function in persons living with and without dementia. *J Appl Gerontol.* 2022;41:441–449.
89. Henry SG, Matthias MS. Patient–clinician communication about pain: A conceptual model and narrative review. *Pain Med.* 2018;19:2154–2165.
90. Meghani SH, Gallagher RM. Disparity vs inequity: Toward reconceptualization of pain treatment disparities. *Pain Med.* 2008;9:613–623.
91. Sleath B, Carpenter DM, Slota C, et al. Communication during pediatric asthma visits and self-reported asthma medication adherence. *Pediatrics.* 2012;130:627–633.
92. Ruben MA, Meterko M, Bokhour BG. Do patient perceptions of provider communication relate to experiences of physical pain? *Patient Educ Couns.* 2018;101:209–213.
93. Kinney M, Seider J, Beaty AF, et al. The impact of therapeutic alliance in physical therapy for chronic musculoskeletal pain: A systematic review of the literature. *Physiother Theory Pract.* 2020;36:886–898.
94. Campbell LC, Robinson K, Meghani SH, et al. Challenges and opportunities in pain management disparities research: Implications for clinical practice, advocacy, and policy. *J Pain.* 2012;13:611–619.

95. Hassett AL, Finan PH. The role of resilience in the clinical management of chronic pain. *Curr Pain Headache Rep*. 2016;20: Article 39.
96. Robinson-Lane SG, Hill-Jarrett TG, Janevic MR. "Ooh, you got to holler sometime": Pain meaning and experiences of Black older adults. In: van Rysewyk S, ed. *Meanings of Pain*. Springer; 2022:45–64.
97. Janevic MR, Mathur VA, Booker SQ, et al. Making pain research more inclusive: Why and how. *J Pain*. 2022;23:707–728.
98. Bassett MT, Galea S. Reparations as a public health priority—A strategy for ending black-white health disparities. *N Engl J Med*. 2020;383:2101–2103.
99. Allen H, Sommers BD. Medicaid expansion and health: Assessing the evidence after 5 years. *JAMA*. 2019;322:1253–1254.
100. Lee J, Callaghan T, Ory M, et al. The impact of Medicaid expansion on diabetes management. *Diabetes Care*. 2020;43:1094–101.
101. Choo EK, Charlesworth CJ, Gu Y, et al. Increased use of complementary and alternative therapies for back pain following statewide Medicaid coverage changes in Oregon. *J Gen Intern Med*. 2021;36:676–682.
102. Thorn BE, Eyer JC, Van Dyke BP, et al. Literacy-adapted cognitive behavioral therapy versus education for chronic pain at low-income clinics. *Ann Intern Med*. 2018;168:471–480.
103. Mathur VA, Trost Z, Ezenwa MO, et al. Mechanisms of injustice: What we (do not) know about racialized disparities in pain. *Pain*. 2022;163:999–1005.
104. Meghani SH, Polomano RC, Tait RC, et al. Advancing a national agenda to eliminate disparities in pain care: Directions for health policy, education, practice, and research. *Pain Med*. 2012;13:5–28.
105. U.S. Department of Health and Human Services. Pain Management Best Practices Inter-Agency Task Force report: Updates, gaps, inconsistencies, and recommendations. U.S. Department of Health and Human Services; 2019. Accessed August 30, 2022. https://www.hhs.gov/sites/default/files/pmtf-final-report-2019-05-23.pdf
106. Dowell D, Haegerich TM, Chou R. CDC guideline for prescribing opioids for chronic pain—United States, 2016. *JAMA*. 2016;315:1624–1645.
107. Corey KL, McCurry MK, Sethares KA, et al. Utilizing internet-based recruitment and data collection to access different age groups of former family caregivers. *Appl Nurs Res*. 2018;44:82–87.
108. Ludwick A, Corey K, Meghani S. Racial and socioeconomic factors associated with the use of complementary and alternative modalities for pain in cancer outpatients: An integrative review. *Pain Manag Nurs*. 2020;21:142–150.
109. United Nations Development Programme. Putting people first: Practice, challenges and innovation in characterizing and mapping social groups: Introduction to social vulnerability. n.d. Accessed August 30, 2022. https://understandrisk.org/wp-content/uploads/Intro-to-social-vulnerability.pdf
110. Whitehead M. The concepts and principles of equity and health. *Health Promot Int*. 1991;6:217–228.
111. Braveman PA, Kumanyika S, Fielding J, et al. Health disparities and health equity: The issue is justice. *Am J Public Health*. 2011;101:S149–S55.
112. Braveman P. What are health disparities and health equity? We need to be clear. *Public Health Rep*. 2014;129(Suppl 2):5–8.
113. Sotto-Santiago S. Time to reconsider the word minority in academic medicine. *J Best Pract Health Professions Diversity*. 2019;12:72–78.
114. Centers for Disease Control and Prevention. Health equity. 2022. Accessed August 30, 2022. https://www.cdc.gov/coronavirus/2019-ncov/community/health-equity/index.html
115. World Health Organization. Social determinants of health. 2022. Accessed August 30, 2022. https://www.who.int/health-topics/social-determinants-of-health#tab=tab_1

2

Insight and Responsibility

Ethical Considerations in the Pain Care of Vulnerable Populations

Rollin M. Gallagher

I imagine there will come a time when my head will say "Enough." Pain takes away your happiness, not only in tennis but in life. And my problem is that many days I live with too much pain.

—Raphael Nadal, winner of 22 major tennis titles, said in Spanish, pursing his lips and shaking his head.[1]

Effective pain management is a moral imperative, a professional responsibility, and the duty of people in the healing professions.

—Institute of Medicine[2]

Introduction

Millennia-old philosophical considerations of morality and values in the practice of medicine have led to the development of the field of bioethics encompassing the domains of clinical care, education and training, clinical and basic research, health administration, and public policy. As "keyholders" to solutions to the universal human problem of pain, the pain field must both provide good care and steward progress in education, science, and health system policy. Success requires insight: the ability to look within—as practitioners, educators, clinical leaders, policymakers, and investigators—to understand our weaknesses, strengths, and opportunities to improve pain care and to steward needed change. Other chapters explore the vulnerability of pain populations shaped by clinical and social conditions throughout the continuum of care. This chapter discusses some ethical challenges of this journey facing clinicians and professional stewards.

The complexity of chronic pain conditions (CPCs) heightens this challenge. The simplicity of managing causes of nociception alone—surgery for injury, steroids for inflamed joints, or analgesics—is appealing. Failures of this "fix it" medical model for CPCs led to pain medicine's emergence as a specialty. For example, chronic low back pain (LBP), once considered a medical diagnosis and often dichotomized as either somatic ("real") or psychosomatic, is now considered a symptom with structural, sensory, affective, cognitive, and behavioral dimensions contributing to pathophysiologic and neurobehavioral expressions of pain chronification. This complexity requires goal-oriented biopsychosocial care within clinical algorithms for precision care increasingly informed by big data and eventually genomics.[3–5]

A sociomedical analysis reveals how disparities in access to effective interdisciplinary pain care persist.[6,7] Structural problems include racism and poverty, discussed in other chapters, and medical education debt which encourages new physicians to choose high-income procedural specialties over primary care. Can a commercialized health system evolve, emphasizing communitarian values and social justice, to enable primary care to focus on maintaining meaningful community lives of patients with CPCs: needed training, reimbursement for clinical time, engagement of community resources, and pain specialty support?[8–13] Can measurement help achieve equity?[14] The potential for reducing rates of disability, substance use disorder (SUD), opioid overdose, depression, and suicide is enormous. Will ethical analysis help us get there?[15]

Ethics in Health Care: A Background

Gregory and Percival outlined the 18th-century tools emphasizing physicians' personal responsibility, such as the "four virtues"[16]: *self-effacement*—avoid nonmedical factors (social class, race, religion, and nationality) from influencing treatment; *self-sacrifice*—assume risk (e.g., communicable diseases)—extra effort the rule; *compassion*—seek to alleviate suffering and stress of illness; and *integrity*—discipline and scientific rigor guide treatment. The sociobiologist E. O. Wilson's observations pertain:

> Science and technology are what we [e.g., medicine] can do; *morality* is what we agree we should or should not do [e.g., ethical rules for clinical practice]. The ethic from which moral decisions spring is a norm or standard of behavior in support of a *value* [e.g., practice personalized, evidence-based medical care] and value in turn depends on *purpose* [e.g., control pain to ease suffering, improve quality of life, return to work rates, depression, etc.]. *Purpose*, whether *personal* [e.g., healthy doctor–patient relationships; satisfaction with clinical practice, teaching, or research] or global [e.g., pain management as a human right], whether urged by *conscience* [e.g., personal values] or graven in "sacred" *script* [e.g., Hippocratic Oath], expresses the image we hold of ourselves [e.g., insight] and our society [e.g., our medical profession]. In short, ethics evolve through discrete steps: from *self-image*, to *purpose*, to *value*, to *ethical precepts*, to *moral reasoning* [applying ethics to clinical, research, and administrative practices].[17(pp130–131)][italics added]

Wilson reflects on how immutable, genetically determined behavioral characteristics of our old-world primate species, such as altruism, evolved within cultures and societies and are modified by other genetically determined characteristics such as tribalism, self-ishness/greed, and aggression.[18] These interacting social instincts through their cultural expression drive human behavior, challenging the ethical care of pain, particularly chronic pain.

Dr. Mark Sullivan introduced a special 2001 issue of *Pain Medicine* dedicated to ethics as follows[19(p106)]:

> While "morality" refers generally to social conventions about right and wrong, "ethics" refers to the more theoretical and systematic understanding of the moral life. Though moral reasoning informs every choice we make about our actions, it becomes particularly important in the face of moral perplexity or uncertainty. Beauchamp and Childress have identified two basic types of moral dilemmas encountered in medicine. In the first, there is evidence that act *x* is morally right *and* there is evidence that act *x* is morally wrong. Abortion might represent this first kind of dilemma. In the second, we have obligations to do *x* and obligations to do *y* but can't do both. Balancing obligations to preserve life and relieve suffering in the decision to terminate life-saving treatment might represent this second kind of dilemma. In dilemmas such as these, our usually reliable sense of moral intuition may not provide adequate guidance. Ethical theory can bring some consistency and rationality to our moral judgments in these kinds of cases by describing what qualifies as relevant and adequate reasons for action.

Dr. Daniel Hamaty, an early leader in pain management with ethics expertise, outlined his observations of ethical challenges practicing in managed care[20(p117)]:

- Today's physician stands alone in the struggle to get the proper care for the patient. Far too often, she or he is stonewalled by inconstant social standards and reigning economic forces.
- Today's physician stands painfully by as controlling health institutions, whose medical directors are not held to the same code of medical ethics, condone the withholding of treatment or allow improper treatment.
- Today's physician is induced to be the titular head of a commercialized, amoral health care institution.
- Today's physician sees the patient's self-direction compromised by captivating media offerings and web page assurances of cure and immortality. That same autonomy is abused by the example of freewheeling assisted suicide flaunting the law.
- Today's physician is faced with the moral implications of progress in genetic engineering, which promises to impose more tension on those responsible for allocating resources.
- In short, today's physician is a lesser professional, a more reluctant entrepreneur. The physician is part of a culture where self-governance is immune to morality and law; part of a society that assigns no value to controlling behavior through a life of virtue and adherence to an oath.

Faced with the ethical conundrums implied by these observations, now complicated by social media, are clinicians managing this stressful environment? More now pursue other opportunities in health care, new careers, or retire early.[11] Clinicians suffer mental health conditions and choose suicide at growing rates.[21] Hamaty's words confront us with our complicity in an "amoral" health care system. Can we balance personal, patient, and community needs to continue our dedication to medical care, teaching, research, and policy? Can hospital ethics boards and primary care discussion forums, such as Balint-type practice management groups, help us?[22]

Insight and Responsibility in Pain Management

Insight about how personal attributes contribute to ethical behavior is important. Evolutionary traits common to social animals, such as altruism, have not changed since hunter–gatherer tribes evolved more than 100,000 years ago.[18] Innate capacity for altruism varies, its expression shaped by life experience. Within a population distribution, high empathy and capacity for caring fall on the opposite end of the trait spectrum from selfishness and aggression—sociopathy their extreme expression. Other personal and social attributes such as resilience and teamwork are important. Can health systems establish the capacity to support helpful traits among caregivers, accounting for the broad spectrum of psychosocial motivations for entering medicine and the multitude of career pathways? Organizational stewardship roles, expressing the collaborative spirit of clinical pain management, are helping the pain field emerge from specialty tribalism that delayed the changes in training and practice organization required to create a competent pain management workforce.[23–25] Can we "bake in" procedures and forums to help providers, practices, and leaders discuss and manage ethical pain care conundrums effectively?

COVID's effects on caregivers and the health system renewed conversations about medical ethics, such as Emanuel and colleagues'[26] outline of how values enter into decision-making

- When explicitly invoking values such as equity, solidarity, trust, and transparency that can form the basis for ethical action.
- When establishing policy objectives which explicitly reflect judgments of what is important or of worth. Science can inform, but not dictate, policy.
- When navigating trade-offs if two or more objectives come in conflict.
- When navigating uncertainty.

As an example of ethical action in pain management, early in COVID some pain specialists were assigned to intensive care units; despite risk of severe illness and high stress, they stepped up.[27] Broad social approbation emerged for their life-saving work. Although waiting lists for pain clinics lengthened temporarily, clinical adaptations such as telemedicine improved access to interdisciplinary care.[27,28]

Business ethics, emphasizing financial success, challenge medical ethics, but coping strategies emerge. Evidence-based guidelines can support patient and physician autonomy, minimize cost-shifting, and incentivize performance-based practice models for clinical decision-making. However, pain specialists often treat outliers—patients who do not conform to the strict selection criteria required in research protocols or even broad categories in clinical guidelines. Daunting complexity may include multiple pain generators (e.g., diabetic neuropathy, osteoarthritis, spinal stenosis, and obesity in a 65-year-old man), inadequate response to conventional treatments in primary care or non-pain specialties, and several comorbidites (e.g., mental illness and substance abuse, other medical diseases, and personal stress [e.g., loss of work, financial insecurity, and family stress]). Any of these, and more together, may influence treatment outcome, and require thoughtful, patient-centered collaboration among clinicians.[3,6,24] Given these realities, the clinical "art" of medicine, informed by but not dictated by evidence-based medicine and grounded in ethical principles, including our responsibilities as professional stewards, should guide our work.[15,19]

Ethical Principles in Pain Management: A Review

The American Medical Association's (AMA) Council on Ethical and Judicial Affairs published the "Code of Medical Ethics." Its nine core ethical "principles" (Box 2.1), as standards of conduct reflecting more than 175 specific ethical issues in medicine,[29(pxiv)] apply to pain management. This volume further codifies how each principle becomes more concretely constructed when physician behavior is interpreted within a court of law. The Council proceeded to publish treatises that address *stewardship* (2012), guiding those holding leadership positions, and *professionalism* (2013), focusing on ethical issues facing practicing physicians.[30,31]

Box 2.1 AMA Ethical Principles in Medicine

1. A physician shall be dedicated to providing competent medical care, with compassion and respect for human dignity and rights.
2. A physician shall uphold the standards of professionalism, be honest in all professional interactions, and strive to report physicians deficient in character or competence, or engaging in fraud or deception, to appropriate entities.
3. A physician shall respect the law and also recognize a responsibility to seek changes in those requirements which are contrary to the best interests of the patient.
4. A physician shall respect the rights of patients, colleagues, and other health professionals, and shall safeguard patient confidences and privacy within the constraints of the law.
5. A physician shall continue to study, apply, and advance scientific knowledge, maintain a commitment to medical education, make relevant information available to patients, colleagues, and the public, obtain consultation, and use the talents of other health professionals when indicated.
6. A physician shall, in the provision of appropriate patient care, except in emergencies, be free to choose whom to serve, with whom to associate, and the environment in which to provide medical care.
7. A physician shall recognize a responsibility to participate in activities contributing to the improvement of the community and the betterment of public health.
8. A physician shall, while caring for a patient, regard responsibility to the patient as paramount.
9. A physician shall support access to medical care for all people

The key question in using a principles-based approach to clinical practice is whether a particular act or course of action is morally right—if it obeys an agreed moral rule or respects an agreed-upon moral principle, either deontological (to do with duties and rights; e.g., "Thou shalt not kill") or consequentialist (concerned with the act's consequences; e.g., "Always do what will produce more good than harm"). Many challenges are posed by this principles-based approach to professionalism and stewardship in pain management. We start with a review of five bioethical principles that are commonly encountered and interact in the clinical process of managing pain: beneficence, nonmaleficence, respect for autonomy, justice, and double effect.[32]

Beneficence, the physician's duty to "take positive steps to help others and not just refrain from harmful acts," was extended to the moral responsibility for easing pain.[33] Established medical, behavioral, and integrative pain therapies can express, but also challenge, beneficence because millions cannot access this care. This disparity shifts our ethical responsibility to stewardship.[30]

Nonmaleficence, the obligation to avoid inflicting harm on patients carelessly or intentionally, is often caused by inadvertent oversights, false information, or unconscious bias:

- Failure to provide adequate analgesia for injuries or procedures, sometimes a manifestation of systemic racism[34] (see Chapters 1, 4, 14, and 33), increases risk of adverse outcomes such as post-traumatic stress, distrusting the medical system, avoiding needed care, or even developmental ramifications for pain processing (see Chapter 4).
- An infant in a world-class pediatric intensive care unit undergoes daily needle punctures during a long hospital stay. Daytime staff routinely utilize analgesic creams; nighttime staff do not, causing the child to cry vigorously. Does omission of nighttime pain prevention indicate clinical or stewardship maleficence: personal decisions of nighttime staff, unclear attending orders, hospital unit policies, or night shift staffing shortages? These are particularly relevant given present health system stresses.[11]
- Managing pain procedurally or with long-term opioid analgesics without screening for and managing comorbidities (depression, anxiety, or SUD) and considering interdisciplinary alternatives increases the probability of treatment failure and/or addiction. If comorbidities are identified and managed, treatment plans can be reconsidered.[35] High 20th-century American surgical rates for LBP (compared to other advanced economies) caused a large population with "failed low back surgery syndrome," with attendant unemployment, family stress, depression/suicide, and SUD costs to society. Interdisciplinary pain rehabilitation, although successful in returning disabled workers to work,[36] became generally unavailable in the 1990s during society's embrace of managed care.[6] It was left up to the surgeons again. An old adage pertains: "Good surgeons know how to operate; better surgeons know when to operate. But only the wisest surgeons know when not to operate."[37(p1325)]
- Thirty years ago, a 19-year-old college rugby player herniates a lumbar disk, causing incapacitating low back and radicular pain. A spine surgeon recommends surgery. There are no indicators for immediate surgery. Instead, a spine rehabilitation program controls pain with epidurals and medications, enabling progressive

physical, behavioral, and occupational therapy. The patient returns to college and a successful career while enjoying vigorous sports. Today, multidisciplinary pain consultation and care are more widely accessible, avoiding unnecessary surgery.[38]

- Opioids can be prescribed inappropriately in terminal illness.
  - Higher doses than required for pain control, with sedation disabling participation in clinical decision-making (autonomy) or conducting personal affairs.
  - Doses too low for pain control, leading to despair, requests for euthanasia, or suicide.
- Opioid analgesics, used episodically in low doses with other medications, carefully supervised with "universal precautions,"[39] may enable rehabilitative activity more safely than regular nonsteroidal anti-inflammatory drugs—for example, in some older patients (see Chapters 6 and 31). However, brief visits required by managed care may not enable the evaluation and follow-up needed to ensure safe opioid management. Care networks that include access to pain and SUD specialty consultation, such as established in the U.S. Department of Veterans Affairs (VA), U.S. Department of Defense (DOD), and the University of New Mexico's Extension for Community Healthcare Outcomes—Pain (Pain ECHO), are needed.[40–45]

These examples reflect Hamaty's[20] observations that personal values, misinformation, organizational values, and related clinical policies all influence clinicians' judgment in pain management. Ethical consultation can consider clinical decisions in the context of societal norms and "rules," balancing "beneficence" and "nonmaleficence."

Aggressive interventions generally represent a compassionate effort to ease suffering; however, judgments might be consciously or unconsciously influenced by factors such as generating income for a hospital, testing the bioethical principle of nonmaleficence. A provider can use "unproven" treatment, where the evidence is weaker for efficacy such as some integrative or interventional therapies, by balancing risks and benefits. Many low-risk, low-cost treatments have undiscovered efficacy because commercial enterprises generally only fund U.S. Food and Drug Administration–required efficacy studies of medications and safety studies of new devices—all very expensive. Psychological, education, transcutaneous electrical nerve stimulation, relaxation exercises, "integrative" therapies, and meditation are examples of generally lower cost, safer therapies, even though some may not yet be "proven." Efficacy studies for many of these therapies are now underway, supported by the National Institutes of Health's (NIH) Helping to End Addiction Long-term Initiative (HEAL Initiative).

Respect for autonomy is based on the Greek *autos nomos*—self-rule, free from controlling interferences that prevent meaningful choice and a capacity for intentional action,[32] such as patient informed consent for a medical or research intervention. Seeking pain relief potentially impedes autonomy of patients dependent on physicians for pain relief or for determining disability or insurance coverage. Ensuring that patients are fully informed and comfortable in the relationship increases the likelihood of autonomous decision-making.

As Hamaty[20] suggests, health systems and insurance frequently constrain physicians' autonomy because they may not be paid for biopsychosocial evaluation, nor their referrals approved. Professional "stewardship" helps health systems develop routine procedures that ensure safety. Adopting universal precautions[39] and other screening/monitoring programs can ensure patient compliance with an agreed-upon therapeutic plan that fits into the organizational care model, such as stepped care in the VA and DOD.[40,41,43–45] These advances support meaningful choices (*autonomy*) by both physician and patients, balancing *beneficence* (providing pain relief while managing opioid risk) against potential *maleficence* (contributing to risk of SUD and overdose).

The concept of *relational autonomy* aligns with these organizational advances.[16] Teamwork improves providers' ability to maintain autonomy in decision-making; similarly, patients' consultations with family and friends or professional "second opinions" support autonomy. Institutional teamwork between VA's pharmacy and primary care, consulting with pain medicine, resulted in a risk screening program in which patients agreeing to universal precautions (autonomy) were maintained on opioids for pain control.[43] Subsequently, the entire VA system developed informed consent, risk-management protocols on the electronic medical record when considering long-term opioid prescribing.[40,41,44,45] Such institutionally sanctioned procedures enable autonomous decision-making for patient and provider, building trust, not suspicion.

When considering intraspinal neuromodulation procedures, routine psychological assessment enables teams to weigh with patients the potential benefits against the risks caused by unmitigated psychosocial factors. Improved success rates spare patients (and society) unnecessary costs and suffering associated with ineffective treatment. The Cleveland Clinic, using multistaged interdisciplinary screening, deemed only 28 of 237 referrals as good candidates for trials of spinal cord stimulation for visceral pain.[46] At 1 year, 19 showed significantly improved pain and lowered opioid doses. Such practices support mutually autonomous decision-making, but they require provider training and health system change.

Justice refers to the fair, equitable, and appropriate distribution of a privilege, benefit, or service in society,[16] such as effective pain management. Disparities based on racial origin, gender, or socioeconomic status are well-established examples of injustice; this vulnerability and its remedies are reviewed in Chapter 14. Our stewardship responsibility includes correction of false stereotypes in preclinical and clinical training, in clinical guidelines, in research, and in policy development. Mathur et al.[47] describe the "socioecological" cascade of injustice, all affecting pain care in a vulnerable population: *cultural beginnings* such as slavery, racism, and the resulting sociopolitical climate; secondary *societal structural injustices* such as reduced access to housing, voting, the health system, and competent pain care; resulting *provider biases leading to interpersonal injustices* such as inadequate analgesia or disbelieving pain and suffering; and, finally, *intrapersonal neuropsychological consequences* such as chronic post-traumatic stress. Interventions at each level require initial awareness followed by training in skills with demonstrable remediating outcomes. Providers must learn how to discuss care with a person of color who has received racially biased care and suffers distrust of the health system.

Double effect occurs when the primary intent (of an intervention), such as raising opioid doses in terminal cancer, may have the desirable effect of pain relief despite the potential of reducing respiratory drive that hastens death, but also the undesirable effect of impairing communication with staff and family. Palliative care programs support insightful ethical input into such decision-making.

Conceptual Issues Affecting Ethical Pain Practices

Several common clinical scenarios in pain management can challenge clinicians' ability to practice ethically. Elaine Scarry's *The Body in Pain*[48] proposes that "having pain" is to "have certainty"; to hear about it (e.g., as a physician looking for a bodily cause) is to "have doubt," sowing the seeds of a "psychosomatic," stigmatizing diagnosis.[49] For example, a flawed diagnostic technique, Waddell's sign, was used widely by insurers and workers' compensation adjusters, abetted by medical authorities, to disprove "organic" etiologies of LBP, thus disqualifying injured workers from receiving unemployment benefits or disability. When carefully studied, Waddell's sign did not prove comorbid psychopathology but, rather, worse spinal pathology.[50,51] Such misattributions stigmatized patients, contributing to self-doubt and social isolation, precursors to anxiety, anger at not being believed, and depression and its risks.[35,49,52] As our field's science has progressed to understand chronification,[53] so has our appreciation of the need for a narrative-based ethics based on our more intimate knowledge of patients' longitudinal experience of pain in their lives.[52]

Common secondary comorbidities of chronic pain, such as depression and anxiety, contribute to physician–patient burden in developing trust. When a physician cannot effectively treat a "real" somatic cause (e.g., below the brain), the onset of clinical depression or an anxiety disorder might reinforce a psychosomatic hypothesis.[35,52,54] The diagnosis of "nociplastic pain" now encompasses cases in which no clear nociceptive or neuropathic cause of persistent pain is easily discoverable. Unfortunately, most primary care and specialty practices are neither trained to delineate these clinical nuances nor provided the time or teamwork to manage them effectively. Screening all patients with chronic pain for depression and anxiety and predictive traits in acute pain such as catastrophizing[54] and treating appropriately will improve response rates to pain therapies.

Carvalho and colleagues[55] describe conflicts in pain care between a "virtue-based ethics" within the provider's character that strictly adheres to evidence-based medicine as emphasized in medical education and training and "care-based ethics" based on the inclusion of person-specific information from the patient–caregiver longitudinal relationship. Patients' desire for pain relief may conflict with providers' focus on finding and eliminating somatic causes or following advised algorithms. Even when the somatic cause of pain is known, often there is no identifiable peripheral "cause" of changes in the patient's pain intensity, leading to an algorithmic solution. Clinicians are thus challenged to apply "evidence-based care" within the narrative of an individual patient whose bodily pain signal to the brain and the intensity of pain suffering are affected by many factors beyond somatic pathology and transmission of pain signals. Factors activating pain at work and home and augmentation of pain by stress and mental health comorbidities also require management that is challenging in a brief clinician encounter. Health systems must support a provider and team's ability to routinely identify predisposing, precipitating, and perpetuating biopsychosocial factors affecting pain intensity and related morbidities and manage them in a goal-directed treatment approach that can be readjusted longitudinally.[3,41]

Stewardship of Pain Care

The AMA's report on physician stewardship reviews causes of high health care costs in the United States (17.6% of gross domestic product in 2009), including physicians' contributions and obligation to manage resources wisely.[30] Many cost-drivers are beyond clinicians' control: administration; trends in population health, such as aging and obesity; public health crises; liability; marketing-driven patient expectations; and hospital services. Stewardship roles are essential: institutional and governmental committees to establish local, regional, and national policy; and specialty organizations that advise such committees and publish clinical guidelines. Coordinated stewardship efforts by professional organizations—for example, the AMA's first national summit on pain[25] that included leaders from all pain-relevant specialties and pain advocacy groups—have helped create societal awareness of pain's impact on public health and promoted coordinated investments in pain research, education, and health policy.[2,23–25,41,56–59] Some of these efforts are listed in Table 2.1.

Two societal events have raised broad cultural awareness of pain's public health significance, encouraging society-wide stewardship. First, during the recent wars in the Middle East, thousands of troops survived terrible battlefield injuries, returning home with disabling combinations of chronic pain, post-concussive brain injury, and post-traumatic stress.[1,41,60,61] Their suffering galvanized Congress to require that the VA and DOD engage the pain field to establish system-wide clinical programming and pain training of clinicians to care for pain from the battlefield[61] to recovery in home communities.[41,44,62,63] The relatively underfunded VA system established a national multidisciplinary group of motivated leaders from diverse backgrounds (addictionology, health psychology, integrative medicine, neurology, nursing, pain medicine, pharmacy, primary care, psychiatry, and rehabilitation medicine) that designed a pain management plan for the entire health system—the biopsychosocial stepped care model.[6,41,58,63] Regional VA pain councils regularly met with national leaders to implement the program system-wide.[41] The DOD adopted the stepped care model. VA and DOD undersecretaries then convened the Pain Management Workgroup of the Health Executive Committee (PMWG), aiming for a seamless pain management from battlefield injury to community reintegration. The PMWG created training modules and clinical support systems to facilitate knowledge acquisition, and it validated the Defense and Veterans Pain Rating Scale, a brief screening tool for pain intensity and factors that, unlike other brief scales, measures factors that affect pain outcomes (sleep, mood, stress, and function).[64] Figure 2.1 was designed to communicate the integration of these activities within the system.[59]

Second, growing awareness of two related national public health problems intersected to galvanize societal attention: the skyrocketing annual cost of chronic pain to the United States, reaching \$580–\$635 billion,[2] and overuse of opioids, with rising rates of opioid addiction and overdoses. Congress' "societal empathy" for this suffering has resulted in the investments in pain training and research that the pain field has sought for decades. Coordinating heretofore independent efforts of government institutions was critical, as listed in Table 2.1. The 2016 Comprehensive Addiction and Recovery Act[65] charged the VA to coordinate interdisciplinary pain specialty care in all hospitals

Table 2.1 Organizational Stewardship of Societal Pain Management

Date	Sample of Pain Management Stewardship Accomplishments—United States
1973	John Bonica in the Department of Anesthesia, University of Washington, founds the interdisciplinary International Association for the Study of Pain (IASP).
1975	American Society of Regional Anesthesia founded.
1977	American Pain Society formed as a national chapter of IASP.
1983	American Academy of Pain Medicine founded (originally American Academy of Algology).
1988	American Academy of Pain Management (Academy of Integrative Pain Management) founded.
1990	American Board of Medical Specialties (ABMS) approves Pain Medicine Fellowships following Anesthesia Residency and established board examination and certification process.
1991	American Board of Pain Medicine founded to examine and certify residency-trained, clinically experienced pain physicians from anesthesiology, neurology, neurosurgery, psychiatry, and rehabilitation medicine.
1991–1992	Acute Pain Management Guideline Panel, Agency for Health Care Policy and Research, Public Health Service, U.S. Department of Health and Human Services, establishes grading system for evidence of effectiveness of treatments.
1998	Australia and New Zealand College of Anesthetists establishes the first 2-year Pain Medicine Fellowship programs and specialty certification, a model for the world.
1998	The National Institutes of Health (NIH) establishes the National Center for Complementary and Alternative Medicine (NCCAM), now renamed the National Center for Complementary and Integrative Health (NCCIH).
2001–2002	The Accreditation Council for Graduate Medical Education (ACGME) Task Force on Pain Management Fellowships establishes multi-specialty pain medicine training programs and certification guidelines for anesthesiology, neurology, physical medicine and rehabilitation, and psychiatry.
2003	The Department of Veterans Affairs (VA) establishes the National Pain Management Strategy Coordinating Committee,
2007	The American Medical Association forms the Pain and Palliative Medicine Specialty Section Council.
2008	Pain ECHO (Extension for Community Healthcare Outcomes—Pain) begins at the University of New Mexico Health Sciences Center, eventually modeled in the VA, Department of Defense (DOD), and internationally.
2009	The VA establishes the biopsychosocial stepped care model of pain management as national policy.
2010	Army Pain Management Task Force report to the DOD adopts the VA's stepped care model.
2010	The VA and DOD establish the Pain Management Work Group, Health Executive Council of the Undersecretaries for Health to establish a system-wide approach to pain care, injury to recovery.
2011	Institute of Medicine (IOM) Committee on Advancing Pain Research, Care, and Education publishes *Relieving Pain in America: A Blueprint for Transforming Prevention, Care, Education, and Research.*

Table 2.1 Continued

Date	Sample of Pain Management Stewardship Accomplishments—United States
2011	"Aches and Gains" radio show begins at Johns Hopkins University, the first national radio show on pain and now a podcast on Sirius XM with more than 500,000 followers.
2013–2014	NIH–Department of Health and Human Services (HHS) Interagency Pain Research Coordinating Committee (IPRCC), Patient Protection and Affordable Care Act: reports on needed care, education, research, and policy change.
2016	Congress passes the Comprehensive Addiction and Recovery Act of 2016 (CARA) with major provisions for pain management, including requiring that VA hospitals establish interdisciplinary pain teams and support regional pain rehabilitation programs.
2017	NIH–VA–DOD Pain Management Collaboratory established to foster nonpharmacologic research.
2018	U.S. Pain Foundation founded.
2018–2019	Pain Management Best Practices Inter-Agency Task Force, HHS convenes relevant public and private professional organizations and patient advocacy groups to review national pain management practices and recommend needed changes.
2018	NIH cross-institute Helping to End Addiction Long-term Initiative (HEAL Initiative) launched.
2020	Centers for Medicare & Medicaid Services (CMS) creates the Integrated Care Resource Center.

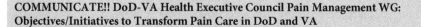

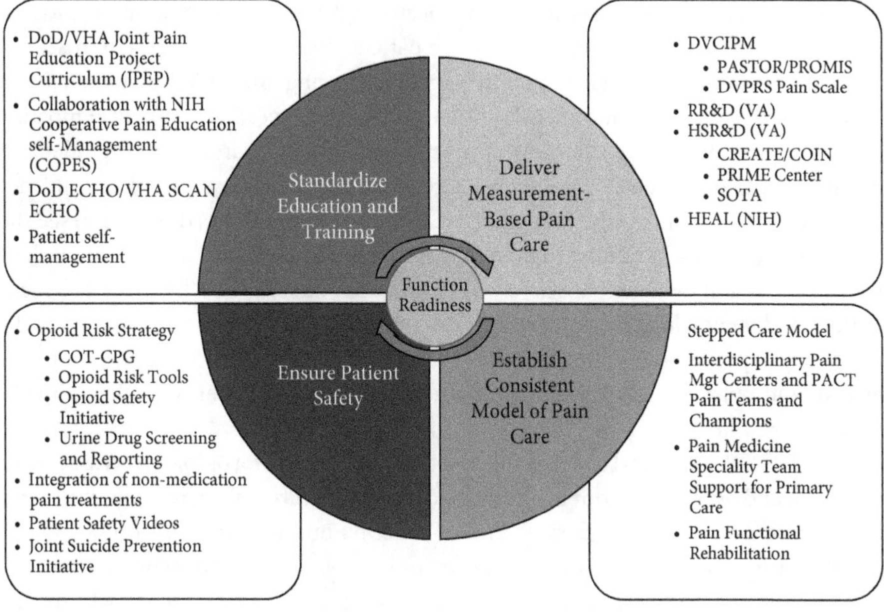

Figure 2.1 VA–DOD pain care system redesign.

Source: Adapted from the Defense and Veterans Center for Integrative Pain Management.[63]

and the Department of Health and Human Services (HSS) to establish an interagency task force on pain management (HHS-PM).[57] This task force convened representatives from organizations within and outside of government related to pain management and included patients with an array of painful conditions. The task force was designed to avoid a more limited focus, such as the 2016 CDC clinical practice guidelines (CPGs) on opioid use and its unanticipated consequences.[66] Cultural changes are needed, including value-based changes in care instituted in organizations such as Kaiser, Mayo Clinic, and Cleveland Clinic.[67] For example, following the HHS's Pain Management Task Force's recommendations for broader access to biopsychosocial care, the Centers for Medicare & Medicaid Services (CMS) created the Integrated Care Resource Center, which helps states develop integrated care programs to coordinate long-term services and supports for eligible individuals.[68,69] Medicare Part B now supports medical care, behavioral health, physical therapy, occupational therapy, spine manipulation, alcohol misuse, depression screening, and acupuncture for LBP. To address growing income disparities between procedural specialties (e.g., anesthesia and surgery) and cognitive-relational specialties (e.g., primary care), CMS is increasing the relative evaluation units for primary care, and potentially more time to manage biopsychosocial components of pain supporting a more effective collaborative stepped model, because primary care has the largest burden of pain care. NIH's HEAL Initiative has made major investments in translational, clinical, and health systems pain research throughout the country. This collective national effort manifests responsible professional stewardship, creating a continuity of public action toward improving pain care. Implementing such advances widely requires policy favoring universal coverage for health care and valuing outcomes over incomes, as occurs in other countries with advanced economies.[70]

How the opioid public health crisis developed and the impact of the CDC's response, the 2016 CPGs for opioid prescribing, provide a cautionary tale about stewardship. Over three decades, managed care's primary care requirements resulted in institutional pressure for both briefer visits and positive patient Press–Gainey satisfaction scores. The 0–10 pain scale, intended to identify patients requiring full clinical pain evaluation, was misused as the evaluation itself, not a full biopsychosocial assessment. Empathic clinicians, encouraged by direct-to-primary-care marketing and clinical guidelines, relied on opioids to lower pain scores across conditions, although opioids did not treat the causes of pain, only the pain itself. Health system leaders did not foresee the consequences of poor training in pain management and SUD risk assessment, lack of time to assess and monitor patient response, and unavailability of other pain treatment options and mental health and addiction resources. The 10–20% of patients with SUD, and a larger proportion with mental health risks, were not identified nor appropriately monitored and treated. A dramatic rise in opioid use disorder (OUD) and opioid overdoses resulted.

The CDC CPGs focused on lowering opioid doses or stopping opioids to avoid opioid addiction and overdoses (nonmaleficence). Consequent directives from employers and health systems caused providers, fearful of sanction and lawsuits, to stop opioids or greatly lower doses, even in patients using opioids responsibly and effectively. However, providers were not trained, nor health systems designed, to achieve this safely and effectively and to manage clinical consequences[66]: difficulty weaning patients from high doses, requiring long and carefully monitored tapers; patients' despair when opioids were stopped or doses dropped precipitously, causing loss of pain control, withdrawal stress, and impaired function; depression and increasing suicide rates; inaccessible SUD treatment; increased exposure to fentanyl-laced street drugs, causing overdose deaths; and sociomedical realities such as limited access to integrative, psychological, pain medicine and SUD care for patients of low income, without insurance, on Medicaid, or with managed care plans. Physicians previously acting under the banner of "beneficence" now, as Elaine Scarry's treatise[48] suggests, risked being perceived by patients as torturing them by withholding available pain relief ("maleficence"), even when the patients did not exhibit risks and had benefited. Doctor–patient trust was fractured. Clinicians now had to balance the risk for causing patient harm by stopping medications versus the risk of an overdose event, but without the tools to manage this balance. Consequences such as licensure loss or lawsuits might follow. These ethical dilemmas have exacted a considerable emotional toll and the potential loss of physicians' practices in a community's health care system.[21,66] Discussion of policies to respond to this secondary crisis rightly focuses on the management of addiction such as access to buprenorphine, which for years has been unreasonably restricted for patients in pain at risk for OUD, and other strategies.[71,72] Until recently, there was little consideration of the larger population seeking pain relief who were exposed to opioids for lack of access to effective options.

Thoughtful stewardship by motivated professionals making changes in health systems for beneficence and justice can make a difference in a population. Australian health systems have long grappled with developing community-based approaches to improve access to good pain care.[73] In one regional system, STEPS, primary care community support groups greatly reduced wait times and costs at public pain medicine units and increased use of active pain management strategies and patient satisfaction.[74] Patients on long-term opioids referred to such pain specialty clinics stopped opioids or reduced doses by more than 50% and also improved their pain scores.[75] This work is a progression of decades-long stewardship of a stepped model of pain care for an Australian province.[73]

The Pain ECHO telementoring program provides another example of professional stewardship to improve pain care for individual patients and an entire health system.[42] Multidisciplinary teams supervise distant primary care providers' direct care of patients with pain conditions over a telehealth network, similar to residency training. Patients obtain specialty-level interdisciplinary consultation; providers gain skills in pain management not learned in residency. Other health systems also challenged by long distances, such as the VA and DOD, instituted this model successfully, increasing the efficiency of stepped care.[76,77] ECHO's and VA–DOD's successes demonstrate how creative stewardship within an organization, when evaluated and disseminated, can serve as a societal model that benefits other organizations' providers, their patients, and the public health more widely.

Conclusion

The current health system in the United States struggles to provide high-quality pain care across the population. For clinicians, achieving success in pain management requires both insight and responsibility. They must understand the needs of their patients and how well they are equipped to provide for those needs. They must strive to achieve clinical competency appropriate to their level of pain care—primary, specialty, or subspecialty—in the biopsychosocial stepped collaborative care model of pain management. They must evaluate how well their health system supports this model and find ways to appropriate resources in the system and community to support good care. When confronted by an ethical conundrum, they must try to understand its dimensions and seek counsel from trusted colleagues or counselors to help them find a moral way forward. To do this well, they must learn effective self-care and prioritize their own physical and mental health.

Health professionals must also provide professional stewardship toward better care in their communities, regions, and nations. This requires recognizing systems' limitations in providing reliable, ethical stepped pain care for patients in their communities—per the Fred Davis model in Michigan; ECHO in New Mexico and beyond; and regionally and nationally as modeled in the VA–DOD, Australian, and some European systems. They must responsibly seek to remediate deficits through teamwork supported by ethical analysis. When confronted by an impasse in the system, health leaders must understand and be willing to overcome sociobiologically determined impediments, such as tribalism and greed, and replace them with healthier instincts such as altruism and teamwork. This will enable them to collaborate more effectively for better pain care and the public good.[78]

References

1. Clarey C. Rafael Nadal falls apart on clay, just in time for the French Open. *The New York Times,* May 12, 2022.
2. Institute of Medicine, Committee on Advancing Pain Research, Care, and Education. *Relieving Pain in America: A Blueprint for Transforming Prevention, Care, Education, and Research.* National Academies Press; 2011.
3. Gallagher RM. Integrating medical and behavioral treatment in chronic pain management. *Med Clin North Am.* 1999;83(5):823–849.
4. Weiner DK. Deconstructing chronic low back pain in the older adult: Shifting the paradigm from the spine to the person. *Pain Med.* 2015;16(5):881–885.
5. Chadwick A, Frazier A, Khan TW, Young E. Understanding the psychological, physiological, and genetic factors affecting precision pain medicine: A narrative review. *J Pain Res.* 2021;14:3145–3161.
6. Gallagher RM. Pain medicine and primary care: A community solution to pain as a public health problem. *Med Clin North Am* 1999;83(5):555–585.
7. Griffiths EP. Revaluing primary care—Going beyond RVU increases. *N Engl J Med.* 2022;387:2302–2303.
8. Juckett DA, Davis FN, Gostine M, et al. Patient-reported outcomes in a large community-based pain medicine practice: Evaluation for use in phenotype modeling. *BMC Med Inform Decis Mak.* 2015;15: Article 41.
9. Bellerose G. *Caring for Our Own: A Portrait of Community Health Care.* Painter House Press, 2006.
10. Parasidis E, Fairchild AL. Closing the public health access gap. *N Engl J Med.* 2022;387(11):961–983.
11. McAneny BL, Byrny RL. The American health care system is broken: It can and must be fixed. *The Pharos* 2022;Spring:2–7

12. Weiner D, Kim Y-S, Bonino P, Wang T. Low back pain in older adults: Are we utilizing healthcare resources wisely? *Pain Med.* 2006;7(2):143–150.
13. Pauly M, Winston F, Naylor M, et al. Index. In *Seemed Like a Good Idea: Alchemy Versus Evidence-Based Approaches to Healthcare Management Innovation.* Cambridge University Press; 2022:409–412.
14. Sandhu S, Liu M, Wadhera RK. Hospitals and health equity—Translating measurement into action. *N Engl J Med.* 2022:387(26):2395–2397.
15. Gallagher RM. Ethics in pain medicine: Good for our health, good for the public health. *Pain Med.* 2001;2(2):87–89.
16. Boyd KM. Medical ethics: Principles, persons, and perspectives: From controversy to conversation. *J Med Ethics.* 2005;31:481–486.
17. Wilson EO. *The Future of Life.* Knopf; 2002.
18. Wilson EO. *On Human Nature.* Harvard University Press; 1978.
19. Sullivan M. Ethical principles in pain medicine. *Pain Med.* 2001;2(2):106–111.
20. Hamaty D. Pain medicine's role in the restoration and reformation of medical ethics. *Pain Med.* 2001;2(2):117–120.
21. Arnold-Forster A, Moses JD, Schotland SV. Obstacles to physicians' emotional health—Lessons from history. *N Engl J Med.* 2022;386:4–7.
22. Gazda T, Gallagher RM, Little DN, Sproul MS. The practice group seminar—A Balint-type group in a family practice setting. *Family Med.* 1984;16(2):54–58.
23. Gallagher RM, Fishman S. Pain medicine: History, emergence as a medical specialty, and evolution of the multidisciplinary approach. In: Cousins MJ, Bridenbaugh PO, Carr D, Horlocker T, eds. *Cousins and Bridenbaugh's Neural Blockade.* 4th ed. Lippincott Williams & Wilkins; 2008:631–643.
24. Dubois M, Gallagher RM, Lippe P. Pain medicine position paper. *Pain Med.* 2009;10(6):972–1000.
25. Lippe PM, Brock C, David J, Crossno R, Gitlow S. The First National Pain Medicine Summit—Final summary report. *Pain Med.* 2010;11(10):1447–1468.
26. Emanuel EJ, Upshur RE, Smith MJ. What Covid has taught the world about ethics. *N Engl J Med.* 2022;387:1542–1545.
27. Cohen SP, Baber ZB, Buvanendran A, et al. Pain management best practices from multispecialty organizations during the COVID-19 pandemic and public health crises. *Pain Med.* 2020;21(7):1331–1346.
28. Driver L. Ethical considerations for chronic pain care during a pandemic. *Pain Med.* 2020;21:1327–1330.
29. AMA Council on Ethical and Judicial Affairs. Principles of medical ethics. In: Code of Medical Ethics: Current Opinions with Annotations. American Medical Association; 2002.
30. AMA Council on Ethical and Judicial Affairs. CEJA Report 1-A-12. Physician stewardship of health care resources. 2012. Accessed October 28, 2022. https://www.ama-assn.org/sites/ama-assn.org/files/corp/media-browser/public/about-ama/councils/Council%20Reports/council-on-ethics-and-judicial-affairs/ceja-1a12.pdf
31. AMA Council on Ethical and Judicial Affairs. CEJA Report 5-I-13. Professionalism in health care systems. 2013. Accessed October 28, 2022. https://www.ama-assn.org/sites/ama-assn.org/files/corp/media-browser/public/about-ama/councils/Council%20Reports/council-on-ethics-and-judicial-affairs/ceja-5i13.pdf
32. Lebovitz A, Gallagher RM. Ethical challenges in pain management. In: Flor H, Kalso E, Dostrovsky J, eds. *Proceedings of the 11th World Congress on Pain.* IASP; 2006:41–48.
33. International Association for the Study of Pain. Declaration that access to pain management is a fundamental human right. 2010. Accessed October 28, 2022. http://www.iasp-pain.org/Advocacy/Content.aspx?ItemNumber=1821
34. Green CR, Anderson KO, Baker TA, et al. The unequal burden of pain: Confronting racial and ethnic disparities in pain. *Pain Med.* 2003;4(3):277–294.
35. Gallagher RM, Moore P, Chernoff I. The reliability of depression diagnosis in chronic low back pain: A pilot study. *Gen Hosp Psychiatry* 1995;17:399–413.

36. Gallagher RM, Myers P: Referral delay in back pain patients on workers' compensation: Costs and policy implications. *Psychosomatics.* 1996;37(3):270–284.
37. Binkley CE, Reynolds JM, Shuman A. From the eyeball test to the algorithm—Quality of life, disability status, and clinical decision-making in surgery. *N Engl J Med.* 2022;387(14):1325–1328.
38. Koes BW, van Tulder M, Lin CW, et al. An updated overview of clinical guidelines for the management of non-specific low back pain in primary care. *Eur Spine J.* 2010;19(12):2075–2094.
39. Gourlay DL, Heit HA, Almahrezi A. Universal precautions in pain medicine: A rational approach to the treatment of chronic pain. *Pain Med.* 2005;6(5):107–112.
40. Sandbrink F, Oliva EM, McMullen TL, et al. Opioid prescribing and opioid risk mitigation strategies in the Veterans Health Administration. *J Gen Intern Med.* 2020;35(Suppl 3):927–934.
41. Gallagher RM. Advancing the pain agenda in the veteran population. *Anesth Clin.* 2016;34:357–378.
42. Katzman JG. ECHO telementoring for pain, palliative care, and opioid management: Progress, challenges, and future goals. *Pain Med.* 2020;21(2):220–225.
43. Wiedemer N, Harden P, Arndt R, Gallagher R. The opioid renewal clinic, a primary care, managed approach to opioid therapy in chronic pain patients at risk for substance abuse. *Pain Med.* 2007;8(7):573–584.
44. Oliva EM, Bowe T, Tavakoli S., et al. Development and applications of the Veterans Health Administration's Stratification Tool for Opioid Risk Mitigation (STORM) to improve opioid safety and prevent overdose and suicide. *Psychol Serv.* 2017;14(1):34–49.
45. Frank JW, Carey E, Nolan C, et al. Increased nonopioid chronic pain treatment in the Veterans Health Administration, 2010–2016. *Pain Med.* 2019;20(5):869–877.
46. Kapural L, Nagem H, Tlucek H, Sessler DI. Spinal cord stimulation for chronic visceral abdominal pain. *Pain Med.* 2012;11(3):347–355.
47. Mathur VA, Trost Z, Ezenwa MO, Sturgeon JA, Hood AM. Mechanisms of injustice: What we (do not) know about racialized disparities in pain. *Pain.* 2022;163(6):999–1005.
48. Scarry E. *The Body in Pain: The Making and Unmaking of the World.* Oxford University Press; 1985.
49. Carr DB. Patients with pain need less stigma, not more. *Pain Med.* 2016;17(8):1391–1393.
50. Fishbain DA, Cole B, Cutler RB, et al. A structured evidence-based review on the meaning of nonorganic physical signs: Waddell signs. *Pain Med.* 2003;4(2):141–181.
51. Fishbain D. Response from Fishbain. *Pain Med.* 2003;4(4):386–387.
52. Dohrenwend B, Marbach J, Raphael K, Gallagher RM. Why is depression co-morbid with chronic facial pain? A family study test of alternative hypotheses. *Pain.* 1999;83:183–192.
53. Gallagher RM. Chronification to maldynia: Biopsychosocial failure of pain homeostasis. *Pain Med.* 2011;12(7):993–995.
54. Darnall BD. Pain psychology and pain catastrophizing in the perioperative setting: A review of impacts, interventions, and unmet needs. *Hand Clin.* 2016;32(1):33–39.
55. Carvalho AS, Pereira SM, Jacomo A, et al. Ethical decision making in pain management: A conceptual framework. *J Pain Res.* 2018;11:967–976.
56. Interagency Pain Research Coordinating Committee, U.S. Department of Health and Human Services. The National Pain Strategy Report: A comprehensive population health-level strategy for pain. 2014. Accessed January 15 2023. https://www.iprcc.nih.gov/node/5/national-pain-strategy-report
57. U.S. Department of Health and Human Services. Pain Management Best Practices Inter-Agency Task Force report: Updates, gaps, inconsistencies, and recommendations. 2019. Accessed October 28, 2022. https://www.hhs.gov/sites/default/files/pmtf-final-report-2019-05-23.pdf
58. Kerns RD, Philip EJ, Lee A, Rosenberger PR. Implementation of the Veterans Health Administration National Pain Management Strategy. *Transl Behav Med.* 2011;1(4):635–643.

59. Defense & Veterans Center for Integrative Pain Management. VA–DoD Joint Pain Education Project. n.d. Accessed October 28, 2022. https://www.dvcipm.org/clinical-resources/joint-pain-education-project-jpep
60. Lew HL, Otis JD, Tun C, et al. Prevalence of chronic pain, posttraumatic stress disorder and post-concussive symptoms in OEF/OIF Veterans: The Polytrauma Clinical Triad. *J Rehab Res Dev.* 2009;46:697–702.
61. Gallagher RM, Polomano R, Giordano N, et al. A prospective cohort study examining the use of regional anesthesia for early pain management after combat-related extremity injury. *Reg Anesth Pain Med.* 2019;44:1045–1052.
62. Pain Management Task Force, Office of the Army Surgeon General. Providing a standardized DoD and VHA vision and approach to pain management to optimize the care for warriors and their families. 2010. Accessed October 28,2022. https://www.dvcipm.org/clinical-resources/pain-management-task-force
63. Defense and Veterans Center for Integrative Pain Management. Stepped care model of pain management [Video]. n.d. Accessed October 28, 2022. https://www.dvcipm.org/clinical-resources/joint-pain-education-project-jpep/pain-educational-videos/#steppedcare
64. Polomano RC, Buckenmaier CC III, Galloway KT, McDuffie M, Kwon N, Gallagher RM. Preliminary validation of the Defense and Veterans Pain Rating Scale (DVPRS) in a military population. *Pain Med.* 2013;14:110–123.
65. CADCA. Comprehensive Addiction and Recovery Act. 2016. Accessed October 28, 2022. https://www.cadca.org/cara/#
66. Hallvik SE, El Ibrahimi S, Johnston K, et al. Patient outcomes after opioid dose reduction among patients with chronic opioid therapy. *Pain.* 2022;163(1):83–90.
67. Nurok M, Lee TH. Transforming culture in health care. *N Engl J Med.* 2023;381(22):2173–2175.
68. Centers for Medicare & Medicaid Services, Department of Health and Human Services. Medicare and Medicaid programs. *Fed Reg.* 2022;87(145):45932–45938. Accessed March 24, 2023. https://www.govinfo.gov/content/pkg/FR-2022-07-29/pdf/2022-14562.pdf
69. Integrated Care Resource Center. n.d. [Home page]. Accessed March 24, 2023. https://www.integratedcareresourcecenter.com
70. Larssen S, Clawson J, Howard R. Value-based health care at an inflection point: A global agenda for the next decade. *N Engl J Med.* February 24, 2023. Accessed March 24, 2023. https://catalyst.nejm.org/doi/full/10.1056/CAT.22.0332
71. Coffin PO, Barreveld AM. Inherited patients taking opioids for chronic pain: Considerations for primary care. *N Engl J Med.* 2022;386(7):611–613.
72. Poorman E. The number needed to prescribe: What would it take to expand access to buprenorphine? *N Engl J Med.* 2021;384:1783–1784.
73. Davies SJ, Hayes C, Quintner JL. System plasticity and integrated care: Informed consumers guide clinical reorientation and system reorganization. *Pain Med.* 2011;12(1):4–8.
74. Antill T, Packer T, Schug SA. Preclinic group education sessions reduce waiting times and costs at public pain medicine units. *Pain Med.* 2011;12(1):59–71.
75. Tardif H, Hayes C, Allingham SF. Opioid cessation is associated with reduced pain and improved function in people attending specialist chronic pain services. *Med J Aust.* 2021;214(9):430–432.
76. Frank JW, Carey EP, Fagan KM, et al. Evaluation of a telementoring intervention for pain management in the Veterans Health Administration. *Pain Med.* 2015;16(6):1090–1100.
77. Katzman JG, Galloway K, Olivas C, et al. Expanding health care access through education: Dissemination and implementation of the ECHO model. Mil Med. 2016;181(3):227–235.
78. Gallagher RM. Pain management in America: Where do we go from here? *EXPLORE* 2019;15:400–403.

3

Pain Genomics

Defining the Vulnerable Patient

Tina Doshi and Arissa Torrie

Despite the universal experience of pain, vulnerability to pain and its manifestations is highly variable across individuals. The biopsychosocial model, the most widely accepted heuristic for pain and its treatment, considers pain as a "dynamic interaction among physiologic, psychological, and social factors."[1(p607)] These interrelated factors include intrinsic (biological) risk factors such as female sex, increasing age, genetic/genomic profile, and changes in molecular signaling pathways, which have been correlated to inter-individual differences in pain sensitivity and susceptibility to developing chronic pain.[2] In addition, extrinsic (environmental) factors, including poor nutrition, substance use, psychological stressors, and physical injury, can induce neurochemical changes that act on intrinsic factors to modify pain perception and vulnerability to painful conditions.[3] Responses to pain treatments also have high inter-individual variability, reflective of an individual's unique intrinsic and extrinsic traits.

Genetic differences that affect disease can range from single base changes called single nucleotide polymorphisms (SNPs) or variants to small insertions or deletions of 1–100 bases and much larger structural variants (e.g., insertions, deletions, duplications, and inversions) up to several hundred kilobases in length.[4] Gene expression can also be influenced by epigenetic (i.e., "beside the genome") changes; these stable, heritable molecular modifications (e.g., DNA methylation and chromatin modification) do not alter the underlying sequence of base pairs and comprise the "epigenome."[5] Other downstream processes or so-called 'omes may also affect disease manifestation; these include RNA expression (transcriptome), protein expression (proteome), metabolites (metabolome), and even the effects of microbial inhabitants in the body (microbiome).[6] At each step from genotype to phenotype, environmental exposures may further modulate disease susceptibility, progression, and recovery.

These collective variations create a unique biochemical profile that influences pain vulnerability and response to pain treatment. Thus, genetic and molecular profiling can provide deeper knowledge of pain mechanisms at the individual-specific and disease-specific levels, aiding in the development of personalized and precision pain therapies.[7] This chapter explores genetic, epigenetic, proteomic, metabolomic, microbiome, and environmental factors that contribute to pain sensitivity, susceptibility, and response to treatment (Figure 3.1).

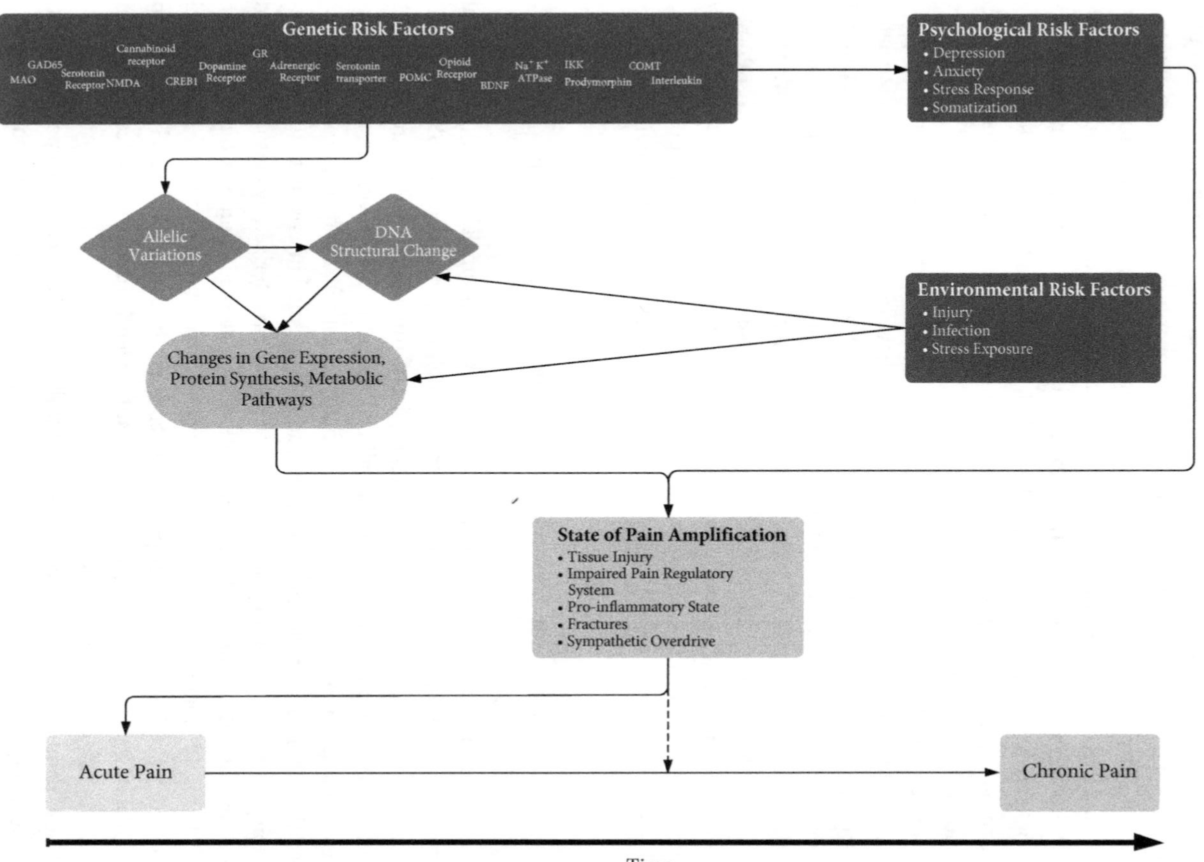

Figure 3.1 Genetic influences along the spectrum of acute to chronic pain.

Hereditary Pain Conditions

Hereditary pain conditions provide a useful framework for understanding the role of genetics in pain and its treatment. Monogenic or single-gene pain conditions that follow Mendelian inheritance (i.e., passed down from parents to offspring) include painful channelopathies affecting the *SCN9A* gene and familial hemiplegic migraine, which are most often caused by mutations in ion channels. Other classic monogenic disorders, such as sickle cell anemia, *HLA-B27* spondyloarthropathies, neurofibromatosis, and Ehlers–Danlos and other connective tissue disorders are also often associated with chronic pain. However, the associations between these monogenic disorders and pain are heterogeneous and not well-defined, with some affected individuals having little or no painful symptoms, reflecting the complex and multifactorial nature of pain development.

More commonly, chronic pain results from a combination of genetic and environmental factors. Multiple genetic variants or alleles have been reported to be associated with chronic pain, most often in genes affecting pain perception, neurotransmitter systems, ion channel function, inflammation, pharmacokinetics, and pharmacodynamics. These alleles typically have variable penetrance—that is, individuals who have putatively pathogenic variants may or may not actually manifest pathology. In addition, environmental factors can lead to changes in the epigenome, gene expression, and/or protein function. Thus, most chronic pain disorders are considered polygenic (i.e., influenced by multiple genes), with substantial contributions from the environment.

Mendelian Inherited Monogenic Pain Conditions

Three classic hereditary pain conditions— primary erythromelalgia (PE), paroxysmal extreme pain disorder (PEPD), and inherited small fiber neuropathy (ISFN)—are intensely painful diseases caused by different gain-of-function mutations in the *SCN9A* gene.[8] *SCN9A* encodes a voltage-gated sodium channel ($Na_v1.7$), which is expressed in sensory and autonomic neurons and plays an important role in nociceptor excitability.[9] Two different loss-of-function mutations lead to congenital insensitivity to pain or hereditary sensory and autonomic neuropathy.[8] PE is characterized by episodic pain and erythema, usually in the hands and feet, with an average age of onset around 20 years. PEPD typically manifests from birth with episodic pain, most frequently in the sacral region and face. ISFN commonly presents in early adulthood as persistent burning pain and, like other small-fiber neuropathies, most frequently occurs in the feet, but it can also affect the upper extremities.

These painful *SCN9A* syndromes are clinically quite severe, autosomal dominant, and have high penetrance. Consequently, prediction of disease susceptibility and diagnosis is straightforward. *SCN9A* testing is available for screening and diagnostic purposes[10]; most are sequence analyses of the entire coding region and used as a confirmatory test for clinical diagnosis. However, testing of asymptomatic individuals without a family history is not recommended for any of the *SCN9A*-related pain syndromes. They are extremely rare, and a number of other mutations in the same gene are associated with different diseases of variable severity and/or clinical significance, such as febrile seizures.[11,12] Thus, routine screening for *SCN9A* mutations would be unlikely to produce a positive diagnosis in patients without clinical features of a painful *SCN9A* channelopathy, and it would also increase the risk of identifying genetic variants of unclear clinical significance, leading to unnecessary additional workup and patient distress. Similarly, prenatal testing for *SCN9A* channelopathies is not recommended for the general population. There are only 80 cases of PEPD in the scientific literature,[13] and the frequencies of PE and ISFN are unknown but believed to be very low,[14,15] so the pretest probability of an individual being a carrier without any family history is also extraordinarily low. However, if one or both parents have a positive family history, prenatal testing for *SCN9A* would be appropriate and can be performed from amniocentesis or chorionic villus sampling.[10] Although these conditions have no cure or preventative treatments, they can be clinically severe, and prenatal diagnostic testing can provide parents with anticipatory guidance.

Another well-known monogenic, Mendelian inherited pain disorder is familial hemiplegic migraine (FHM), a rare disease characterized by severe migraine and aura symptoms of motor weakness or numbness (usually hemiparesis), often with other neurologic symptoms, including visual, sensory, or speech disturbances; confusion; seizures; memory loss; and coma.[16] It is caused by mutations in one of at least three genes—*CACNA1A* (classified as FHM1), *ATP1A2* (FHM2), or *SCN1A* (FHM3)—each of which encodes an ion channel or ion transport protein, although a few very rare pathogenic variants in other genes have also been reported.[16] Although the subtypes are clinically indistinguishable, there is variable penetrance, and clinical phenotypes can differ widely even among patients with identical mutations, indicating likely polygenic or environmental contributions.

The first causative gene identified for FHM was *CACNA1A*, a brain-specific voltage-gated calcium channel subunit.[17] More than 25 variants of the gene have been reported to cause FHM1, usually with gain-of-function effects leading to enhanced glutamatergic activity and neuronal hypexcitability.[16] Similarly, numerous variants of the *ATP1A2* gene have been implicated in the development of FHM2; the gene encodes a catalytic subunit of the Na^+/K^+ ATPase ion transport pump.[18] In general, the pathogenic variants of *ATP1A2* lead to dysfunctional ion transport, increasing synaptic K^+ concentrations and glutamate. These changes in turn predispose the brain to cortical spreading depression (CSD), the phenomenon behind migraine aura, in which a wave of depolarization spreads across the cortex and is followed by neuronal suppression.[16] In FHM3, mutations in the *SCN1A* gene, which encodes the $Na_v1.1$ voltage-gated sodium channel, usually cause gain-of-function effects that also enhance glutamate release and trigger CSD.[19] Interestingly, some loss-of-function mutations in the same gene are associated with (typically nonpainful) epilepsy syndromes.[20] De novo mutations in these same genes have also been associated with sporadic (nonfamilial) hemiplegic migraine, which comprises approximately one-third of cases.[21]

A variety of other much less common pathogenic variants in other genes have also been reported to cause either familial or sporadic hemiplegic migraine.[16] However, these same genes are often associated with other neurological disorders, making the diagnosis of hemiplegic migraine particularly challenging in the absence of any *CACNA1A*, *ATP1A2*, and *SCN1A* mutations, or when a complex patient presents with symptoms that are atypical or overlap with other conditions. Newer DNA sequencing approaches may be instrumental in resolving these difficult cases and provide a paradigm that could be applied to other complex pain disorders. *CACNA1A*, *ATP1A2*, and *SCN1A* were all identified using traditional DNA sequencing methods that are time-consuming and expensive, often focused on selected exons. By contrast, next-generation sequencing (NGS) technologies have allowed for faster, cheaper profiling of larger coding regions of interest or even the entire genome. In the case of hemiplegic migraine, NGS techniques have led to improved diagnostic success, identification of novel mutations, and testing for overlapping neurological disorders, and the ability to examine large portions of the genome using NGS could facilitate the discovery of new migraine-related genes and provide deeper understanding of migraine pathophysiology.[16]

Non-Mendelian Inherited (Polygenic) Pain Conditions

Numerous genetic risk factors have been identified for all of the most common chronic pain disorders, including migraine, fibromyalgia, and low back pain (LBP). Unlike the monogenic pain disorders, which have distinctive clinical effects, most genetic variants associated with chronic pain are SNPs, which typically have only minor phenotypic effects in isolation. However, SNPs can manifest as increased or decreased susceptibility to disease, particularly in conjunction with other genetic/genomic changes or environmental factors.[22] In general, SNPs implicated in chronic pain and response to pain treatment have been located in genes that affect key aspects of the pain experience, including pain perception, neurotransmitter systems, ion channel function, and analgesic or placebo response.

The chronic pain condition with the largest body of evidence for genetic association is migraine.[22] Migraine is a primary headache disorder associated with photophobia and phonophobia or nausea/vomiting. Worldwide prevalence of migraine is approximately 10%, and it is a leading pain-related cause of disability.[23] Studies of twins have found the heritability of migraine to be approximately 30–50% or more.[24,25] Approximately 40 different genetic loci have been associated with migraine susceptibility.[26] These loci are located in genes associated with endothelial function, neurotransmission, and inflammatory markers, which is consistent with our contemporary understanding of migraine as a disorder of cerebrovascular dysregulation and neuronal hyperexcitability, modulated by inflammation.[22]

The most reported genetic association in migraine is methylenetetrahydrofolate reductase (*MTHFR*), which encodes an enzyme responsible for amino acid metabolism and folate processing; as such, it affects DNA synthesis and repair, neurotransmitter synthesis, vascular endothelial integrity, and immune function. MTHFR deficiency causes elevated plasma homocysteine levels, which in turn are associated with endothelial injury, and studies have identified *MTHFR* variants as risk factors for developing migraine and other vascular disorders (e.g., stroke and heart disease).[27] An estimated 20–40% of White and Hispanic Americans are heterozygous for the most common variant (*C677T*), whereas 8–20% of North Americans, Europeans, and Australians are homozygous, although the prevalence of *C677T* in Blacks is much lower (1–2%).[28] Heterozygotes for the *MTHFR C677T* allele have 65% enzyme function, whereas homozygotes have only 30% function, and other common *MTHFR* variants causing decreased function have also been identified.[28]

Because *MTHFR* variants are so common, often asymptomatic, and present in a diverse range of clinical pathology, there is little utility in routine genetic testing for *MTHFR* mutations. However, in patients who have clinical conditions associated with *MTHFR* deficiency, testing may be helpful to guide potential treatments based on MTHFR function. In one small study, migraine patients receiving vitamin supplementation to support MTHFR function and mitigate elevated homocysteine levels had decreased headache frequency and severity compared to placebo.[29] Interestingly, homozygotes for *C677T* had the weakest clinical response, suggesting that they may require higher doses than heterozygotes or homozygotes without the variant. Stratified dosing based on genotype exemplifies a personalized medicine approach to pain treatment.

Fibromyalgia is another common chronic pain condition with substantial evidence for genetic contributions, with various studies noting heritability of 15–50%.[30,31] Chronic widespread musculoskeletal pain and associated fatigue, sleep disturbances, and cognitive and somatic symptoms are hallmarks of the condition, which has an estimated prevalence of 2–4% of the general population.[32] Genetic variants associated with fibromyalgia have been identified in genes involved in monoaminergic pathways (e.g., dopamine, norepinephrine, serotonin, and histamine), neuronal inhibition and excitation (including *SCN9A*), and inflammation; these findings suggest fibromyalgia as a disorder of altered nociceptive signaling and heightened stress response.[22]

An understanding of genetic associations in fibromyalgia may also have implications for pain treatment strategies. The enzyme catechol-*O*-methyltransferase (COMT) plays an important role in catecholamine metabolism, which in turn influences sympathetic tone and pain inhibition.[33] Multiple *COMT* variants have been associated with fibromyalgia diagnosis and symptom severity.[33] One of the most common is the *Val158Met* polymorphism, which encodes a protein with lower enzymatic activity, leading to decreased catecholamine metabolism.[33,34] Fibromyalgia patients with one or two copies of this variant have been shown to have increased sensitivity to thermal and pressure pain compared to those with two copies of the normal gene.[34] Fibromyalgia has also been associated with multiple variants in different serotonin- and dopamine-related genes, including *HTR2A* for a serotonin receptor, *SLC6A4* for a serotonin transporter, and the dopamine D2 and D4 receptors.[33] Given the key role of antidepressants in the management of fibromyalgia, additional research in the genetics of this condition may provide insights on recommended dosing and predicting treatment response based on genotype, applying a precision medicine approach to pain.

Back pain, particularly LBP, is another common debilitating condition with significant impact on well-being.[35] Known clinical risk factors for LBP include age, female gender, and increased body mass index,[35] but evidence obtained during the past decade suggests that genetic factors may be significantly responsible for wide interindividual variations seen in disc degeneration and other spinal pathology among adults.[36] Although there is no single genetic variant responsible for LBP, there are several proposed genetic variants that may be associated with susceptibility to developing spinal pathology and pain. Genetic studies of LBP characterize it as a disease of disrupted tissue remodeling with overactive inflammatory signaling. Variants in genes associated with disc integrity, such as the apoptosis-mediating caspase CASP9, protein degradation enzymes MMP1 and MMP2, and the chondrogenesis transcription factor SOX5, have all been linked to increased susceptibility to disc degeneration and LBP.[22,37] Disc degeneration has also been associated with increased pro-inflammatory cytokines. Genetic variants of the chemotactic factor CCL2, the skeletal tissue differentiation growth factor GDF5, interleukin (IL)-1A, IL-1 receptor antagonist, and IL-18 receptor subunits are correlated with LBP susceptibility and response to LBP treatment.[22,37]

As with other chronic pain conditions discussed above, the development of LBP may also have contributions from genes related to neurotransmission and pain perception. LBP has also been associated with an SNP in the gene *DCC* (deleted in colorectal carcinoma) encoding the receptor Netrin-1, which contributes to the development of cortical and spinal commissural neurons.[37,38] Both *DCC* and Netrin-1 have high expression in degraded discs, suggesting an association with degenerative back pain. Interesting, the same Val158Met polymorphism in the *COMT* gene that has been linked to fibromyalgia has also been associated with disc herniation.[22,37] As noted above, the COMT enzyme regulates adrenergic, noradrenergic, and dopaminergic signaling, and low COMT levels are associated with attenuated spinal nociceptive activity and central sensitization.[37,39] The opioid receptor system also appears to contribute to the development of LBP, although the mechanism has not been proven and remains poorly understood. An SNP at position 118 on the μ-opioid receptor 1 gene that converts an A to a G (i.e., *OPRM1 A118G*) has been linked to decreased pain improvement and worsened subjective health complaints following disc herniation and radicular pain compared to those with the A allele, but only in women compared to men.[40] These results suggest a sex-linked component to the role of *OPRM1 A118G* in LBP; however, results from other subsequent studies have been inconsistent.[22,37] It has been suggested that the *OPRM1 A118G* genotype may impart sensitivity to pro-inflammatory, immune, and stress responses, potentially in a way that is modulated by sex and/or age.[37,41]

There is also evidence for a genetic component to treatment response for these and other polygenic pain conditions, to be discussed below. A tailored approach using genetics for pain would be to identify patients at risk of developing chronic pain and then use genetic profiles to guide treatment in a mechanism-based fashion. Implementation of gene-based pharmacotherapy may therefore offer more efficacious drugs for the chronic pain patient.

The Genetics of Chronic Overlapping Pain Conditions

Many patients with chronic pain conditions often have other coexisting pain conditions with similar symptomatology, including migraine, fibromyalgia, LBP, temporomandibular disorder, irritable bowel syndrome, interstitial cystitis, and vulvodynia.[42] Collectively known as chronic overlapping pain conditions, these disorders are paradigmatic of chronic pain in general and are characterized as states of heightened pain amplification and psychological distress resulting from the interaction of genetic determinants and environmental exposures.[43] Genetic factors can therefore increase vulnerability to chronic pain by enhancing pain sensitivity and predisposing patients to conditions that increase psychological distress (e.g., depression, anxiety, and somatization), which intensifies the experience of pain.[43]

The significant heterogeneity in pain manifestations, even within a single pain diagnosis, makes it challenging to identify specific genes corresponding to chronic pain vulnerability. However, genome-wide association studies have identified variants corresponding to generally increased pain sensitivity, including some of the genes discussed in specific pain conditions above. Genes for ion channels affecting neuronal excitation (*SCN9A*, *KCNS1*, and multiple voltage-gated Ca^{2+} channels) and genes associated with neurotransmission (*COMT*, *SLC6A4*, and *HTR2A*) are the two most common categories of polymorphisms that may increase susceptibility to pain.[44] Clearly, chronic pain is polygenic and subject to significant environmental effects, but further elucidation of genetic determinants of pain will allow us to better identify individuals at increased risk of developing chronic pain and employ possible preventative or mitigating treatment strategies.

"Omic" Changes Associated with Chronic Pain

Epigenetics

There is a small but growing body of literature examining epigenetic targets of chronic pain, including microRNAs (miRNAs), DNA methylation, and histone modification.[45] These epigenetic modifications occur in cells of the central or peripheral nervous system and have the phenotypic effect of inducing changes in sensory thresholds, changes in neuronal ion channels (leading to alterations in pain signaling), altering neuronal response to injury and inflammation, and modifying the body's natural pain-relieving mechanisms (i.e., the endogenous opioid system).[45]

Methylation patterns have been associated with differences in pain sensitivity. A study of pain sensitivity in 25 pairs of twins identified nine genes with differential methylation that were associated with differences in pain thresholds in response to heat; the researchers also found that these same genes were associated with pain sensitivity in 50 unrelated individuals.[46] The strongest signal of differential methylation was in the promoter region of the *TRPA1* gene, which encodes a membrane ion channel on pain-detecting neurons.[46] Further evidence of the role of methylation in pain sensitivity is the fact that mutations in *MECP2*, which encodes an enzyme that binds to methylated CG sites, can lead to abnormal pain sensations.[47] *MECP2* has been postulated to be a global regulator of chromatin remodeling.[48]

Histone acetylation may also play a role in the development of pain. Animal models of neuropathic pain have found that increased histone deacetylase expression and decreased histone acetylation contribute to nociceptor sensitization.[45] It has also been observed that histone deacetylase inhibitors modulate expression of glutamate receptors to decrease inflammatory pain.[49] Because glutamate is the main excitatory neurotransmitter in the central nervous system, activation of glutamate receptors plays a key role in pain processing.

Finally, various miRNAs linked to inflammatory regulation, nociceptive signaling, and protein kinase function have all been found to differ significantly between pain patients with conditions such as fibromyalgia, complex regional pain syndrome, and migraine and healthy controls.[50] However, no single miRNA or group of miRNAs has been causally associated with increased pain sensitivity.

Transcriptomics

The transcriptomic changes that occur in pain states are poorly understood and not well-characterized, with few human transcriptomic studies available. Because pain sensation is conducted through the sensory nervous system, and the cell bodies of the first-order neurons along the pathway from the peripheral to central nervous system are located in the dorsal root ganglia (DRG), the DRG is one of the most frequently investigated targets for pain research.[51,52] One study compared healthy human DRG transcriptomes to those of other human and mouse tissues, identifying 13 unique transcription factors and 202 differentially expressed genes, which fell into categories that are functionally important in the DRG: ion channels, receptors, kinases, and RNA binding proteins.[51] A subsequent study in patients with neuropathic (nerve-related) pain identified sex-specific differential expression in genes and signaling pathways related to immune response and neuronal plasticity.[52] Analyses of less invasive peripheral nerve and skin punch biopsies in patients with neuropathic pain have found increased expression of the cytokines IL-6 and IL-10 and decreased expression of neurotrophic factors NGF and NT3,[53] consistent with the above studies identifying immune response and neuronal growth as important processes in pain. A study of psychiatric patients, who are at high risk for comorbid pain disorders, identified several blood biomarkers that were predictive of pain and future emergency department visits for pain.[54] Decreased expression of *MFAP3* (microfibril associated protein 3), a component of elastin-associated microfibrils in the extracellular matrix, was found to be the most robust predictor for increased pain in this study, despite any previous known relationship to pain in the previous literature.[54] Other differentially expressed genes identified in this study (*GNG7*, *CNTN1*, *LY9*, *CCDC144B*, and *GBP1*) are involved in signal transduction, cell motility, and immunomodulation.[54] Another study, evaluating blood of patients with LBP compared to mouse models of nerve pain and inflammatory pain, found an overrepresentation of differentially expressed genes corresponding to SNPs in extracellular matrix proteins (i.e., cell–cell structure).[55] Taken together, these transcriptomic findings support the genetic evidence that changes occur in multiple molecular pathways in the setting of pain, including immune modulation, signal transduction, nerve growth, and extracellular structure.

Proteomics

Voltage-gated sodium (Na_v) channels have a pivotal role in the transmission of pain signals, and post-translational modification of these channels can affect pain signaling.[56] In particular, the addition of small molecules (e.g., peptides, phosphoryl groups, ubiquitin moieties, and carbohydrates) can either physically interfere with Na_v signaling or direct where Na_v is trafficked in the cell.[56] Proteomic changes can also occur in chronic pain beyond the Na_v channels. One study of the cerebrospinal fluid of fibromyalgia patients identified increased activity of multiple pain-related proteins involved in inflammatory responses, neuropeptide signaling, and hormonal activity.[57] Another study used a semi-automated text mining approach to aggregate 93,271 molecular interactions from 765,692 publications to build a network of 1,002 protein–protein interactions associated with inflammatory and neuropathic pain.[58] Both types of pain were associated with increased activity of $Na_v1.8$, as well as neurotrophic factors (NGF and BDNF) and the ephrin receptor (EPHB1), which are important in neuronal growth and axon guidance.[58] As with the transcriptomic studies, proteomic analyses of pain clearly associated it with changes in inflammation, cell signaling, and nerve growth.

Metabolomics

Metabolites found to differ between pain patients and healthy controls include amino acids (glutamine, serine, and phenylalanine) and intermediate products of macromolecule metabolism (succinate, citrate, acetylcarnitine, and *N*-acetylornithine).[59] A very large—albeit very nonspecific—study of 17,834 patient blood samples analyzed at a national reference laboratory found that chronic pain was associated with elevated levels of quinolinic acid, pyroglutamate, xanthurenic acid, 3-hydroxypropyl mercapturic acid, and methylmalonic acid and low levels of neurotransmitter metabolites.[60] These metabolites are associated with diverse biological processes, including inflammatory response, detoxification, oxidative stress response, and neurotransmission, indicating the broad scope of changes occurring throughout the body during pain. Magnetic resonance spectroscopy studies of the brain have found *increased* levels of the main inhibitory (γ-aminobutyric acid [GABA]) and excitatory (glutamate) neurometabolites,[61] as well as other metabolites suggestive of increased neuronal activity, such as elevated total creatine and myoinositol.[62,63]

Microbiome

Nearly all published studies on the effect of the microbiome on pain pertain to the gut microbiome. The gut microbiome appears to play a role beyond abdominal pain and may affect inflammatory pain, headache, neuropathic pain, and opioid (pain medication) tolerance.[64] Gut microbiota can increase mediators, such as pathogen-associated molecular patterns (e.g., lipopolysaccharide, peptidoglycan, and β-glucan) and short-chain fatty acids, to affect processes such as neuroinflammation and the excitability of pain-sensing neurons.[64] A study of fibromyalgia patients found significant differences in microbiome compositions of patients versus healthy controls, and furthermore these changes were correlated with symptom severity.[65] Interestingly, many of these differentially abundant microbes were butyrate-metabolizing species, and the researchers found increased levels of butyric acid in patients.[65] Butyrate is believed to increase levels of the inhibitory neurotransmitter GABA compared to the excitatory neurotransmitter glutamate. Similarly, gut microbiota can affect tryptophan metabolism; tryptophan is a precursor to serotonin, another neurotransmitter important in the control of pain sensation, suggesting another mechanism by which the microbiome can influence pain.[66]

Environmental Modifiers of Pain

Environmental factors can be a significant contributor to chronic pain and include lifestyle choices, psychological distress, and social stressors. The interrelationship between environmental factors, social support, physical stress, and injuries may modulate genetic predisposition to pain amplification.[43] Persistent low-grade inflammation ("meta-inflammation") caused by persistent external and internal stressors has been linked to chronic illness, including chronic pain.[43,67] Consequently, addressing modifiable environmental influences has been an attractive targets for the treatment of chronic pain.

Nutrition, one of the best-studied environmental influences on pain, can affect gene expression that influences nervous, immune, and endocrine function. Poor nutrition, such as a high-fat diet, upregulates genes related to metabolic and mitochondrial stress, leading to increased pro-inflammatory cytokines and enhanced nociceptive responses.[68] Dietary choices also directly impact excess weight, which increases pain by imposing mechanical and structural stress on the body; adipose tissue can also generate pro-inflammatory cytokines, leading to increased pain sensitivity.[69]

Exercise is considered an important part of a healthy lifestyle, but it is also considered an effective chronic pain management modality by producing exercise-induced hypoalgesia (EIH).[70] EIH is the phenomenon of generalized pain relief following a single episode of exercise, and it may persist for a period time afterward. However, the acute effect of exercise on pain sensitivity is variable in chronic pain populations, with some chronic pain patients having an increased pain sensitivity, locally and globally, to pain after exercising.[70] The mechanism of EIH was initially theorized to be activation of the endogenous opioid system; however, non-opioid hypoalgesia has also been proposed via the endocannabinoid system and interactions between opioid and serotonin SNP variations.[70] Several models have been proposed, with SNPs in the *OPRM1* gene activating the μ-opioid receptor gene and/or the *HTR1a* gene regulating serotonin 1A receptor expression, to produce either stronger or weaker EIH responses.[70] EIH has also been shown to influence perceived pain by altering inflammatory cytokines, neurotrophins, neurotransmitters, endogenous opioids, and histone acetylation.[71]

Sleep and pain present a multidimensional relationship characterized as a cycle of reciprocal relationships whereby poor sleep quality increases pain, and increased pain reduces quality of sleep.[72] The GG genotype of the *OPRM1 A118G* polymorphism, noted above to be associated with worse subjective health complaints and increased pain sensitivity,[40,41] has also been found to be significantly correlated with increased pain symptoms and lower sleep adequacy in patients with chronic pain treated with opioids.[73] The neurobiological mechanism that has been suggested to explain the relationship between chronic pain and sleep disturbances is that serotonin receptor modulation causes intrusion of alpha waves (i.e., brain activity consistent with wakefulness) into non–rapid eye movement sleep, leading to feelings of malaise, fatigue, and waking unrefreshed.[74] As discussed previously, serotonin pathways play a major role in pain processing and can be influenced by genetic variations, demonstrating how gene–environment interactions can exacerbate pain vulnerability.

Social stressors, including discrimination based on race, ethnicity, and gender, can also have profound effects on health.[75] Originally proposed by Arline Geronimus et al.[75] after studying health care disparities between Blacks and Whites in the United States, the weathering hypothesis posits that race-related adversity rooted in cultural conditions serves to accelerate biological decline, resulting in premature health deterioration. Numerous subsequent studies on the impact of discrimination on health outcomes have substantiated this hypothesis.[76] The putative genetic mechanism underlying the weathering hypothesis is "allostatic load," which is conceptualized as the cumulative physiologic burdens imposed by stress, as indicated by two categories of biomarkers: (1) primary molecular mediators released in response to stress (e.g., norepinephrine, epinephrine, cortisol, and dehydroepiandrosterone sulfate) and (2) the physiological effects of those primary mediators (e.g., elevated systolic and diastolic blood pressures, increased glycated hemoglobin levels, and high waist-to-hip ratio).[75,77] As humans age, the effects of the allostatic load accumulate at both the molecular level (epigenetically) and the whole-person level (phenotypically), and individuals who have been exposed to greater or more persistent stressors have older epigenetic profiles.[78] Older epigenetic age has been found to be associated with greater pain during daily activities and anatomical pain sites, although not necessarily pain frequency or duration.[78] Reciprocally, it has also been posited that chronic pain is associated with accelerated epigenetic aging, even in otherwise healthy individuals.[78] Thus, vulnerability to pain may also be a risk factor for other negative health consequences through shared molecular mechanisms activating stress response pathways associated with premature physiologic aging.

Last, environmental factors, social support, physical stress, and injuries may modulate genetic predisposition to psychological distress and pain amplification. For example, polymorphisms in the promoter region of the serotonin transporter (*5-HTT*) gene are associated with the effect of stress on development of depression, a major risk factor for chronic pain.[79] Similarly, an SNP in the vasopressin-1A receptor can affect experimentally induced pain in humans, but only in male subjects reporting stress.[80] These findings illustrate how gene–environmental interactions can also be influenced by other biological determinants, such as sex.

Pharmacogenomics of Pain Treatment

Most research on drug–gene interactions in chronic pain focuses on the cytochrome P450 system, although variants in numerous other genes have also been investigated for their role in analgesic response. The PharmGKB database (https://www.pharmgkb.org) is a comprehensive pharmacogenomics resource supported by the National Institutes of Health that provides information on the impact of human genetic variation on drug response, including clinical guidelines, drug labels, potential gene–drug interactions, and genotype–phenotype relationships. Table 3.1 shows some examples of potentially clinically relevant gene–drug relationships in chronic pain.

Cytochrome P450 Polymorphisms

The cytochrome P450 (CYP450 or CYP) family of enzymes is responsible for the initial metabolism of approximately 80% of all drugs, and they represent one of the most important classes of molecules responsible for individual differences in drug metabolism.[81] CYP biosynthesis is controlled by a substantial number of genes, with changes in those genes resulting in alterations to enzyme activity and function, thereby altering drug metabolism.[81] One CYP isoform that has been extensively studied with respect to pain and

Table 3.1 Selected Examples of Clinically Relevant Drug–Gene Interactions in Analgesics

Drug	Variants	Effect on Drug Metabolism	Effect on Side Effects
Acetaminophen	No moderate/high evidence	No moderate/high evidence	No moderate/high evidence
Celecoxib/ NSAIDs	CYP2C9*1 CYP2C9*2, *3, *13	Homozygotes may have increased metabolism. Homo-/heterozygotes may have decreased metabolism.	Higher risk of adverse effects (i.e., gastrointestinal bleed)
Duloxetine	CYP2D6 poor metabolizers	Limited data suggest higher plasma levels of drug, but no evidence of clinical effects.	None
Carbamazepine/ oxcarbazepine	HLA-A*31:01:01, HLA-B*15:02:01	None	Homo-/heterozygotes for either variant may have increased risk of severe cutaneous adverse reactions (e.g., Stevens–Johnson syndrome, toxic epidermal necrolysis).
Codeine	CYP2D6*1 CYP2D6*1xN, CYP2D6*2, CYP2D6*2xN CYP2D6*3, CYP2D6*4, CYP2D6*5, CYP2D6*6, CYP2D6*10, CYP2D6*17, CYP2D6*40, CYP2D6*41	Increased metabolism/ clearance, increased likelihood of response Increased formation of morphine (active metabolite) Decreased metabolism/ clearance, decreased likelihood of response	Decreased risk of side effects compared to patients with non/ reduced function alleles Higher risk of toxicity (central nervous system/respiratory depression, death) Poor pain control
TCAs	CYP2C19 poor metabolizer	Limited data suggest higher drug–drug interaction.	None

NSAIDs, nonsteroidal anti-inflammatory drugs; TCAs, tricyclic antidepressants.

genetic variation is CYP2D6, with 80 gene variations identified.[37,81] Functionally, these variants are classified into four general phenotypes: extensive metabolizer (normal), intermediate metabolizer (IM), poor metabolizer (PM), and ultra-rapid metabolizer (UM).[82] CYP450 polymorphisms affect the metabolism of many opioid drugs, including codeine, tramadol, hydrocodone, oxycodone, hydromorphone, and morphine.[37] In particular, the CYP2D6 isozyme is pivotal for metabolizing the prodrug codeine into morphine, tramadol into *O*-desmethyltramadol, oxycodone into oxymorphone, and hydrocodone into hydromorphone, with each of these metabolites having substantially more affinity and potency for the μ-opioid receptor.[82] An individual's CYP2D6 genetic variants and phenotype may therefore affect vulnerability to decreased analgesic efficacy or increased adverse events in response to certain opioids. For example, PM individuals can have significantly reduced codeine metabolism, leading to insufficient pain relief and lower drug clearance, requiring a dose reduction to avoid undesired adverse effects. In the extreme case, individuals possessing a *CYP2D6* mutation that results in a completely nonfunctional enzyme experience no pain relief with codeine administration.[83] Conversely, UM patients have a substantially elevated risk of opioid toxicity with codeine due to increased formation of morphine. These observations have led several international pharmacogenetics professional societies to recommend *CYP2D6* genotype testing prior to administration of codeine or tramadol,[82,84,85] although such testing is not typically covered by insurance and has yet to be implemented into routine clinical practice.[86]

In addition to opioids, CYP polymorphisms also have an influence on the metabolism of nonsteroidal anti-inflammatory drugs (NSAIDs).[81] Many NSAIDs are metabolized by CYP2C9, which has been shown to have two allelic variants of the normal enzyme, CYP2C9*2 and CYP2C9*3.[81,87] The *2 and *3 alleles have 50% and 15% of the activity of the wild-type enzyme, respectively, resulting in poor metabolism and prolonged action of NSAIDs in affected individuals.[81] The selective COX-2 inhibitor celecoxib is metabolized by CYP2C9. In a study of rheumatoid and osteoarthritis patients prescribed celecoxib, those with the *2 or *3 genotypes showed an increased elimination half-life compared to patients with the wild-type genotype.[88] Another study of patients prescribed celecoxib, ibuprofen, and naproxen found that the *2 and *3 genotypes were significantly associated with a higher risk of gastrointestinal bleeding.[89]

CYP enzymes are also involved in the metabolism of antidepressants used in chronic pain treatment, with the major isozymes being CYP1A2, CYP2D6, and CYP2C19.[37,81] However, other isoforms are also involved, as evidenced by the metabolism of amitriptyline (1A2, 2C9, 2C19, 2D6, and 3A), bupropion (2B6), imipramine (1A2, 2C19, 2D6, and 3A), and venlafaxine (2D6 and 3A).[37,81] Understanding a patient's *CYP* genotype and associated phenotype may therefore inform antidepressant treatment selection and dosing. For example, some experts recommend avoiding venlafaxine in patients with PM and IM CYP2D6 phenotypes and selecting an alternate drug (e.g., citalopram or sertraline) or adjusting the venlafaxine dose.[90] In contrast, for the UM phenotype, it has been recommended to select an alternative or titrate venlafaxine to a maximum of 150% of the normal dose.[90]

Opioid Receptor Polymorphisms

Pain sensitivity, perception, and opioid analgesia are reported to be heritable as the result of polymorphisms of pain-relevant genes.[91] The three opioid receptor subtypes—mu (μ), kappa (κ), and delta (δ)—differ in their function and drug-binding specificity. The μ-opioid receptor is the primary site of action for many endogenous opioids, as well as the exogenously administered opioids most commonly used for analgesia. Thus, the human μ-opioid receptor encoded by the *OPRM1* gene is a primary candidate for the pharmacogenetic variability of the clinical effects of opioid analgesics.[91] The most common SNP of *OPRM1* is substitution of adenine (A) to guanine (G) at position 118

(A118G) of exon 1[91]; this is the same variant discussed above that has been associated with LBP, increased pain sensitivity, and sleep disturbances in chronic pain.[40,41,73] The mutation leads to an amino acid substitution that reduces receptor binding affinity, with a decrease in opioid potency by a factor of two or three.[92,93] This mechanism is consistent with the observation that *A118G* heterozygotes and GG homozygotes both have increased pain sensitivity and require higher opioid doses compared to AA homozygotes (wild-type).[91,93] It has also been theorized that more copies of the G allele may confer greater protection from the effects of endogenous opioid activation and persistent hyperalgesia after trauma.[93] Thus, the significance of the *A118G* polymorphism for chronic pain vulnerability is complex and closely related to the administration of μ-opioid analgesics.

Catechol-*O*-Methyltransferase Polymorphisms

In addition to their association with fibromyalgia and LBP as discussed above, variants in the COMT enzyme may also influence response to analgesics. The common $Val^{158}Met$ variant that is associated with some chronic pain disorders is characterized by decreased thermal stability and reduced enzymatic activity of COMT.[81] The reduced COMT activity has been proposed to result in upregulation of the μ-opioid receptor, thus increasing the efficacy of opioid analgesics.[94] Studies of cancer patients have found that patients homozygous for the wild-type Val^{158} required higher doses of morphine for analgesia compared to heterozygotes or those homozygous for the Met^{158} variant.[95,96] In addition, other COMT variants have been associated with increased susceptibility to the central side effects of morphine, including drowsiness, confusion, and hallucinations.[97] However, there is insufficient evidence to support COMT testing for analgesics, with the major pharmacogenetics guidelines for opioids providing no recommendation for COMT testing.[82,84]

Serotonin Receptor Polymorphisms

Serotonin or 5-hydroxytryptamine (5-HT) is a key neurotransmitter in the central nervous system and has an anti-nociceptive role in the dorsal horn of the descending tract of the spinal cord.[98] Both serotonin–norepinephrine reuptake inhibitors and selective serotonin reuptake inhibitors are commonly used agents in the treatment of pain and comorbid depression. Polymorphisms of the serotonin receptor genes—most notably the 2A receptor encoded by *HRT2A*—have been associated with susceptibility to chronic pain conditions such as fibromyalgia, chronic widespread pain, and chronic LBP.[37,98,99] However, there is little evidence that genetic variations in serotonin receptor subtypes are associated with clinically actionable differences in analgesic response for chronic pain patients. One small study found that the SNP rs6318 in the *HTR2C* gene (but none in the *HTR2A* gene) was associated with significantly improved analgesic response to escitalopram in patients with painful polyneuropathy.[100] Importantly, pharmacogenetic studies of genetic variants and antidepressant response for major depressive disorder have not identified any reliable genetic predictors for treatment response.[101] Nevertheless, because antidepressant medications likely have analgesic properties through mechanisms independent of their effects on depression,[102] serotonin receptor polymorphisms may still be a potential source of pharmacogenetic variability in analgesic response.

Anticonvulsants

Anticonvulsants are common analgesics that promote membrane stabilization and suppress the neuronal hyperexcitability that is characteristic of chronic (usually neuropathic) pain.[103] The anticonvulsant carbamazepine and its analog, oxcarbazepine, are used in neuropathic pain conditions such as trigeminal neuralgia to decrease neuronal excitability via blockade of voltage-gated sodium channels.[104] Side effects of these drugs include somnolence, dizziness, and unsteadiness.[104] The U.S. Food and Drug Administration (FDA) labeling for carbamazepine carries a black box warning regarding the increased risk of serious and potentially fatal cutaneous hypersensitivity reactions, including Stevens–Johnson syndrome and toxic epidermal necrolysis in individuals carrying a specific allele of human leukocyte antigen B (*HLA-B*).[105] *HLA-B* and the related *HLA-A* encode cell surface proteins that present intracellular antigens to the immune system.[105] The risk of serious cutaneous adverse reactions is significantly increased in individuals carrying the *HLA-B*15:02* allele, most frequently seen in Asian populations, or the *HLA-A*31:01* allele, which is found in high frequencies in some Caucasian, Hispanic/South American, and East Asian populations.[106,107] Thus, the FDA labeling for carbamazepine and oxcarbazepine recommends *HLA-B*15:02* testing be considered prior to initiation of therapy in genetically at-risk populations.[105]

Other anticonvulsant medications for pain include the gabapentinoids (gabapentin and pregabalin), which are commonly used in the treatment of diabetic neuropathy, post-herpetic neuralgia, trigeminal neuralgia, multiple sclerosis, migraine, and other chronic pain conditions. Gabapentin binds to voltage-gated calcium channels, leading to a reduction in the release of the neurotransmitter glutamate and substance P.[37] Unlike most other drugs, the gabapentinoids are not metabolized by the liver but, instead, by the organic cation transporters *OCTN1* and *OCT2*, encoded by the *SLC22A4* and *SLC22A2* genes, respectively.[37] Interestingly, polymorphisms in these genes have negligible effects on gabapentin metabolism, with clearance affected more by renal function.[37]

Role of Genetic Testing

There are no recommended newborn screening tests and no routine genetic or genomic tests recommended for screening, carrier testing, or family planning for chronic pain. Most data on preconception carrier screening and prenatal testing for pain focus on the monogenic hereditary pain conditions, such as *SCN9A*. Preconception carrier testing for mutations is not appropriate due to the low prevalence and low specificity of genetic testing for this disease. Prenatal *SCN9A* testing would be indicated in cases in which one or both parents have a positive family history because it may affect clinical care of

Table 3.2 Examples of Commercially Available Genetic Tests Marketed for Pain Treatment

Text (Reference)	Genes Tested	Availability
ClarityX Mindwell and Max Rx[109]	Not all listed; website focuses on cytochrome P450 variants *CYP2D6*, *CYP3A4*, and *CYP2C9*	No doctor's order required; works with network of physicians licensed in all 50 states to review and authorize order
Inagene Personalized Insights Pain & Mental Health Test Kit[110]	Not all listed; website states prediction of response to more than 140 medications based on 58 genes tested	No doctor's referral needed
GX Sciences chronic pain panel[111]	Not listed; website states 21 selected SNPs associated with inflammation, detoxification, metabolism, and neurotransmitters	Patients referred to licensed, registered providers via internal directory
PMCDx Pain Management PGx Test Panel[112]	*CYP2C19, CYP2D6, CYP2C9, CYP3A4, CYP3A5, CYP1A2, CYP2B6, COMT, OPRM1*	Order from licensed provider required

SNPs, single nucleotide polymorphisms.

the newborn. These conditions may influence pregnancy through use of maternal pain medications or if the parents are considering termination should the fetus be diagnosed with a defect in the *SCN9A* gene. There is evidence in favor of pharmacogenomic testing, with some pharmacogenomics professional societies advocating for genetic testing in selected clinical scenarios (e.g., *CYP2D6* testing prior to codeine administration).[82,84,85] Importantly, however, clinical pain studies have yet to demonstrate definitive benefit from routine genetic testing for analgesic drugs, and it is not currently a part of standard clinical practice.

Given the clear evidence of heritability in chronic pain and the improved accessibility and affordability of genetic testing, there has been marked interest in genetic testing for chronic pain. Marketed to both pain patients and their health care providers, there are several commercially available tests that screen for multiple genes or variants to create a complex risk profile of pain sensitivity and/or response to pain treatments (Table 3.2). These tests claim to improve pain management by creating pain "risk" profiles that are based on genes associated with increased pain sensitivity, susceptibility to pain disorders, altered analgesic treatment response, adverse drug reactions, and tolerance or abuse potential. However, the genes tested—and the scientific literature supporting their association with pain—can vary widely, and genetic testing for pain has not been clinically validated. Consequently, genetic testing for pain is not typically covered by insurance and would be an out-of-pocket expense with unclear potential benefit. Tests typically cost $200–$500, depending on the laboratory and specific testing panel ordered. In addition, nonspecific genetic testing without a clear link to clinical significance can risk overinterpretation of positive findings. Unclear clinical significance is also the primary reason that epigenetic, transcriptomic, and other 'omic testing have remained predominantly confined to the research setting.

Conclusion

Although there remains much to be explored regarding the genetic and genomic aspects of pain, there are clear links between heritable individual variations and the experience of chronic pain. Genetic, genomic, and other 'omic profiling may help screen patients vulnerable to chronic pain, inform pain treatment recommendations, and suggest novel therapeutic targets. In addition, pharmacogenomic profiles can predict response to different pain medications, and various genetic and genomic markers could identify specific pathological processes that would be responsive to different therapies. Although genetic testing currently offers limited utility in pain management, further investigation may allow us to identify patients vulnerable to pain and offer optimized, personalized pain treatment.

References

1. Gatchel RJ, Peng YB, Peters ML, Fuchs PN, Turk DC. The biopsychosocial approach to chronic pain: Scientific advances and future directions. *Psychol Bull.* 2007;133(4):581–624. doi:10.1037/0033-2909.133.4.581
2. Denk F, McMahon SB, Tracey I. Pain vulnerability: A neurobiological perspective. *Nat Neurosci.* 2014;17(2):192–200. doi:10.1038/nn.3628
3. Mills SEE, Nicolson KP, Smith BH. Chronic pain: A review of its epidemiology and associated factors in population-based studies. *Br J Anaesth.* 2019;123(2):e273–e283. doi:10.1016/j.bja.2019.03.023
4. Snyder M. Genome fundamentals. In: *Genomics and Personalized Medicine: What Everyone Needs to Know.* Oxford University Press; 2016:5–20.
5. Snyder M. Effects of the environment on the genome and epigenetics. In: *Genomics and Personalized Medicine: What Everyone Needs to Know.* Oxford University Press; 2016:87–94.
6. Snyder M. Other 'omes. In: *Genomics and Personalized Medicine: What Everyone Needs to Know.* Oxford University Press; 2016:95–100.
7. Sexton JE, Cox JJ, Zhao J, Wood JN. The genetics of pain: Implications for therapeutics. *Annu Rev Pharmacol Toxicol.* 2018;58:123–142. doi:10.1146/annurev-pharmtox-010617-052554
8. Bennett DLH, Woods CG. Painful and painless channelopathies. *Lancet Neurol.* 2014;13(6):587–599. doi:10.1016/S1474-4422(14)70024-9
9. Toledo-Aral JJ, Moss BL, He Z-J, et al. Identification of PN1, a predominant voltage-dependent sodium channel expressed principally in peripheral neurons. *Proc Natl Acad Sci USA.* 1997;94:1527–1532.
10. National Center for Biotechnolgy Information, National Library of Medicine. SCN9A. GTR: Genetic Testing Registry. n.d. Accessed December 8, 2020. https://www.ncbi.nlm.nih.gov/gtr/all/tests/?term=scn9a
11. Dib-Hajj SD, Yang Y, Waxman SG. Genetics and molecular pathophysiology of Nav1.7-related pain syndromes. *Adv Genet.* 2008;63:85–110. doi:10.1016/S0065-2660(08)01004-3
12. Klein CJ, Wu Y, Kilfoyle DH, et al. Infrequent SCN9A mutations in congenital insensitivity to pain and erythromelalgia. *J Neurol Neurosurg Psychiatry.* 2013;84:386–391.
13. Paroxysmal extreme pain disorder. MedlinePlus Genetics. n.d. Accessed October 20, 2020. https://medlineplus.gov/genetics/condition/paroxysmal-extreme-pain-disorder/#synonyms
14. Erythromelalgia. MedlinePlus Genetics. n.d. Accessed October 20, 2020. https://medlineplus.gov/genetics/condition/erythromelalgia/#inheritance
15. Small fiber neuropathy. MedlinePlus Genetics. n.d. Accessed October 20, 2020. https://medlineplus.gov/genetics/condition/small-fiber-neuropathy

16. Sutherland HG, Albury CL, Griffiths LR. Advances in genetics of migraine. *J Headache Pain.* 2019;20(1): Article 72. doi:10.1186/S10194-019-1017-9
17. Ophoff RA, Terwindt GM, Vergouwe MN, et al. Familial hemiplegic migraine and episodic ataxia type-2 are caused by mutations in the Ca^{2+} channel gene CACNL1A4. *Cell.* 1996;87(3):543–552. doi:10.1016/S0092-8674(00)81373-2
18. De Fusco M, Marconi R, Silvestri L, et al. Haploinsufficiency of ATP1A2 encoding the Na^+ /K^+ pump $alpha_2$ subunit associated with familial hemiplegic migraine type 2. *Nat Genet.* 2003;33(2):192–196. doi:10.1038/NG1081
19. Dichgans M, Freilinger T, Eckstein G, et al. Mutation in the neuronal voltage-gated sodium channel SCN1A in familial hemiplegic migraine. *Lancet.* 2005;366(9483):371–377. doi:10.1016/S0140-6736(05)66786-4
20. Meng H, Xu HQ, Yu L, et al. The SCN1A Mutation Database: Updating information and analysis of the relationships among genotype, functional alteration, and phenotype. *Hum Mutat.* 2015;36(6):573–580. doi:10.1002/humu.22782
21. Thomsen LL, Eriksen MK, Romer SF, et al. An epidemiological survey of hemiplegic migraine. *Cephalalgia.* 2002;22(5):361–375. doi:10.1046/J.1468-2982.2002.00371.X
22. Zorina-Lichtenwalter K, Meloto CB, Khoury S, Diatchenko L. Genetic predictors of human chronic pain conditions. *Neuroscience.* 2016;338:36–62. doi:10.1016/J.NEUROSCIENCE.2016.04.041
23. Stovner LJ, Hagen K, Jensen R, et al. The global burden of headache: A documentation of headache prevalence and disability worldwide. *Cephalalgia.* 2007;27(3):193–210. doi:10.1111/j.1468-2982.2007.01288.x
24. Mulder EJ, Van Baal C, Gaist D, et al. Genetic and environmental influences on migraine: A twin study across six countries. *Twin Res.* 2003;6(5):422–431. doi:10.1375/136905203770326420
25. Honkasalo M-L, Kaprio J, Winter T, Heikkilä K, Sillanpää M, Koskenvuo M. Migraine and concomitant symptoms among 8167 adult twin pairs. *Headache J Head Face Pain.* 1995;35(2):70–78. doi:10.1111/J.1526-4610.1995.HED3502070.X
26. De Boer I, Van Den Maagdenberg AMJM, Terwindt GM. Advance in genetics of migraine. *Curr Opin Neurol.* 2019;32(3):413. doi:10.1097/WCO.0000000000000687
27. Stuart S, Cox HC, Lea RA, Griffiths LR. The role of the MTHFR gene in migraine. *Headache.* 2012;52(3):515–520. doi:10.1111/J.1526-4610.2012.02106.X
28. Moll S, Varga EA. Homocysteine and MTHFR mutations. *Circulation.* 2015;132(1):e6–e69. doi:10.1161/CIRCULATIONAHA.114.013311
29. Lea R, Colson N, Quinlan S, MacMillan J, Griffiths L. The effects of vitamin supplementation and MTHFR (C677T) genotype on homocysteine-lowering and migraine disability. *Pharmacogenet Genomics.* 2009;19(6):422–428. doi:10.1097/FPC.0B013E32832AF5A3
30. Markkula R, Järvinen P, Leino-Arjas P, Koskenvuo M, Kalso E, Kaprio J. Clustering of symptoms associated with fibromyalgia in a Finnish twin cohort. *Eur J Pain.* 2009;13(7):744–750. doi:10.1016/J.EJPAIN.2008.09.007
31. Dutta D, Brummett CM, Moser SE, et al. Heritability of the fibromyalgia phenotype varies by age. *Arthritis Rheumatol.* 2020;72(5):815. doi:10.1002/ART.41171
32. Bair MJ, Krebs EE. In the clinic: fibromyalgia. *Ann Intern Med.* 2020;172(5):ITC33–ITC48. doi:10.7326/AITC202003030
33. Ablin JN, Buskila D. Update on the genetics of the fibromyalgia syndrome. *Best Pract Res Clin Rheumatol.* 2015;29(1):20–28. doi:10.1016/J.BERH.2015.04.018
34. Martínez-Jauand M, Sitges C, Rodríguez V, et al. Pain sensitivity in fibromyalgia is associated with catechol-*O*-methyltransferase (*COMT*) gene. *Eur J Pain.* 2013;17(1):16–27. doi:10.1002/J.1532-2149.2012.00153.X
35. Freidin MB, Tsepilov YA, Palmer M, et al. Insight into the genetic architecture of back pain and its risk factors from a study of 509,000 individuals. *Pain.* 2019;160(6):1361–1373. doi:10.1097/j.pain.0000000000001514
36. Battié MC, Videman T, Levalahti E, Gill K, Kaprio J. Heritability of low back pain and the role of disc degeneration. *Pain.* 2007;131(3):272–280. doi:10.1016/j.pain.2007.01.010

37. Suntsov V, Jovanovic F, Knezevic E, Candido KD, Knezevic NN. Can implementation of genetics and pharmacogenomics improve treatment of chronic low back pain? *Pharmaceutics*. 2020;12(9): Article 894. doi:10.3390/pharmaceutics12090894
38. Finci L, Zhang Y, Meijers R, Wang J-H. Signaling mechanism of the netrin-1 receptor DCC in axon guidance. *Prog Biophys Mol Biol*. 2015;118(3):153–160. doi:10.1016/j.pbiomolbio.2015.04.001
39. Jacobsen LM, Eriksen GS, Pedersen LM, Gjerstad J. Catechol-*O*-methyltransferase (COMT) inhibition reduces spinal nociceptive activity. *Neurosci Lett*. 2010;473(3):212–215. doi:10.1016/j.neulet.2010.02.049
40. Hasvik E, Iordanova Schistad E, Grøvle L, Julsrud Haugen A, Røe C, Gjerstad J. Subjective health complaints in patients with lumbar radicular pain and disc herniation are associated with a sex–OPRM1 A118G polymorphism interaction: A prospective 1-year observational study. *BMC Musculoskelet Disord*. 2014;15(1): Article 161. doi:10.1186/1471-2474-15-161
41. Matsunaga M, Isowa T, Murakami H, et al. Association of polymorphism in the human μ-opioid receptor OPRM1 gene with proinflammatory cytokine levels and health perception. *Brain Behav Immun*. 2009;23(7):931–935. doi:10.1016/j.bbi.2009.03.007
42. Maixner W, Fillingim RB, Williams DA, Smith SB, Slade GD. Overlapping chronic pain conditions: Implications for diagnosis and classification. *J Pain*. 2016;17(9):T93–T107. doi:10.1016/j.jpain.2016.06.002
43. Diatchenko L, Nackley AG, Slade GD, Fillingim RB, Maixner W. Idiopathic pain disorders—pathways of vulnerability. *Pain*. 2006;123(3):226–230.
44. Young EE, Lariviere WR, Belfer I. Genetic basis of pain variability: Recent advances. *J Med Genet*. 2012;49(1):1–9. doi:10.1136/JMEDGENET-2011-100386
45. Descalzi G, Ikegami D, Ushijima T, Nestler EJ, Zachariou V, Narita M. Epigenetic mechanisms of chronic pain. *Trends Neurosci*. 2015;38(4):237–246. doi:10.1016/j.tins.2015.02.001
46. Bell JT, Loomis AK, Butcher LM, et al. Differential methylation of the TRPA1 promoter in pain sensitivity. *Nat Commun*. 2014;5(1): Article 2978. doi:10.1038/ncomms3978
47. Downs J, Géranton SM, Bebbington A, et al. Linking MECP2 and pain sensitivity: The example of Rett syndrome. *Am J Med Genet Part A*. 2010;152(5):1197–1205. doi:10.1002/ajmg.a.33314
48. Skene PJ, Illingworth RS, Webb S, et al. Neuronal MeCP2 is expressed at near histone-octamer levels and globally alters the chromatin state. *Mol Cell*. 2010;37(4):457–468. doi:10.1016/j.molcel.2010.01.030
49. Chiechio S, Zammataro M, Morales ME, et al. Epigenetic modulation of mGlu2 receptors by histone deacetylase inhibitors in the treatment of inflammatory pain. *Mol Pharmacol*. 2009;75(5):1014–1020. doi:10.1124/mol.108.054346
50. Polli A, Godderis L, Ghosh M, Ickmans K, Nijs J. Epigenetic and miRNA expression changes in people with pain: A systematic review. *J Pain*. 2020;21(7–8):763–780. doi:10.1016/j.jpain.2019.12.002
51. Ray P, Torck A, Quigley L, et al. Comparative transcriptome profiling of the human and mouse dorsal root ganglia: An RNA-seq-based resource for pain and sensory neuroscience research. *Pain*. 2018;159(7):1325–1345. doi:10.1097/j.pain.0000000000001217
52. North RY, Li Y, Ray P, et al. Electrophysiological and transcriptomic correlates of neuropathic pain in human dorsal root ganglion neurons. *Brain*. 2019;142(5):1215–1226. doi:10.1093/brain/awz063
53. Üçeyler N, Riediger N, Kafke W, Sommer C. Differential gene expression of cytokines and neurotrophic factors in nerve and skin of patients with peripheral neuropathies. *J Neurol*. 2015;262(1):203–212. doi:10.1007/s00415-014-7556-8
54. Niculescu AB, Le-Niculescu H, Levey DF, et al. Towards precision medicine for pain: Diagnostic biomarkers and repurposed drugs. *Mol Psychiatry*. 2019;24(4):501–522. doi:10.1038/s41380–018-0345-5
55. Parisien M, Samoshkin A, Tansley SN, et al. Genetic pathway analysis reveals a major role for extracellular matrix organization in inflammatory and neuropathic pain. *Pain*. 2019;160(4):932–944. doi:10.1097/j.pain.0000000000001471

56. Laedermann CJ, Abriel H, Decosterd I. Post-translational modifications of voltage-gated sodium channels in chronic pain syndromes. *Front Pharmacol.* 2015;6: Article 263. doi:10.3389/fphar.2015.00263
57. Khoonsari PE, Ossipova E, Lengqvist J, et al. The human CSF pain proteome. *J Proteomics.* 2019;190:67–76. doi:10.1016/j.jprot.2018.05.012
58. Jamieson DG, Moss A, Kennedy M, et al. The pain interactome: Connecting pain-specific protein interactions. *Pain.* 2014;155(11):2243–2252. doi:10.1016/j.pain.2014.06.020
59. Aroke EN, Powell-Roach KL. The metabolomics of chronic pain conditions: A systematic review. *Biol Res Nurs.* 2020;22(4):458–471. doi:10.1177/1099800420941105
60. Gunn J, Hill MM, Cotton BM, Deer TR. An analysis of biomarkers in patients with chronic pain. *Pain Physician.* 2020;23(1):E41–E49.
61. Peek AL, Rebbeck T, Puts NA, Watson J, Aguila MER, Leaver AM. Brain GABA and glutamate levels across pain conditions: A systematic literature review and meta-analysis of ^{1}H-MRS studies using the MRS-Q quality assessment tool. *NeuroImage.* 2020;210:116532. doi:10.1016/j.neuroimage.2020.116532
62. Ito T, Tanaka-Mizuno S, Iwashita N, et al. Proton magnetic resonance spectroscopy assessment of metabolite status of the anterior cingulate cortex in chronic pain patients and healthy controls. *J Pain Res.* 2017;10:287–293. doi:10.2147/JPR.S123403
63. Chang L, Munsaka SM, Kraft-Terry S, Ernst T. Magnetic resonance spectroscopy to assess neuroinflammation and neuropathic pain. *J Neuroimmune Pharmacol.* 2013;8(3):576–593. doi:10.1007/s11481-013-9460-x
64. Guo R, Chen LH, Xing C, Liu T. Pain regulation by gut microbiota: Molecular mechanisms and therapeutic potential. *Br J Anaesth.* 2019;123(5):637–654. doi:10.1016/j.bja.2019.07.026
65. Minerbi A, Gonzalez E, Brereton NJB, et al. Altered microbiome composition in individuals with fibromyalgia. *Pain.* 2019;160(11):2589–2602. doi:10.1097/j.pain.0000000000001640
66. O'Mahony SM, Clarke G, Borre YE, Dinan TG, Cryan JF. Serotonin, tryptophan metabolism and the brain-gut-microbiome axis. *Behav Brain Res.* 2015;277:32–48. doi:10.1016/j.bbr.2014.07.027
67. Naylor R, Hayes C, Egger G. The relationship between lifestyle, metaflammation, and chronic pain: A systematic review. *Am J Lifestyle Med.* 2013;7(2):130–137. doi:10.1177/1559827612451710
68. Brandão AF, Bonet IJM, Pagliusi M, et al. Physical activity induces nucleus accumbens genes expression changes preventing chronic pain susceptibility promoted by high-fat diet and sedentary behavior in mice. *Front Neurosci.* 2020;13:1453. doi:10.3389/fnins.2019.01453
69. Okifuji A, Hare BD. The association between chronic pain and obesity. *J Pain Res.* 2015;8:399–408. doi:10.2147/JPR.S55598
70. Rice D, Nijs J, Kosek E, et al. Exercise-induced hypoalgesia in pain-free and chronic pain populations: State of the art and future directions. *J Pain.* 2019;20(11):1249–1266. doi:10.1016/j.jpain.2019.03.005
71. Senba E, Kami K. A new aspect of chronic pain as a lifestyle-related disease. *Neurobiol Pain.* 2017;1:6–15. doi:10.1016/j.ynpai.2017.04.003
72. Godfrey KM, Strachan E, Mostoufi S, Poeschla B, Succop A, Afari N. Familial contributions to self-reported sleep and pain in female twins. *Pain Med.* 2016;17(1):33–39. doi:10.1111/pme.12894
73. Peiró AM. OPRM1 gene interaction with sleep in chronic pain patients treated with opioids. *Pain Physician.* 2019;1(22;1):97–107. doi:10.36076/ppj/2019.22.97
74. Menefee LA, Cohen MJM, Anderson WR, Doghramji K, Frank ED, Lee H. Sleep disturbance and nonmalignant chronic pain: A comprehensive review of the literature. *Pain Med.* 2000;1(2):156–172. doi:10.1046/j.1526-4637.2000.00022.x
75. Geronimus AT, Hicken M, Keene D, Bound J. "Weathering" and age patterns of allostatic load scores among Blacks and Whites in the United States. *Am J Public Health.* 2006;96(5):826–833. doi:10.2105/AJPH.2004.060749
76. Simons RL, Lei M-K, Klopack E, Beach SRH, Gibbons FX, Philibert RA. The effects of social adversity, discrimination, and health risk behaviors on the accelerated aging of African

Americans: Further support for the weathering hypothesis. *Soc Sci Med.* 2021;282:113169. doi:10.1016/j.socscimed.2020.113169
77. McEwen BS, Stellar E. Stress and the individual: Mechanisms leading to disease. *Arch Intern Med.* 1993;153(18):2093–2101. doi:10.1001/ARCHINTE.1993.00410180039004
78. Cruz-Almeida Y, Sinha P, Rani A, Huo Z, Fillingim RB, Foster T. Epigenetic aging is associated with clinical and experimental pain in community-dwelling older adults. *Mol Pain.* 2019;15:1744806919871819. doi:10.1177/1744806919871819
79. Caspi A, Sugden K, Moffitt TE, et al. Influence of life stress on depression: Moderation by a polymorphism in the 5-HTT gene. *Science.* 2003;301(5631):386–389. doi:10.1126/science.1083968
80. Mogil JS, Sorge RE, Lacroix-Fralish ML, et al. Pain sensitivity and vasopressin analgesia are mediated by a gene–sex–environment interaction. *Nat Neurosci.* 2011;14(12):1569–1573. doi:10.1038/nn.2941
81. Kapur BM, Lala PK, Shaw JLV. Pharmacogenetics of chronic pain management. *Clin Biochem.* 2014;47(13–14):1169–1187. doi:10.1016/j.clinbiochem.2014.05.065
82. Crews KR, Monte AA, Huddart R, et al. Clinical Pharmacogenetics Implementation Consortium guideline for CYP2D6, OPRM1, and COMT genotypes and select opioid therapy. *Clin Pharmacol Ther.* 2021;110(4):888–896. doi:10.1002/CPT.2149
83. Lötsch J, Geisslinger G. Are μ-opioid receptor polymorphisms important for clinical opioid therapy? *Trends Mol Med.* 2005;11(2):82–89. doi:10.1016/j.molmed.2004.12.006
84. Matic M, Nijenhuis M, Soree B, et al. Dutch Pharmacogenetics Working Group (DPWG) guideline for the gene–drug interaction between CYP2D6 and opioids (codeine, tramadol and oxycodone). *Eur J Hum Genet.* 2023 [Online ahead of print]. doi:10.1038/S41431-021-00920-Y
85. Madadi P, Amstutz U, Rieder MJ, et al. Clinical practice guideline: CYP2D6 genotyping for safe and efficacious codeine therapy. *J Popul Ther Clin Pharmacol.* 2013;20(3):e369–e396.
86. Taylor C, Crosby I, Yip V, Maguire P, Pirmohamed M, Turner RM. A review of the important role of CYP2D6 in pharmacogenomics. *Genes.* 2020;11(11):1–23. doi:10.3390/GENES11111295
87. Blanco G, Martínez C, García-Martín E, Agúndez JAG. Cytochrome P450 gene polymorphisms and variability in response to NSAIDs. *Clin Res Regul Aff.* 2005;22(2):57–81. doi:10.1080/10601330500214559
88. Kirchheiner J, Störmer E, Meisel C, Steinbach N, Roots I, Brockmöller J. Influence of CYP2C9 genetic polymorphisms on pharmacokinetics of celecoxib and its metabolites. *Pharmacogenetics.* 2003;13(8):473–480. doi:10.1097/00008571-200308000-00005
89. Pilotto A, Franceschi M, Vitale DF, et al. Upper gastrointestinal symptoms and therapies in elderly out-patients, users of non-selective NSAIDs or coxibs. *Aliment Pharmacol Ther.* 2005;22(2):147–155. doi:10.1111/j.1365-2036.2005.02537.x
90. Swen JJ, Nijenhuis M, De Boer A, et al. Pharmacogenetics: From bench to byte—An update of guidelines. *Clin Pharmacol Ther.* 2011;89(5):662–673. doi:10.1038/CLPT.2011.34
91. Janicki PK, Schuler G, Francis D, et al. A genetic association study of the functional A118G polymorphism of the human mu-opioid receptor gene in patients with acute and chronic pain. *Anesth Analg.* 2006;103(4):1011–1017. doi:10.1213/01.ane.0000231634.20341.88
92. Lötsch J, Geisslinger G. Current evidence for a genetic modulation of the response to analgesics. *Pain.* 2006;121(1):1–5. doi:10.1016/j.pain.2006.01.010
93. Linnstaedt SD, Hu J, Bortsov A V, et al. μ-Opioid receptor gene A118 G variants and persistent pain symptoms among men and women experiencing motor vehicle collision. *J Pain.* 2015;16(7):637–644. doi:10.1016/j.jpain.2015.03.011
94. Tammimäki A, Männistö PT. Catechol-*O*-methyltransferase gene polymorphism and chronic human pain: A systematic review and meta-analysis. *Pharmacogenet Genomics.* 2012;22(9):673–691. doi:10.1097/FPC.0B013E3283560C46
95. Rakvåg TT, Klepstad P, Baar C, et al. The Val158Met polymorphism of the human catechol-*O*-methyltransferase (COMT) gene may influence morphine requirements in cancer pain patients. *Pain.* 2005;116(1–2):73–78. doi:10.1016/J.PAIN.2005.03.032

96. Reyes-Gibby CC, Shete S, Rakvåg T, et al. Exploring joint effects of genes and the clinical efficacy of morphine for cancer pain: OPRM1 and COMT gene. *Pain*. 2007;130(1–2):25–30. doi:10.1016/J.PAIN.2006.10.023
97. Ross JR, Riley J, Taegetmeyer AB, et al. Genetic variation and response to morphine in cancer patients: Catechol-*O*-methyltransferase and multidrug resistance-1 gene polymorphisms are associated with central side effects. *Cancer*. 2008;112(6):1390–1403. doi:10.1002/CNCR.23292
98. Tander B, Gunes S, Boke O, et al. Polymorphisms of the serotonin-2A receptor and catechol-*O*-methyltransferase genes: A study on fibromyalgia susceptibility. *Rheumatol Int*. 2008;28(7):685–691. doi:10.1007/s00296-008-0525-8
99. Yildiz SH, Ulaşli AM, Özdemir Erdoğan M, et al. Assessment of pain sensitivity in patients with chronic low back pain and association with HTR2A gene polymorphism. *Arch Rheumatol*. 2016;32(1):3–9. doi:10.5606/ArchRheumatol.2017.5846
100. Brasch-Andersen C, Møller MU, Christiansen L, et al. A candidate gene study of serotonergic pathway genes and pain relief during treatment with escitalopram in patients with neuropathic pain shows significant association to serotonin receptor2C (HTR2C). *Eur J Clin Pharmacol*. 2011;67(11):1131–1137. doi:10.1007/S00228-011-1056-X/TABLES/2
101. Uher R, Tansey KE, Rietschel M, et al. Common genetic variation and antidepressant efficacy in major depressive disorder: A meta-analysis of three genome-wide pharmacogenetic studies. *Am J Psychiatry*. 2013;170(2):207–217. doi:10.1176/APPI.AJP.2012.12020237/ASSET/IMAGES/LARGE/207F3.JPEG
102. Urits I, Peck J, Orhurhu MS, et al. Off-label antidepressant use for treatment and management of chronic pain: Evolving understanding and comprehensive review. *Curr Pain Headache Rep*. 2019;23(9):1–10. doi:10.1007/S11916-019-0803-Z/TABLES/3
103. Wiffen PJ, Derry S, Moore RA, et al. Antiepileptic drugs for neuropathic pain and fibromyalgia: An overview of Cochrane reviews. *Cochrane Database Syst Rev*. 2013;2013(11):CD010567. doi:10.1002/14651858.CD010567.PUB2
104. Wiffen PJ, Derry S, Moore RA, Kalso EA. Carbamazepine for chronic neuropathic pain and fibromyalgia in adults. *Cochrane Database Syst Rev*. 2014;2014(4):CD005451. doi:10.1002/14651858.CD005451.PUB3
105. Phillips EJ, Sukasem C, Whirl-Carrillo M, et al. Clinical Pharmacogenetics Implementation Consortium guideline for HLA genotype and use of carbamazepine and oxcarbazepine: 2017 update. *Clin Pharmacol Ther*. 2018;103(4):574–581. doi:10.1002/CPT.1004
106. McCormack M, Alfirevic A, Bourgeois S, et al. HLA-A*3101 and carbamazepine-induced hypersensitivity reactions in Europeans. *N Engl J Med*. 2011;364(12):1134–1143. doi:10.1056/NEJMoa1013297
107. Dean L. Carbamazepine therapy and HLA genotype. National Center for Biotechnology Information; 2012. Accessed July 25, 2019. http://www.ncbi.nlm.nih.gov/pubmed/28520367
108. Genelex. Pharmacogenetics and chronic pain. n.d. Accessed June 30, 2022. https://www.genelex.com/patients/conditions/chronic-pain
109. ClarityX. Genetic testing for pain management medication. 2021. Accessed June 30, 2022. https://www.clarityxdna.com/genetic-testing-for-pain-management
110. Inagene Diagnostics. Personalized Insights Precision Pain & Mental Health Test Kit. n.d. Accessed June 30, 2022. https://inagene.com/products/the-inagene-personalized-insights%E2%84%A2-pharmacogenetics-cheek-swab-kit
111. GX Sciences. Chronic pain panel. n.d. Accessed June 30, 2022. https://gxsciences.com/nutrigenomics/chronic-pain-panel
112. PMCDx. Pain Management PGx Test Panel. n.d. Accessed June 30, 2022. https://pmcdx.com/pain-management-pgx-test-panel

4
The Vulnerable Patient
Pain Throughout the Life Span

Jana M. Mossey

Introduction

This chapter focuses on the occurrence, consequences, and risk factors for pain across the life course. Pain is seen as both a generator and a consequence of a person's vulnerability. Although acute pain is inevitable, chronic pain, defined as lasting 3 months or more and classified as nociceptive, nociplastic, and/or neuropathic, receives special emphasis. This chapter traces the experiences and consequences of pain and pain risk across the life course and provides the reader with an evidence-based context from which to appreciate how vulnerability to chronic pain begins at birth and accumulates over time. Such knowledge should inform development of actionable frameworks for primary prevention of chronic pain and development of effective intervention strategies.

The chapter's content reflects past decades of scholarship that addresses definitions and assessments of pain in human populations and ways individuals respond to their and others' pain. Pain research is occurring at a time of substantial scientific and societal change. Those older than age 80 years are the fastest growing population segment,[1] and the proportion of "vital" elders is increasing. The age boundaries of different life-stage groups are being modified. For example, "old age" is divided into "young old" and "old old," and "young adults" now comprise a separate life-stage period.[2,3] Recent events, such as the COVID-19 pandemic, climate change consequences (e.g., devastating storms and wildfires), and interpersonal and societal violence expose populations to unimaginably numerous noxious stressors. Viewed from the biopsychosocial[4] model of pain, such exposures increase vulnerability to physiological and emotional consequences of high allostatic loads and, concurrently, to development of chronic pain conditions.

The chapter is organized into three sections:

1. The first section addresses (1) challenges to interpreting published pain research, (2) difficulties understanding subjective pain self-reports, (3) incongruences of using the U.S. Census Bureau/U.S. Office of Management and Budget (OMB) race/ethnicity classification, and (4) influences of structural/systemic racism and chronic stress exposures for chronic pain. Although important, a comprehensive presentation of each topic is beyond this chapter's scope.

2. The second section summarizes research findings for age-defined groups pertinent to the occurrence, risk factors, and consequences of chronic pain.
3. The third section presents main conclusions and recommendations for improving the rigor and relevance of pain research.

Background Material

Challenges to Interpreting and Synthesizing the Published Pain Literature

World Health Organization (WHO) Global Burden of Disease scientists have identified low back pain and headaches/migraines as the top causes of disability worldwide, affecting millions and costing billions of dollars in health care and productivity[5]; however, no single definition or assessment tool for chronic pain is consistently used by pain researchers.[6,7] When diverse scientists study the same pain condition, conceptual and/or operational pain definitions differ,[8] and incidence or prevalence rates vary widely (e.g., adult chronic low back pain [CLBP] prevalence is 22–75%,[9] and childhood pain prevalence is 26–69%[10]). Moreover, findings pertinent to pain epidemiology often are derived from secondary analyses of data collected for an unrelated purpose.[6,10] Lack of study rigor and/or ability to compare within and across populations seriously limits the development of a coherent, accurate epidemiology of chronic pain.

Interpretation of Subjective Pain Reports

Although subjective self-report is the recognized approach to assessing pain,[11] interpretations of a person's pain reports inherently are difficult. Various sociomedical factors influence pain assessments—for example, sensitivity to painful stimuli, current level of stress, prior pain experiences, and trust in the questioner.[12,13] Pain care providers unaware of such factors risk misinterpretation and/or incorrect clinical recommendations. For example, the frequently observed lower chronic pain prevalence reported by non-Hispanic Blacks (NHB; e.g., 19.3% vs. 23.6% for non-Hispanic Whites [NHW])[14] could support the conclusion that fewer NHB experience chronic pain. However, such NHB pain prevalence may reflect the reticence of historically marginalized individuals to accurately acknowledge their pain and vulnerability. Alternatively, higher NHW pain prevalence may reflect greater medical care access and/or greater trust in their care provider.

U.S. Census Bureau "Race/Ethnicity" Categories for Population Classification

Pain studies frequently have used the OMB race/ethnicity classification system: non-Hispanic Whites (NHW), non-Hispanic Blacks (NHB), Hispanics (HISP), American Indians or Alaska Natives (AI/AN), Asians, and Native Hawaiian or other Pacific

Islanders (NHPI).[15] Yearby[16] argues that this race/ethnicity classification only represents a "social indicator." Since the Human Genome Project[17] confirmed humans share more than 99.5% of their genetic material, claims of distinct "races" are simply false. Distinction of a "Hispanic" ethnicity fails to acknowledge the geographic, philosophical/religious, and lifestyle heterogeneity of group members. Mora[18] provides compelling evidence that the term "Hispanic" did not represent ethnicity but, rather, was adopted in approximately 1967 through negotiations between U.S. Census Bureau officials, Chicano organizers in Chicago, and leaders of a Spanish-language television network to (1) legitimize a census designation for Spanish-speaking groups and (2) justify "Hispanic" population statistic required for accessing government funds. While agreeing with Yearby[16] that the OMB racial/ethnic classification perpetuates discrimination, absent alternatives, it is used here.

Systemic/Structural Racism, Chronic Stress, and Their Relationships to Chronic Pain

Brown and Homan[19] described "systemic racism" as "institutionalized with interconnected, multifaceted elements that are overtly and covertly designed to perpetuate systems of racial subordination and racial inequalities."[19(p6),20] Persistent in the United States for centuries, systematic racism has been directed toward NHB, AI/AN, and, to a lesser extent, Spanish-speaking immigrants. Racism-driven policies created segregated residential neighborhoods (characterized by poverty, substandard housing and schools, limited health care access, and violence). Unfair legal and judicial systems and intergenerational poverty have negatively impacted the well-being and life opportunities of minoritized groups.[21,22] The consequences of inequity and discrimination are implicated in striking health disparities in which NHW groups enjoy better health than NHB, AI/AN, and Spanish-speaking populations (HISP).[23] Life expectancy at birth in 2019 (NHW 80.1 years, NHB 75.4 years, AI/AN 67.1 years, HISP 77.9 years)[24] and pregnancy-related death rates per 100,000 births, 2007–2016 (NHW 13.7, NHB 40.8, AI/AN 29.7, HISP 11.2)[25] highlight health discrepancies especially for AI/AN and NHB groups.

Compelling evidence identifies chronic exposures to noxious stimuli/stressors associated with systemic racism as important risk factors for chronic pain (see Abdallah and Geha[26] and Lindell and Grimby-Ekman[27]). The implications for chronic pain risk of chronic exposure to noxious stimuli are briefly addressed. *Stress* has been defined as "a dynamic [unpleasant/aversive] state within the organism" resulting from exposure to stimuli perceived as noxious and/or threatening[28(p340)] (e.g., the death of a loved one, job loss, physical attack, abuse, and/or exposure to discrimination). Upon experiencing a situation considered noxious and/or dangerous, a complex physiological "stress" response is evoked. The "fight or flight response"[29(p109)] is designed to mitigate the perceived danger, promote adaptation, and regain stability. Characteristic sympathetic nervous system activation is accompanied by parallel hypothalamic–pituitary–adrenal (HPA) axis responses. With resolution of the acute noxious exposure, the neurophysiologic systemic changes should return to baseline levels. When exposures to noxious stimuli become chronic, return to baseline neurophysiologic status does not

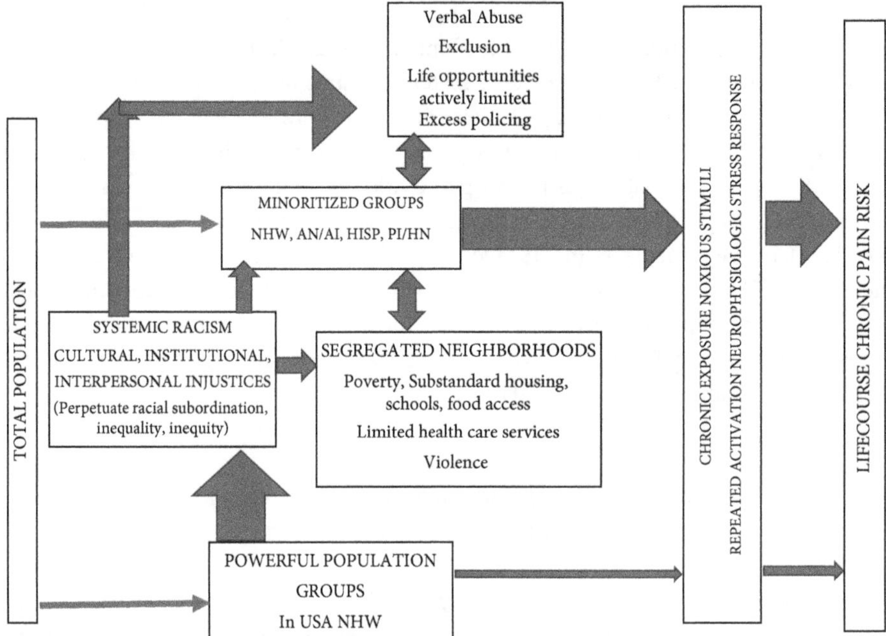

Figure 4.1 Effects of systemic racism on chronic pain risk: minoritized groups versus non-Hispanic Whites. AN/AI, Alaska Natives or American Indians; HISP, Hispanics; NHW, non-Hispanic Whites; PI/HN, Pacific Islanders or native Hawaiians.

occur. Prolonged attempts to deal with the persistent stress often are maladaptive.[30,31] Figure 4.1 provides a visual description of the path through systemic racism to exposure to chronic noxious stimuli and chronic pain risk.

Chronic pain and chronic stress are distinct phenomena, but multiple conceptual and physiological components overlap.[26(p1),32] HPA axis dysfunction and changes in higher brain centers consequent to chronic stress exposure are thought to contribute to changes in somatosensory pain processing at central nervous system levels. Such alterations, termed *central sensitization* (CS),[33,34] are characterized by chronic amplification of pain (hyperalgesia) and lowered pain thresholds (allodynia). Fibromyalgia, complex regional pain syndrome, and tension-type headaches emerge in the absence of apparent injury or disease etiology and are considered to reflect CS.

Pain Experiences According to Age Groupings

Descriptive information is presented for six age groups: (1) newborns (pre- and full-term), (2) preschool (children younger than age 6 years), (3) preadolescent–adolescent (ages 6–18 years), (4) young adult (ages 19–34 years), (5) middle age (ages 35–64 years), and (6) elderly (ages 65–79 years and 80 years or older). These groups represent developmental periods during which individuals experience important social and environmental life events and challenges.

Table 4.1 Age Group–Specific Prevalence Rates for Low Back Pain and Injuries Resulting in Nonfatal Emergency Department Visits

Age Group (Years)	2019 Low Back Pain Prevalence (WHO Highest Socio-Demographic Index Regions)	Age Group (Years)	All Injuries: Nonfatal Emergency Room Visits: 2020 Crude rate/ 100,000 Males/Females
<5	0.9/100	00–04	7,262/5,883
		05–09	4,768/3,728
5–19	4.2/100	10–19[a]	6,109/5,165
20–39	10.5/100	20–39[a]	9,465/6,676
40–64	17.6/100	40–64[a]	8,006/5,320
65–84	20.0/100	65–74[a]	6,194/5,554
≥85	23.4/100	≥75[a]	9,723/9,002

[a] Crude rate represents average of 5-year age groups.

To enable age group comparisons of the same pain condition and the likelihood of injury-related pain, data were accessed from the 2019 WHO Burden of Disease Low Back Pain (LBP) project[35] and the CDC surveillance data (2020) on injuries resulting in nonfatal emergency department (ED) visits.[36] As shown in Table 4.1, LBP prevalence rates increase with age through the oldest group. Discrepant cross-sectional findings showing declining chronic pain after age 60 years are considered due to early, selective mortality.[37] As a proxy for serious acute pain experiences, the ED data suggest higher rates for those younger than age 5 years and more injury-related pain for males than females.

Many factors relevant to all age groups that directly or indirectly increase an individual's risk for chronic pain are shown in Box 4.1. Some, such as age, are unchanging; the majority are amenable to primary prevention or modification. For example, children who experience maltreatment experience long-term increased chronic pain risk.[38] Other pain risk factors, such as obesity, are implicated in the later development of risk factors such as type 2 diabetes and musculoskeletal stress/injury. Although evidence is limited, effects of different risk factors are thought to be additive and/or interactive.

Newborns (Pre- and Full-Term)

In 2020, 3,613,847 U.S. births were registered.[39] Newborn infants, pre- and full-term, represent the most vulnerable population group; however, even at birth, vulnerability is not equally distributed. Although routine postnatal procedures such as a heel prick or an injection are painful, newborns differ according to their (1) subsequent pain exposure, (2) pain processing capacities, and (3) risk of developing later life chronic pain.

Box 4.1 Chronic Pain Risk Factors Relevant to Most Age Groups

Advancing age
Sex: Females all age groups
Genes: Other family members (especially parents) chronic pain history
Low household socioeconomic status; chronic poverty
Preterm birth; neonatal intensive care unit admission
Previous episode(s) chronic pain
Absent or low physical activity
Weight—obesity
Nonrestorative sleep
Addictive behaviors: alcohol, drugs, smoking
Falling and fear of falling
Chronic medical conditions: e.g., diabetes, hypertension, asthma, heart disease, arthritic conditions
Internalizing disorders: depression, anxiety, post-traumatic stress disorder
Chronic exposure noxious stressors: e.g., discrimination/marginalization, abuse, poverty, food and/or housing insecurity, violence
Negative, fearful attitudes regarding pain; pain catastrophizing
Especially dependent age individuals, parent(s) with internalizing disorders
Especially dependent age individuals, parents with negative fearful attitudes regarding pain, pain catastrophizing

To review sources that identify chronic pain risk factors, see references 4, 7, 9, 10, 56, 59, 75, 122, 130, and 136.

Some full-term infants have birth defects (e.g., clubfoot), genetic conditions (e.g., sickle cell disease), or conditions such as cerebral palsy[40,41] that increase their vulnerability and lifetime pain experiences.[42] The most vulnerable newborns are those delivered preterm (<37 weeks gestational age [GA]). In the U.S. 2020 birth cohort, 10.09% of live births were preterm[43]; of these, more than 90% were admitted to a neonatal intensive care unit (NICU).[44] NICU-admitted preterm infants are exposed to a large number of medically necessary, painful procedures (5–27 daily), including heel lances, venipuncture, and intramuscular injections,[45] and noninvasive, often painful, care activities such as turning, bathing, etc.[46] Although newborns feel pain, across hospitals, effective analgesia is not consistently administered.[47] At birth, peripheral and central nervous system pain processing components of full-term infants are intact but immature. In contrast, the preterm infant brain, especially extremely preterm (<28 weeks GA or ≤1,500 g birth weight), is not fully developed.[48] The descending inhibitory pain pathways are incomplete; preterm infants are unable to suppress afferent pain signals from reaching and overwhelming higher levels of the somatosensory pain processing system. The reactive adjustments by the preterm brain can be maladaptive. White and gray matter injuries and decreases in the size of brain components (e.g., thalamus, cerebellum, and hippocampus) have been documented. Hyperalgesia and allodynia may develop.[49] Substantial evidence exists that such central nervous somatosensory pain processing system changes may have lifelong, debilitating impacts. At 18 months, preterm infants were less sensitive to "everyday" pains, had lower cognitive function scores, and manifest more internalizing behaviors than full-term controls.[50] Depression rates were substantially higher for adolescents, aged 17 years, born preterm (female = 15.2, male = 1.0) than full-term classmates (female = 1.8, male = 0.25).[51] When questioned, middle-age and older age chronic pain patients have confirmed their preterm birth.[52]

Maternal age younger than age 25 years or older than age 39 years, not married, previous preterm birth or interpregnancy less than 18 months, multiple births, unhealthy behaviors, chronic poverty, and inadequate prenatal care are risk factors for preterm birth.[53] NHB and AI/AN, historically marginalized groups, disproportionately deliver preterm infants.[54]

Children: Preschool or Age 6 Years or Younger

Preterm and full-term children with a birth defect or genetic condition enter this age group with vulnerabilities that impact their subsequent development. Cerebral palsy,[55] associated with chronic pain, occurs in 2–2.6% of newborns. The U.S. sickle cell disease incidence is 1/365 NHB and 1/16,500 Hispanic births.[56] Pain crises increase with age, and pain often becomes chronic.[57] Documenting pain felt by cognitively immature children younger than age 6 years is challenging. Due to their own experiences and biases, the often used parents/caregivers' reports of their child's pain have mixed accuracy.[58,59]

As shown in Table 4.1, children younger than age 6 years have considerable opportunity for serious injury-related pain. Fearon et al.[60] observed the daily frequency of milder painful events (e.g., bumps, scrapes, and cuts) experienced by 3- to 7-year-olds (one or two each preschool day). "Functional" pains in preschool children (headache, abdominal, and nonspecific musculoskeletal pain) are characterized by chronicity, absent or unclear etiology,[61] and unfavorable impacts on life quality. Chronic pain prevalence of 25% was seen in one study of preschool children,[62] with "functional" abdominal pain most common. At school enrollment, chronic functional pain for headache (3.6%), abdominal pain (31.9%), and headache and abdominal pain (48.6%) was observed.[63] In another study, chronic pain was seen in 13.6% and 9.9%, respectively, of boys and girls younger than age 3 years, and at ages 4–7 years, it was seen in 15.8% of boys and 22.7% of girls.[64] Chronic musculoskeletal pain,[65] juvenile idiopathic arthritis,[66] and chronic post-surgical pain occur in 3–5% of those aged 6 years or younger.[67,68] Extensive moderate to severe chronic pain is seen in preschoolers; not necessarily reflecting central sensitization; a substantial proportion of such pain is of "unknown etiology."

During critical preschool years, chronic pain limits active play, social interactions, and activities requiring concentration. Motor and social skills, positive peer comments/behaviors, curiosity to explore, and confidence to act independently are compromised. Chronic pain vulnerability and limited mastery of future adolescent and adult challenges increase.

Children Ages 7–9 Years and Adolescents Ages 10–19 Years

Many pain studies group together individuals ages 7–19 years; the majority are ages 10–19 years, the designated WHO age of "adolescence."[69] Viner et al. describe adolescence as "one of the central dramas of the human life course . . . accompanied by . . . major central nervous system changes, and dramatic psychosocial change."[70(p719)] Puberty-related hormonal fluctuations affect personal and social relationships; questions regarding gender identity and/or sexual preference may arise. School participation requires attentive, cooperative, and appropriately responsive students. Such expectations can overwhelm vulnerable individuals. Health problems emerge and risky behaviors that influence chronic pain incidence develop. Due to early exposures and medical conditions, at age 7 years, a substantial proportion of children are already vulnerable to chronic pain.[71] During adolescence, many develop new chronic pain risks. Obesity is seen in 29.7% of AI/AN aged 19 years or younger[72] and 21% of other adolescents.[73] Up to 30% of U.S. adolescents have a diagnosed chronic disease,[74] including hypertension (11%),[75] major depressive disorder (boys 8.6%, girls 23.4%),[76] and neurodevelopmental disorders (1.3–12.9%).[77] NHB, AI/AN, and low-income adolescents are at disproportionately higher risk for these chronic diseases.[78] Increasing pain risk, addictive behaviors often begin during adolescence. Violence-related injuries[79] and workplace accidents[80] expose youth aged 7–19 years to many potentially painful events.

Reported pain rates for those aged 7–19 years range from 4% to 83%.[7,64,81] A 2013–2014 WHO, 42-country study of 10- to 17-year-olds observed 44.2% reported chronic headache, abdominal, or low back pain, with 20.6% endorsing two or more pain sites.[82] The Norwegian HUNT youth study (2006–2008) reported that 33.4% endorsed chronic idiopathic musculoskeletal pain unrelated to illness or injury and 11% indicated another idiopathic pain location.[83] Rabbitts and Groenewald[67] reported that 38% of 6- to 18-year-old surgical patients experienced moderate to severe chronic post-surgical pain. Among those aged 15–19 years, chronic widespread pain or fibromyalgia were reported by 7–15% and 3.5–6.2%, respectively.[84]

Adolescents with chronic pain experience delays in achieving developmental milestones, disturbed sleep, frequent absenteeism, limited physical activity, reduced age-appropriate social and educational activities,[85,86] bullying, and restricted opportunities to explore.[18,64,87] Depression, substance abuse, and/or suicidal feelings/behaviors may be observed.[88,89] Moreover, adolescent chronic pain often persists into young adulthood or re-emerges later.[90,91]

Young Adults (Ages 20–39 Years)

As Furstenberg and colleagues[3] noted, the life stage, "young adult," emerged in the 1990s when marriage and childbearing were no longer the only legitimate signs of adulthood. Replaced by education, employment, and financial independence, young adulthood is a stressful life stage with high personal and societal expectations to successfully transition to full autonomy, financial self-reliance, and/or committed partnership/family.[92] Compared to pain-free age-mates, individuals entering young adulthood with cumulative pain-related vulnerabilities (e.g., central nervous system injury, developmental delays, and negative interpersonal interactions) are disadvantaged. Murray et al.[93] reported substantial deficits in educational attainment, employment income, and more frequent receipt of public assistance for young adults aged 24–32 years who had previously reported adolescent chronic pain. Findings from the National Longitudinal Study on Adolescent to Adult Health revealed disproportionately higher rates of persistent anxiety among young adults with adolescent chronic pain histories.[94] For many, young adulthood brings new challenges, including work-related injuries. Yang et al.[95] reported disabling work-related injury claims rates for those aged 19–21 and 22–24 years of 119/10,000 and 116/10,000, respectively.[95] Among military enlistees aged 18–39 years, adjusted odds of serious pain were 3.2 times those observed in non-military age-mates.[96]

Using young adult, longitudinal data, Angst et al.[97] observed annual lumbar and cervical pain incidence rates of 5.8–13.3% and 7.8–12.6%, respectively. Meta-analysis of data from 43 studies generated a pooled chronic pain prevalence rate of 11.6% for young adults.[98] The 2018 U.S. National Health Interview Survey (NHIS) analyses of those aged 18–29 years yielded chronic pain without limitations prevalence of 8.5% and high-impact chronic pain prevalence of 2.2%.[99] Chronic pain risk variables most salient to young adults include past chronic pain, childhood trauma, nonrestorative sleep, and low socioeconomic status. Chronic pain prevalence is also higher in those who self-describe "not always heterosexual."[100]

Middle-Aged Adults (Ages 40–64 Years)

Historically, "middle age" has been described as "the golden age of adulthood."[101(p163)] In contrast, Lachman et al. suggest midlife is a time of "growth" in terms of "knowledge, experience, and emotional regulation" and "decline" in "functional health, speed of [cognitive] processing, working memory."[102(Fig.4, p24)] Citing others, Lachman and colleagues indicate that with diligent attention to lifestyle factors (e.g., smoking and physical exercise), middle-age adults can reverse accumulated losses in resilience, cognition, and physical capacity. Without such attention, chronic pain prevalence increases. Middle-aged adults sustain higher rates of chronic medical conditions (CMCs) than young adults (e.g., type 2 diabetes, 129/1,000 [ages 45–64 years] vs. 33/1,000 [ages 18–44 years]; hypertension, 524/1,000 [ages 40–59 years] vs. 234/1,000 [ages 20–39 years];and arthritis, 303/1,000 [ages 45–64 years] vs. 70/1,000 [ages 18–44 years]).[103] Many middle-agers engage in unhealthy lifestyle habits (e.g., current smokers [11%] and physical inactivity [not meeting 2008 federal physical activity guidelines; 80%]) and other behaviors resulting in 44% meeting criteria for obesity.[104]

A substantial proportion of middle-aged individuals experience chronic pain, and, for many, such pain already is of long duration. Seven percent of middle-aged Canadian residents reporting high-severity chronic pain indicated their pain lasted 10 years or more, and 22.5% indicated persistent pain for 20 years or more.[105] Prevalence of chronic pain without limitations and high-impact chronic pain rates for individuals aged 45–64 years were 25.8% and 10.3%, respectively.[14] Analysis of data obtained at ages 49 or 50 years from community dwellers who were aged 20 or 21 years at study enrollment revealed the 23-year cumulative incidence of lumbar back pain (52.3%) and the cumulative prevalence (66.9%).[97] A five-wave, 28-year longitudinal study[106] (individuals aged 44–58 years in 1981 and 72–86 years in 2009) allowed examination of LBP trajectories. By ages 60–74 years, three LBP trajectories were identified: (1) persistently low pain (21%), (2) stable moderate pain (60%), and (3) high/severe slightly decreasing pain

(19%). Fewer high/severe LBP trajectory individuals reported high physical activity levels (48% vs. 59% low pain trajectory). More had a "blue-collar" job (57% vs. 25%); currently smoked (14% vs. 10%); and/or had reported respiratory, cardiovascular, and/or musculoskeletal disease. At ages 72–86 years, high LBP trajectory members reported activity of daily living and/or mobility limitations three times more often than low LBP trajectory members.[106] Chronic pain during middle age has been implicated in memory impairment and cognitive decline,[107,108] losses that reduce independence and life quality.

Although falls are considered problematic for "old people," middle-agers also sustain increased fall incidence and related injuries.[109] Based on the 2008 NHIS, 12-month falls incidence rates were 37.9% for ages 35–44 years, 40.2% for ages 45–54 years, 43.8% for ages 55–64 years, and 42.6% for ages 65–74 years.[110] Falling during middle age, irrespective of injury or chronic pain, is traumatic.[111] Out of fear, fallers often reduce physical activities, even walking. The diminished activity and heightened fear can precipitate loss of reserve, lowered sense of efficacy, and increased chronic pain vulnerability.

Older Adults: Ages 65–74 Years ("Young Old") and Ages 75 Years or Older ("Old Old")

Although not universal, evidence suggests a high percentage of individuals aged 65 years or older have compromised physical resilience. Estimated CMC prevalence (high-income country residents aged 65 years or older) exceeds 80%. Hypertension affects 60.6%, followed by dyslipidemia (51.2%), diabetes (25.2%), etc.[112] Many elders experience "multimorbidity" (≥2 or ≥3 CMC).[113] In one study, such prevalence rates were 73.7% (ages 60–74 years), 84.3% (ages 75–89 years), and 63.3% (age 90 years or older).[114(Table 1)] Multimorbidity severity increases chronic pain risk, functional decline, and mortality risk.[115]

Chronic pain among community-dwelling elders ranges between 21% and 75%,[9] reflecting osteoarthritic LBP or neck pain (65%), other musculoskeletal pain (40%), peripheral neuropathic pain (35%), and chronic joint pain (15–25%).[116] Nonspecific CLBP is the most prevalent pain diagnosis (36.1–42.9%).[117] Diabetic neuropathies occur in 21–50% of older type 2 diabetics.[118] Fibromyalgia prevalence of 5.5% has been reported.[119] High-impact chronic pain prevalence estimates (2016 NHIS data) are respectively 10.7% and 15.8% for ages 65–84 years and 85 years or older.[120] Due to age-related changes in somatosensory systems, elders typically experience increased pain thresholds; they show greater pain acceptance and express less pain catastrophizing.[121] Often believing pain is "normative" with aging, many elders underreport their pain or its severity.[122]

With aging, reductions in vision, hearing, balance, cognitive integrity, etc.[123] appear to accelerate. Falls and fear of falling gain importance; they diminish physical and social activities. Elderly falls precipitate injury-related chronic pain and increase mortality. In 2018, 12-month falling rates in the United States for those aged 65 years or older ranged between 26% and 34%[124]; 2016 mortality per 100,000 due to falling were 15.5 for ages 65–74 years, 61.4 for ages 75–84 years, and 257.9 for ages 85 years or older.[125] Chronic pain diminishes elders' abilities to navigate "growing older." Physical and mental health, social activities, and quality of life are negatively impacted. Moreover, persons aged 65 years or older experiencing chronic pain are at increased risk of dementing illnesses[126] and earlier death.[127]

Summary, Conclusions, and Recommendations

Published findings from diverse research studies have been assembled to describe the occurrences, risks, and consequences of pain for six age groups. The paucity of risk estimates and incidence or prevalence rates comparable across studies and between age groups and the many "chronic pain" definitions and assessment approaches have hindered development of a concise picture of pain over the life span. Despite the many challenges, several conclusions have emerged with unexpected clarity. Presented below, these are accompanied by recommended "next steps" designed to advance prevention efforts, mitigate existing risks, and/or provide effective clinical interventions.

Chronic Pain Conditions: Conclusions and Recommendations

1. Disabling chronic pain, especially idiopathic pain, is not an inevitable life experience even among those who appear most vulnerable. Despite existing evidence that prevention and recovery are possible, public understanding regarding pain epidemiology and/or clinical management is limited, erroneous, or nonexistent. Remedies exist, such as the following:
   a. Global, accurate public health information documents and education programs geared to distinct age groups that (1) describe chronic pain epidemiology; (2) identify and relate biological, psychological, behavioral, and experiential factors to pain risk; and (3) provide operational prevention/early intervention strategies for fast-track development and wide dissemination in all media formats.
2. For some, chronic pain vulnerability begins in the NICU. Central nervous system injuries from painful or chronic noxious stimuli can occur at any age, accumulate over time, and negatively influence a person's current and future experiences and pain risk. Remedies include the following:
   a. Ongoing work to develop and guarantee universal delivery of effective and safe analgesia protocols across all NICU settings must be expanded.
   b. Like existing pediatric physician office autism screening programs, pediatricians and elementary school nurses could routinely screen for and monitor pain risks (e.g., preterm birth, internalizing disorders, adverse childhood events, and physical inactivity). Such programs require development and worldwide implementation.
   c. Societal- and individual-level protocols that inform the development and implementation of risk prevention and/or management programs geared to the youngest at-risk individuals must be developed.

3. Of many identified chronic pain risk factors, only a few (e.g., age, genes, and sex) are "immutable." Most chronic pain risk factors, including young age chronic pain conditions and inactivity, are preventable or modifiable.
   a. Insightful, creative, publicly accessible, and age-appropriate programs addressing preventable risk behaviors (e.g., physical inactivity, smoking, and substance abuse) and/or preventable/treatable internalizing disorders (e.g., depression and anxiety) require development and implementation, at earliest appropriate ages, within all educational settings, workplaces, faith organizations, senior centers, etc.
4. Chronic pain conditions thought to reflect central sensitization CS occur in every age group. The prevention and treatment of functional abdominal disorders, fibromyalgia, widespread chronic pain, etc. appear distinct from those of other chronic pain conditions.
   a. CS requires further elucidation regarding its etiology, course, and relationships to chronic noxious stressor exposures and chronic pain occurrence and recovery. Additional research focusing on all age groups is required.
5. Across ages, NHB and AI/AN individuals and those born poor are at high risk of chronic exposures to noxious stimuli associated with systemic racism and/or poverty-related disadvantages.
   a. Despite health and pain care disparities, chronic pain rates of NHB are typically lower than those of NHW groups. Research is required to determine the actual drivers of NHB, NHW, and others' pain reports and to identify assessment approaches that yield unbiased estimates.
   b. As advocated in other chapters in this book, efforts by all individuals, including pain care providers, to eliminate the perverse attitudes, government and social policies, and individual biases that perpetuate systemic racism are essential.
6. An individual's biological age when a pain risk factor transitions from protective/neutral to positive influences its strength and impact on chronic pain occurrence (e.g., type 2 diabetic neuropathy occurrence reflects diabetes duration, and adolescent incidence increases probability of lower limb neuropathies). Chronic obesity, an important risk factor for type 2 diabetes, is increasingly seen in children.
   a. Obesity prevention/management protocols are essential. Rigorous research on its pathophysiology, genetic, behavioral, nutritional, and psychological aspects is required to develop scientifically informed obesity prevention and intervention protocols. All protocols need to clearly explain the relationships between obesity, diabetes onset, and chronic pain.
7. Irrespective of age, reactions to those with disabling chronic pain appear similarly indifferent or unpleasant. The impact of negative feedback to preschoolers through elders with chronic pain can be devastating and result in feeling shame, anxiety, and/or depression and social withdrawal. For younger, less emotionally mature sufferers, the impact on their nascent life course may be catastrophic.
   a. Programs to educate individuals at all ages regarding chronic pain etiology, course, and personal suffering could increase empathy and diminish the negative, insensitive reactions to chronic pain sufferers.

The global incidence, prevalence, and suffering of chronic pain conditions and consequences should be diminished by continuous, repetitive implementation of widely distributed, age-appropriate educational programs addressing the epidemiology and significance of chronic pain; rigorous, universal pain risk screening and monitoring programs to identify and reverse preventable risks and manage nonpreventable conditions; and scientifically informed risk prevention and early intervention programs as recommended above.

Recommendations to Improve Epidemiological and Clinical Rigor of Pain Research

1. In a recent meta-analysis, Wong et al.[117] lamented that because the available evidence was of such poor quality, conclusions regarding CLBP epidemiology were not possible. Their criticisms reflected the absence of standard conceptual and operational definitions of pain used by public health and clinical researchers.
   a. Agreement on standard pain definitions requires consensus among pain scientists, clinicians, and national/international professional organizations (e.g., the American Academy of Pain Medicine, the International Association for the Study of Pain, the European Pain Federation, and the South Asian Regional Pain Society). Although difficult to achieve, such consensus would allow the development of a coherent body of knowledge regarding pain epidemiology and the scientifically informed development of pain prevention and targeted intervention strategies.
2. Given consensus-developed conceptual and operational pain definitions, further descriptive research is required regarding pain etiology, course, and consequences across age and diverse population groups. Longitudinal trajectories of nociplastic chronic pain are needed to better elucidate the neurophysiologic links and interrelationships between depression, anxiety, chronic pain, chronic diseases, and CS. Sophisticated approaches for the dissemination of "user-friendly" evidence-based findings regarding pain and prevention/intervention protocols require development.

Achievement of the above will not be simple. Concentrated effort and funding resources will need to be marshaled, but the alternatives of "do nothing" and "continue to piece things together" are unacceptable.

References

1. U.S. Census Bureau. Population and housing units estimates tables: National population by characteristics. 2020–2021. Accessed September 12, 2022. https://www.census.gov/programs-surveys/popest/data/tables.html
2. National Institute on Aging, National Institutes of Health. Why population aging matters: A global perspective. 2007. Publication No. 07-6134. Accessed September 12, 2022. https://www.nia.nih.gov/sites/default/files/2017-06/WPAM.pdf

3. Furstenberg FF Jr, Kennedy S, McLoyd VC, et.al. Growing up is harder to do. *Contexts.* 2004;3(3):33–41.
4. Bolton D. Looking forward to a decade of the biopsychosocial model. *Br J Psych Bull.* 2022;46(4):228–232.
5. GBD 2017 Disease and Injury Incidence and Prevalence Collaborators. Global, regional, and national incidence, prevalence, and years lived with disability for 354 diseases and injuries for 195 countries and territories, 1990–2017: A systematic analysis for the Global Burden of Disease Study 2017. *Lancet.* 2018;392:1789–1858.
6. Centers for Disease Control and Prevention. Prevalence of chronic pain and high-impact chronic pain among adults—United States, 2016. *MMWR Morb Mortal Wkly Rep.* 2018;67:1001–1006.
7. Tutelman PR, Langley CL, Chambers CT, et al. Epidemiology of chronic pain in children and adolescents: A protocol for a systematic review update. *BMJ Open.* 2021;11:e043675. doi:10.1136/bmjopen-2020-043675
8. Steingrímsdóttir ÓA, Landmark T, Macfarlane GJ, et al. Defining chronic pain in epidemiological studies: A systematic review and meta-analysis. *Pain.* 2017;158:2092–2107.
9. de Souza IMB, Sakaguchi TF, Yuan SLK, et al. Prevalence of low back pain in the elderly population: A systematic review. *Clinics.* 2019;74:e789.
10. King S, Chambers CT, Huguet A, et al. The epidemiology of chronic pain in children and adolescents revisited. *Pain.* 2011;157:2729–2738.
11. Fillingim RB, Loeser JD, Baron R, et al. Assessment of chronic pain: Domains, methods, and mechanisms. *J Pain.* 2016;17(9):T10–T20.
12. Scott W, Jackson SE, Hackett RA. Perceived discrimination, health, and well-being among adults with and without pain: A prospective study. *Pain.* 2022;163:258–266.
13. Chan JY, von Baeyer CL. Cognitive developmental influences on the ability of preschool-aged children to self-report their pain intensity. *Pain.* 2016;157(5):997–1001.
14. Zelaya CE, Dahlhamer JM, Lucas JW, Connor EM. Chronic pain and high-impact chronic pain among U.S. adults, 2019. *NCHS Data Brief.* 2020;(390):1–8.
15. Office of Management and Budget. Revisions to the standards for the classification of federal data on race and ethnicity. *Fed Reg.* 1977;62(210):58782–58790. Accessed March 15, 2022. https://www.govinfo.gov/content/pkg/FR-1997-10-30/pdf/97-28653.pdf
16. Yearby R. Race medicine, colorblind disease: How racism in medicine harms us all. *Am J Bioeth.* 2021;21(2):19–27.
17. Maglo KN, Mersha TB, Martin LJ. Population genomics and the statistical values of race: An interdisciplinary perspective on the biological classification of human populations and implications for clinical genetic epidemiological research. *Front Genet.* 2016;7:Article 22.
18. Mora GC. Cross-field effects and ethnic classification: The institutionalization of Hispanic panethnicity, 1965–1990. *Am Sociol Rev.* 2014;79(2):183–210.
19. Brown T, Homan P. Structural racism and health stratification in the US: Connecting theory to measurement. Zoom talk. March 20, 2022.
20. Krieger N. Discrimination and health inequities. In: Berkman LF, Kawachi I, Glymour M, eds. *Social Epidemiology.* 2nd ed. Oxford University Press; 2014:63–124.
21. Braveman P, Arkin E, Proctor D, et al. Systemic and structural racism: Definitions, examples, health damages, and approaches to dismantling. *J Health Aff.* 2022;41:171–178.
22. Murry VM, Bradley C, Cruden G, et al. Re-envisioning, retooling, and rebuilding prevention science methods to address structural and systemic racism and promote health equity. *Prev Sci.* 2022 [Epub ahead of print].
23. Bailey BD, Krieger N, Agénor M, et al. Structural racism and health inequities in the USA: Evidence and interventions. *Lancet.* 2017;389:1453–1463.
24. Arias E, Xu JQ. United States life tables, 2020. *Natl Vital Stat Rep.* 2022;71(1):1–64.
25. Petersen EE, Davis NL, Goodman D, et al. Racial/ethnic disparities in pregnancy-related deaths—United States, 2007–2016. *MMWR Morb Mortal Wkly Rep.* 2019;68:762–765. http://dx.doi.org/10.15585/mmwr.mm6835a3

26. Abdallah CG, Geha P. Chronic pain and chronic stress: Two sides of the same coin? *Chronic Stress*. 2017;1:1–10.
27. Lindell M, Grimby-Ekman A. Stress, non-restorative sleep, and physical inactivity as risk factors for chronic pain in young adults: A cohort study. *PLoS One*. 2022;17(1):e0262601.
28. Wolff HG. Personal Communication as quoted in: The Concept of "Stress" in the Biological and Social Sciences. Lawrence E. Hinkle, Jr. *Int J Psychiatry Med*. 1974;4:335–357.
29. Goldstein DS, Kopin IJ. Evolution of concepts of stress. *Stress*. 2007;10(2):109–120. doi:10.1080/10253890701288935
30. McEwen BS. Neurobiological and systemic effects of chronic stress. *Chronic Stress*. 2017;10:1–11. https://doi.org/10.1177/2470547017692328
31. Woolf CJ. Central sensitization: Implications for the diagnosis and treatment of pain. *Pain*. 2011;152(3 Suppl):S2–S15. doi:10.1016/j.pain.2010.09.030
32. Blackburn-Munro G. Hypothalamo–pituitary–adrenal axis dysfunction as a contributory factor to chronic pain and depression. *Curr Pain Headache Rep*. 2004;8:116–124.
33. Harte J. The neurobiology of central sensitization. *Appl Behav Res*. 2018;23(2):e12137.
34. Bazzari FH. Advances in targeting central sensitization and brain plasticity in chronic pain. *Egypt J Neurol Psychiatry Neurosurg*. 2022;58:Article 38.
35. Global Burden of Disease Collaborative Network. Global Burden of Disease Study 2019 (GBD 2019) data resources. 2020. Accessed June 5, 2022. https://ghdx.healthdata.org/gbd-2019
36. Centers for Disease Control and Prevention. Unintentional all injury causes nonfatal emergency department visits and rates per 100,000, 2020, United States [Table]. *Non Fatal Injury Reports 2000–2020: WISQARS*. Accessed May 5, 2022. https://www.cdc.gov/injury/wisqars/nonfatal.html
37. Grol-Prokopczyk H. Sociodemographic disparities in chronic pain, based on 12-year longitudinal data. *Pain*. 2017;158(2):313–322.
38. Barnett KA, Mara CA, King C, et al. Does exposure to maltreatment in childhood contribute to differences in pain outcomes in adulthood? *J Pain*. 2022;23(5):54.
39. Martin JA, Hamilton BE, Osterman MJK. Births in the United States, 2020. *NCHS Data Brief*. 2021;(418):1–8.
40. Center for Disease Control and Prevention. World Birth Defects Day 2022: Global effort to prevent birth defects and support families. 2022. Last reviewed March 2, 2022. Accessed June 2, 2022. https://www.cdc.gov/globalhealth/stories/2022/world-birth-defects-day-2022.html#
41. Maenner MJ, Blumberg SJ, Kogan MD, et al. Prevalence of cerebral palsy and intellectual disability among children identified in two U.S. National Surveys, 2011–2013. *Ann Epidemiol*. 2016;26(3):222–226.
42. Hankerson SH, Moise N, Wilson D, et al. The intergenerational impact of structural racism and cumulative trauma on depression. *Am J Psychiatry*. 2022;179:434–440.
43. March of Dimes. Prematurity profile United States. 2022. Accessed May 15, 2022. https://www.marchofdimes.org/peristats/reports/united-states/prematurity-profile
44. Zhao T, Griffith T, Zhang Y, et al. Early-life factors associated with neurobehavioral outcomes in preterm infants during NICU hospitalization. *Pediatr Res*. 2022;*92*(6):1695–1704.
45. Cong X, Wu J, Vittner D, et al. The impact of cumulative pain/stress on neurobehavioral development of preterm infants in the NICU. *Early Hum Dev*. 2017;108:9–16.
46. Fitzgerald M. What do we really know about newborn infant pain? *Exp Physiol*. 2015;100(12):1451–1457.
47. Lake ET, Staiger D, Edwards EM, et al. Nursing care disparities in neonatal intensive care units. *Health Serv Res*. 2018;53:3007–3026.
48. Volpe JJ. Dysmaturation of premature brain: Importance, cellular mechanisms and potential interventions. *J Pediatr Neurol*. 2019;95:42–66.
49. Duerden EG, Grunau RE, Guo T, et al. Early procedural pain is associated with regionally-specific alterations in preterm neonates thalamic development in preterm neonates. *J Neurosci*. 2018; 38(4):878–886.

50. Grunau RE. Neonatal pain in very preterm infants: Long-term effects on brain neurodevelopment and pain reactivity. *Rambam Maimonides Med J*. 2013;4(4):e0025.
51. Patton GC, Coffey C, Carlin JB, et al. Cognitive trajectories from infancy to early adulthood. *Br J Psychiatry*. 2004;184:446–447.
52. Mills SE, Nicolson KP, Smith BH. Chronic pain: A review of its epidemiology and associated factors in population-based studies. *Br J Anaesth*. 2019;123(2):e273–e283.
53. Li J, Shen J, Zhang X. Risk factors associated with preterm birth after IVF/ICSI. *Sci Rep*. 2022;12:7944.
54. Margerison-Zilko, CE, Talge NM, Holzman, C. Preterm delivery trends by maternal race/ethnicity in the United States, 2006–2012. *Ann Epidemiol*. 2017;27:689–694.
55. McKinnon C, Meeham EM, Harvey AR, et al. Prevalence and characteristics of pain in children and young adults with cerebral palsy: A systematic review. *Dev Med Child Neurol*. 2019;61:305–314.
56. Centers for Disease Control and Prevention. Sickle cell disease (SCD). National Center on Birth Defects and Developmental Disabilities, Centers for Disease Control and Prevention. Last reviewed August 18, 2022. Accessed September 1, 2022. https://www.cdc.gov/ncbddd/sicklecell/facts.html
57. Dampier C, Ely E, Brodecki D, et al. Pain characteristics and age-related pain trajectories in infants and young children with sickle cell disease. *Pediatr Blood Cancer*. 2014;61(2):291–296.
58. Brooke E, Lifland BA, Mangione-Smith R, et al. Agreement between parent proxy- and child self-report of pain intensity and health-related quality of life after surgery. *Acad Pediatr*. 2018;18(4):376–383.
59. Craiga KD, Versloota J, Goubertb L, et al. Perceiving pain in others: Automatic and controlled mechanisms. *J Pain*. 2010;11(2):101–108.
60. Fearon P, McGrath J, Achat H. "Booboos": The study of everyday pain among young children. *Pain*. 1996;68(1):55–62.
61. Korterink JJ, Diederen K, Benninga MA, et al. Epidemiology of pediatric functional abdominal pain disorders: A meta-analysis. *PLoS One*. 2015;10(5):e0126982. doi:10.1371/journal.pone.0126982
62. Roth-Isigkeit A, Ute T, Hartmut S, et al. Pain among children and adolescents: Restrictions in daily living and triggering factors. *Pediatrics*. 2005;115(2):e152–e162.
63. Ostkirchen GG, Andler F, Hammer F, et al. Prevalences of primary headache symptoms at school-entry: A population-based epidemiological survey of preschool children in Germany. *J Headache Pain*. 2006;7:331–340.
64. Perquin C, Hazebroek-Kampschreurb AA, Hunfeld JM, et al. Pain in children and adolescents: A common experience. *Pain*. 2000;87:51–58.
65. van den Heuvela M, Jansenc PW, Bindelsa PJE, et al. Musculoskeletal pain in 6-year-old children: The Generation R Study. *Pain*. 2020;161:1278–1285.
66. Harrold HR, Salman C, Shoor S. Incidence and prevalence of juvenile idiopathic arthritis among children in a managed care population, 1996–2009. *J Rheumatol*. 2013;40(7):1218–1225.
67. Rabbitts JA, Groenewald CB. Epidemiology of pediatric surgery in the United States. *Paediatr Anaesth*. 2020;30(10):1083–1090.
68. Kristensen AD, Ahlburg P, Lauridsen MC, et al. Chronic pain after inguinal hernia repair in children. *Br J Anaesth*. 2012;109(4):603–608.
69. World Health Organization. Health topics/WHO: Adolescent health. n.d. Accessed May 20, 2022. World Health Organization. https://www.who.int/health-topics/adolescent-health#tab=tab_1
70. Viner RM, Ross D, Hardy R. Life course epidemiology: Recognizing the importance of adolescence. *J Epidemiol Commun Heath*. 2015;69:719–720.
71. Walker LS, Sherman AL, Bruehl S, et al. Functional abdominal pain patient subtypes in childhood predict functional gastrointestinal disorders with chronic pain and psychiatric comorbidities in adolescence and adulthood. *Pain*. 2012;153(9):1798–1806.

72. Bullok A, Sheff K, Moore K, et al. Obesity and overweight in American Indian and Alaska Native children, 2006–2015. *Am J Public Health*. 2017;107(9):1502–1506.
73. National Center for Health Statistics. Table 27. Obesity among children and adolescents aged 2–19 years, by selected characteristics: United States, selected years 1988–1994 through 2015–2018. *Health United States*. 2019. Accessed May 15, 2022. https://www.cdc.gov/nchs/data/hus/2019/027-508.pdf
74. Russo R. Assessment and treatment of adolescents with chronic medical conditions. *J Health Serv Psychol*. 2022;48:69–78.
75. Anderson E, Durstine JL. Physical activity, exercise, and chronic diseases: A brief review. *Sports Med Health Sci*. 2019;1:3–10.
76. Daly M. Prevalence of depression among adolescents in the U.S. from 2009 to 2019: Analysis of trends by sex, race/ethnicity, and income. *J Adolesc Health*. 2022;70(3):496–499.
77. U.S. Environmental Protection Agency. America's children and the environment: Health-neurodevelopmental disorders. Last updated May 11, 2022. Accessed February 10, 2023. https://www.epa.gov/americaschildrenenvironment/health-neurodevelopmental-disorders
78. Price JH, Khubchandani J, McKinney M. Racial/ethnic disparities in chronic diseases of youths and access to health care in the United States. *BioMed Res Int*. 2013;2013:787616.
79. Centers for Disease Control and Prevention. Unintentional all injury causes nonfatal emergency department visits and rates per 100,000, 2020, United States [Table]. *Non Fatal Injury Reports 2000–2020: WISQARS*. Accessed May 5, 2022. https://www.cdc.gov/injury/wisqars/nonfatal.html
80. Sámano-Ríosa ML, Ijaz S, Ruotsalainen S. Occupational safety and health interventions to protect young workers from hazardous work—A scoping review. *Saf Sci*. 2019;113:389–403.
81. Holstein BE, Damsgaard MT, Madsen KR, et al. Chronic back pain among adolescents in Denmark: Trends 1991–2018 and association with socioeconomic status. *Eur J Pediatr*. 2022;181:691–699.
82. Gobina I, Villberg J, Välimaa R, et al. Prevalence of self-reported chronic pain among adolescents: Evidence from 42 countries and regions. *Eur J Pain*. 2019;23(2):316–326.
83. Hoftun GB, Romundstad PR, Zwart AJ, et al. Chronic idiopathic pain in adolescence—High prevalence and disability: The young HUNT study 2008. *Pain*. 2011;152:2259–2266.
84. Tan AC, Jaaniste T, Champion D. Chronic widespread pain and fibromyalgia syndrome: Life-course risk markers in young people. *Pain Res Manag*. 2019;2019:6584753.
85. Jones A, Caes L, McMurtry M, et al. Socio-developmental challenges faced by young people with chronic pain: A scoping review. *J Pediatr Psychol*. 2021;46(2):219–230.
86. Wager J, Brown J, Kupitz A, et al. Prevalence and associated psychosocial and health factors of chronic pain in adolescents: Differences by sex and age. *Eur J Pain*. 2020;4:761–772.
87. Jill, TJM, Hayden A, Lewinson R. A systematic review of the prospective relationship between bullying victimization and pain. *J Pain Res*. 2021;14:1875–1885.
88. Luntamo T, Lempinen L, Sourander A. Secular trends in childhood pain and comorbid psychiatric symptoms: A population-based study. *Soc Psychiatry Psychiatr Epidemiol*. 2022;57:1017–1026.
89. Hinze V, Crane C, Ford T. The relationship between pain and suicidal vulnerability in adolescence: A systematic review. *Lancet Child Adolesc Health*. 2019;3(12):899–916.
90. Larsson B, Sigurdson FS, Sund AM. Long-term follow-up of a community sample of adolescents with frequent headaches. *J Headache Pain*. 2018;19: Article 79.
91. Noel M, Groenewald CB, Beals-Erickson SE, et al. Chronic pain in adolescence and internalizing mental health disorders: A nationally representative study. *Pain*. 2016;157(6):1333–1338.
92. Hochberg Z, Konner M. Emerging adulthood, a pre-adult life style stage. *Front. Endocrinol*. 2020;10: Article 918.
93. Murray CB, Groenewald CB, de la Vega R. Long-term impact of adolescent chronic pain on young adult educational, vocational, and social outcomes. *Pain*. 2020;161(2):439–445.

94. Kashikar-Zuck S, Cunningham N, James Peugh J. Long-term outcomes of adolescents with juvenile-onset fibromyalgia into adulthood, and impact of depressive symptoms on functioning over time. *Pain*. 2019;160(2):433–441.
95. Yang L, Branscum A, Bovbjerg V. Assessing disabling and non-disabling injuries and illnesses using accepted workers compensation claims data to prioritize industries of high risk for Oregon young workers. *J Safety Res*. 2021;77:241–254.
96. Nahin RL. Severe pain in veterans: The impact of age and sex, and comparisons to the general population. *J Pain*. 2017;18(3):247–254.
97. Angst F, Angst J, Ajdacic-Gross V. Epidemiology of back pain in young and middle-aged adults: A longitudinal population cohort survey from age 27–50 years. *Psychosomatics*. 2017;58(6):604–613.
98. Murray CB, de la Vega R, Murphy LK, Kashikar-Zuck S, Palermo TM. The prevalence of chronic pain in young adults: A systematic review and meta-analysis. *Pain*. 2022;163(9):e972–e984.
99. Pitcher MH, Von Korff M, Bushnell MC, et al. Prevalence and profile of high-impact chronic pain in the United States. *J Pain*. 2019;20(2):146–160.
100. Wallace B, Varcoe C, Holmes C. Towards health equity for people experiencing chronic pain and social marginalization. *Int J Equity Health*. 2021;20: Article 53.
101. Colarusso CA. Middle adulthood (ages 40–60). In: *Child and Adult Development: A Psychoanalytic Introduction for Clinicians*. Springer; 1992:163–182.
102. Lachman ME, Teshale S, Agrigoroaei S. Midlife as a pivotal period in the life course: Balancing growth and decline at the crossroads of youth and old age. *Int J Behav Dev*. 2015;39(1): 20–31.
103. Stierman B, Afful J, Carroll MD, et al. National Health and Nutrition Examination Survey 2017–March 2020 prepandemic data files—Development of files and prevalence estimates for selected health outcomes. National Health Statistics Reports No 158. National Center for Health Statistics; 2021.
104. Villarroel MA, Blackwell DL, Jen A. Table A-14a: Age adjusted percent distributions (with standard errors) of participation in leisure-time aerobic and muscle-strengthening activities that meet the 2008 federal physical activity guidelines among adults aged 18 and over, by selected characteristics: United States, 2018. 2018 National Health Interview Survey. National Center for Health Statistics. 2019. Accessed April 24, 2022. http://www.cdc.gov/nchs/nhis/SHS/tables.htm
105. Schopenflocker D, Taenzer P, Jovey R. The prevalence of chronic pain in Canada. *Pain Res Manage*. 2011;16(6):445–452.
106. Kyrönlahti SM, Nygård CH, Neupane S. Trajectories of low back pain from midlife to retirement and functional ability at old age. *Eur J Public Health*. 2022;32(3):497–503.
107. Cao S, Fisher DW, Yu T, et al. The link between chronic pain and Alzheimer's disease. *J Neuroinflammation*. 2019;16: Article 204.
108. Ferreira KdS, Velly AM. Cognitive decline over time in patients with chronic pain and headache: How can different outcomes be explained? *J Pain*. 2022;163(8):e966–e967.
109. Cai Y, Leveille SG, Shi L, et al. Chronic pain and risk of injurious falls in community-dwelling older adults. *J Gerontol A Biol Sci Med Sci*. 2021;76(9):e179–e186.
110. Verma SK, Willetts JL, Corns HL, et al. Falls and fall-related injuries among community-dwelling adults in the United States. *PLoS One*. 2016;11(3):e0150939.
111. Ganz DA, Bao Y, Shekelle PG, et al. Will my patient fall? *JAMA*. 2007;297(1):77–86.
112. Ofori-Asenso R, Chin KL, Curtis AJ, et al. Recent patterns of multimorbidity among older adults in high-income countries. *Popul Health Manag*. 2019;22(2):127–137.
113. Scherer M, Hansen H, Gensichen J, et al. Association between multimorbidity patterns and chronic pain in elderly primary care patients: A cross-sectional observational study. *BMC Fam Pract*. 2016;17:1–8.
114. Ioakeim-Skoufa I, Poblador-Plou B, Carmona-Pírez J, et al. Multimorbidity patterns in the general population: Results from the EpiChron cohort study. *Int J Environ Res Pub Health*. 2020;17(12):4242.

115. Lee ES, Koh HL, Ho EQ-Y, et al. Systematic review on the instruments used for measuring the association of the level of multimorbidity and clinically important outcomes. *BMJ Open* 2021;11:e041219.
116. Molton IR, Terrill AL. Overview of persistent pain in older adults. *Am Psychol.* 2014;69(2):197–207.
117. Wong CK, Mak RY, Kwok TS, et al. Prevalence, incidence, and factors associated with non-specific chronic low back pain in community-dwelling older adults aged 60 years and older: A systematic review and meta-analysis. *J Pain.* 2022;23(4):509–534.
118. Iqbal Z, Azmi S, Yadav R, et al. Diabetic peripheral neuropathy: Epidemiology, diagnosis, and pharmacotherapy. *Clin Ther.* 2018;40(6):828–849.
119. Santos AM, Burti JS, Lopes JB, et al. Prevalence of fibromyalgia and chronic widespread pain in community-dwelling elderly subjects living in São Paulo, Brazil. *Maturitas.* 2010;67(3):251–255.
120. Dahlhamer J, Lucas J, Zelaya C, et al. Prevalence of chronic pain and high-impact chronic pain among adults—United States, 2016. *MMWR Morbid Mortal Wkly Rep.* 2018;9;67(36):1001.
121. Lautenbacher S, Peters JH, Heesen M, et al. Age changes in pain perception: A systematic-review and meta-analysis of age effects on pain and tolerance thresholds. *Neurosci Biobehav Rev.* 2017;75:104–1013.
122. Murray CB, Patel KV, Twiddy H, Sturgeon JA, Palermo TM. Age differences in cognitive-affective processes in adults with chronic pain. *Eur J Pain.* 2021;25(5):1041–1052.
123. Ferrucci L, Gonzalez-Freire M, Fabbri E, et al. Measuring biological aging in humans: A quest. *Aging Cell.* 2020;19(2):e13080.
124. Blanton H, Reddy PH, Benamar K. Chronic pain in Alzheimer's disease: Endocannabinoid system. *Exp Neurol.* 2023;360:114287.
125. Burns E, Kakara R. Deaths from falls among persons aged ≥65 years—United States, 2007–2016. *MMWR Morb Mortal Wkly Rep.* 2018;67:509–514.
126. Whitlock EL, Diaz-Ramirez LG, Glymour MM, Boscardin WJ, Covinsky KE, Smith AK. Association between persistent pain and memory decline and dementia in a longitudinal cohort of elders. *JAMA Intern. Med.* 2017;177:1146–1153.
127. Macfarlane GJ, Barnish MS, Jones GT. Persons with chronic widespread pain experience excess mortality: Longitudinal results from UK Biobank and meta-analysis. *Ann Rheum Dis.* 2017;76:1815–1822.

5
Pain in Infants and Children

Denise Harrison, Mariana Bueno, and Nicole Marie Pope

Introduction

This chapter focuses on pain in newborns, infants, and children. Sick and preterm newborns and hospitalized infants and children are especially vulnerable to pain. Vulnerabilities relate not only to the large number of painful procedures required during the course of an illness and hospitalization but also to their respective immature developmental stages, parental separation, lack of known effective pain treatment strategies at different ages, and, where evidence exists, lack of consistent use of the evidence. In addition, as infants and children develop, they are at risk of developing fears of different environments and of medical procedures, especially if they have experienced pain during procedures in the past. Finally, increasing evidence demonstrates long-term consequences of untreated or poorly managed pain in these populations.

Three main sections in this chapter discuss (1) evidence for vulnerability, (2) illness models for this population and its subpopulations, and (3) treatment relating to remediation of the vulnerability itself within a social context and treatment strategies both available and used.

The first section outlines the evidence for vulnerability in preterm, sick, and healthy newborns, infants, young children, and school-aged children. These subpopulations are at different developmental stages, and there are variable known effective pain treatment strategies and inconsistent use of such pain strategies.

What Makes Infants and Children More Vulnerable to Pain?

Evidence for vulnerability in these populations includes the following factors:

1. The burden of pain—multiple painful procedures spanning over days, weeks, and months of hospitalization[1–5]
2. Inconsistent use of known effective pain management strategies, including strategies involving parents/caregivers[6,7]
3. Separation of parental role/inability to comfort during painful procedures[6]
4. Association between the number of painful procedures and poorer neurocognitive outcomes[8,9]

Burden of Pain

Multiple studies during the past 25 years have highlighted the large number of painful procedures to which sick and preterm infants are exposed. The first such study was published in 1995,[10] in which a cohort of 54 newborns in a single neonatal intensive care unit (NICU) were reported on. A total of 3,283 invasive procedures were recorded for the 54 newborns, averaging 61 painful procedures per infant. More than half (n = 1,849) of the procedures were heel lances. Despite these large numbers of documented procedures, it is likely that they underestimated the true number of episodes of invasive, painful, and distressing procedures, given that procedures such as nasogastric tube insertion and repeat attempts at each procedure were not included. In 2016, Cruz et al.[3] published the first systematic review of observational studies of painful procedures performed in neonates. Eighteen studies from 13 different countries were included from 1995 to 2014. Data for a total of 3,156 infants were included. The total number of painful procedures recorded ranged from 6,832 up to 42,413, a mean of 7.5–17.3 painful procedures per neonate per day. Heel lance procedures were the most frequently recorded, followed by airway suctioning and venipuncture. Studies published more recently show little change from those reported almost 30 years ago. For example, Kassab et al.[4] reported on a cohort of 150 neonates in a NICU and found that heel lancing was the most commonly performed needle-related painful procedure. A total of 1,199 heel lances were recorded with an average of 8 heel lances per neonate during their first 7 days of life. Despite these large numbers, the authors acknowledged that these data might underrepresent the true number of painful procedures because repeat procedures were not captured. Courtois et al.[1] included 562 neonates in a European-wide study examining the epidemiology of heel lance procedures and reported a total of 8,995 heel lances, with a mean (SD) of 16 (14.4), ranging from 1 to 86 per neonate. The same team reported on venipuncture procedures and found that 84% (495 of the 589 newborns included) underwent at least one venipuncture and a mean (SD) number of procedures per newborn of 3.8 (2.8), up to 19 per infant.[2] In another study, Orovec et al.[5] reported on 242 neonates who underwent a total of 11,191 procedures, which included 722 repeat attempts at procedures. As per previous reports, most procedures were heel lances. Extremely preterm infants spend an average of 81 days in neonatal intensive care,[11] these large numbers of painful procedures during hospitalization, which occur during a critical period of neurodevelopment, therefore make neonates especially vulnerable to pain-induced damage that can result in sustained changes to pain perception and neurodevelopmental and behavioral consequences.

Numerous pain prevalence studies have included hospitalized infants and children of all ages.[12–18] Similar to the studies of sick and preterm neonates, these reports from throughout the world also highlight the substantial numbers of painful procedures being performed throughout hospitalization and high levels of pain reported by children or their families.[13,15,17–20] Needle-related venipuncture procedures and peripheral line insertion are the most commonly reported painful procedures by children or their parents.[13,15–18]

Inconsistent Use of Pain Management Strategies

Many studies published throughout the years have highlighted inconsistent use of evidence-based effective pain management strategies for newborns and hospitalized infants and children. For example, high-quality synthesized evidence exists for analgesic effects of breastfeeding during procedures when feasible and culturally acceptable,[21] skin-to-skin care,[22] and sucrose or other sweet-tasting solutions for preterm and term newborns.[23,24] However, studies consistently show infrequent use of these effective pain management strategies. For example, Orovec et al.[5] reported that approximately 58% of procedures in their cohort of 242 neonates were performed without pain management interventions. Sucrose was most commonly used (34% of procedures), while skin-to-skin care was used for only 9.8% of procedures, and breastfeeding was rarely used. Similarly, Courtois et al.[1] reported that most painful procedures in newborns were performed with no pain treatment; sucrose with or without sucking was used during less than 40% of heel lances, breastfeeding was only used during 16 (0.2%) procedures, and skin-to-skin care was not reported at all.

For children, evidence-based strategies such as distraction (e.g., bubbles, toys, virtual reality games, breathing techniques, relaxation, etc.), in which the purpose is to draw children's attention toward non-distressing or pleasant stimuli, have been shown to be effective,[25] as have topical anesthetics for needle-related procedures.[26] Yet studies of hospitalized children's pain management have shown minimal documentation of psychological strategies[13,14,18,27–29] and minimal documentation of pharmacological strategies such as sucrose and topical anesthetics.[13,18,30]

Separation of Parental Role/Inability to Comfort During Painful Procedures

The 1959 Platt report titled "The Welfare of Children in Hospital"[31] set the scene for the development of the philosophy of family-centered care (FCC) for hospitalized children, with a key premise being avoiding separation of children from their parents.[32] This significantly changed the face of hospitalized care for children, with parents given more opportunities and, in many cases, expected to be involved in all aspects of care, including during routine painful procedures. However, a large body of literature continues to report parents being separated from their hospitalized newborns.[33] This is despite many hospitals having a philosophy of FCC[6] and the importance of parental and comforting roles in parent–infant attachment.[34] Parents and their preterm and sick newborns are typically separated. Despite concentrated efforts around various philosophies of care aimed at minimizing separation and promoting parental involvement in care, most neonatal units throughout the world do not have the facilities or organizational structures to enable parents to stay with their sick newborn.[6,35] For example, a study of NICU nurses' perceived beliefs about "necessary" FCC practices and their own current practices showed that practice scores were all lower than "necessary" FCC practices.[35] This highlights that although NICU nurses believed that FCC aspects were essential and necessary, FCC was not being practiced in the clinical settings. In addition, societal structures do not sufficiently enable parents to stay with their hospitalized newborns over long periods.[6] Parents are therefore excluded from much of the care of their sick newborns, including during painful procedures, despite wishing to be involved.[7,36] Parents report feeling guilty, traumatized, and angry that they are not informed of, nor supported to, comfort their infants.[7,36] Even in a cohort of mothers of healthy newborns ($N = 99$), despite most parents' preference to breastfeed or hold their newborns skin-to-skin during newborn screening, these methods were rarely used (4 [4%] and 2 [2%], respectively).[37] Sucrose, however, was used for 59 (60%) newborns during newborn screening. Although this use of sucrose for more than half of the newborns is promising, the fact remains that 40% of the newborns did not receive effective pain management. Breastfeeding and skin-to-skin care, which are also effective and feasible in healthy infant populations and preferred by parents, were rarely used.

Adverse Effects of Pain

A crucial aspect of vulnerability for preterm and sick neonates is the growing evidence of the association between the number of painful procedures with long-term adverse outcomes on brain development and developmental and cognitive outcomes in premature infants.[8,9,38] Cumulative pain exposure from tissue-breaking procedures has been shown to have the strongest association with adverse early and later developmental outcomes.[8,38] Strategies are therefore urgently needed to improve pain treatment during painful procedures for premature and sick newborns.

The problem is not confined to neonates only. Older hospitalized infants and children also require numerous painful procedures and inconsistent use of known effective pain management strategies have been reported for these age groups.[12,13,27,29,39,40] Undertreatment of pain is associated with the development of fears of painful procedures and escalation of distress during procedures. For young children aged 1–3 years, the situation is complicated by fewer known effective pain management strategies for this age group and high levels of distress exhibited in young children, which may not necessarily directly relate to the painful procedures. Fears associated with unfamiliar environments and unfamiliar people, parental separation, and being positioned lying down during procedures all contribute to high levels of distress. For example, in a randomized controlled trial (RCT) of sucrose for children aged 12–36 months, most of the children were already crying at baseline, before the insertion of the cannula.[41] Similarly, in an RCT evaluating 2% lidocaine compared to normal saline via nebulizer for pain and distress during nasogastric tube insertion in young children, most children were extremely distressed in both groups prior to the procedure due to the nebulizer.[42] School-aged children are also particularly vulnerable to pain. As per younger populations, underrecognized, undertreated, and poorly treated pain can lead to long-lasting consequences, which can continue into adulthood.[39] Consequences of poorly managed pain include psychological effects, such as developing a fear of needles. In a systematic review of 119 studies, fear of needles was greatest in young children, yet still estimated to be present in 20–50% of adolescents.[43] The establishment or exacerbation of needle fears, avoidance of medical procedures, and vaccine hesitancy can have serious long-term consequences for children and surrounding communities. Vaccine hesitancy was named one of the top 10 public health threats by the World Health

Organization.[44] This high prevalence of fear of needles highlights the imperative to consistently use known effective pain management strategies in diverse settings in which infants and children receive health care and needle-related procedures.

Children are also vulnerable to the persistent effects of poorly controlled pain. Studies of childhood cancer survivors who undergo repeated procedures show a high prevalence of somatosensory abnormalities, such as hyperalgesia and allodynia, years after their treatment.[45] In addition to somatosensory changes, undertreated pain in hospitalized children is associated with prolonged hospital admissions, medical complications, and functioning difficulties. Persistent, unrelieved pain in children has been strongly linked with developing persistent and chronic pain conditions. However, the mechanisms underlying the transition from acute to persistent and chronic pain following injury, surgery, or other events are not fully understood.[46] In a systematic review published in 2011, which included 41 studies, the prevalence of chronic pain in children was estimated to range from 8% to 83% for headaches and from 4% to 53% for abdominal pain.[47] Children with chronic pain often suffer comorbid health problems, including depression, anxiety, post-traumatic stress, and insomnia. There is also evidence that chronic childhood pain persists into adulthood.[47] Such multiple sequelae underscore the vulnerabilities of infants and children arising from pain exposure and poor pain management.

To further understand vulnerability to pain in infants and children, the underlying biological and socioecological aspects of the pain experience must be understood. During the past 20 years, there has been a proliferation of conceptual models concerning pediatric pain. Many share similar explanatory purposes in understanding the interplay between biological, psychological, and social processes during children's painful events. The social communication model of pain (SCM)[48] and the model of parent involvement in infant pain management[34] are two models designed to understand acute pain from a biopsychosocial perspective. An overview of these models is provided in the following section. Factors contributing to vulnerability across a child's life span ensuing from these models are then examined from neurobiological, psychosocial, and contextual perspectives.

Discussion

The Social Communication Model of Pain

Understanding the impact of the social environment on a child's pain is critical in planning pain prevention and intervention strategies for sick, hospitalized children and their families. The SCM provides a developed biopsychosocial formulation for understanding acute and chronic pediatric pain.[48] Although this model applies to adults, it has been extensively used in examining childhood pain. It integrates an understanding of the biological and psychological processes of pain and directs attention to social determinants as causes and consequences of how pain is experienced and expressed. There is also an explicit focus on the dyadic communication between the child and other people in the context of the broader social–ecological systems within which pain is experienced. This attention to the impact of the child's socialization on pain experience is important because infants and children rely on others, such as their family and health care professionals, for care, including assessing and treating their pain.[49]

The SCM is differentiated into four stages following an initial painful event:

Stage 1: The child's internal pain experience is encoded in expressive behaviors (e.g., facial reactions and vocalizations).
Stage 2: The child's expressive behaviors are subsequently decoded (interpreted) by the caregiver.
Stage 3: Action is taken (i.e., comforting) or not.
Stage 4: The caregiver's reaction to pain, in turn, impacts the child's pain experience and expression.

The dyadic process is embedded in a broader social context, including culture. The model draws attention to the impact of the child's socialization on pain experience and expression, and it highlights how intra- and interpersonal factors of the child and caregiver are critical to understanding the reciprocal social relationship between the child and the caregiver in the context of pediatric pain. At Stage 1, in addition to autonomic and reflexive responses, pain perception is influenced by the child's biological and environmental history and higher level brain processes. Pain manifestations are expressed vocally, through crying, or nonvocally, through facial expressions and body actions. As the child develops verbal skills, they are more able to express their pain through language; children as young as age 4 years can provide detailed verbal accounts of their pain experiences when asked.[50] At Stages 3 and 4, the reciprocal relationship between the child's pain expression and caregiver pain assessment is seen; how the child expresses pain influences the caregiver's assessment, informing their reactions and responses to the child, which subsequently impacts the child's pain experience and expression. This component emphasizes the social phenomenon of pain, drawing attention to the role of parents and clinicians in being attuned to children's pain expressions.[51] The model provides clinicians with conceptual guidance on the intra- and interpersonal factors influencing pain, from its cause to treatment. However, a limitation of the model is that it does not consider the unique developmental stages of childhood, which is an essential component of understanding pain and children's particular vulnerabilities.[48]

The Model of Parent Involvement in Infant Pain Management

The principles of FCC emphasize that family and health care staff share responsibility for the child's care. Understanding the influence of parental presence and participation in their child's pain care is critical to moderating vulnerability in sick infants, children, and their families. The model of parent involvement in infant pain care (Figure 5.1) offers a conceptual representation of the dynamic trajectories for parental involvement during painful procedures.[34] Although the model was developed for and applies specifically to NICU settings, it also provides a valuable framework for examining parents' involvement in the comfort of older infants and children cared for across health care clinical settings. The model is presented as three discs (see Figure 5.1), each representing a domain of contextual facilitators and barriers to parental involvement in pain care. Holes in each of the

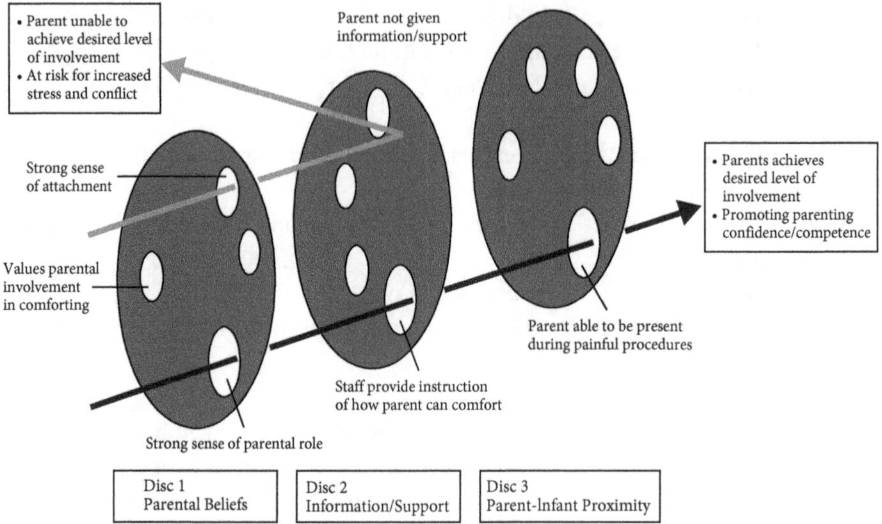

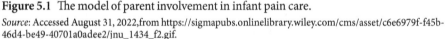

Figure 5.1 The model of parent involvement in infant pain care.
Source: Accessed August 31, 2022,from https://sigmapubs.onlinelibrary.wiley.com/cms/asset/c6e6979f-f45b-46d4-be49-40701a0adee2/jnu_1434_f2.gif.

three discs depict opportunities for parental engagement in each domain, and the size of each hole represents the degree of opportunity. Parents can achieve their desired level of involvement when the roles are lined up. Disc 1 represents parental belief factors and relates to parents' views about their role, their values about being involved in comforting their child, and parent–infant attachment. Disc 2 concerns parental access to information and support. Access is influenced by various setting-specific contextual and social factors. For example, the role of clinical staff in facilitating and supporting parental engagement in their infants' pain care is a critical determinant of their involvement. Disc 3 depicts factors that influence parents' proximity to their child. Parents who face visitation restriction limitations or do not feel welcome to stay with their child during painful procedures, and those who feel too emotionally overwhelmed, may not be able to actualize their intended involvement with their child's comfort. The model offers conceptual guidance to clinical practices related to supporting parents' involvement in their child's pain care.

Summary

Both the SCM and the model of parent involvement in infant pain management demonstrate concordance regarding central dimensions of early childhood pain and reflect advances in our understanding of how, in addition to biological mechanisms, psychosocial factors impact pain experiences, pain management, and responses to pain. Importantly, they direct attention to the multidirectional forces between the child and caregivers and the surrounding systems that ultimately influence pain outcomes. To add to this understanding, further discussions of psychosocial and contextual dimensions provide frameworks for examining the vulnerabilities of sick hospitalized children, including conditions for vulnerability across the child's life span.

Psychosocial Factors

In addition to fostering a secure attachment, the soothing actions of parents can help minimize children's pain and pain-related distress. Comfort positioning with parents, such as allowing the child to sit upright on their parent's lap during painful needle procedures, helps give children a sense of control and decreases fear and distress.[25] Parents' presence also helps children feel safe and confident to express their pain to others, such as clinicians, and what they need to help with their pain.[50] Although a significant developmental outcome of youth is achieving separateness from parents and autonomy in making decisions, parents still play an essential role in advocating for and supporting their older children in pain.[52,53] This is especially true for children with chronic and persistent pain conditions. The effective management of chronic pain in children relies on bidirectional influences between youth and their parents. For example, parental distress, overly protective behaviors, and parental pain catastrophizing can reinforce and encourage pain and functional disability and contribute to worse pain outcomes in children.[54]

Contextual Factors

The psychosocial determinants of pain posited in models emphasize that young children's pain cannot be understood outside the caregivers' context. The way children express pain and their caregivers' interpretations and reactions to pain are also influenced by various sociocultural systems. Children learn how to express and react to pain through family norms and wider society. Unfortunately, societal views of pain are often narrow, evidenced by the pervasive misconception that pain is self-limited, physical, and to be endured.[39] Coping well with pain is esteemed as a strength, perpetuated by phrases such as "boys don't cry" and "no pain, no gain." These sentiments are bolstered through media and social media, including children's cartoons. This social insensitivity to pain predisposes sick and hospitalized infants and children to suffer repeated painful procedures without analgesia.[39] Furthermore, when pain does not follow typical acute pain trajectories or there is no apparent organic cause of pain, pain is dismissed or devalued by others.[55] Children and adolescents with chronic pain are particularly vulnerable to having their pain devalued by peers, family, and clinicians. This contributes to poor outcomes for children.

The next section outlines specific treatment strategies and organizational, nationwide, and global knowledge translation initiatives aimed at widely disseminating pain management information.

Treatment Relating to Remediation of Vulnerability

As the focus on children's pain has been brought to the forefront, there has been an exponential increase in research regarding the effectiveness of treatment interventions as well as broader organizational-wide and global initiatives aimed at implementing evidence into practice to improve pain management.[56] Such specific effective strategies and broader initiatives, if globally adopted, have the potential to remediate the effects of vulnerabilities across the age spectrum of childhood as a result of pain exposure. Here, a summary of synthesized evidence for strategies shown to be effective for specific populations of hospitalized children is presented, followed by a discussion of broader organizational-wide strategies. Because a large body of research focuses on needle-related procedures, the most common sources of pain in hospitalized children, the systematic reviews highlighted focus on treatment for needle procedures across the pediatric age span.

High-quality synthesized evidence exists for breastfeeding,[21] skin-to-skin care,[22] and small volumes of sweet solutions[23,24] for needle-related procedures in newborn and young infants. In addition, other strategies shown to have some benefits include facilitated tucking, swaddling, rocking, and holding,[25] especially when used in combination with sweet solutions.[57] In a systematic review of breastfeeding beyond the neonatal period up to age 12 months, breastfeeding during vaccinations was also shown to be effective, although 8 of the 10 studies included infants only up to age 6 months.[58] Similarly, a systematic review of 20 trials found that sweet solutions (sucrose and glucose) reduced crying duration in infants beyond the neonatal period up to age 12 months.[59] However, most studies included infants aged 6 months or younger and during vaccination only. Strategies focused on children during needle-related procedures include psychological, physical, and pharmacological interventions. Evidence supports psychological strategies, including distraction, hypnosis, combined cognitive–behavioral therapy, and breathing interventions for reducing children's needle-related pain and/or distress.[60] There is also evidence to support physical strategies such as vibratory stimulation; however, topical anesthetics were more effective when used as the standard of care.[61] Topical anesthetics were also strongly recommended for children with cancer and for major procedures (lumbar puncture and bone marrow aspiration); deep sedation or general anesthetic were also recommended.[62] The combination of sucrose (up to age 12–18 months), topical anesthetics, age-appropriate distraction, and positioning—including upright positioning for children aged 6 months and older, with parents holding them on their lap or sitting nearby—is strongly recommended when possible.[40] When these strategies are ineffective or not feasible, or for children with needle phobia, conscious sedation using nitrous inhalation is recommended. In addition, support by hospital play therapists and/or referral to pediatric psychologists for children with needle phobia should be considered.[40]

For all strategies, involving and facilitating the engagement of parents/caregivers in pain management practices is a crucial factor in moderating vulnerability in hospitalized infants and children. This includes facilitating parents' role in neonatal care[6,63,64] and in the care of hospitalized children of all ages.[39,65,66] Facilitating families' involvement in care is critical in promoting optimal health outcomes in the short and long term, in hospital and beyond.[67] For example, parental presence in the NICU may lead to increased use of analgesic strategies during painful procedures,[3,68] and parents can play a vital part in recognizing their child's pain. Likewise, they can take on the role of advocating for, and supporting the management of, their child's pain.[69] It is crucial, however, to be flexible with regard to the ways in which to support parents to be involved in pain-management processes.[63] Because infants and children have an innate need for a parent's presence and nurturing actions, especially when sick or in an unfamiliar hospital environment, a parent's constant presence and responsiveness are

Table 5.1 Examples of Knowledge Translation Resources for Parents of Newborns

Initiative	Focus	URL	Details
"Be Sweet to Babies" (Canada)	Breastfeeding, skin-to-skin, and sweet solutions during heel lance and venipuncture	https://www.youtube.com/watch?v=L43y0H6XEH4&feature=youtu.be	4-min video posted on YouTube, 2016 Available in 10 languages: English, French, Spanish, Arabic, Inuktitut, Farsi, Mandarin, German, Hindi, Swiss Italian
"The Power of a Parent's Touch" (Canada)	Skin-to-skin care and breastfeeding during painful procedures	https://m.youtube.com/watch?v=3nqN9c3FWn8&feature=youtu.be	2-min 40-s video posted on YouTube, 2014 Includes information about burden of pain, risk of adverse outcomes of poorly treated pain, and benefits of skin-to-skin care and breastfeeding during painful procedures
Comfy booklet (United States)	Parents' role in the NICU and strategies to use in reducing stress and in comforting sick newborns	https://familynursing.ucsf.edu/sites/familynursing.ucsf.edu/files/wysiwyg/Comfy%20PDF%20ENGLISH%20Dec%2017.pdf	40-page multimedia booklet (2013) with information for parents, and embedded brief (<40 s) video clips

essential to promote positive biopsychological outcomes for children suffering pain or illness.[70] Most parents wish to be involved as much as possible and to receive appropriate and timely information; have more opportunities to be involved in their child's care; and learn, use, and be supported to use effective pain-reducing interventions.[7,34,36,71] To support parents, knowledge translation strategies co-produced with parents and targeted at parents have been developed and widely disseminated to inform parents and help them advocate for their involvement.[69,72–74] Three specific examples focused on parents of newborns are presented here and summarized in Table 5.1:

1. A publicly available video titled "Be Sweet to Babies" demonstrates newborns undergoing heel lance and venipuncture procedures and the use and effectiveness of breastfeeding, skin-to-skin care, and sweet solutions.[73] The video, posted on YouTube, has been translated into multiple languages and shown to be useful, feasible, and persuasive, with parents and staff reporting that they plan to use the strategies in the future.[72,75–78]
2. A publicly available video titled "The Power of a Parent's Touch" demonstrates breastfeeding and skin-to-skin care.[74] Evaluation by parents and clinicians demonstrated the acceptability and usefulness of the video. Respondents reported that after viewing the video, they felt more confident and were more likely to use skin-to-skin care and breastfeeding during future painful procedures.
3. The "Comfy" booklet is a multimedia booklet with embedded short video clips, targeted at parents to help them recognize signs of pain and distress.[79] Brief video

clips are interspersed throughout, focused on demonstrating to parents how to use strategies such as reducing noise and light, facilitated tucking, swaddling, skin-to-skin care, sucrose, and pacifiers during painful procedures.

Whereas much of this chapter has focused on acute procedural pain, identifying risks of development of chronic pain and recognizing and treating chronic pain in infants and children is also important. For instance, an art- and narrative-based electronic book (e-book) for pediatric chronic pain targeted at parents was developed and evaluated by Reid and colleagues.[80] Parental evaluation of this e-book resource was positive, with the authors reporting an increase in parents' knowledge and understanding that chronic pain is a disease involving the nervous system and also an increase in parents' confidence in managing pain. This single study highlights the positive role of parents being actively involved and informed. Because there is little evidence of the effectiveness of pharmacological strategies in managing chronic pain in children,[81] focusing on the whole family with the support of multidisciplinary teams is essential in remediating adverse outcomes of chronic pain in children.

Institution-wide or national and international initiatives to improve pain management, focusing on prevention, assessment, and treatment, have also been reported. Four initiatives are presented in Table 5.2: Children's Comfort Promise, ChildKind

Table 5.2 Examples of Organizational, National, and Global Child Pain Initiatives

Initiative	Focus	URL	Details
Children's Comfort Promise (Children's Minnesota Hospital)	Hospitalized children's needle pain and parent education and engagement	https://www.childrensmn.org/services/care-specialties-departments/pain-program/childrens-comfort-promise	Organizational promise to minimize needle pain using four strategies: (1) topical anesthetics, (2) sucrose or breastfeeding for infants aged 0–12 months, (3) comfort positioning (including swaddling, skin-to-skin, or facilitated tucking for infants; sitting upright for children), and (4) age-appropriate distraction
ChildKind International	Accreditation of hospitals caring for children	https://childkindinternational.org	Recognition of institutional commitment to incorporate child pain management as a value
Help Eliminate Pain in Kids & Adults (HELP)	Vaccination pain	http://phm.utoronto.ca/helpinkids/resources1.html	Produce knowledge translation products showcasing evidence-based pain management during vaccination; involves partnership with universities, hospitals, and governmental and nongovernmental organizations throughout Canada
Solutions for Kids in Pain (SKIP)	Raising public awareness of child pain	https://kidsinpain.ca	Brings together pediatric pain specialists, knowledge users, consumers, and patient–caregiver partners across various sectors (e.g., charities, governments, businesses, and health care); goal is to increase awareness of children's pain in Canada

International, Help Eliminate Pain in Kids & Adults (HELP), and Solutions for Kids in Pain (SKIP).

Conclusion

As stated in the *Lancet Child & Adolescent Health* Commission for pediatric pain,[39] four goals need to be actioned for improving pain management in all populations of children globally: (1) make pain matter, (2) make pain understood, (3) make pain visible, and (4) make pain better. Using these broad goals as a starting point, and prioritizing pain management, children's vulnerabilities related to poorly managed pain can be minimized.

We have come a long way since parents' were not allowed to visit their hospitalized children[31] and preterm newborns had surgery without analgesia.[82] We now have evidence of effective pain treatment strategies, and large-scale organizations involving clinicians, parents, caregivers, and children and youth are publicly advocating for best pain management.[66] Recommendations are included in the recently produced Canadian pediatric pain management standards. The challenges for all lie in consistently utilizing best practices across diverse settings in which sick newborns, infants, and children are cared for. We must continue the journey to ensure the prevention of pain, where possible, and prioritize the minimization of pain in vulnerable populations.

References

1. Courtois E, Droutman S, Magny JF, et al. Epidemiology and neonatal pain management of heelsticks in intensive care units: EPIPPAIN 2, a prospective observational study. *Int J Nurs Stud.* 2016;59:79–88. doi:10.1016/j.ijnurstu.2016.03.014
2. Courtois E, Cimerman P, Dubuche V, et al. The burden of venipuncture pain in neonatal intensive care units: EPIPPAIN 2, a prospective observational study. *Int J Nurs Stud.* 2016;57:48–59. doi:10.1016/j.ijnurstu.2016.01.014
3. Cruz M, Fernandes A, Oliveira C. Epidemiology of painful procedures performed in neonates: A systematic review of observational studies. *Eur J Pain.* 2016;20(4):489–498. doi:10.1002/ejp.757
4. Kassab M, Alhassan AA, Alzoubi KH, Khader YS. Number and frequency of routinely applied painful procedures in university neonatal intensive care unit. *Clin Nurs Res.* 2019;28(4):488–501. doi:10.1177/1054773817744324
5. Orovec A, Disher T, Caddell K, Campbell-Yeo M. Assessment and management of procedural pain during the entire neonatal intensive care unit hospitalization. *Pain Manag Nurs.* 2019;20(5):503–511. doi:10.1016/j.pmn.2018.11.061
6. Larocque C, Peterson WE, Squires JE, Mason-Ward M, Harrison D. Family-centered care in the neonatal intensive care unit: A concept analysis and literature review. *J Neonatal Nurs.* 2021;27(6):402–411. https://doi.org/10.1016/j.jnn.2021.06.014
7. Bujalka H, Cruz M, Ingate V, et al. Be Sweet to Babies: Consumer evaluation of a parent-targeted video aimed at improving pain-management strategies in newborn infants undergoing painful procedures. *Adv Neonatal Care.* 2023;23(1):E2–E13.
8. Valeri BO, Holsti L, Linhares M. Neonatal pain and developmental outcomes in children born preterm: A systematic review. *Clin J Pain.* 2015;31(4):355–362. doi:10.1097/AJP.0000000000000114

9. Walker SM. Long-term effects of neonatal pain. *Semin Fetal Neonatal Med.* 2019;24(4):101005. doi:10.1016/j.siny.2019.04.005
10. Barker DP, Rutter N. Exposure to invasive procedures in neonatal intensive care unit admissions. *Arch Dis Child.* 1995;72(1):F47–F48.
11. Rolnitsky A, Unger SL, Urbach DR, Bell CM. Cost of neonatal intensive care for extremely preterm infants in Canada. *Transl Pediatr.* 2021;10(6):21–36. doi:10.21037/tp-21-36
12. Birnie KA, Chambers CT, Fernandez CV., et al. Hospitalized children continue to report undertreated and preventable pain. *Pain Res Manag.* 2014;19(4):198–204. doi:10.1155/2014/614784
13. Wilding J, Scott H, Suwalska V, et al. A quality improvement project on pain management at a tertiary pediatric hospital. *Can J Nurs Res.* 2022;54(3):357–368. doi:10.1177/08445621211047716
14. Stevens B, Abbott L, Yamada J, et al. Epidemiology and management of painful procedures in hospitalized children across Canada. *C Can Med Assoc J.* 2011;183(7):E403–E410. doi:10.1503/cmaj.101341
15. Harrison D, Joly C, Chretien C, et al. Pain prevalence in a pediatric hospital: Raising awareness during Pain Awareness Week. *Pain Res Manag.* 2014;19(1):e24–e30. doi:10.1155/2014/737692
16. Taylor EM, Boyer K, Campbell FA. Pain in hospitalized children: A prospective cross-sectional survey of pain prevalence, intensity, assessment and management in a Canadian pediatric teaching hospital. *Pain Res Manag.* 2008;13(1):25–32. doi:10.1016/j.acpain.2008.05.042
17. Walther-Larsen S, Pedersen MT, Friis SM, et al. Pain prevalence in hospitalized children: A prospective cross-sectional survey in four Danish university hospitals. *Acta Anaesthesiol Scand.* 2017;61(3):328–337. doi:10.1111/aas.12846
18. Velazquez Cardona C, Rajah C, Mzoneli YN, et al. An audit of paediatric pain prevalence, intensity, and treatment at a South African tertiary hospital. *Pain Reports.* 2019;4(6):1–7. doi:10.1097/PR9.0000000000000789
19. Vejzovic V, Bozic J, Panova G, Babajic M, Bramhagen AC. Children still experience pain during hospital stay: A cross-sectional study from four countries in Europe. *BMC Pediatr.* 2020;20(1):1–6. doi:10.1186/s12887-020-1937-1
20. Kozlowski LJ, Kost-Byerly S, Colantuoni E, et al. Pain prevalence, intensity, assessment and management in a hospitalized pediatric population. *Pain Manag Nurs.* 2014;15(1):22–35. doi:10.1016/j.pmn.2012.04.003
21. Benoit B, Martin-Misener R, Latimer M, Campbell-Yeo M. Breast-feeding analgesia in infants. *J Perinat Neonatal Nurs.* 2017;31(2):145–159. doi:10.1097/JPN.0000000000000253
22. Johnston C, Campbell-Yeo M, Disher T, et al. Skin-to-skin care for procedural pain in neonates. *Cochrane Database Syst Rev.* 2017;2:CD008435. doi:10.1002/14651858.CD008435.pub3
23. Stevens B, Yamada J, Ohlsson A, Haliburton S, Shorkey A. Sucrose for analgesia in newborn infants undergoing painful procedures. *Cochrane Database Syst Rev.* 2016;7(7):CD001069. doi:10.1002/14651858.CD001069.pub5
24. Harrison D, Larocque C, Bueno M, et al. Sweet solutions to reduce procedural pain in neonates: A meta-analysis. *Pediatrics.* 2017;139(1):e20160955. doi:10.1542/peds.2016-0955
25. Pillai Riddell RR, Bucsea O, Shiff I, et al. Non-pharmacological management of infant and young child procedural pain. *Cochrane Database Syst Rev.* 2023(6). doi:10.1002/14651858.CD006275.pub4
26. Shah V, Taddio A, McMurtry CM, et al. Pharmacological and combined interventions to reduce vaccine injection pain in children and adults. *Clin J Pain.* 2015;31(10):S38–S63. doi:10.1097/AJP.0000000000000281
27. Stevens BJ, Yamada J, Promislow S, Barwick M, Pinard M. Pain assessment and management after a knowledge translation booster intervention. *Pediatrics.* 2016;138(4):e20153468. doi:10.1542/peds.2015-3468
28. Stevens BJ, Yamada J, Promislow S, Stinson J, Harrison D, Victor JC. Implementation of multidimensional knowledge translation strategies to improve procedural pain in hospitalized children. *Implement Sci.* 2014;9: Article 120. doi:10.1186/s13012-014-0120-1

29. Stevens BJ, Yamada J, Estabrooks CA, et al. Pain in hospitalized children: Effect of a multidimensional knowledge translation strategy on pain process and clinical outcomes. *Pain.* 2014;155(1):60–68. doi:10.1016/j.pain.2013.09.007
30. Rosenberg RE, Klejmont L, Gallen M, et al. Making comfort count: Using quality improvement to promote pediatric procedural pain management. *Hosp Pediatr.* 2016;6(6):359–368. doi:10.1542/hpeds.2015-0240
31. Lightwood R. Welfare of children in hospital. *Health Educ J.* 1959;16(3):168–181. doi:10.1177/001789695801600303
32. O'Connor S, Brenner M, Coyne I. Family-centred care of children and young people in the acute hospital setting: A concept analysis. *J Clin Nurs.* 2019;28(17–18):3353–3367. doi:10.1111/jocn.14913
33. Power NM, North N, Leonard AL, Bonaconsa C, Coetzee M. A scoping review of mother-child separation in clinical paediatric settings. *J Child Heal Care.* 2021;25(4):534–548. doi:10.1177/1367493520966415
34. Franck L, Oulton K, Bruce E. Parental involvement in neonatal pain management: An empirical and conceptual update. *J Nurs Scholarsh.* 2012;44(1):45–54.
35. Franck LS, Cormier DM, Hutchison J, et al. A multisite survey of NICU healthcare professionals' perceptions about family-centered care. *Adv Neonatal Care.* 2021;21(3):205–213. doi:10.1097/ANC.0000000000000805
36. McNair C, Chinian N, Shah V, et al. Metasynthesis of factors that influence parents' participation in pain management for their infants in the NICU. *J Obstet Gynecol Neonatal Nurs.* 2020;49(3):263–271. doi:10.1016/j.jogn.2020.02.007
37. Lavin Venegas C, Taljaard M, Reszel J, et al. A parent-targeted and mediated video intervention to improve uptake of pain treatment for infants during newborn screening: A pilot randomized controlled trial. *J Perinat Neonatal Nurs.* 2019;33(1):74–81. doi:10.1097/JPN.0000000000000386
38. Duerden EG, Grunau RE, Guo T, et al. Early procedural pain is associated with regionally-specific alterations in thalamic development in preterm neonates. *J Neurosci.* 2017;38(4):878–886. doi:10.1523/JNEUROSCI.0867-17.2017
39. Eccleston C, Fisher E, Howard RF, et al. Delivering transformative action in paediatric pain: A *Lancet Child & Adolescent Health* Commission. *Lancet Child Adolesc Health.* 2021;5(1):47–87. doi:10.1016/S2352-4642(20)30277-7
40. Friedrichsdorf SJ, Goubert L. Pediatric pain treatment and prevention for hospitalized children. *Pain Rep.* 2020;5(1):E804. doi:10.1097/PR9.0000000000000804
41. Modanloo S, Barrowman N, Martelli B, et al. Be sweet to hospitalized toddlers during venipuncture. *Clin J Pain.* 2022;38(1):41–48. doi:10.1097/AJP.0000000000000998
42. Babl FE, Goldfinch C, Mandrawa C, et al. Does nebulized lidocaine reduce the pain and distress of nasogastric tube insertion in young children? A randomized, double-blind, placebo-controlled trial. *Pediatrics.* 2009;123(6):1548–1555.
43. McLenon J, Rogers MAM. The fear of needles: A systematic review and meta-analysis. *J Adv Nurs.* 2019;75(1):30–42. doi:10.1111/jan.13818
44. World Health Organization. Ten threats to global health in 2019. 2020. Accessed July 28, 2022. https://www.who.int/news-room/spotlight/ten-threats-to-global-health-in-2019
45. Tutelman PR, Chambers CT, Cornelissen L, et al. Long-term alterations in somatosensory functioning in survivors of childhood cancer. *Pain.* 2022;163(6):1193–1205. doi:10.1097/j.pain.0000000000002486
46. Vania Apkarian A, Baliki MN, Farmer MA. Predicting transition to chronic pain. *Curr Opin Neurol.* 2013;26(4):360–367. doi:10.1097/WCO.0b013e32836336ad
47. King S, Chambers CT, Huguet A, et al. The epidemiology of chronic pain in children and adolescents revisited: A systematic review. *Pain.* 2011;152(12):2729–2738.
48. Hadjistavropoulos T, Craig KD, Duck S, et al. A biopsychosocial formulation of pain communication. *Psychol Bull.* 2011;137(6):910–939. doi:10.1037/A0023876
49. Goubert L, Pillai Riddell R, Simons L, Borsook D. Theoretical basis of pain. In: Stevens BJ, Hathway G, Zempsky WT, eds. *Oxford Textbook of Pediatric Pain.* 2nd ed. Oxford University Press; 2021:89–100. doi:10.1093/med/9780198818762.001.0001

50. Pope N, Tallon M, Leslie G, Wilson S. Ask me: Children's experiences of pain explored using the draw, write, and tell method. *J Spec Pediatr Nurs.* 2018;23(3):e12218. doi:10.1111/jspn.12218
51. Craig KD. A child in pain: A psychologist's perspective on changing priorities in scientific understanding and clinical care. *Paediatr Neonatal Pain.* 2020;2(2):40–49. doi:10.1002/pne2.12034
52. Psihogios AM, Daniel LC, Tarazi R, Smith-Whitley K, Patterson CA, Barakat LP. Family functioning, medical self-management, and health outcomes among school-aged children with sickle cell disease: A mediation model. *J Pediatr Psychol.* 2018;43(4):423–433. doi:10.1093/jpepsy/jsx120
53. Lee S, Dick BD, Jordan A, McMurtry CM. Psychological interventions for parents of youth with chronic pain: A scoping review. *Clin J Pain.* 2021;37(11):825–844. doi:10.1097/AJP.0000000000000977
54. Higgins KS, Chambers CT, Rosen NO, et al. Child catastrophizing about parent chronic pain: A potential child vulnerability factor. *Br J Health Psychol.* 2020;25(2):339–357. doi:10.1111/BJHP.12410
55. Wakefield EO, Puhl RM, Litt MD, Zempsky WT. "If it ever really hurts, I try not to let them know": The use of concealment as a coping strategy among adolescents with chronic pain. *Front Psychol.* 2021;3(12):666275. doi:10.3389/fpsyg.2021.666275
56. Caes L, Boerner KE, Chambers CT, et al. A comprehensive categorical and bibliometric analysis of published research articles on pediatric pain from 1975 to 2010. *Pain.* 2016;157(2):302–313. doi:10.1097/j.pain.0000000000000403
57. McNair C, Campbell-Yeo M, Johnston C, Taddio A. Nonpharmacologic management of pain during common needle puncture procedures in infants: Current research evidence and practical considerations: An update. *Clin Perinatol.* 2019;46(4):709–730. doi:10.1016/j.clp.2019.08.006
58. Harrison D, Reszel J, Bueno M, et al. Breastfeeding for procedural pain in infants beyond the neonatal period. *Cochrane Database Syst Rev.* 2016;2016(10):CD011248. doi:10.1002/14651858.CD011248.pub2.
59. Chen SL, Harrison D, Huang RR, Zhang Q, Xie RH, Wen SW. Efficacy of sweet solutions in relieving pain caused by vaccination in infants aged 1 to 12 months: A systematic review. *Chinese J Contemp Pediatr.* 2016;18(6):534–540. doi:10.7499/j.issn.1008-8830.2016.06.013
60. Birnie K, Noel M, Chambers C, Uman L, Parker J. Psychological interventions for needle-related procedural pain and distress in children and adolescents. *Cochrane Database Syst Rev.* 2018;2018(10):CD005179. doi:10.1002/14651858.CD005179.pub4
61. Ueki S, Yamagami Y, Makimoto K. Effectiveness of vibratory stimulation on needle-related procedural pain in children: A systematic review. *JBI Database Syst Rev Implement Rep.* 2019;17(7):1428–1463. doi:10.11124/JBISRIR-2017-003890
62. Loeffen EAH, Mulder RL, Font-Gonzalez A, et al. Reducing pain and distress related to needle procedures in children with cancer: A clinical practice guideline. *Eur J Cancer.* 2020;131:53–67. doi:10.1016/j.ejca.2020.02.039
63. Haward MF, Lantos J, Janvier A, Janvier A. Helping parents cope in the NICU. *Pediatrics.* 2020;145(6):e20193567. doi:10.1542/PEDS.2019-3567
64. Waddington C, van Veenendaal NR, O'Brien K, Patel N. Family integrated care: Supporting parents as primary caregivers in the neonatal intensive care unit. *Pediatr Investig.* 2021;5(2):148–154. doi:10.1002/ped4.12277
65. Friedrichsdorf SJ, Eull D, Weidner C, Postier A. A hospital-wide initiative to eliminate or reduce needle pain in children using lean methodology. *Pain Rep.* 2018;3(Suppl 1):e671. doi:10.1097/PR9.0000000000000671
66. Schechter NL, Finley GA, Bright NS, Laycock M, Forgeron P. ChildKind: A global initiative to reduce pain in children. *Pediatr Pain Lett.* 2010;12(3):26–30.
67. Franck LS, O'Brien K. The evolution of family-centered care: From supporting parent-delivered interventions to a model of family integrated care. *Birth Defects Res.* 2019;111(15):1044–1059. doi:10.1002/BDR2.1521

68. Johnston C, Barrington KJ, Taddio A, Carbajal R, Filion F. Pain in Canadian NICUs: Have we improved over the past 12 years? *Clin J Pain.* 2011;27(3):225–232. doi:10.1097/AJP.0b013e3181fe14cf
69. Gagnon MM, Hadjistavropoulos T, McAleer LM, Stopyn RJN. Increasing parental access to pediatric pain-related knowledge. *Clin J Pain.* 2020;36(1):47–60. doi:10.1097/ajp.0000000000000770
70. Fearon P, Belsky J. Attachment in infancy and childhood. In: Cassidy J, Shaver P, eds. *Handbook of Attachment: Theory, Research, and Clinical Applications.* 3rd ed. Guilford; 2016:271–396.
71. Gates A, Shave K, Featherstone R, et al. Procedural pain: Systematic review of parent experiences and information needs. *Clin Pediatr.* 2018;57(6):672–688. doi:10.1177/0009922817733694
72. Harrison D, Larocque C, Reszel J, Harrold J, Aubertin C. Be Sweet to Babies: Pilot evaluation of a brief parent-targeted video to improve pain management practices. *Adv Neonatal Care.* 2017;17(5):372–380. doi:10.1097/ANC.0000000000000425
73. Harrison D, Reszel J, Dagg B, et al. Pain management during newborn screening: Using YouTube to disseminate effective pain management strategies. *J Perinat Neonatal Nurs.* 2017;31(2):172–177. doi:10.1097/JPN.0000000000000255
74. Campbell-Yeo M, Dol J, Disher T, et al. The power of a parent's touch: Evaluation of reach and impact of a targeted evidence-based YouTube Video. *J Perinat Neonatal Nurs.* 2017;31(4):341–349. doi:10.1097/JPN.0000000000000263
75. Bueno M, Nogueira Costa R, de Camargo PP, Costa T, Harrison D. Evaluation of a parent-targeted video in Portuguese to improve pain management practices in neonates. *J Clin Nurs.* 2018;27(5–6):1153–1159. doi:10.1111/jocn.14147
76. Modanloo S, Hu J, Reszel J, Larocque C, Harrison D. Be sweet to babies during painful procedures: Evaluation of a parent-targeted and mediated video in Farsi. *J Neonatal Nurs.* 2021;27(6):419–425. doi:10.1016/j.jnn.2021.06.002
77. Hu J, Xue F, Zhou Y, et al. Using social media to disseminate effective pain treatments for newborns during needle-related painful procedures in China. *J Perinat Neonatal Nurs.* 2021;35(4):E50–E57. doi:10.1097/JPN.0000000000000602.
78. Labaky D, Joly C, Reszel J, et al. Petite douceur pour bébé: Using YouTube to disseminate effective pain management strategies. *Pediatr Pain Lett.* 2018;23(2):2019–2022.
79. Franck LS. Comforting your baby in intensive care (multimedia edition). 2013. http://familynursing.ucsf.edu/sites/familynursing.ucsf.edu/files/wysiwyg/Comfy PDF ENGLISH Dec 17.pdf
80. Reid K, Hartling L, Ali S, Le A, Norris A, Scott SD. Development and usability evaluation of an art and narrative-based knowledge translation tool for parents with a child with pediatric chronic pain: Multi-method study. *J Med Internet Res.* 2017;19(12):e412. doi:10.2196/JMIR.8877
81. Eccleston C, Fisher E, Cooper TE, et al. Pharmacological interventions for chronic pain in children: An overview of systematic reviews. *Pain.* 2019;160(8):1698–1707. doi:10.1097/j.pain.0000000000001609
82. Lawson J. Letter to the editor. *N Engl J Med.* 1986;318(21):1398.

6
Pain in Older Adults

Lauren A. Kelly, Caitlyn Kuwata, Suzanne Goldhirsch, and Helen M. Fernandez

Introduction

Pain Vulnerability in Older Adults

Among older adults (aged 65 years and older), pain is a highly prevalent, disabling, and underrecognized condition that can be challenging to manage. Chronic pain, usually defined as pain that extends for a duration of at least 3–6 months or beyond expected healing time, affects an estimated 18–57% of community-dwelling older adults.[1] Older people living in nursing homes have an even greater burden of chronic pain, with estimates of chronic pain as high as 83–93%.[2] Pain should not be considered an expected complication of aging, as many older adults live without significant pain. However, pain that impairs daily functioning occurs at higher frequencies among older adults. Many chronic nonmalignant pain conditions affect older adults, including generalized osteoarthritis, chronic back pain, myofascial pain, peripheral neuropathy, and fibromyalgia syndrome.[3] Older adults, in whom surgery is twice as common, are at risk for more severe pain and disability after surgery.[4] Injuries related to falls are another common source of pain in older adults, including fractures of hip, pelvis, vertebrae, and extremities.

Extensive data support the conclusion that older adults are more vulnerable to severe or persistent pain and are less able to tolerate pain.[5,6] The biological basis of this vulnerability is termed "homeostenosis," or the diminishing physiologic capacity for the organ systems of the body to adapt to stressors.[7] Aging affects every organ system, most notably the cardiovascular, renal, hepatic, musculoskeletal, and nervous systems.[8] Older adults have a decline in glomerular function, decreased liver mass and blood flow, and decreased muscle mass. Adverse medication effects are more common in older adults due to these changes, which impact drug distribution, concentration, and metabolism. With regard to the neurological system, regardless of the presence of clinically apparent cognitive impairment, the aging brain becomes increasingly sensitive to psychoactive medications and prone to the development of delirium, both of which complicate pain assessment and treatment.

The usual homeostatic mechanisms of pain signaling are also altered. Older adults appear to have an increased pain threshold and may be less sensitive to pain. However, when they do experience pain, they tolerate it less well than younger individuals, possibly due to reduced inhibitory pain signaling and fewer neurochemicals necessary for pain modulation, resulting in more severe, persistent, and prolonged pain after tissue injury.[6] Changes in pain sensing also underlie the differences in how older adults with visceral pain may present. For example, an older adult with myocardial infarction or perforated viscus may not exhibit overt signs of pain, and so a high index of suspicion for a serious condition must be maintained when older adults present with vague complaints.

Due to the diminished capacity to adapt to changes combined with a high burden of comorbid illness, painful conditions may become very consequential for older adults. Pain can negatively affect physical and mental well-being, accelerate physical debility, impair focus and sleep, and make it difficult to cope with even the most basic stressors of life.[9] Pain also contributes to a cycle of frailty, whereby deconditioning, immobility, and poor nutrition beget more sarcopenia and frailty. Pain must therefore be taken very seriously as a threat to the older adult, and relief of pain is imperative. When pain is properly addressed, it is associated with improved mobility and function, better rehabilitation potential, less health care utilization, and lower incidence of developing chronic or persistent pain.[4,10]

The Complexities of Treating Pain in Older Adults

Concerningly, pain in older adults is underidentified and undertreated.[8] Ageism and therapeutic nihilism play a role because pain is often underreported by patients and even minimized by providers as an expected feature of growing old.[11] Due to the presence of multiple comorbidities, presentations of pain are atypical in that they depend on the most vulnerable organ system(s). For example, patients experiencing pain related to a wide range of conditions may present similarly with acute confusion or delirium, particularly if they have underlying neurocognitive impairment. Pain is often undertreated even when it is identified, as providers may view pain medications as unsafe for older adults, citing adverse side effects and the addictive potential of opioids. The collective toll of unrelieved chronic pain represents a significant public health concern and leads to diminished quality of life for patients, greater caregiver burden, and increased health care utilization and costs.[5,8,12]

Although many studies have indicated a relationship between pain and aging, the direction of this relationship (e.g., pain accelerating aging or aging begetting pain) remains equivocal due to the many factors that interact with and mediate pain.[1,12] Various aspects of physical, mental, and social functioning have complex bidirectional relationships with pain. Along the physical domain, pain has been associated with a greater degree of chronic conditions, impaired mobility, gait disturbances, falls, lower rehabilitation potential, and malnutrition. From a mental and cognitive health standpoint, depression, anxiety, cognitive impairment, poor sleep, and social isolation may both affect and be affected by pain, deepening the pain experience and reducing tolerability to painful stimuli.

Acknowledging the multifaceted nature of pain in older adults, a key principle of pain management becomes especially relevant: Targets for pain treatment may be directed at multiple risk factors that may not seem immediately causative, such as untreated depression. Because many individual physical, psychosocial, and economic risks can act together to contribute to pain, the most effective interventions involve a multimodal approach to achieving improvements across several risk categories, rather than large improvements in a single risk category.[13]

Pain and the Geriatric Assessment

To navigate the complexities in identifying, characterizing, and effectively treating pain, geriatricians depend on a whole-person approach to patient care. By conducting a comprehensive geriatric assessment, providers develop a tailored intervention that accounts for the unique risk factor profiles and health care needs of older adults. Rather than focusing on piecemeal recommendations for individual conditions, geriatricians conduct a multicomponent evaluation that routinely includes functional status (i.e., activities of daily living [ADLs], instrumental ADLs [IADLs]), neurocognitive issues (i.e., dementia and delirium), mood disorders (i.e., depression and anxiety), visual and hearing impairments, urinary incontinence, nutritional status, gait, balance, falls, polypharmacy, social support, financial concerns, and environmental issues (e.g., home safety evaluation).[11] Not every patient aged 65 years and older requires a comprehensive geriatric assessment; however, higher risk patients with multiple comorbidities including pain and those with functional impairment will significantly benefit from this approach.

The framework for geriatric assessment that we utilize for this chapter is the 5 Ms of Geriatrics (5Ms).[14] The 5Ms model captures a broad spectrum of physical and psychosocial aspects of patient assessment, including "mobility," "medication," "mind and mood," "multicomplexity," and "matters most." Using the 5Ms framework, we examine how each assessment domain relates to the multiple dimensions of the pain experience, including etiologies of pain, clinical features, and pain management. Common geriatric syndromes, such as mobility impairment, cognitive impairment, and frailty, are reviewed with attention to the characteristics of these conditions that are associated with pain. We also review the psychosocial, socioeconomic, and health system–level factors that contribute to the pain experience in older adults, providing practical tips for comprehensive pain management and insight into achieving equity for pain care in this population.

Mobility

Pain and Mobility

The first of the 5Ms is mobility. Patients frequently complain about pain as an inability to "move" through the world. Pain and function are inextricably linked in this way. Data have shown that older adults with pain have a substantially higher prevalence of mobility disability than those without pain, suggesting that pain is an accelerator of functional decline.[15] Pain puts patients at greater risk for falls, poorer physical performance, and onset of progression of disability, further compounding the pain experience.[15] Immobility even for shorter durations, such as for an acute hospitalization, can have significant effects on function. When patients suffer acute-on-chronic worsening of their pain, such as after orthopedic surgery, this must be aggressively managed. Allowing acute pain to go unchecked can lead to changes in central nervous system processing of pain, making older adults vulnerable to persistent pain and further decline in functional baseline.[16]

Mobility Assessment

Geriatric assessment of mobility offers added insight into the mechanisms and potential treatments for pain. Geriatric mobility assessment typically involves evaluation of mobility-related ADLs and IADLs (e.g., the ability to dress and bathe oneself, perform household tasks, take public transportation, etc.), gait, posture, balance, and visual/auditory assessment. Pain treatment is inextricably linked with supportive care to promote mobility function. For example, when abnormal gait or balance problems are identified, this can inform which is the most appropriate mobility device to aid the patient and if the patient would benefit from home hazard modification and/or targeted physical therapy. Mobility screening also helps identify patients who are at higher risk for adverse effects from medications that increase fall risk. Visual or hearing deficits may exacerbate incoordination, injury, and fall, and thus they should be corrected to the extent possible as a preventive measure.[17]

Although pain may not be completely eliminated, significant improvement in function is often realistic and frequently a key priority for patients. Understanding the ways that pain can affect function can inform a problem-focused approach. For example, pain that builds up in the evening and prevents sleep can inform the recommendation for a bedtime dose of pain medication. Assessing pain in relationship to function can be more challenging for patients with cognitive impairment. Examining changes in activity level (e.g., willingness to walk to the bathroom or go outside) is often more informative than relying on commonly administered graded pain scales.

Mobility screening additionally offers prognostic value that can inform treatment, such as when a patient is deemed high risk for falls or if a patient is facing a terminal decline as they near the end of life. Treatment priorities in a patient receiving hospice care may be more oriented toward comfort and maximal pain relief, with acknowledgment that function will continue to deteriorate.

Conditions That Impact Mobility

Conditions that impair mobility are often painful. Unsurprisingly, pain prevalence is substantially higher in older adults with musculoskeletal conditions, including arthritis, low back pain, other rheumatologic joint disease, osteoporosis, hip fracture, and obesity.[3,15] Pain related to osteoarthritis can be particularly disabling as it progresses to bone-on-bone disease for which there are few effective medications and interventions short of joint replacement. Patients with chronic low back pain often have degenerative discs and facets, although they may also have spinal stenosis that can lead to severe pain and mobility impairment. Although surgical repair may be an option for some, many older adults have comorbidities that put them at high risk for surgical complication and must be managed conservatively. A stepped approach to pain management involves patient education, use of assistive devices, physical and/or occupational therapy (PT/OT), joint and/or spinal injections, and analgesics. Rehabilitative therapies including PT and/or OT are foundational to any pain intervention because they help stabilize the primary disorder, prevent secondary injury, and promote adaptations to current disabilities.[18] Other nonpharmacologic treatments can be especially helpful, low cost, and can minimize the need for medications. These include tai chi, acupuncture, chiropractic manipulation, massage, meditation, and cognitive–behavioral therapy.[2,19]

In cases in which nonpharmacologic and pharmacologic treatments are insufficient, surgery may be a consideration. Those who choose surgery should be counseled on reasonable expectations for relief, in which cure is the exception and improvement in pain or function is more likely. Failed back surgery syndrome can occur in up to nearly half of older adults when treatment decisions are based on advanced imaging alone, because degenerative pathology is seen in virtually 100% of older adults regardless of the presence of pain.[3] Judicious ordering of imaging tests is therefore advised among older adults with musculoskeletal complaints and should focus on ruling out serious disease (e.g., compression fracture, bony metastasis, and disc space infection) rather than diagnosing a cause of pain. Of note, more than two-thirds of vertebral compression fractures occur nontraumatically in older adults.[20] In cases in which acute or subacute back pain is not responding to treatment, plain films of the spine may be cost-effective and diagnostically helpful when they lead to the diagnosis and subsequent treatment of osteoporosis.

Myofascial pain and fibromyalgia may also affect mobility. Myofascial pain is broadly defined as pain in physiologically abnormal muscles, characterized by taut muscle bands and reproducible pain with firm palpation of trigger points.[3] Treatment includes physical therapy with stretching exercises, as well as trigger point deactivation with "dry needling" and trigger point injections. Patients with fibromyalgia often have prominent axial pain elicited with characteristic pressure point testing on exam. Although patients frequently present with a chief complaint of low back pain, many sites are often involved. Thought to be related to central nervous system dysregulation, fibromyalgia treatment involves increasing levels of physical activity and utilizing neuropathic agents. Treatment may also be directed toward associated mood and sleep disorders. Motivational interviewing, a style of skilled communication that helps build trust between patients and providers, can be a useful tool to promote adaptive coping mechanisms for patients with central pain syndromes.

Broader Implications of Mobility Impairment

Patients who suffer mobility impairment in association with pain may face substantial long-term disability that can have profound psychological effects and be financially costly for patients, families, and the health system. Mobility impairment can put a great deal of stress on the older adult, require purchase of non-reimbursed durable medical equipment for home safety, and necessitate expensive and inefficient transportation services to and from office visits. Acclimating to new levels of functional impairment is especially difficult for older adults who live alone or have little psychosocial support.

Decreased mobility can be a barrier to seeking care, resulting in severe decline, hazardous home environment, and acute decompensation that requires emergency care. Older adults who were previously independent may suddenly require hospitalization or placement in a nursing home. If patients do not have financial resources to maintain independence at home, they may exhaust allotted days of facility-based post-acute care and face high out-of-pocket nursing home costs.

What may begin as a post-acute care plan to "get stronger" before returning home, a commonly stated goal by patients and providers alike, often ends in systematic institutionalization of older adults.[21] Patients most at risk for this trajectory are those who have suffered the cumulative effects of poverty, lower levels of education, work-related injury, and other social disadvantages over the life course.[15] In addition, patients with cognitive impairment or severe mental health disorders who struggle to participate in the structured activities of rehabilitation face further decline and need for facility placement. Efforts under the Affordable Care Act to rebalance Medicaid funding away from nursing home care to increase long-term services and supports in the home and community have fallen short, and more recent federal efforts to similarly meet this aim have yet to yield progress.

Medications

Medication Treatment for Pain

Medication therapy, the second of the 5Ms, is an essential component to multimodal pain treatment. Older adults have a high prevalence of complex medication regimens and multimorbidity. Polypharmacy, commonly defined as five or more chronic medications, can lead to consequential drug–drug and drug–disease interactions, as well as adverse drug-related reactions and events, including falls, fractures, renal impairment, functional decline, cognitive decline, hospitalization, and even death.[22] Approximately 10% of hospitalizations in older adults are due to adverse drug reactions.[22] Polypharmacy results from many factors, including care based on single-disease–focused guidelines among patients with fragmented multispecialist care, as well as a "prescribing cascade" when an adverse drug reaction is misinterpreted as a new condition that triggers addition of more medication.[23] Although systems have been implemented for safe prescribing of controlled substances, such as local prescription drug monitoring programs, there is no routinely utilized approach for noncontrolled medications.

The second "M" of the geriatric assessment focuses on medications, providing a framework to safely evaluate and navigate a patient's medication regimen to optimize pain prescribing. The key assessment components include medication reconciliation, review of adherence, and frequent reassessment. Medication reconciliation with attention to drug–drug and drug–disease effects ideally involves review of the actual bottles of medication that patients are using, including prescribed and nonprescribed medications and supplements.[24] This allows the provider to see how patients are taking medications, with what frequency, and if they understand why they are taking each one. This review is particularly relevant for medications that are taken on an "as needed" basis and may have variable usage during the day. When there is concern for cognitive impairment, it is strongly advised to reconcile medications with caregivers and/or with the patient's pharmacy.

Effective medication reconciliation informs deprescribing of medications that may contribute to adverse reactions and events, and it also promotes appropriate prescribing guided by geriatric physiology and pharmacology. A tool that is commonly used to assess medication regimens in older adults is the Beer's Criteria. This tool does not advise blanket deprescribing of high-risk agents but, rather, informs a cautious balance of risks and benefits when new medications are added.

If nonadherence is identified during medication assessment, modifications such as blister-packing pills or utilizing pill organizers that can be prefilled by caregivers are commonly employed. Modifications to support adherence to the treatment regimen can be especially helpful for patients with cognitive impairment, visual impairment, and those who struggle with manual dexterity to self-administer medications. Patients with difficulty tolerating oral medications due to dysphagia or other conditions also benefit from rotation to liquid or patch formulations. More fundamentally, adherence can be promoted with improved communication about the purpose and side effects of medications, simplified dosing regimens, and regular follow-ups to identify treatment barriers and fine-tune the treatment regimen. Frequent patient assessment allows the prescriber to adjust the medication dosage to the desired effect and discontinue medications that have proven harmful or ineffective after adequate trial.

Key Medication Considerations in Older Adults

As a general principle in geriatrics, the lowest risk therapies are used initially to avoid toxicities and side effects. Nonpharmacologic treatments including physical therapy often form the backbone of pain treatment regimens. Local therapies, such as lidocaine patches or corticosteroid joint injections, should be utilized prior to systemic therapies. When additional medication is required, the appropriate drug class and lowest effective dose should be initiated. Choice of an analgesic agent is guided by the degree of pain acuity, etiology of the pain (i.e., nociceptive vs. neuropathic), pain severity, and the presence of age-associated physiological changes.[5,25] Treatment should begin with over-the-counter analgesics, then escalate with addition of non-opioid adjuvants such as antidepressants and anticonvulsants as clinically indicated (Table 6.1). Of note, nonsteroidal anti-inflammatory drugs are not recommended for routine use in older adults due to the risk of both drug–drug and drug–disease related adverse effects, and acetaminophen should be preferentially utilized.[26] Opioids are generally reserved for pain that is refractory to these treatments.

The choice to initiate opioids should be balanced with risks, including side effects (e.g., cognitive, gastrointestinal, and mobility-related), adverse events (e.g., ability of patient or caregiver to responsibly manage the medication), and potential for risky opioid use. As with all medications in older adults, opioids must be introduced slowly and at reduced doses. A reasonable dose reduction may range from 25% to 50% of the starting dose for an opioid-naive adult. Opioids with short half-lives and without active or toxic metabolites are preferred. When using opioid therapy, the goals of

Table 6.1 Commonly Used Pain Medications with Key Considerations for Older Adults

Drug Class	Select Examples	Key Considerations for Older Adults
OTC Topical Medications: Use in mild pain		
NSAIDs	Topical diclofenac	Considered a safer alternative compared to oral NSAIDs due to lower systemic absorption Can provide relief for localized pain due to osteoarthritis
	Topical lidocaine	Can provide relief for localized neuropathic pain
OTC Medications: Use in mild/moderate pain		
Acetaminophen (paracetamol)		Maximum daily dose 4 g/day; reduce by 50–70% in those with hepatic dysfunction ± malnutrition, low body weight, advanced age Counsel patients on presence of acetaminophen in other combination medications to prevent unintentional overdose
NSAIDs	Naproxen Ibuprofen Celecoxib	Increased risk of gastrointestinal bleeding and renal injury in older adults Consider only for short-term use Avoid if history of chronic kidney disease or heart failure
Adjuvant Analgesics: Use in neuropathic pain		
SNRIs	Duloxetine Venlafaxine	Common adverse effects include hyponatremia, dizziness, abdominal pain, nausea Avoid duloxetine in renal impairment creatinine clearance <30 mL/min
Tricyclic antidepressants	Nortriptyline Desipramine	Caution with use given risk for QTc prolongation and anticholinergic effects (e.g., confusion, falls, constipation)
Anti-seizure medications	Gabapentin Pregabalin	Decreased doses recommended in renal impairment Common adverse effects include sedation, dizziness, edema, constipation
Opioids: Use in moderate/severe pain unresponsive to alternative agents Caution using opioids with other sedating medications (e.g., benzodiazepines, gabapentinoids) All opioid use should be frequently monitored for adverse effects, including Constipation (of note, laxatives are routinely co-prescribed with opioids) Sedation Respiratory depression		
Use in normal renal function (eGFR > 30)	Morphine	Available in liquid preparations that can allow for low doses Potentially lower cost compared to other opioids
Use in renal impairment and normal renal function	Buprenorphine	Lower risk of respiratory depression, sedation, and constipation compared to other opioids Available formulations are suited for those with dysphagia (i.e., transdermal, buccal, sublingual) Cost of co-payments can be prohibitive
	Methadone	Use with caution in those with cardiac history as can prolong QTc, requires ECG monitoring
	Fentanyl (transdermal)	Not recommended for opioid naive patients

(continued)

Table 6.1 Continued

Drug Class	Select Examples	Key Considerations for Older Adults
	Oxycodone	- long-acting sprinkle formulations are available for those with dysphagia or feeding tubes
	Hydromorphone	Limited access to long-acting formulations due to cost and insurance barriers
Consider avoiding	Tramadol	Avoid use in those with seizure disorder or renal impairment Risk of SIADH/hyponatremia Unpredictable analgesic effect due to individual variability in metabolism to active metabolite
	Codeine	Avoid use in renal impairment Unpredictable analgesic effect due to individual variability in metabolism to active metabolite
	Muscle relaxants	Avoid use given risk for sedation, dizziness, and anticholinergic effects
Other Analgesics		
Cannabinoids		Limited clinical trials for efficacy and safety in older adults Use with caution given adverse effects (e.g., motor impairment, dysphoria, sedation)

ECG, electrocardiogram; eGFR, estimated glomerular filtration rate; NSAIDs, nonsteroidal anti-inflammatory drugs; OTC, over-the-counter; QTc, corrected QT interval; SIADH, syndrome of inappropriate antidiuretic hormone secretion; SNRIs, serotonin–norepinephrine reuptake inhibitors.

Sources: References 2, 9, 26, 27, 29, and 40.

treatment should be linked to specific functional goals, such as improving mobility or increasing participation in therapy. This allows for optimization of dosing, including rotating or tapering the opioid when clinically appropriate. It is also important to note that the guiding geriatric principle of "start low and go slow" is not equivalent to "start low and stay low," which can lead to undertreatment of pain.[27] Frequent assessment and documentation of medication impact on pain and function are imperative to determine the degree of pain relief, associated side effects, and potential for risky opioid use.

Risky Opioid Use in Older Adults

An estimated 21–29% of patients taking long-term opioids for chronic pain develop risky opioid use, and 8–12% develop opioid use disorder (OUD).[28] Risky opioid use, also referred to as "opioid misuse" or "aberrant use," is characterized by taking opioids in a way other than prescribed or by patient behaviors that may indicate a patient has an OUD, such as taking opioids for symptoms other than pain, using more than prescribed, making frequent requests for early fills, and illicit drug use. OUD, distinct from risky use, is characterized by a problematic pattern of opioid use leading to problems or distress. Adults with OUD who are over 50 years of age have increased all-cause mortality compared to younger adults, and the prevalence of OUD and risky opioid use among older adults is rising steadily.[29]

It is important to collect a thorough substance use and mental health history for all geriatric patients, as the presence of current or past history of substance use disorder and certain mental health conditions is associated with increased risky opioid use. Urine toxicology screening is a practice that, when employed, should be universally administered to minimize bias. It is important to note that concern for risky opioid use does not mean that opioids should not be prescribed or be stopped abruptly. Strategies for managing older adults with concern for risky opioid use who require opioid medications include shorter medication refills (e.g., 1 or 2 weeks), frequent assessment, and consideration of the type of opioid (e.g., buprenorphine).

Buprenorphine is a safer opioid in older adults because it can be used in renal and hepatic impairment, has lower risk of respiratory depression and adverse cognitive effects, and has multiple formulations suitable for patients with dysphagia and cognitive impairment.[29] Buprenorphine is increasingly being initiated for older adults who cannot tolerate full agonist opioids as well as for patients with either history of OUD or concerns for risky opioid use. The efficacy of buprenorphine for pain, its favorable safety profile, and its status as a life-saving medication for OUD make it a powerful tool that geriatricians are increasingly utilizing.

Medication Access and Equity

Maintaining a pain medication routine can be a challenging task for older adults with mobility impairment, cognitive impairment, and/or lack of social support. Medications require retrieval from the pharmacy, which may be difficult for mobility-impaired patients. Patients with cognitive impairment require caregiver support for medication dispensing, particularly for as-needed medications when breakthrough pain occurs.[30] Lack of clear communication from providers that is tailored to the needs and health literacy of the patient regarding the intended medication use and instructions can also lead to adverse drug events and adherence issues. Teach-back about medication with patients and involvement of caregivers are reliable approaches to improve pain treatment outcomes. The period of transition in care, such as from hospital to facility or home setting, is especially vulnerable, and careful attention to medication reconciliation during these transitions is needed.

Equity in pain medication access is particularly challenging for older adults who have high rates of poverty. Many older adults depend on income from savings or social security, and because the majority are no longer working, this corresponds to fewer sources of income.[30] The need for multiple medications due to higher comorbidity also contributes to lack of affordability. Prescription drug coverage under Medicare can be limited, and the opaque landscape of supplemental insurance plans for older adults may lead to even greater financial strain. Patients on opioids also face unique challenges to medication access, specifically those residing in low-income and racially and ethnically diverse geographic locations where medications may not be routinely stocked in pharmacies.[31]

Older adults with OUD taking buprenorphine and methadone also face unique challenges in access to appropriate pain treatment. The presence of significant opioid tolerance often requires larger doses of added opioids for patients with uncontrolled pain, which providers may not feel comfortable administering for fear of adverse effects or worsening the OUD. This can result in suboptimal pain treatment. Patients taking medications for OUD who require relocation to nursing home settings for rehabilitation or long-term care also may face systematic discrimination in the admission process, resulting in gaps in access to medication, opioid withdrawal, and increased requirements for pain medications.

Mind and Mood

Pain and Neuropsychology

The third of the 5Ms is mind and mood and focuses on assessment of the neuropsychological state of a patient. Pain is itself a complex neuropsychological phenomenon. As such, other commonly encountered conditions, including psychiatric disorders, cognitive impairment, and delirium, interrelate with the pain experience. Recognition and treatment of these conditions are essential to the overall success of pain management.

Both mood and cognition can contribute to maladaptations in the central pain pathway. Like other age-related changes in physiologic systems, central pain pathway functioning may decline with age, making it more difficult for older adults to modulate and respond to new or higher levels of pain input.[16] Mood is a modulator of the areas of the brain that are involved in descending inhibition of pain, which damp down the effect of afferent nociceptive pain signals. Depressed mood can predispose older adults to pain and exacerbate the pain intensity, duration, and associated disability.[32] In turn, the experience of living with significant pain can contribute to depressed mood and anxiety, as well as negative attitudes, beliefs, and expectations about pain.[5] Other negative affective associations with pain, such as pain catastrophizing and fear avoidance, can potentiate adverse cognitive modulation of pain.[33] Pain catastrophizing, a style characterized by rumination and sense of helplessness about pain, is more strongly associated with pain intensity among older adults than younger adults,[34] and it predicts less physical activity and more sedentary behavior, exacerbating pain and disability.[35]

Dementia changes how pain sensations are interpreted and is characterized by difficulties recalling and communicating about pain.[5] Evidence suggests that people with certain types of dementia are more susceptible to the development of central and neuropathic pain.[36] Other studies have shown that chronic pain is associated with increased risk of developing cognitive impairment,[37] and effective pain treatment has been associated with a lower rate of cognitive decline.[37] In older adults with dementia, challenges around communication about pain as well as different, more subtle pain manifestations put them at high risk for underrecognition and undertreatment of pain.

Identifying and Treating Mood and Memory Conditions

When conducting a geriatric assessment, it is helpful to consider mood, memory, and delirium on separate but related axes, as distinguishing between these three main drivers of altered cognition helps direct pain assessment and treatment. Depression can be difficult to diagnose in older adults, who often present atypically with more somatic or functional symptoms, such as poor sleep, fatigue, decreased enjoyment or interest in activities, and a sense of helplessness.[32,38] A validated tool designed for detecting depression in older adults is the Geriatric Depression Scale (GDS).[39] The GDS utilizes "yes" or "no" questions and may be easier to complete compared to other depression screening tools.

Medications for depression must be selected cautiously in the older adult based on the side effect profile. Although tricyclic antidepressants are often considered for dual treatment of neuropathic pain and depression, they are not recommended due to their anticholinergic properties and risk for QTc prolongation and arrhythmias. Instead, serotonin and norepinephrine reuptake inhibitors should be considered first for concomitant treatment of pain and depression, due to a safer side effect profile.[40] Nonpharmacologic psychological therapies employed for pain treatment, such as cognitive–behavioral therapy, may also offer some benefit for reducing pain and catastrophizing beliefs, leading to improved self-efficacy for managing pain.[2,27,32]

There are various screening tests routinely used for cognitive assessment, including the Mini-Mental Status Exam and the Montreal Cognitive Assessment. The identification of any degree of cognitive impairment has important implications for pain management. Awareness of a patient's limitations in taking medication or verbalizing symptoms allows providers to craft a pain regimen tailored to the patient's needs and fortify the care plan with appropriate counseling and caregiver support.[13]

Delirium is another neuropsychological condition that can complicate pain care. Defined as an abrupt change in cognition associated with inattention and reduced awareness of the environment, delirium tends to have a fluctuating course. Seen commonly in hospitalized patients, it can usually be linked to an underlying acute process, the successful treatment of which alleviates the delirium. Delirium is formally assessed with tools such as the Confusion Assessment Method.[41] Numerous underlying processes can contribute to delirium in older adults, including uncontrolled pain.[4] Review of data including verbal and nonverbal expressions of pain (e.g., grimacing, moaning, and restlessness), the presence of tachycardia and/or hypertension, and inadequate receipt of analgesics may reveal pain as the likely driver of delirium compared to other causes.

Interventions for delirium should be informed by geriatric treatment principles, including nonpharmacological techniques to improve patient orientation and mobility safety, as well as careful medication review for agents that may contribute to confusion. It is also important to distinguish between delirium and behavioral disturbance among patients with dementia. Patients with dementia who have documented behavior disturbance at baseline may have breakthrough delirium related to pain that is disregarded as usual behavior, rather than treated as an acute change in medical status. For this reason, it is always necessary to confer with caregivers about a patient's baseline.

Social Connectedness as Pain Treatment

Although expanding access to behavioral health care is a crucial part of efforts to relieve the burden of pain for all patients, we must also consider loneliness and social isolation as key modifiable variables that can impact the pain experience for older adults. Social isolation is highly prevalent among older adults, as aging is often associated with a decreasing size of social networks, fewer surviving family members, and fewer friends. Loneliness and social isolation predict negative outcomes, including higher pain intensity and even increased mortality.[11] Improving a patient's social environment should therefore be considered as a pain treatment strategy. Programs that increase connectivity between older adults and their communities such as senior centers and local case management services can provide patients with additional caregiving resources, improve their functioning, and strengthen their ability to cope with persistent pain.[42] Streamlined care for older adults that consolidates medical, behavioral, and social service resources is another way to offer robust wrap-around care for the most vulnerable patients. One such approach is the Program for All-Inclusive Care for the Elderly, which provides a system of care that allows adults aged 55 and older who are eligible for nursing home care to remain at home.[43]

Multicomplexity

Multicomplexity and Pain

The most fundamental of the 5Ms of geriatrics is multicomplexity, which describes older adults living with multiple chronic conditions, advanced illness, and/or with complex biopsychosocial needs. Nearly half of Medicare beneficiaries have at least four chronic medical conditions, and approximately one-third have functional impairment and/or cognitive impairment,[44] resulting in an increased burden of symptoms, the need for multiple medications, and a reduced tolerance to medical and surgical treatments. The presence of multicomplexity, also referred to in the literature as multimorbidity, has been associated with poorer quality of life; higher rates of death, disability, and institutionalization; and increased pain severity and frequency.[15,45]

Most clinical practice guidelines focus on the management of single diseases, but among older adults with multimorbidity, this kind of care can be cumulatively impractical or even harmful.[45] Older adults with multimorbidity are routinely underrepresented in clinical trials and observational studies, which translates to less focus and relevancy of clinical guidelines for the older adult population. Providers therefore should employ a multimodal pain management approach that considers the patient's unique risk profile; interactions between their diseases and medications; patient preferences, goals, and prognosis; and the feasibility of each management decision.

Multimodal interventions can be challenging to implement because they are complex; require patient and caregiver motivation; necessitate frequent follow-up with providers; and depend on the use of interdisciplinary team members such as social workers, physical and occupational therapists, psychotherapists, and care coordinators to be successful.

Common Comorbidities That Contribute to Pain

Common conditions frequently associated with both pain and functional impairment in older adults include cancer, chronic neuropathic pain from diabetes and herpes zoster, osteoarthritis, compression fractures, vascular disease, heart failure, and chronic obstructive pulmonary disease.[46,47] In addition to those individual disease processes, older adults can develop pain related to "geriatric syndromes," which are clinical conditions that are the end result of the collective effects of multiple disease processes.[48] Frailty is a very common geriatric syndrome that has a major relationship to pain. Frailty is characterized by decreased function across multiple organ systems leading to a state of reduced physiologic reserve and increased vulnerability to stressors that can then increase the risk of adverse health outcomes.[49] Frailty has a bidirectional relationship with pain: The presence of frailty increases the risk of more severe pain, and the presence of pain increases an individual's risk of developing frailty.[49,50]

Overcoming Barriers to Pain Care for Patients with Multicomplexity

The current health care infrastructure is not designed to support patients with multiple medical conditions and instead silos the care of individual conditions, leading to care fragmentation.[51] The average Medicare patient sees five specialists a year,[52] which can lead to multiple conflicting and burdensome treatment plans, increased adverse drug events due to polypharmacy, and increased health expenditures. Patients with multimorbidity may also be forced to prioritize more symptomatic conditions such as pain at the expense of their less symptomatic but potentially life-limiting conditions, such as uncontrolled hypertension or diabetes.

In order to deliver high-quality pain care for patients, providers need an effective interdisciplinary team, caregiver resources and supports, models of care that are patient-centered, and a reimbursement structure that incentivizes meaningful health outcomes for older adults. There have been increasing efforts to develop community care coordination services and high-risk patient programs to improve care quality and integration of services for the most vulnerable patients. Transitions of care are another key area for intervention. An estimated 2 million older adults annually are initiated on opioids for the first time after hospitalization, which can lead to drug-related adverse events.[53] To improve safety during this tenuous period, critically needed programs have been developed that incorporate self-management education, telephone follow-up, and medication reconciliation.[54]

Matters Most

Pain and Patient Values

Pain is a uniquely personal experience. Across the life span, pain and pain treatment are influenced by patient-specific factors, including values; preferences; health beliefs; cultural, religious, and spiritual beliefs; personality; readiness to engage in management;

availability of social supports; prior health care experiences; and information from the internet and media.[1] Experiences of trauma, abuse, strain related to work and living environments, or other stressful life events such as divorce, incarceration, or death of a family member can accumulate with age and significantly affect physical and mental health among older adults, shaping their ability to process and cope with painful conditions. Individual patient expectations about pain management also vary considerably, from the belief that doctors can solve or cure nearly any medical problem to the view that pain medications are dangerous and should be avoided.

When formulating pain management strategies, it is crucial to understand the psychosocial milieu of the patient, as well as patient values and goals, including nontraditional outcomes such as effect on caregivers. The fifth of the 5Ms is aptly titled matters most. Broadly, this domain involves examining goals of care, coordinating advance care planning, and ensuring that important priorities and preferences become part of treatment plans. There are important benefits and harms that result from various pain treatment options (e.g., surgery, medication therapy, intensive physical therapy, etc.) that need to be weighed in relation to the patient's values, expectations, and goals.

In geriatrics, there is an often understated recognition that much of the care we provide goes beyond evidence-based medicine and ventures into a realm where we acknowledge that what we *can* do may not be what we *should* do when considering broader goals. The best option for pain treatment thus involves shared decision-making between the patient, the provider, and very often the caregiver(s), taking into account the patient's value system to determine what patients are able and willing to undertake to achieve their desired outcomes. For pain treatment, it is especially relevant to address outcomes for each treatment strategy. There are few treatment approaches that offer total relief of pain, some that prevent pain progression and support function, and others that aim to provide symptom relief or comfort only.

Health Outcome Priorities Can Guide Pain Treatment

It can no doubt be a challenge to arrive prepared for an encounter where we absorb the storied depths from which our patients and their families meet us. When patients describe pain, language often does not come easily, and dialogue can be emotionally laden and intense. Thoughtful attention is needed on the part of providers to locate salience and to direct a plan of care. The field of geriatrics has multiple guidelines and care planning protocols to help elucidate a patient's priorities and values to facilitate a plan of care that directly responds to their needs and concerns. One such useful framework is called health outcomes prioritization.[55] This approach considers treatment in terms of its effects on a set of universal, cross-disease outcomes, including length of life, physical and cognitive function, and symptoms. In a study of prioritization of health outcomes, older adults were asked to prioritize in rank order four universal health outcomes: "keeping you alive," "maintaining independence," "reducing or eliminating pain," and "reducing or eliminating other symptoms." Maintaining independence was the highest ranked priority (76%, $n = 270$), followed by staying alive (11%), pain relief (7%), and other symptom relief (6%). The variability observed in preferences suggests that getting a sense of an older person's prioritization of these key outcomes can be a fruitful starting point for conversation.

Given the variable priorities among patients, it becomes necessary for a provider to develop and explain a range of treatment options, rather than a "one-size-fits-all" approach to managing a problem. For example, a patient with dementia who is residing in a subacute rehabilitation facility after a hospital admission for a hip fracture has become progressively immobilized and malnourished due to pain and debility. In addition to implementing pain treatment, prioritizing pain and symptom management may involve a transition to comfort-focused care with hospice, whereas prioritizing length of life may involve more intensive physical rehabilitation and nutritional optimization. Risks and benefits of different approaches should be explored, including expectations from the provider about the potential trajectory for each option.

Broader Implications of Pain and Loss of Independence

Maintaining independence is the chief priority for the majority of older adults, and pain frequently compromises independence, as we have described in this chapter. The magnitude of the impact of functional loss on patients, caregivers, and the health system cannot be overstated. The effects of functional loss for caregivers can also be far reaching, necessitating new and often unfamiliar ways of relating, giving, and receiving with respect to the dependent patient. Although this can deepen and strengthen connectivity, it can also be a source of great relationship strain and caregiver burden. Some patients may be reluctant to relinquish roles and insist on remaining independent despite needing assistance, which can lead to concealing pain to avoid overburdening caregivers.[42] There is wide variability in how patients and caregivers deal with functional loss, ranging from caregivers assuming greater direct patient-care responsibilities to depending more heavily on the health system to navigate the patient's needs. Often what patients and families desire most, such as costly home health aide support, is financially untenable, and so they are faced with difficult decisions about facility placement. However, significant patient and family concerns exist around poor care quality, health care disparities, elder abuse, and neglect in nursing homes—all concerns corroborated by data.[56,57]

In nursing homes, pain is more common compared to that in the community, and it contributes to significant morbidity among patients. Undertreatment of pain among patients from racial and ethnic minority groups is especially troubling. Black patients residing in nursing homes are less likely to have reported pain documentation and are less likely to receive pain management than White patients.[58] Black patients are also at higher risk of developing pressure sores than White patients, which was linked to the fact that nursing homes serving a high concentration of Black patients have lower staffing levels and tend to be larger, for-profit, and urban facilities.[59] Early funding and policy decisions shaped by racism, such as government certification of facilities that participate in Medicare and Medicaid but continue to use discriminatory practices to deny admission to members of racial and ethnic minority groups, continue to perpetuate these inequities.[59]

Despite a large population of patients in nursing homes in the United States (approximately 700,000 residents), an estimated 10–20% have only modest levels of need for personal care assistance and can thus be cared for at home with minimal support.[60] Home-based care is cheaper than nursing home care for patients who need more minimal assistance, such as those who need help getting out of bed, starting the day, and tending to personal care. However, the extent to which Medicaid programs fund home care varies significantly by state, and patients are often faced with long waiting periods for services. The future remains uncertain as the need for long-term care grows with an aging population met by an underfunded nursing home infrastructure.

Conclusion

Bringing It All Together

Despite the many challenges in identifying, characterizing, and effectively treating pain in older adults, exceptional pain management is well within reach. The 5Ms geriatric assessment tool presented in this chapter is a mechanism to guide providers and interdisciplinary team members in the development of multifactorial interventions that address the unique risk factor profiles and patterns of health care needs encountered in older adults with multimorbidity, frailty, and disability. Integrated geriatric assessment can be performed in the clinical setting over a series of visits. To demonstrate the 5Ms model at work, a case example of an older adult patient with chronic pain is presented in the Case Example. Over the course of several clinic visits, implementation of multiple pain treatment modalities, and involvement of interdisciplinary team members to address patient needs, the patient is able to remain in her home living independently with adequate pain control despite significant symptom burden and multiple barriers to care. Biopsychosocially complex cases are the rule and not the exception in geriatrics, and when we can meet patients' goals in the face of these challenges, the benefits are that much more profound.

Case Example: Pain Assessment Utilizing the 5Ms of Geriatrics

Case details: Mrs. Woods is a 78-year-old female with a past medical history of obesity, hypertension, hypothyroidism, sleep apnea, opioid use disorder in remission, chronic low back pain due to lumbar stenosis on opioids, polyarticular osteoarthritis, fibromyalgia, and depression. She presents to the geriatrics clinic for routine follow-up with complaints of poorly controlled pain in her lower back and knees that is limiting her ability to ambulate. The pain is dull and aching in quality, and it is fairly constant but worse with any mobility. She suffered a recent mechanical fall with resultant injury to her left knee, which is now swollen. Mrs. Woods is tearful, explaining she "cannot go on like this any longer" and feels that "life with so much pain is not worth living." She asks for your help with pain relief.

Mobility: Mrs. Woods explains that she has been using a cane inside her small two-bedroom apartment instead of the walker that was prescribed due to significant clutter. You observe that when walking into your clinic room, she is wincing and hunched forward with an antalgic gait and is using the cane in her left hand. She seems out of breath when she reaches her chair and takes more than 20 s to stand up and walk to the exam table. She explains that grooming herself has been challenging and that although she does have a shower chair, she fears she may fall when stepping into her tub. She has been frequently eating frozen dinners to avoid doing dishes. She relies on a friend in her building who helps bring groceries once weekly because she can no longer do this on her own. She gets to appointments using a ride service through her insurance, but she seldom leaves her home otherwise. She has normal hearing and wears corrective lenses that are up-to-date. She had bilateral cataracts that were surgically treated.

Medication: She takes oxycodone 10 mg approximately five or six times daily and has been on this for nearly 10 years since her decompressive lumbar back surgery. She is worried because she has feelings of withdrawal when she misses a dose and also feels she has lost some control over how she takes the oxycodone. She occasionally uses two tabs even when the pain is not severe. She has never run out of medication early because she "stretches" the medication over the course of the month. The oxycodone provides some relief when her pain is severe, from approximately 9/10 to 7/10. She has not used heroin in more than 30 years and does not drink alcohol or use other nonprescribed drugs. She is not using acetaminophen because she does not think it works. When asked how she took it in the past, she says she tried a 650 mg dose one or two times daily with no effect. She also tried an adequate dose of gabapentin for radicular back pain but stopped using it because she believed it stopped working. Mrs. Woods also takes five other medications for blood pressure, depression, thyroid, and low vitamin D.

Mind and mood: Mrs. Woods shares that her mood has been very low because she can no longer do the things she enjoys, such as leaving her home and spending time with friends. Her closest friend is very ill and now living in a nursing home. She has some friends in her apartment building; however, the usual senior programming was suspended due to the COVID-19 pandemic and has not resumed. Her sister calls her nearly every day to check in, but Mrs. Woods does not want to upset her sister with her problems because her sister is caring for her husband, who has dementia. Mrs. Woods feels very lonely. Although she feels her life has little meaning, she is future-oriented and is hopeful that as the weather gets warmer, she may be able to spend more time outside of her home. Mrs. Woods has had normal cognitive screening and has no concerns about her memory. She manages her own medications and is able to handle her finances.

Multicomplexity: Mrs. Woods has multiple medical issues, including the need for continuous positive airway pressure (CPAP) machine nightly. She did not wear her CPAP for almost 6 months because it was uncomfortable, so the device was reclaimed. Since stopping her CPAP, she has felt more tired due to disrupted sleep and is frequently taking daytime naps. She also takes a diuretic for her blood pressure and requires frequent nighttime trips to the bathroom. She has experienced urge incontinence and has had several near falls when ambulating in her dark apartment overnight.

Matters most: Mrs. Woods lives alone in an elevator building in an urban neighborhood. She was never married, has no children, and worked as a teacher in the public school system. She has a sister who lives out of state whom she keeps in close touch with, and she has appointed her sister as her health care proxy. She cannot afford home health care and is not eligible for Medicaid due to receiving a modest monthly pension. She has Medicare with a supplemental plan with multiple coverage limitations, and she has had difficulty finding a physical therapy facility that accepts her plan. Mrs. Woods worries about what will happen if her function declines further. When reflecting on her sister's difficult experience with caregiving for her husband with dementia, Mrs. Woods says, "I can't imagine how difficult life would be if I didn't have my mind, if I couldn't recognize the people around me." She shares that her mother died of pancreatic cancer and had a difficult prolonged hospitalization before being discharged to a nursing home, where she died. "I would never want to be on machines the way my mother was. She was in so much pain. When it's my time, I want to go in peace."

Assessment/plan: You acknowledge the key goal for today's visit by summarizing all that Mrs. Woods has shared, namely the goals for improved pain relief, physical functioning, and social connectedness. You share concern for her use of oxycodone and discuss the alternative of buprenorphine as a safer opioid with fewer side effects. After a discussion about risks and benefits, she agrees to rotate from oxycodone to buprenorphine. You also review pain adjuvants, including a 1-week course of celecoxib for her acute knee pain with a plan to transition to standing acetaminophen up to 3 g daily thereafter. You prescribe diclofenac gel for bilateral knees, which she has never tried. You explain that physical therapy will be important for her deconditioning, gait instability, strengthening, and fall prevention. You refer her to the local visiting nurse service for home physical therapy, home safety evaluation, and evaluation for a home health aide. You instruct her to use her cane in the hand opposite to her painful knee, and you adjust the height of the cane to align the top with the crease of her wrist. Based on your assessment, she would benefit from a shower chair, shower bar, and raised toilet seat. You recommend follow-up with Sleep Medicine to get her CPAP reinstated because poor sleep may be contributing to low mood, energy, and pain tolerance. In addition, you refer Mrs. Woods to your social worker to discuss the option of transitioning to Medicaid. You review advance care planning and resolve to address this more in depth at her next visit. You will see her in follow-up at 1 week to determine how she is tolerating the transition to buprenorphine and check in about her pain.

Geriatric assessment is increasingly being incorporated across multiple specialities, including in primary care, surgery, mental health, and addiction care, and it has great potential to inform and enhance pain management in addition to many other aspects of whole-person care. There is a growing need to standardize, measure, and report on pain outcomes among older adults. Research is needed to define the impact of both individual and overlapping pain conditions, characterize with more granularity which risk factors increase risks of pain in older adults, and better characterize the longitudinal trajectories of pain across various settings of care. Significant reform is required at the health system level to reimagine and rebuild long-term care systems for patients among whom pain is highly prevalent and a driver of functional decline and disability. Long-term care systems face considerable challenges and will look very different in a post-pandemic world in ways that we cannot yet know. Nevertheless, it is abundantly clear that the imperative to address the burden of pain is inextricably linked with our larger efforts to support the independence and quality of life of older adults.

References

1. Simon LS. Relieving pain in America: A blueprint for transforming prevention, care, education, and research. *J Pain Palliat Care Pharmacother.* 2012;26(2):197–198. doi:10.3109/15360288.2012.678473
2. Abdulla A, Adams N, Bone M, et al. Guidance on the management of pain in older people. *Age Ageing.* 2013;42(Suppl 1):i1–i57. doi:10.1093/ageing/afs200
3. Weiner DK. Office management of chronic pain in the elderly. *Am J Med.* 2007;120(4):306–315. doi:10.1016/j.amjmed.2006.05.048
4. Esses G, Deiner S, Ko F, Khelemsky Y. Chronic post-surgical pain in the frail older adult. *Drugs Aging.* 2020;37(5):321–329. doi:10.1007/s40266-020-00761-2
5. Horgas AL. Pain management in older adults. *Nurs Clin North Am.* 2017;52(4):e1–e7. doi:10.1016/j.cnur.2017.08.001
6. Tinnirello A, Mazzoleni S, Santi C. Chronic pain in the elderly: Mechanisms and distinctive features. *Biomolecules.* 2021;11(8):1256. doi:10.3390/biom11081256
7. Resnick NM, Marcantonio ER. How should clinical care of the aged differ? *Lancet.* 1997;350(9085):1157–1158. http://dx.doi.org/10.1016/S0140-6736(05)63817-2
8. Rajan J, Behrends M. Acute pain in older adults. *Anesthesiol Clin.* 2019;37(3):507–520. doi:10.1016/j.anclin.2019.04.009
9. Robeck I. Chronic pain in the elderly: Special challenges. *Pract Pain Manag.* 2014;12(2). https://www.practicalpainmanagement.com/pain/chronic-pain-elderly-special-challenges
10. Morrison RS, Flanagan S, Fischberg D, Cintron A, Siu AL. A novel interdisciplinary analgesic program reduces pain and improves function in older adults after orthopedic surgery. *J Am Geriatr Soc.* 2009;57(1):1–10. doi:10.1111/j.1532-5415.2008.02063.x
11. Miaskowski C, Blyth F, Nicosia F, et al. A biopsychosocial model of chronic pain for older adults. *Pain Med.* 2020;21(9):1793–1805. doi:10.1093/pm/pnz329
12. Henschke N, Kamper SJ, Maher CG. The epidemiology and economic consequences of pain. *Mayo Clin Proc.* 2015;90(1):139–147. doi:10.1016/j.mayocp.2014.09.010
13. Leipzig RM, Whitlock EP, Wolff TA, et al. Reconsidering the approach to prevention recommendations for older adults. *Ann Intern Med.* 2010;153(12):809–814. doi:10.7326/0003-4819-153-12-201012210-00007
14. Molnar F, Frank CC. Optimizing geriatric care with the GERIATRIC 5Ms. *Can Fam Physician.* 2019;65(1): Article 39.

15. Patel KV, Phelan EA, Leveille SG, et al. Prevalence and impact of pain among older adults in the United States: Findings from the 2011 National Health and Aging Trends Study. *Pain*. 2013;154(12):2649–2657. doi:10.1016/j.pain.2013.07.029
16. Blyth FM, Rochat S, Cumming RG, et al. Pain, frailty and comorbidity on older men: The CHAMP study. *Pain*. 2008;140(1):224–230. doi:10.1016/j.pain.2008.08.011
17. Cobbs EL, Duthie EH, Murphy JB. *Geriatrics Review Syllabus: A Core Curriculum in Geriatric Medicine*. Wiley; 2002.
18. Kaye AD, Baluch A, Scott JT. Pain management in the elderly population: A review. *Ochsner J*. 2010;10(3):179–187.
19. Park J, Hughes AK. Nonpharmacological approaches to the management of chronic pain in community-dwelling older adults: A review of empirical evidence. *J Am Geriatr Soc*. 2012;60(3):555–568.
20. Jarvik JG, Deyo RA. Diagnostic evaluation of low back pain with emphasis on imaging. *Ann Intern Med*. 2002;137(7):586–597. doi:10.7326/0003-4819-137-7-200210010-00010
21. Flint LA, David DJ, Smith AK. Rehabbed to death. *N Engl J Med*. 2019;380(5):408–409. doi:10.1056/NEJMp1809354
22. Wastesson JW, Morin L, Tan ECK, Johnell K. An update on the clinical consequences of polypharmacy in older adults: A narrative review. *Expert Opin Drug Saf*. 2018;17(12):1185–1196. doi:10.1080/14740338.2018.1546841
23. Nunnari P, Ceccarelli G, Ladiana N, Notaro P. Prescribing cascades and medications most frequently involved in pain therapy: A review. *Eur Rev Med Pharmacol Sci*. 2021;25(2):1034–1041. doi:10.26355/eurrev_202101_24673
24. Hoel RW, Giddings Connolly RM, Takahashi PY. Polypharmacy management in older patients. *Mayo Clin Proc*. 2021;96(1):242–256. doi:10.1016/j.mayocp.2020.06.012
25. Schofield P, Dunham M, Martin D, et al. Evidence-based clinical practice guidelines on the management of pain in older people: A summary report. *Br J Pain*. 2022;16(1):6–13. doi:10.1177/2049463720976155
26. 2019 American Geriatrics Society Beers Criteria Update Expert Panel. American Geriatrics Society 2019 updated AGS Beers Criteria for potentially inappropriate medication use in older adults. *J Am Geriatr Soc*. 2019;67(4):674–694. doi:10.1111/jgs.15767
27. Makris UE, Abrams RC, Gurland B, Reid MC. Management of persistent pain in the older patient: A clinical review. *JAMA*. 2014;312(8):825–837. doi:10.1001/jama.2014.9405
28. Merlin JS, Patel K, Thompson N, et al. Managing chronic pain in cancer survivors prescribed long-term opioid therapy: A national survey of ambulatory palliative care providers. *J Pain Symptom Manage*. 2019;57(1):20–27. doi:10.1016/j.jpainsymman.2018.10.493
29. Dufort A, Samaan Z. Problematic opioid use among older adults: Epidemiology, adverse outcomes and treatment considerations. *Drugs Aging*. 2021;38(12):1043–1053. doi:10.1007/s40266-021-00893-z
30. Yap AF, Thirumoorthy T, Kwan YH. Systematic review of the barriers affecting medication adherence in older adults. *Geriatr Gerontol Int*. 2016;16(10):1093–1101. doi:10.1111/ggi.12616
31. Morrison RS, Wallenstein S, Natale DK, Senzel RS, Huang LL. "We don't carry that": Failure of pharmacies in predominantly nonwhite neighborhoods to stock opioid analgesics. *N Engl J Med*. 2000;342(14):1023–1026. doi:10.1056/NEJM200004063421406
32. Zis P, Daskalaki A, Bountouni I, Sykioti P, Varrassi G, Paladini A. Depression and chronic pain in the elderly: Links and management challenges. *Clin Interv Aging*. 2017;12:709–720. doi:10.2147/CIA.S113576
33. Quartana PJ, Campbell CM, Edwards RR. Pain catastrophizing: A critical review. *Expert Rev Neurother*. 2009;9(5):745–758. doi:10.1586/ERN.09.34
34. Ruscheweyh R, Nees F, Marziniak M, Evers S, Flor H, Knecht S. Pain catastrophizing and pain-related emotions: Influence of age and type of pain. *Clin J Pain*. 2011;27(7):578–586. doi:10.1097/AJP.0b013e31820fde1b

35. Zhaoyang R, Martire LM, Darnall BD. Daily pain catastrophizing predicts less physical activity and more sedentary behavior in older adults with osteoarthritis. *Pain.* 2020;161(11):2603–2610. doi:10.1097/j.pain.0000000000001959
36. Scherder EJA, Plooij B. Assessment and management of pain, with particular emphasis on central neuropathic pain, in moderate to severe dementia. *Drugs Aging.* 2012;29(9):701–706. doi:10.1007/s40266-012-0001-8
37. Pan X, Meng H. Pain management and cognitive function among older adults: An exploratory study of the China Health and Retirement Longitudinal Study. *Aging Clin Exp Res.* 2020;32(12):2611–2620. doi:10.1007/s40520-020-01491-6
38. Reynolds CF, Lenze E, Mulsant BH. Assessment and treatment of major depression in older adults. *Handb Clin Neurol.* 2019;167:429–435. doi:10.1016/B978-0-12-804766-8.00023-6
39. Krishnamoorthy Y, Rajaa S, Rehman T. Diagnostic accuracy of various forms of geriatric depression scale for screening of depression among older adults: Systematic review and meta-analysis. *Arch Gerontol Geriatr.* 2020;87:104002. doi:10.1016/j.archger.2019.104002
40. Schwan J, Sclafani J, Tawfik VL. Chronic pain management in the elderly. *Anesthesiol Clin.* 2019;37(3):547–560. doi:10.1016/j.anclin.2019.04.012
41. Milisen K, Braes T, Fick DM, Foreman MD. Cognitive assessment and differentiating the 3 Ds (dementia, depression, delirium). *Nurs Clin North Am.* 2006;41(1):1–22. doi:10.1016/j.cnur.2005.09.001
42. Hadjistavropoulos T, Gallant N. Pain in older adults: Caregiver challenges. In: Vervoort T, Karos K, Trost Z, Prkachin KM, eds. Social and Interpersonal Dynamics in Pain: We Don't Suffer Alone. Springer; 2018:415–429. doi:10.1007/978-3-319-78340-6_19
43. Gyurmey T, Kwiatkowski J. Program of All-Inclusive Care for the Elderly (PACE): Integrating health and social care since 1973. *R I Med J.* 2019;102(5):30–32.
44. Altman D, Frist WH. Medicare and Medicaid at 50 years: Perspectives of beneficiaries, health care professionals and institutions, and policy makers. *JAMA.* 2015;314(4):384–395. doi:10.1001/jama.2015.7811
45. American Geriatrics Society Expert Panel on the Care of Older Adults with Multimorbidity. Patient-centered care for older adults with multiple chronic conditions: A stepwise approach from the American Geriatrics Society. *J Am Geriatr Soc.* 2012;60(10):1957–1968. doi:10.1111/j.1532-5415.2012.04187.x
46. Baker TA, Clay OJ, Johnson-Lawrence V, et al. Association of multiple chronic conditions and pain among older Black and White adults with diabetes mellitus. *BMC Geriatr.* 2017;17(1): Article 255. doi:10.1186/s12877-017-d0652-8
47. Feder SL, Canavan ME, Wang S, et al. Patterns of opioid prescribing among Medicare Advantage beneficiaries with pain and cardiopulmonary conditions. *J Palliat Med.* 2021;24(2):195–204. doi:10.1089/jpm.2020.0193
48. Thapa S, Shmerling RH, Bean JF, Cai Y, Leveille SG. Chronic multisite pain: Evaluation of a new geriatric syndrome. *Aging Clin Exp Res.* 2019;31(8):1129–1137. doi:10.1007/s40520-018-1061-3
49. Guerriero F, Reid MC. Linking persistent pain and frailty in older adults. *Pain Med.* 2020;21(1):61–66. doi:10.1093/pm/pnz174
50. Esses GJ, Liu X, Lin HM, Khelemsky Y, Deiner S. Preoperative frailty and its association with postsurgical pain in an older patient cohort. *Reg Anesth Pain Med.* 2019;44(7):695–699. doi:10.1136/rapm-2018-100247
51. Aggarwal P, Woolford SJ, Patel HP. Multi-morbidity and polypharmacy in older people: Challenges and opportunities for clinical practice. *Geriatr Basel.* 2020;5(4): Article 85. doi:10.3390/geriatrics5040085
52. Tinetti ME, Esterson J, Ferris R, Posner P, Blaum CS. Patient priority-directed decision making and care for older adults with multiple chronic conditions. *Clin Geriatr Med.* 2016;32(2):261–275. doi:10.1016/j.cger.2016.01.012
53. Herzig SJ, Anderson TS, Jung Y, Ngo L, Kim DH, McCarthy EP. Relative risks of adverse events among older adults receiving opioids versus NSAIDs after hospital discharge: A nationwide cohort study. *PLoS Med.* 2021;18(9):e1003804. doi:10.1371/journal.pmed.1003804

54. Tomlinson J, Cheong VL, Fylan B, et al. Successful care transitions for older people: A systematic review and meta-analysis of the effects of interventions that support medication continuity. *Age Ageing*. 2020;49(4):558–569. doi:10.1093/ageing/afaa002
55. Fried TR, Tinetti ME, Iannone L, O'Leary JR, Towle V, Van Ness PH. Health outcome prioritization as a tool for decision making among older persons with multiple chronic conditions. *Arch Intern Med.* 2011;171(20):1856–1858. doi:10.1001/archinternmed.2011.424
56. Rivera-Hernandez M, Rahman M, Mukamel DB, Mor V, Trivedi AN. Quality of post-acute care in skilled nursing facilities that disproportionately serve Black and Hispanic patients. *J Gerontol A Biol Sci Med Sci.* 2019;74(5):689–697. doi:10.1093/gerona/gly089
57. Yon Y, Ramiro-Gonzalez M, Mikton CR, Huber M, Sethi D. The prevalence of elder abuse in institutional settings: A systematic review and meta-analysis. *Eur J Public Health.* 2019;29(1):58–67. doi:10.1093/eurpub/cky093
58. Mack DS, Hunnicutt JN, Jesdale BM, Lapane KL. Non-Hispanic Black–White disparities in pain and pain management among newly admitted nursing home residents with cancer. *J Pain Res.* 2018;11:753–761. doi:10.2147/JPR.S158128
59. Yearby R, Clark B, Figueroa JF. Structural racism in historical and modern US health care policy. *Health Aff.* 2022;41(2):187–194. doi:10.1377/hlthaff.2021.01466
60. Long-Term Services & Supports State Scorecard. AARP Foundation, The Commonwealth Fund, The SCAN Foundation, and AARP Foundation. 2022. Accessed July 9, 2022. https://www.longtermscorecard.org

7
Pain in Women

*Keisha G. Dodman, Allison M. Berken, and Antje M. Barreveld**

Introduction

Although gender equality has significantly evolved over centuries, sociocultural disparities as well as important biological differences persist between women and men. Recognizing biological differences as well as potential biases toward women is essential to providing optimal health care. This is especially evident in women's acute and chronic pain experiences and treatment.

Many barriers to pain care in this vulnerable population exist.[1] Over the long history of medicine and medical research, women have been largely excluded as subjects but also as physicians, scientists, and researchers. The result has been a great deficiency in our understanding of many female-predominant diseases. Providers often do not address or manage women's pain, both acute and chronic, in the same way as they do men's pain, and women with chronic pain often feel psychologically dismissed.[1] This chapter highlights the genetic, biological, and psychosocial differences for women with pain and emphasizes pain care vulnerabilities in this population. The chapter provides a brief review of pain states specific to the female sex and chronic pain diseases more commonly seen in women. It is important for the health care community to recognize biases, gendered norms, and barriers to pain care in women to guarantee improved access to contemporary, informed, and compassionate diagnosis and treatment.

What Makes Women More Vulnerable to Pain?

Evidence is mounting that female patients experience pain differently than their male counterparts. Women are more likely to suffer from chronic pain, self-report higher levels of pain, endure pain of longer duration, and report pain more frequently than men.[2] Although this may have do with their predisposition to uniquely female pain syndromes (i.e., endometriosis and child birth), there are also data emerging that women feel painful stimuli more intensely. For instance, regarding acute surgical pain, current data support that women have higher levels of pain after cardiac surgery and total knee arthroplasty.[3,4] An analysis of a large electronic medical record database showed that women report more pain for almost every diagnosis than men—including musculoskeletal, circulatory, respiratory, digestive, and infectious diseases, among

These authors contributed equally to this work.

* Keisha G. Dodman and Allison M. Berken contributed equally to this work.

others.[5] Other groups have previously reported sex differences in neuropathic pain, musculoskeletal pain, abdominal pain, and migraines, with women consistently reporting higher pain levels than men. However, for certain conditions such as cancer pain, no such difference appears to exist.[6] In addition to clinical differences in reported pain, research suggests that women experience higher sensitivity to experimentally induced pain as well. Several studies have examined various types of pain, including pressure, heat, cold, and electrical stimuli, and found that women have higher sensitivity to almost all inputs.[6] Proposed mechanisms for these differences in the pain experience have included biological sex differences such as genetic, hormonal, and immunological factors, as well as cultural and psychosocial factors.

Discussion

Genetics and Chronic Pain in Women

Genetics plays a prominent role in the vulnerability of women to chronic pain conditions, including chronic pelvic pain and chronic widespread pain.[7–9] More than 150 genes associated with chronic pain states have been identified.[10] Twin studies indicate that as much as 40% of the variance in chronic pelvic pain prevalence is genetically based.[9,11] Twin studies have also implicated genetics as the substrate for a range of other chronic pain syndromes, including chronic widespread musculoskeletal pain and irritable bowel syndrome (IBS).[9]

Research has also focused on identifying single nucleotide polymorphisms (SNPs) that confer sex-specific vulnerability to chronic pain. A 2021 sex-stratified genome-wide association study of multisite chronic pain (MCP) found more than 100 SNPs associated with MCP in men and nearly 300 SNPs associated with MCP in women—evidence that sex differences in SNPs are reflected in pain susceptibility.[12]

Two of the most extensively studied pain-related SNP variants are for polymorphic catechol-*O*-methyltransferase (*COMT*) and the opioid receptor μ_1 (*OPRM1*) genes, both of which have been implicated in chronic pelvic pain.[13,14] *COMT* is a neuromodulator involved in the breakdown of catecholamines, including dopamine, epinephrine, and norepinephrine, that appears to play a role in the perception of and sensitivity to pain.[13] *OPRM1* encodes the μ-opioid receptor, a protein that mediates the analgesic effects of opioids in the central nervous system.[7,15]

Hormones and Chronic Pain in Women

Population-based studies across multiple geographic regions have demonstrated a greater prevalence of chronic pain conditions among women than men. Evidence suggests that gonadal steroid hormones are, at least in part, responsible for some of the observed differences. A similar pain prevalence has been shown for prepubescent boys and girls, with a shift to female predominance during and following puberty.[16] Data relating phases of the menstrual cycle to pain threshold have shown increased pain responses to higher estradiol levels.[17] Testosterone, on the other hand, seems to be anti-nociceptive. Testosterone levels appears to be inversely correlated with the risk of chronic pain.[18] Interesting data relating to the differential effects of sex hormones on pain response comes from a study of transgender individuals undergoing hormonal treatment. Nearly 30% of males transitioning to female and receiving estradiol and anti-androgen treatment developed a chronic pain condition, whereas more than 60% of females transitioning to men, treated with testosterone, experienced a reduction in their pretreatment chronic pain (mostly headache) symptoms.[19] These findings support the notion that the administration of estrogens increases vulnerability to pain, whereas the withdrawal of estrogens decreases the risk.[19,20]

The Immune System and Chronic Pain in Women

Immune mechanisms also play a role in chronic pain states. Microglia, macrophage-derived cells that are involved in many pain processing pathways, have been implicated in the establishment of neuropathic allodynia through their effects on synaptic plasticity.[21–23] Investigations have determined that mast cells in the central and peripheral nervous system also play a role in the development of chronic neuropathic pain and are believed to interact with microglia.[24] This communication appears to be through toll-like receptor (TLR) signaling pathways, especially TLR2 and TLR4. TLRs are transmembrane receptors that recognize pathogens and patterns of ligands associated with tissue damage and cell death.[25]

Psychology and Chronic Pain in Women

Clinical and neuroimaging studies of pain in women and men have provided strong evidence of greater pain sensitivity and reduced pain inhibition in women.[26] Although the exact role of sex differences in the experience of pain has yet to be established, psychosocial mechanisms, including sociocultural perspectives relating to masculine and feminine behavioral stereotypes, appear to influence pain perception.[26,27] Studies of pain sensitivity across cultures suggest that different valences of gender roles are reflected in the degree to which male versus female pain sensitivity manifests.[28] In addition, the prevalence and severity of chronic pain are associated with coexisting affective disorders, most commonly anxiety, depression, and post-traumatic stress disorder (PTSD).[29,30] It is likely that depression and/or anxiety promotes the establishment of a chronic pain syndrome and that the inverse is true as well.[29,31] It is estimated that, on average, 65% of patients diagnosed with depression have chronic pain as a comorbidity.[32] PTSD following a history of physical or sexual abuse, assault, or major trauma is a type of anxiety disorder that is highly associated with chronic pain.[33,34] Adverse childhood experiences are associated with an increased incidence of chronic pain in adulthood.[34]

Cultural Inequities and Chronic Pain in Women

The societal and cultural perception of women's pain has also led to significant inequities in research, treatment, and barriers to care. These disparities date back many thousands of years to the origin of the word "hysteria," from the Greek word for "uterus"—*hystera*. Throughout history, many unexplainable or mysterious female medical maladies have been attributed to "hysteria" and believed to be more psychiatric in nature rather than truly medical. In the late 1800s, Sigmund Freud developed his now famous hypothesis that hysteria was a primarily female disorder related to a " 'psychological scar produced through trauma or repression." Hysteria continued to be a diagnosis and concept recognized by the medical community until the 1980s, when the word was removed from the *Diagnostic and Statistical Manual of Mental Disorders*.[35]

Evidence that the medical community persistently treats women's pain differently than their male counterparts continues to build. In Karen Calderone's[36] 1990 study, she examined postoperative pain management after cardiac surgery. She found that female patients were significantly more likely to be prescribed sedatives than male patients, and male patients were significantly more likely to be prescribed analgesics than their female counterparts. Even when controlled for age and surgery, medical professionals were more likely to view female complaints of pain as anxiety or other psychological symptoms, whereas men with the same symptoms were treated for pain. A more recent study in the emergency department setting found that among patients presenting with abdominal pain, women were significantly less likely to receive any analgesia and significantly less likely to receive opioids despite similar baseline pain scores reported in men.[37] Women also had a longer wait time to receive any analgesia.[37]

Historically, both bench and clinical research studies have vastly excluded women. Including female subjects requires coordination and controlling for hormonal fluctuations, menstruation, the possibility of pregnancy or lactation, and accounting for possible sex and gender differences in eventual analyses of findings. As a result, most research efforts have exclusively enrolled male subjects, leading to a further disparity in our ability to understand and better treat women's acute and chronic pain conditions. In 1993, Congress wrote the National Institute of Health Inclusion Policy mandating inclusion of women in clinical trials as federal law.[38] Unfortunately, much of what we know and understand about pain processing and pain syndromes comes from studies completed long before the inclusion of women in most research efforts. Ethical considerations regarding inclusion of pregnant or lactating women in experimental trials usually result in their exclusion to this day.

An Illness Model for Pain in Women

Various pain states specific to the female sex or seen more commonly in women are reviewed below and summarized in Table 7.1.

Dysmenorrhea

Primary dysmenorrhea, the most common gynecological pain syndrome, is defined as menstrual pain in the absence of an identifiable pelvic pathology.[39–42] Symptoms begin before or at the onset of menses, with crampy lower abdominal pain, often radiating to

Table 7.1 Important Pain States in Women

Pain Diagnoses Specific to Females	Pain Diagnoses More Commonly Seen in Women versus Men
Dysmenorrhea	Pelvic floor muscle pain
Endometriosis	Post-mastectomy pain
Adenomyosis	Fibromyalgia
Vaginal pain/Vulvodynia	Interstitial cystitis/painful bladder syndrome
	Pudendal neuralgia
	Migraine headache Irritable bowel syndrome

the lower back or thighs, with a duration of less than 72 h. Nausea and vomiting, headache, and dizziness are often associated symptoms.[39–42] Its prevalence ranges from 17% to as high as 81% depending on the definition and severity.[40] It is likely underreported because many women consider pelvic pain as part of the normal menstrual cycle.[39–41] Secondary dysmenorrhea presents clinically like primary dysmenorrhea, and associated pathologies include endometriosis, adenomyosis, pelvic inflammatory disease, and the use of some intrauterine contraceptive devices.[43]

The diagnosis of primary and/or secondary dysmenorrhea is based on history and pelvic examination.[44] The etiology of primary dysmenorrhea is believed to be due in large part to the hypersecretion of prostaglandin F2α ($PGF_2α$) and prostaglandin FGF2 by the uterine endometrium, which increase uterine tone and contractions and lower the threshold for pain perception.[39]

Nonsteroidal anti-inflammatory drugs (NSAIDs) are the first-line treatment of dysmenorrhea.[45] Oral contraceptives have shown efficacy in adolescents, presumably by reducing the production of prostaglandins.[46]

Endometriosis

Endometriosis is defined as the presence of endometrial glands and stroma outside of the uterine cavity. This ectopic tissue chiefly occurs in the pelvis but may occur in other areas, such as the ovary (endometrioma), bowel and bladder serosa, and pleural cavity.[47] Endometriosis predominantly affects women during their reproductive years, peaking between ages 25 and 35 years.[48] The associated inflammation can result in significant pelvic pain, dyspareunia, and infertility.[47] The prevalence in reproductive-age females is approximately 10%.[49] Although the pathogenesis of endometriosis has not firmly been elucidated, the most prevalent theory is that of retrograde menstruation, where endometrial cells enter the peritoneal cavity via the fallopian tubes.[50,51]

The pain of endometriosis can be debilitating, with the predominant symptoms being dysmenorrhea and deep dyspareunia.[52] The type of pain experience correlates with the loci of endometrial implants. The diagnosis of endometriosis can be made clinically in some instances, especially if nodularity can be felt on pelvic exam in the case of vaginal involvement.[47] However, histologic diagnosis requires laparoscopic surgery, although noninvasive methods, such as transvaginal ultrasound and biomarkers, are being evaluated.[53]

The treatment of endometriosis pain depends on a woman's symptomology and treatment goals. Endometriomas of significant size are generally excised, and peritoneal implants can be laser coagulated or excised.[54] Nonsurgical therapies involve the inhibition of ovulation and menstruation. Gonadotropin-releasing hormone agonists, androgens, and hyperprogestogenic oral contraceptives have all been shown to suppress endometrial cell proliferation.[47] Targeted therapies aimed at suppressing the signaling pathways of endometriosis are being evaluated.[55]

Note that the treatment of the endometriosis pain is not just hormonal. A multimodal interdisciplinary approach that is tailored to each patient's symptom complex is advantageous. Complementary therapies may include pelvic floor physical therapy, trigger point injections, massage, and muscle relaxant suppositories. Psychosocial therapy, including cognitive–behavioral therapy focusing on coping Mechanisms, and biofeedback are often helpful adjuncts.[56]

Adenomyosis

Adenomyosis is a benign disorder of the uterus characterized by the infiltration of the uterine myometrium by endometrial glands.[57] This invasion manifests as a diffusely enlarged uterus, chronic pelvic pain, dysmenorrhea, infertility, and abnormal uterine bleeding. Heavy menstrual bleeding occurs in 40–60% of patients, with dysmenorrhea in up to 30%.[58] The severity of symptoms depends on the degree of myometrial involvement and the depth of endometrial infiltration. Studies have revealed an increased production of prostaglandins by the endometrial tissue within the myometrium, a factor that may in part be responsible for symptoms of dysmenorrhea.[59]

The prevalence of this disorder is approximately 20–25% of women, with the majority of cases occurring in those aged between 40 and 50 years.[58] It is estimated that one-third of patients are asymptomatic.[58] Transvaginal ultrasound and pelvic magnetic resonance imaging (MRI) are useful nonsurgical diagnostic adjuncts and have accuracy, sensitivity, specificity, and positive predictive value in the 80% range.[60,61]

The therapeutic management of adenomyosis pain is broad, with hormonal therapies being prominent. Continuous-use oral contraceptives are often used to decrease menses and increase decidualization of the endometrium.[47] As with the approach to endometriosis, adjunctive treatments, including pelvic physical therapy and cognitive–behavioral therapy focusing on coping mechanisms, can be beneficial.[56]

Vaginal Pain, Vulvodynia, and Dyspareunia

Vaginal pain syndromes encompass all causes of vaginal and vulvar pain, whereas vulvodynia specifically refers to "vulvar discomfort, most often described as burning pain, occurring in the absence of relevant visible findings or a specific, clinically identifiable, neurologic disorder."[62] Dyspareunia refers to pain with penetrative sexual intercourse, and vaginal pain syndrome or vulvodynia can be a subtype of dyspareunia. The incidence of vulvodynia is estimated at approximately 8–10% of all women, it can occur at any age, and it has a significant negative impact on quality of life.[63]

Diagnosis of vulvodynia involves a thorough history, ruling out other medical causes, and a physical exam. Vaginal pain and/or vulvodynia can be further classified by the locations of pain and by whether symptoms are provoked by physical contact versus unprovoked or spontaneous.[64]

Treatment is aimed at multidisciplinary management, including vulvar care modifications (change in underwear and hygiene), pelvic floor physical therapy/biofeedback, cognitive–behavioral therapy, intravaginal medications (i.e., lidocaine, baclofen, and amitriptyline), or oral medications (i.e., neuropathic agents such as gabapentin, amitriptyline, and duloxetine).[62,65–67] Options with less definitive evidence but still some possibility of providing pain relief include injections such as intralesional injection, pudendal nerve blocks, and botulinum toxin injection. In rare cases, surgery such as vestibulectomy may be indicated.[62]

Fibromyalgia

Fibromyalgia is a syndrome of chronic multifocal pain with nonspecific findings such as fatigue, cognitive dysfunction, and sleep disturbance.[68] Frequently dismissed in the past as a psychosomatic disorder, fibromyalgia is now believed to be due to abnormalities in central pain processing leading to central sensitization to pain.[68–70] Its prevalence is estimated at 2–8% of the population.[71]

The diagnosis of fibromyalgia requires multisite pain (greater than six of nine body regions), duration of at least 3 months, sleep disturbance, and fatigue.[72] There is characteristic increased sensitivity to pressure and light touch that is perceived as allodynia and hyperalgesia.[68]

A multimodal approach is often used for patients with fibromyalgia. As the first-line approach, nonpharmacologic treatments are often considered as the most effective treatments for fibromyalgia and include exercise, relaxation techniques, massage therapy, and acupuncture.[73]

Although no medication is effective in all cases, many U.S. Food and Drug Administration (FDA)-approved medications and alternative therapies are part of the therapeutic armamentarium. To date, only the anticonvulsive pregabalin and the serotonin–norepinephrine reuptake inhibitors (SNRIs) duloxetine and milnacipran have been approved.[73,74]

Interstitial Cystitis/Bladder Pain Syndrome

Interstitial cystitis/bladder pain syndrome is a chronic pelvic pain disorder associated with painful urination. The prevalence is estimated to be approximately 1% or 2% in women.[75,76] Interstitial cystitis/bladder pain syndrome has a 5:1 to 10:1 female-to-male preponderance in most studies.[3] The pathophysiology remains unknown, but inflammation, mast cell activation, autoimmune mechanisms, and defects in abnormalities in the mucus layer of the bladder have all been implicated.[77,78] There is a strong genetic predisposition and a markedly increased prevalence of interstitial cystitis/bladder pain syndrome among first-degree female relatives.[79]

Diagnostic criteria include an increased sense of urgency and/or frequency, with chronic pain for at least 6 months, and a pressure sensation emanating from the bladder.[80] Conservative treatment is initially warranted, including the elimination of caffeine, carbonated beverages, and spicy foods because they may irritate the bladder wall.[81] Pentosan polysulfate sodium, a synthetic polysaccharide used to replace the defective glucosaminoglycans of patients with interstitial cystitis/bladder pain syndrome, has been shown to decrease symptoms.[82] Intravesical treatment with dimethyl sulfoxide and chondroitin sulfate have shown some positive effect.[81] Minimally invasive procedures such as intertrigonal injection of botulinum toxin A have also shown promise in refractory cases.[83] Sacral neuromodulation is FDA-approved for urinary frequency and urgency but may not be effective for treating bladder pain.

Pudendal Neuralgia

Pudendal neuralgia is a relatively rare neuropathic condition, generally presenting as a burning hyperalgesic pain in the dermatome of the pudendal nerve.[84] Although the prevalence is unknown, it has been estimated at approximately 1% of the population.[85] It occurs more commonly in woman than in men. The pain of pudendal neuralgia in women localizes to the vulva, vagina, clitoris, perineum, and rectum, whereas in men pain is experienced in the glans penis, scrotum, perineum, and rectum.[84] The pain distribution may be localized to one branch of the pudendal nerve dermatome or may extend over the entire nerve field.[85] Pudendal neuralgia is generally unilateral and is described as unremitting perineal pain that is significantly exacerbated by sitting, improved by lying down or standing, and worsening as the day progresses.[86,87] The condition is most often due to nerve entrapment by pelvic floor muscles, ligaments, or scar tissue following trauma.[87,88] In women, the most common antecedents are gynecological surgery, especially for prolapse, pelvic trauma, and vaginal childbirth.[89,90] Other causes include herpes simplex infection, chemoradiation, and intensive cycling or prolonged squatting.[84,91–93]

The Nantes criteria (Labat) are widely used for the diagnosis of pudendal neuralgia. They include pain in the pudendal nerve distribution, pain more severe when sitting, pain that awakens the patient from sleep, absence of sensory impairment, and pain relieved by a pudendal nerve block with local anesthetic.[85]

Initial management of pudendal neuralgia is nonpharmacologic, with physical therapy with stretching and muscle lengthening exercises.[86,89] Neuropathic agents, such as gabapentin and pregabalin, as well as tricyclic antidepressants have been effective in some instances, as has botulinum toxin type A.[89,94] Pudendal nerve block under fluoroscopy, computed tomography, or MRI guidance with local anesthetic and methylprednisolone or triamcinolone can be effective when more conservative measures have not been successful.[95,96] For refractory cases in which pudendal nerve entrapment is likely, surgical decompression is an alternative.[97]

Pelvic Floor Pain

Pelvic floor pain is a broad diagnosis that encompasses many different causes and symptoms of pelvic and perineal pain. The reported incidence of pelvic pain ranges widely from 3% to 24%, probably in part due to the lack of specific diagnostic criteria or recognized symptomology.[98] Pain can be acute or chronic in nature and may involve a neuropathic component or central sensitization. Pelvic floor–related pain can coexist with other diagnoses, including interstitial cystitis, pudendal neuralgia, endometriosis, IBS, and vulvodynia.[99,100] In some cases, it may also be an isolated musculoskeletal pain syndrome with no discernable cause. There does appear to be some association with history of sexual trauma or PTSD.[34]

The mainstay of treatment involves pelvic floor physical therapy. In some cases, interventional options may be helpful, such as pudendal nerve block, pelvic floor trigger point injections, pelvic floor botulinum toxin injection, or obturator internus muscle injection.[102,103] Oral medications have mixed efficacy, but a trial of oral NSAIDs and/or neuropathic medications (gabapentin, pregabalin, SNRI, or tricyclic antidepressant) may be worthwhile.[103] Vaginal or rectal muscle relaxants such as valium or baclofen suppositories also may provide meaningful pain relief in some cases.[104] Involvement of pain psychology can be helpful in all cases, but particularly in cases with concurrent anxiety, depression, or trauma history. Psychological treatment strategies vary but may include cognitive–behavioral therapy, mindfulness, or biofeedback to reduce pain-related fear, anxiety, and catastrophizing.[105,106]

Post-Mastectomy Pain

Post-mastectomy pain syndrome is defined as chronic pain after mastectomy that "persists beyond the normal healing time of 3 months."[107] It involves aching, burning, or shooting pain or other unpleasant sensation in the region of the anterior chest wall, thorax, or arm on the ipsilateral side.[107,108] Although it was previously considered uncommon, the incidence is now estimated to be approximately 20–50%.[107–109] The presentation is becoming increasingly more common as breast cancer survival rates increase and genetic testing allows for prophylactic mastectomies.[108] Studies suggest that many factors are associated with development of post-mastectomy pain syndrome, including younger age, axillary lymph node dissection, adjunctive treatment (radiation and chemotherapy), racial minority status, pre-existing pain condition, psychological factors such as depression and anxiety, and acute post-procedure pain after surgery.[108] Although direct damage to the intercostobrachial nerve has been previously implicated, recent evidence is less clear on whether nerve injury might play a role.[108]

Treatment for post-mastectomy pain typically begins with nonpharmacological or interventional options such as physical therapy and pain psychology. Pain psychology strategies are theorized to reduce centrally mediated mechanisms of pain.[110] First-line pharmacological treatment is similar to that for other neuropathic pain conditions and includes acetaminophen, NSAIDs, gabapentin/pregabalin, tricyclic antidepressants, selective serotonin reuptake inhibitors, and SNRIs.[111] Randomized control trials support gabapentin, amitriptyline, and venlafaxine in particular.Click or tap here to enter text.[110] There is evidence that venlafaxine reduces chronic post-mastectomy pain when administered perioperatively.[112] Second-line therapy may include topicals such as capsaicin and lidocaine. Surgical treatment of post-mastectomy pain syndrome with autologous fat grafting has been found in some studies to provide significant pain relief, whereas in other studies it has been found to provide no improvement over sham surgery.[111,113] Studies have also found that regional anesthesia (i.e., paravertebral block) at the time of mastectomy surgery results in lower chronic pain at 1 year following the operation.[114,115]

Migraine Headaches

Although migraines and other severe headaches can affect both men and women, their female predominance cannot be ignored. Prevalence in women is approximately 19% across all ages, whereas male prevalence is 9%. Among females of reproductive age (ages 18–44 years), the prevalence is closer to 24%.[116] In addition, women report longer headaches and worse symptomology, such as a higher chance of having nausea and vomiting.[117] Although the exact mechanism is yet to be elucidated, there appears to be an association between hormonal fluctuations and severe headaches. Accordingly, these headaches tend to fluctuate with menstrual cycle, pregnancy, and other variations in hormone levels.[117]

Although much of migraine treatment is the same across male and female patients, a few differences are important to highlight. First, the role of aforementioned hormonal fluctuations means that hormonal birth control plays a role in both the treatment and the potential cause of migraines. Some women experience new-onset migraines after beginning exogenous hormonal therapy. These headaches tend to decline and resolve over time on the medication, but in a small proportion of patients they do not, and hormonal medications may need to be discontinued.[118] In other cases, headaches are linked to estrogen withdrawal or specifically to menstruation. In these patients, continuous combined oral contraceptives may be indicated as part of treatment.[118] In general, treatment of women with migraines or other severe headaches requires special consideration of the patient's hormonal fluctuations and how these may contribute to or impact their pain.

Temporomandibular Disorders and Orofacial Pain

Another syndrome with significant female predominance comprises temporomandibular disorders (TMDs) and orofacial pain. TMD is defined as "pain and dysfunction of the masticatory syndrome" and encompasses a wide spectrum of clinical symptomology and pathology.[119] Among those with TMD, pain is the most common symptom.Click or tap here to enter text.[120] TMDs are estimated to be 1.5 to 2 times more prevalent in women than in men, and the highest prevalence in women is of those of reproductive age, approximately ages 20–40 years.[119] Women are also more likely to seek treatment for these disorders, and one study estimated that approximately 80% of patients seeking treatment are women.[119] Many have posited a role of hormones and hormonal fluctuations in TMD symptoms. At least one study has found a link between serum estrogen and progesterone levels and the severity of TMD.[121]

Irritable Bowel Syndrome

Irritable bowel syndrome is yet another disease state that is much more prevalent in women. It is a functional disorder defined as "abdominal pain and abnormal bowel habits with no detectable organic disease."[122] It is estimated that IBS has a female-to-male ratio of 2–2.5:1—at least among those who seek care. Women with IBS also have a lower quality of life than their male counterparts, and they are more likely to experience non-gastrointestinal side effects such as depression, anxiety, and fatigue.[122] Although there are several FDA-approved medications for the treatment of IBS, its diagnosis and treatment are still a work in progress. The female predominance of this disease process may prove to play an important role in these areas in the future.

Conclusion

Despite recent attempts to increase awareness of women as a vulnerable population in medicine, there is still much work to be done. Women's pain remains underrecognized, undertreated, understudied, and underfunded, resulting in significant discomfort, distress, and disability to one-half of the world's population. One glaring area of needed improvement is the baseline lack of knowledge for health care providers and general society regarding women's pain issues. This chapter aims to provide a baseline knowledge of the genetic, biological, and psychosocial differences for women with pain as well as pain states and chronic diseases specific to the female sex so that we may break down the barriers to improving pain care in this vulnerable population.

Equally important to improving knowledge of pain in women is recognizing gendered norms and bias toward women with pain. Realizing bias in the medical community will help identify solutions to pain care barriers and equitable treatment access for women. Increased research and education around pain care issues in women will allow for the creation of treatment guidelines that prevent editorialization and allow for standardized, evidence-based care.

Pain care in women must emphasize interdisciplinary and multimodal approaches to pain management. Treatment of complex pain issues often requires the collaboration of multiple disciplines, including gynecology, urology, pain management, physiatry, gastroenterology, physical therapy, and psychology. Wherever possible, a collaborative women's pain treatment team should be established in order to review complex cases and share expertise. In general, a better understanding of and compassion for women's pain will decrease deficiencies, alleviate suffering, and improve access to care for this vulnerable population.

References

1. Samulowitz A, Gremyr I, Eriksson E, Hensing G. "Brave men" and "emotional women": A theory-guided literature review on gender bias in health care and gendered norms towards patients with chronic pain. *Pain Res Manag.* 2018;2018:6358624. doi:10.1155/2018/6358624
2. Unruh AM. Gender variations in clinical pain experience. *Pain.* 1996;65(2–3):123–167. doi:10.1016/0304-3959(95)00214-6
3. Bjørnnes AK, Parry M, Lie I, et al. Pain experiences of men and women after cardiac surgery. *J Clin Nurs.* 2016;25(19–20):3058–3068. doi:10.1111/JOCN.13329
4. Singh JA, Gabriel S, Lewallen D. The impact of gender, age, and preoperative pain severity on pain after TKA. *Clin Orthop Relat Res.* 2008;466(11):2717–2723. doi:10.1007/S11999-008-0399-9
5. Ruau D, Liu LY, Clark JD, Angst MS, Butte AJ. Sex differences in reported pain across 11,000 patients captured in electronic medical records. *J Pain.* 2012;13(3):228–234. doi:10.1016/J.JPAIN.2011.11.002
6. Fillingim RB, King CD, Ribeiro-Dasilva MC, Rahim-Williams B, Riley JL. Sex, gender, and pain: A review of recent clinical and experimental findings. *J Pain.* 2009;10(5):447–485. doi:10.1016/J.JPAIN.2008.12.001
7. Till SR, As-Sanie S, Schrepf A. Psychology of chronic pelvic pain: Prevalence, neurobiological vulnerabilities, and treatment. *Clin Obstet Gynecol.* 2019;62(1):22–36. doi:10.1097/GRF.0000000000000412
8. Descalzi G, Ikegami D, Ushijima T, Nestler EJ, Zachariou V, Narita M. Epigenetic mechanisms of chronic pain. *Trends Neurosci.* 2015;38(4):237–246. doi:10.1016/J.TINS.2015.02.001
9. Vehof J, Zavos HMS, Lachance G, Hammond CJ, Williams FMK. Shared genetic factors underlie chronic pain syndromes. *Pain.* 2014;155(8):1562–1568. doi:10.1016/J.PAIN.2014.05.002
10. Mills SEE, Nicolson KP, Smith BH. Chronic pain: A review of its epidemiology and associated factors in population-based studies. *Br J Anaesth.* 2019;123(2):e273–e283. doi:10.1016/J.BJA.2019.03.023
11. Zondervan KT, Cardon LR, Kennedy SH, Martin NG, Treloar SA. Multivariate genetic analysis of chronic pelvic pain and associated phenotypes. *Behav Genet.* 2005;35(2):177–188. doi:10.1007/S10519-004-1017-6
12. Johnston KJA, Ward J, Ray PR, et al. Sex-stratified genome-wide association study of multisite chronic pain in UK Biobank. *PLoS Genet.* 2021;17(4):e1009428. doi:10.1371/JOURNAL.PGEN.1009428
13. Sexton JE, Cox JJ, Zhao J, Wood JN. The genetics of pain: Implications for therapeutics. *Annu Rev Pharmacol Toxicol.* 2018;58:123–142. doi:10.1146/ANNUREV-PHARMTOX-010617-052554
14. Zorina-Lichtenwalter K, Meloto CB, Khoury S, Diatchenko L. Genetic predictors of human chronic pain conditions. *Neuroscience.* 2016;338:36–62. doi:10.1016/J.NEUROSCIENCE.2016.04.041
15. Wei SY, Chen LF, Lin MW, et al. The *OPRM1* A118G polymorphism modulates the descending pain modulatory system for individual pain experience in young women with primary dysmenorrhea. *Sci Rep.* 2017;7:39906. doi:10.1038/SREP39906
16. LeResche L, Mancl LA, Drangsholt MT, Saunders K, Von Korff M. Relationship of pain and symptoms to pubertal development in adolescents. *Pain.* 2005;118(1–2):201–209. doi:10.1016/J.PAIN.2005.08.011
17. Fillingim RB, Maixner W, Girdler SS, et al. Ischemic but not thermal pain sensitivity varies across the menstrual cycle. *Psychosom Med.* 1997;59(5):512–520. doi:10.1097/00006842-199709000-00008
18. Bragdon EE, Light KC, Costello NL, et al. Group differences in pain modulation: Pain-free women compared to pain-free men and to women with TMD. *Pain.* 2002;96(3):227–237. doi:10.1016/S0304-3959(01)00451-1
19. Aloisi AM, Bachiocco V, Costantino A, et al. Cross-sex hormone administration changes pain in transsexual women and men. *Pain.* 2007;132(Suppl 1):S60–S67. doi:10.1016/J.PAIN.2007.02.006

20. Craft RM, Mogil JS, Maria Aloisi A. Sex differences in pain and analgesia: The role of gonadal hormones. *Eur J Pain*. 2004;8(5):397–411. doi:10.1016/J.EJPAIN.2004.01.003
21. Malcangio M. Role of the immune system in neuropathic pain. *Scand J Pain*. 2019;20(1):33–37. doi:10.1515/SJPAIN-2019-0138
22. Clark AK, Gruber-Schoffnegger D, Drdla-Schutting R, Gerhold KJ, Malcangio M, Sandkühler J. Selective activation of microglia facilitates synaptic strength. *J Neurosci*. 2015;35(11):4552–4570. doi:10.1523/JNEUROSCI.2061-14.2015
23. Zhou LJ, Peng J, Xu YN, et al. Microglia are indispensable for synaptic plasticity in the spinal dorsal horn and chronic pain. *Cell Rep*. 2019;27(13):3844–3859. doi:10.1016/J.CELREP.2019.05.087
24. Skaper SD, Facci L, Giusti P. Mast cells, glia and neuroinflammation: Partners in crime? *Immunology*. 2014;141(3):314–327. doi:10.1111/IMM.12170
25. Schäfers M, Brinkhoff J, Neukirchen S, Marziniak M, Sommer C. Combined epineurial therapy with neutralizing antibodies to tumor necrosis factor-alpha and interleukin-1 receptor has an additive effect in reducing neuropathic pain in mice. *Neurosci Lett*. 2001;310(2–3):113–116. doi:10.1016/S0304-3940(01)02077-8
26. Bartley EJ, Fillingim RB. Sex differences in pain: A brief review of clinical and experimental findings. *Br J Anaesth*. 2013;111(1):52–58. doi:10.1093/BJA/AET127
27. Robinson ME, Riley JL, Myers CD, et al. Gender role expectations of pain: Relationship to sex differences in pain. *J Pain*. 2001;2(5):251–257. doi:10.1054/JPAI.2001.24551
28. Defrin R, Shramm L, Eli I. Gender role expectations of pain is associated with pain tolerance limit but not with pain threshold. *Pain*. 2009;145(1–2):230–236. doi:10.1016/J.PAIN.2009.06.028
29. Tsang A, Von Korff M, Lee S, et al. Common chronic pain conditions in developed and developing countries: Gender and age differences and comorbidity with depression–anxiety disorders. *J Pain*. 2008;9(10):883–891. doi:10.1016/J.JPAIN.2008.05.005
30. Kind S, Otis JD. The interaction between chronic pain and PTSD. *Curr Pain Headache Rep*. 2019;23(12): Article 91. doi:10.1007/S11916-019-0828-3
31. Gorczyca R, Filip R, Walczak E. Psychological aspects of pain. *Ann Agric Environ Med*. 2013;Spec no. 1:23–27.
32. Bair MJ, Robinson RL, Katon W, Kroenke K. Depression and pain comorbidity: A literature review. *Arch Intern Med*. 2003;163(20):2433–2445.
33. Siqveland J, Hussain A, Lindstrøm JC, Ruud T, Hauff E. Prevalence of posttraumatic stress disorder in persons with chronic pain: A meta-analysis. *Front Psychiatry*. 2017;8: Article 164. doi:10.3389/FPSYT.2017.00164/FULL
34. Meltzer-Brody S, Leserman J, Zolnoun D, Steege J, Green E, Teich A. Trauma and posttraumatic stress disorder in women with chronic pelvic pain. *Obstet Gynecol*. 2007;109:902–910.
35. McVean A. The history of hysteria. Office for Science and Society, McGill University. 2017. Accessed May 27, 2022. https://www.mcgill.ca/oss/article/history-quackery/history-hysteria
36. Calderone KL. The influence of gender on the frequency of pain and sedative medication administered to postoperative patients. *Sex Roles*. 1990;23(11):713–725. doi:10.1007/BF00289259
37. Chen EH, Shofer FS, Dean AJ, et al. Gender disparity in analgesic treatment of emergency department patients with acute abdominal pain. *Acad Emerg Med*. 2008;15:414–418. doi:10.1111/j.1553-2712.2008.00100.x
38. National Institutes of Health, Office of Research on Women's Health. History of women's participation in clinical research. n.d. Accessed May 27, 2022. https://orwh.od.nih.gov/toolkit/recruitment/history
39. Ferries-Rowe E, Corey E, Archer JS. Primary dysmenorrhea: Diagnosis and therapy. *Obstet Gynecol*. 2020;136(5):1047–1058. doi:10.1097/AOG.0000000000004096
40. Ju H, Jones M, Mishra G. The prevalence and risk factors of dysmenorrhea. *Epidemiol Rev*. 2014;36(1):104–113. doi:10.1093/EPIREV/MXT009

41. Guimarães I, Póvoa AM. Primary dysmenorrhea: Assessment and treatment. *Rev Bras Ginecol Obstet*. 2020;42(8):501–507. doi:10.1055/S-0040-1712131
42. Iacovides S, Avidon I, Baker FC. What we know about primary dysmenorrhea today: A critical review. *Hum Reprod Update*. 2015;21(6):762–778. doi:10.1093/HUMUPD/DMV039
43. *Am Fam Physician*. See page 225 for definitions of strength-of-recommendation labels. 2005. Accessed June 27, 2022. www.aafp.org/afp
44. Latthe PM, Champaneria R. Dysmenorrhoea. *BMJ Clin Evid*. 2014;2014:0813.
45. Doty E, Attaran M. Managing primary dysmenorrhea. *J Pediatr Adolesc Gynecol*. 2006;19(5):341–344. doi:10.1016/J.JPAG.2006.06.005
46. Marjoribanks J, Ayekele R, Farquhar C, Proctor M. Nonsteroidal anti-inflammatory drugs for dysmenorrhoea. *Cochrane Database Syst Rev*. 2015;2015(7):CD001751. doi:10.1002/14651858.CD001751.PUB2/INFORMATION/EN
47. Vercellini P, Viganò P, Somigliana E, Fedele L. Endometriosis: Pathogenesis and treatment. *Nat Rev Endocrinol*. 2013;10(5):261–275. doi:10.1038/nrendo.2013.255
48. Viganò P, Parazzini F, Somigliana E, Vercellini P. Endometriosis: Epidemiology and aetiological factors. *Best Pract Res Clin Obstet Gynaecol*. 2004;18(2):177–200. doi:10.1016/J.BPOBGYN.2004.01.007
49. Shafrir AL, Farland L V., Shah DK, et al. Risk for and consequences of endometriosis: A critical epidemiologic review. *Best Pract Res Clin Obstet Gynaecol*. 2018;51:1–15. doi:10.1016/J.BPOBGYN.2018.06.001
50. Sampson JA. Peritoneal endometriosis due to the menstrual dissemination of endometrial tissue into the peritoneal cavity. *Am J Obstet Gynecol*. 1927;14(4):422–469. doi:10.1016/S0002-9378(15)30003-X
51. Burney RO, Giudice LC. Pathogenesis and pathophysiology of endometriosis. *Fertil Steril*. 2012;98(3):511–519. doi:10.1016/J.FERTNSTERT.2012.06.029
52. Vercellini P. Endometriosis: What a pain it is. *Semin Reprod Endocrinol*. 1997;15(3):251–261. doi:10.1055/S-2008-1068755/BIB
53. Eskenazi B, Warner M, Bonsignore L, Olive D, Samuels S, Vercellini P. Validation study of nonsurgical diagnosis of endometriosis. *Fertil Steril*. 2001;76(5):929–935. doi:10.1016/S0015-0282(01)02736-4
54. Healey M, Ang WC, Cheng C. Surgical treatment of endometriosis: A prospective randomized double-blinded trial comparing excision and ablation. *Fertil Steril*. 2010;94(7):2536–2540. doi:10.1016/J.FERTNSTERT.2010.02.044
55. Hung SW, Zhang R, Tan Z, Chung JPW, Zhang T, Wang CC. Pharmaceuticals targeting signaling pathways of endometriosis as potential new medical treatment: A review. *Med Res Rev*. 2021;41(4):2489–2564. doi:10.1002/MED.21802
56. Shahhosseini Z, Hamzehgardeshi Z, Soleimani S. A review of non-pharmacological interventions in pain management associated with endometriosis. *J Res Dev Nurs Midw*. 2020;17. https://nmj.goums.ac.ir/article-1-1248-en.html
57. Pontis A, D'Alterio MN, Pirarba S, de Angelis C, Tinelli R, Angioni S. Adenomyosis: A systematic review of medical treatment. *Gynecol Endocrinol*. 2016;32(9):696–700. doi:10.1080/09513590.2016.1197200
58. Struble J, Reid S, Bedaiwy MA. Adenomyosis: A clinical review of a challenging gynecologic condition. *J Minim Invasive Gynecol*. 2016;23(2):164–185. doi:10.1016/J.JMIG.2015.09.018
59. Koike H, Egawa H, Ohtsuka T, Yamaguchi M, Ikenoue T, Mori N. Correlation between dysmenorrheic severity and prostaglandin production in women with endometriosis. *Prostaglandins Leukot Essent Fatty Acids*. 1992;46(2):133–137. doi:10.1016/0952-3278(92)90219-9
60. Reinhold C, Atri M, Mehio A, Zakarian R, Aldis AE, Bret PM. Diffuse uterine adenomyosis: Morphologic criteria and diagnostic accuracy of endovaginal sonography. *Radiology*. 1995;197(3):609–614. doi:10.1148/RADIOLOGY.197.3.7480727
61. Reinhold C, Tafazoli F, Mehio A, et al. Uterine adenomyosis: Endovaginal US and MR imaging features with histopathologic correlation. *RadioGraphics*. 1999;19(Suppl 1). doi:10.1148/RADIOGRAPHICS.19.SUPPL_1.G99OC13S147

62. Haefner HK, Collins ME, Davis GD, et al. The vulvodynia guideline. *J Low Genit Tract Dis.* 2005;9(1):40–51. doi:10.1097/00128360-200501000-00009
63. Bergeron S, Reed BD, Wesselmann U, Bohm-Starke N. Vulvodynia. *Nat Rev Dis Primers.* 2020;6(1):1–21. doi:10.1038/s41572-020-0164-2
64. Bornstein J, Preti M, Simon JA, et al. Descriptors of vulvodynia: A multisocietal definition consensus (International Society for the Study of Vulvovaginal Disease, the International Society for the Study of Women Sexual Health, and the International Pelvic Pain Society). *J Low Genit Tract Dis.* 2019;23(2):161–163. doi:10.1097/LGT.0000000000000461
65. Ventolini G, Barhan S, Duke J. Vulvodynia, a step-wise therapeutic prospective cohort study. *J Obstet Gynaecol.* 2009;29(7):648–650. doi:10.1080/01443610903095882
66. Bates CM, Timmins DJ. Vulvodynia: New and more effective approaches to therapy. *Int J STD AIDS.* 2002;13(3):210–212. doi:10.1258/0956462021924802
67. Ben-David B, Friedman M. Gabapentin therapy for vulvodynia. *Anesth Analg.* 1999;89(6):1459–1460. doi:10.1213/00000539-199912000-00026
68. Chinn S, Caldwell W, Gritsenko K. Fibromyalgia pathogenesis and treatment options update. *Curr Pain Headache Rep.* 2016;20(4):1–10. doi:10.1007/S11916-016-0556-X
69. Inanici F, Yunus MB. History of fibromyalgia: Past to present. *Curr Pain Headache Rep.* 2004;8(5):369–378. doi:10.1007/S11916-996-0010-6
70. Hadler NM. "Fibromyalgia" and the medicalization of misery. *J Rheumatol.* 2003;30(8):1668–1670.
71. Clauw DJ. Fibromyalgia: A clinical review. *JAMA.* 2014;311(15):1547–1555. doi:10.1001/JAMA.2014.3266
72. Bair MJ, Krebs EE. Fibromyalgia. *Ann Intern Med.* 2020;172(5):ITC33–ITC48. doi:10.7326/AITC202003030
73. Koçyiğit BF, Akaltun MS. Kinesiophobia levels in fibromyalgia syndrome and the relationship between pain, disease activity, depression. *Arch Rheumatol.* 2020;35(2):214–219. doi:10.46497/ArchRheumatol.2020.7432
74. Maffei ME. Molecular sciences fibromyalgia: Recent advances in diagnosis, classification, pharmacotherapy and alternative remedies. *Int J Mol Sci.* 2020;21(21):7877. doi:10.3390/ijms21217877
75. Clemens JQ, Link CL, Eggers PW, Kusek JW, Nyberg LM, McKinlay JB. Prevalence of painful bladder symptoms and effect on quality of life in Black, Hispanic and White men and women. *J Urol.* 2007;177(4):1390–1394. doi:10.1016/J.JURO.2006.11.084
76. Marcu I, Campian EC, Tu FF. Interstitial cystitis/bladder pain syndrome. *Semin Reprod Med.* 2018;36(2):123–135. doi:10.1055/S-0038-1676089/ID/JR001132-40
77. Vij M, Srikrishna S, Cardozo L. Interstitial cystitis: Diagnosis and management. *Eur J Obstet Gynecol Repro Biol.* 2012;161(1):1–7. doi:10.1016/J.EJOGRB.2011.12.014
78. Lokeshwar VB, Selzer MG, Cerwinka WH, et al. Urinary uronate and sulfated glycosaminoglycan levels: Markers for interstitial cystitis severity. *J Urol.* 2005;174(1):344–349. doi:10.1097/01.JU.0000161599.69942.2E
79. Warren JW, Jackson TL, Langenberg P, Meyers DJ, Xu J. Prevalence of interstitial cystitis in first-degree relatives of patients with interstitial cystitis. *Urology.* 2004;63(1):17–21. doi:10.1016/J.UROLOGY.2003.08.027
80. Hanno PM, Burks DA, Clemens JQ, et al. AUA guideline for the diagnosis and treatment of interstitial cystitis/bladder pain syndrome. *J Urol.* 2011;185(6):2162–2170. doi:10.1016/J.JURO.2011.03.064
81. Davis NF, Brady CM, Creagh T. Interstitial cystitis/painful bladder syndrome: Epidemiology, pathophysiology and evidence-based treatment options. *Eur J Obstet Gynecol Reprod Biol.* 2014;175(1):30–37. doi:10.1016/J.EJOGRB.2013.12.041
82. Mulholland SG, Sant GR, Hanno P, Staskin DR, Parsons L. Pentosan polysulfate sodium for therapy of interstitial cystitis: A double-blind placebo-controlled clinical study. *Urology.* 1990;35(6):552–558. doi:10.1016/0090-4295(90)80116-5
83. Pinto R, Lopes T, Frias B, et al. Trigonal injection of botulinum toxin A in patients with refractory bladder pain syndrome/interstitial cystitis. *Eur Urol.* 2010;58(3):360–365. doi:10.1016/J.EURURO.2010.02.031

84. Robert R, Prat-Pradal D, Labat JJ, et al. Anatomic basis of chronic perineal pain: Role of the pudendal nerve. *Surg Radiol Anat.* 1998;20(2):93–98. doi:10.1007/BF01628908
85. Labat JJ, Riant T, Robert R, Amarenco G, Lefaucheur JP, Rigaud J. Diagnostic criteria for pudendal neuralgia by pudendal nerve entrapment (Nantes criteria). *Neurourol Urodyn.* 2008;27(4):306–310. doi:10.1002/NAU.20505
86. Khoder W, Hale D. Pudendal neuralgia. *Obstet Gynecol Clin North Am.* 2014;41(3):443–452. doi:10.1016/J.OGC.2014.04.002
87. Ramsden CE, McDaniel MC, Harmon RL, Renney KM, Faure A. Pudendal nerve entrapment as source of intractable perineal pain. *Am J Phys Med Rehabil.* 2003;82(6):479–484. doi:10.1097/01.PHM.0000069196.15353.7D
88. Campbell JN, Meyer RA. Mechanisms of neuropathic pain. *Neuron.* 2006;52(1):77–92. doi:10.1016/J.NEURON.2006.09.021
89. Hibner M, Desai N, Robertson LJ, Nour M. Pudendal neuralgia. *J Minim Invasive Gynecol.* 2010;17(2):148–153. doi:10.1016/J.JMIG.2009.11.003
90. Lien KC, Morgan DM, Delancey JOL, Ashton-Miller JA. Pudendal nerve stretch during vaginal birth: A 3D computer simulation. *Am J Obstet Gynecol.* 2005;192(5):1669–1676. doi:10.1016/J.AJOG.2005.01.032
91. Delmas V. Anatomical risks of transobturator suburethral tape in the treatment of female stress urinary incontinence. *Eur Urol.* 2005;48(5):793–798. doi:10.1016/J.EURURO.2005.02.002
92. Howard EJ. Postherpetic pudendal neuralgia. *JAMA.* 1985;253(15):2196–2196. doi:10.1001/JAMA.1985.03350390038023
93. Amarenco G, Lanoe Y, Ghnassia RT, Goudal H, Perrigot M. [Alcock's canal syndrome and perineal neuralgia]. *Rev Neurol.* 1988;144(8–9):523–526. https://europepmc.org/article/med/3187310
94. Abbott JA, Jarvis SK, Lyons SD, Thomson A, Vancaille TG. Botulinum toxin type A for chronic pain and pelvic floor spasm in women: A randomized controlled trial. *Obstet Gynecol.* 2006;108(4):915–923. doi:10.1097/01.AOG.0000237100.29870.CC
95. Choi SS, Lee PB, Kim YC, Kim HJ, Lee SC. C-arm-guided pudendal nerve block: A new technique. *Int J Clin Pract.* 2006;60(5):553–556. doi:10.1111/J.1742-1241.2006.00836.X
96. Filler AG. Diagnosis and treatment of pudendal nerve entrapment syndrome subtypes: Imaging, injections, and minimal access surgery. *Neurosurg Focus.* 2009;26(2):1–14. doi:10.3171/FOC.2009.26.2.E9
97. Beco J, Climov D, Bex M. Pudendal nerve decompression in perineology: A case series. *BMC Surg.* 2004;4: Article 15. doi:10.1186/1471-2482-4-15
98. Prather H, Spitznagle TM, Dugan SA. Recognizing and treating pelvic pain and pelvic floor dysfunction. *Phys Med Rehabil Clin North Am.* 2007;18(3):477–496. doi:10.1016/J.PMR.2007.06.004
99. Gyang A, Hartman M, Lamvu G. Musculoskeletal causes of chronic pelvic pain: What a gynecologist should know. *Obstet Gynecol.* 2013;121(3):645–650. doi:10.1097/AOG.0B013E318283FFEA
100. Prather H, Camacho-Soto A. Musculoskeletal etiologies of pelvic pain. *Obstet Gynecol Clin North Am.* 2014;41(3):433–442. doi:10.1016/J.OGC.2014.04.004
101. Meister MR, Sutcliffe S, Badu A, Ghetti C, Lowder JL. Pelvic floor myofascial pain severity and pelvic floor disorder symptom bother: Is there a correlation? *Am J Obstet Gynecol.* 2019;221(3):235.e1–235.e15. doi:10.1016/J.AJOG.2019.07.020
102. Moldwin RM, Fariello JY. Myofascial trigger points of the pelvic floor: Associations with urological pain syndromes and treatment strategies including injection therapy. *Cur Urol Rep.* 2013;14(5):409–417. doi:10.1007/S11934-013-0360-7
103. Hwang SK. Advances in the treatment of chronic pelvic pain: A multidisciplinary approach to treatment. *Mo Med.* 2017;114(1):47–51.

104. Hong MK, Ding DC. Current treatments for female pelvic floor dysfunctions. *Gynecol Minim Invasive Ther*. 2019;8(4):143–148. doi:10.4103/GMIT.GMIT_7_19
105. Alappattu MJ, Bishop MD. Psychological factors in chronic pelvic pain in women: Relevance and application of the fear-avoidance model of pain. *Phys Ther*. 2011;91(10):1542–1550. doi:10.2522/PTJ.20100368
106. Champaneria R, Daniels JP, Raza A, Pattison HM, Khan KS. Psychological therapies for chronic pelvic pain: Systematic review of randomized controlled trials. *Acta Obstet Gynecol Scand*. 2012;91(3):281–286. doi:10.1111/J.1600-0412.2011.01314.X
107. Nogueira Fabro EA, Bergmann A, do Amaral e Silva B, et al. Post-mastectomy pain syndrome: Incidence and risks. *The Breast*. 2012;21(3):321–325. doi:10.1016/J.BREAST.2012.01.019
108. Tait RC, Zoberi K, Ferguson M, et al. Persistent post-mastectomy pain: Risk factors and current approaches to treatment. *J Pain*. 2018;19(12):1367–1383. doi:10.1016/J.JPAIN.2018.06.002
109. Smith WCS, Bourne D, Squair J, Phillips D), Chambers WA. A retrospective cohort study of post mastectomy pain syndrome. *Pain*. 1999;83(1):91–95. doi:10.1016/S0304-3959(99)00076-7
110. Chappell AG, Yuksel S, Sasson DC, Wescott AB, Connor LM, Ellis MF. Post-mastectomy pain syndrome: An up-to-date review of treatment outcomes. *JPRAS Open*. 2021;30:97–109. doi:10.1016/J.JPRA.2021.07.006
111. Larsson IM, Ahm Sørensen J, Bille C. The post-mastectomy pain syndrome: A systematic review of the treatment modalities. *Breast J*. 2017;23(3):338–343. doi:10.1111/TBJ.12739
112. Amr YM, Yousef AAAM. Evaluation of efficacy of the perioperative administration of venlafaxine or gabapentin on acute and chronic postmastectomy pain. *Clin J Pain*. 2010;26(5):381–385. doi:10.1097/AJP.0B013E3181CB406E
113. Sollie M, Toyserkani NM, Bille C, Thomsen JB, Sørensen JA. Autologous fat grafting as treatment of postmastectomy pain syndrome: A randomized controlled trial. *Plast Reconstr Surg*. 2022;149(2):295–305. doi:10.1097/PRS.0000000000008705
114. Ilfeld BM, Madison SJ, Suresh PJ, et al. Persistent postmastectomy pain and pain-related physical and emotional functioning with and without a continuous paravertebral nerve block: A prospective 1-year follow-up assessment of a randomized, triple-masked, placebo-controlled study. *Ann Surg Oncol*. 2015;22(6):2017–2025. doi:10.1245/S10434-014-4248-7
115. Lin ZM, Li MH, Zhang F, et al. Thoracic paravertebral blockade reduces chronic postsurgical pain in breast cancer patients: A randomized controlled trial. *Pain Med*. 2020;21(12):3539–3547. doi:10.1093/PM/PNAA270
116. Burch RC, Loder S, Loder E, Smitherman TA. The prevalence and burden of migraine and severe headache in the United States: Updated statistics from government health surveillance studies. *Headache*. 2015;55(1):21–34. doi:10.1111/HEAD.12482
117. U.S. Department of Health & Human Services, Office on Women's Health. Migraine. n.d. Accessed June 13, 2022. https://www.womenshealth.gov/a-z-topics/migraine
118. Edlow AG, Bartz D. Hormonal contraceptive options for women with headache: A review of the evidence. *Rev Obstet Gynecol*. 2010;3(2):55–65.
119. Warren MP, Fried JL. Temporomandibular disorders and hormones in women. *Cells Tissues Organs*. 2001;169(3):187–192. doi:10.1159/000047881
120. Bagis B, Ayaz EA, Turgut S, Durkan R, Özcan M. Gender difference in prevalence of signs and symptoms of temporomandibular joint disorders: A retrospective study on 243 consecutive patients. *Int J Med Sci*. 2012;9(7):539–544. doi:10.7150/IJMS.4474
121. Patil SR, Yadav N, Mousa MA, et al. Role of female reproductive hormones estrogen and progesterone in temporomandibular disorder in female patients. *J Oral Res Rev*. 2015;7(2): Article 41. doi:10.4103/2249-4987.172492
122. Kim YS, Kim N. Sex-gender differences in irritable bowel syndrome. *J Neurogastroenterol Motil*. 2018;24(4):544–558. doi:10.5056/JNM18082

8
Pain in the LGTBQ+ Population

Noelle Marie Javier

Introduction

Sexual and gender minorities (SGMs), also called the LGBTQI+ community (lesbian, gay, bisexual, transgender, queer, intersex, plus all types of sexual orientations and gender identities), comprise approximately 7.1% of the U.S. population based on a 2021 Gallup poll.[1] This is a 2.6% increase from the 2016 data. In the Human Rights Commission Household Pulse Survey, the estimated proportion of LGBTQI+ people approaches 20 million, with bisexuals as the most prevalent cohort.[2] In 2011, the National Academy of Medicine (formerly Institute of Medicine) identified gaps in research toward the needs, concerns, and priorities in the provision of optimal health care for the LGBTQI+ community.[3] This was further reinforced in 2016 when the National Institute on Minority Health and Health Disparities designated that LGBTQI+ community as a health disparity population for ongoing research.[4] As a whole, the LGBTQI+ community has experienced multiple societal barriers to living life fully and safely. Over their lifetime, members of the LGBTQI+ community have experienced significant stressors, including various forms of trauma, widespread oppression, outright prejudice, perpetual victimization, and blatant abuse.[5,6] A 2019 U.S. poll showed that the LGBTQI+ community has been subjected to intolerance and oppression by society at large and therefore has faced heightened discrimination, including vicious hate crimes.[7] Multiple internal and external stressors contribute to the marginalized identities of this community. These have led to disparate and inequitable access to health care. Furthermore, these stressors also serve as triggers for ongoing physical and psychological trauma, resulting in members of the LGBTQI+ community further delaying and avoiding medical care by not disclosing their sexual orientation and gender identity to health care providers. Hence, this unfortunate reality has led to further invisibility impacting the early identification of their unique health care needs as well as timely and appropriate high-quality medical care, including pain management.

What Makes the LGTBQI+ Population More Vulnerable to Pain?

Illness Model

The approach to pain assessment and management for an LGBTQI+ adult with a major illness does not have a definitive template that is well studied in the literature. However, there are some guiding principles that can be used to provide inclusive and affirming care for this minority. One conceptual framework is using the biopsychosocial model for pain assessment and management. This could be further expanded to include the cultural and spiritual aspects in diagnosing and treating pain. Hence, for the purpose of this chapter, I refer to and propose a biopsychosocial, cultural, and spiritual framework to pain assessment and management. Well known in the palliative care literature, this multidimensional framework is a highly regarded and widely accepted heuristic approach. This model posits that there are multiple dimensions to pain assessment and management. It pertains to the interplay between the neurobiology of pain and the associated psychological, social, cultural, and spiritual factors that distinguish disease from illness and how they all intersect.[8] Moreover, this model focuses on both disease and illness. The former is defined as an objective biological event involving the disruption of specific body structures or organ systems caused by anatomical, pathological, or physiological changes, whereas the latter is the subjective experience or self-attribution that a disease is present and how a sick person and their family members live with and respond to symptoms of disability.[8]

The proposed biopsychosocial, cultural, and spiritual framework of pain assessment and management fits well in the provision of a holistic and humane approach to vulnerable and marginalized groups such as the LGBTQI+ community. They have been subjected to a long-standing history of societal oppression. Furthermore, intrinsic to the individuals themselves, the experience of self-oppression and stigmatization adds more complexity to how this vulnerable community thrives and adapts in society over time. Hence, the lasting and aggregate impact of multiple stressors affecting this community is exemplified clearly in the minority stress model conceptualized by the American psychiatric epidemiologist and policy scholar Ilan Meyer in 2003.[9] This model refers to the excess stress to which individuals from stigmatized social categories are exposed to as a result of their social and minority position. Moreover, this construct is further described in three categories: (1) *additive* to general stressors that are experienced by all people and therefore require adaptations above and beyond those required of the non-stigmatized, (2) *chronic* in that they are related to relatively stable social structures such as laws and social policies, and (3) *socially based* in that they stem from social and structural forces rather than individual events or conditions.[9]

Complementary to the minority stress model is the effect of *allostatic load* on the lived experiences of this population. In essence, this pertains to the cumulative burden of chronic stress and life events affecting an individual or groups of individuals. Furthermore, this involves the interaction of various physiological systems at varying levels of activity. The phenomenon of allostatic overload occurs when external challenges exceed the threshold of the coping resources of the individual.[10] The existence of these stressors may result in significant physical and mental health outcomes that could either be positive or negative. There are good data to support that allostatic load (and overload) may lead to poorer health outcomes. What is also evident in this model is the emphasis on internal and external resources in coping with these stressors while allowing the minority adult to thrive and survive in an otherwise oppressive society.

As a whole, the LGBTQI+ community has developed supportive and affirming strategies in the context of resilience and robustness. *Resilience* is defined as a person's ability to mitigate the adverse impact of stress while successfully thriving in society.[11]

Robustness pertains to the individual's or system's ability to resist disruption from external stressors.[12] The impacts of these stressors in the context of internal and external resources for resiliency and robustness intertwine in the construct of *intersectionality*. This in turn is a theoretical framework that describes how individuals have multiple overlapping identities while understanding of their interconnectedness allows for the detection of systemic injustice and social inequities.[13] For the LGBTQI+ community, the disparities in health care stemming from discrimination and prejudice are related and influenced by racism, sexism, classism, religion, disability, homophobia, transphobia, literacy, employment, and other determinants of a person's identity as a whole. Although most of these factors affect the general population at large, these are especially magnified in this minority population. These can then lead to further marginalization and oppression. The implication of understanding these constructs as they relate to sexual and gender minorities can lead to the practice of *cultural humility*. This approach recognizes the power imbalance between a health care provider and a patient, especially if that person is marginalized. Cultural humility is a shift from the more traditional paternalistic paradigm. It is further described as a self-reflective, open-minded, egoless, and supportive approach to patient care that integrates self-appraisal and reflection in daily interactions.[14]

Discussion

The following sections describe the proposed biopsychosocial, cultural, and spiritual model in more detail.

Biological Domain

The literature is clear that there are existing physical health care disparities that affect the LGBTQI+ community as a whole. Gay and bisexual men have higher rates of cardiovascular disease, hypertension, diabetes, and physical disability compared to their heterosexual cohort.[15,16] Women who identify as LGBTQI+ have higher rates of obesity, cardiovascular disease, and gynecologic and breast neoplasms compared to straight women.[17] Implicated risk factors for these sexual and gender minority women include nulliparity, unopposed estrogen from a lack of progesterone and breastfeeding, and higher body mass indices. A higher prevalence of cardiovascular disease can also lead to other types of illnesses, including neurocognitive disorders. There are data to support that gay and bisexual men as well as transgender women have higher rates of HIV infection as well.[6] HIV seropositive sexual and gender minority men have greater risks for development of anal cancer.[18,19] Commonly cited reasons for these health care disparities include lack of medical insurance, fear of being stigmatized by medical providers and the health care system at large, lack of protective policies ensuring equitable access, structural gaps in sexual orientation and gender identity (SOGI) disclosure, and low cultural competency and sensitivity training among various providers.

Pain in the LGTBQI+ Community

The data on the prevalence of pain among LGBTQI+ adults compared to non-LGBTQI+ individuals is not well-defined in the literature. There is no precedent that the experience of physical nociceptive pain is worse among LGBTQI+ people. To my knowledge and based on a review of the existing literature, there is no distinction in the neural and somatosensory pathways for the transmission of pain signals and the experience of pain in members of this population compared to their cisgender heterosexual counterparts. Two striking pathophysiologic models of pain tie in well with the concept of the biopsychosocial, cultural, and spiritual framework of pain assessment and management: the gate control theory of pain and the neuromatrix theory of pain. In 1996, Melzack and Wall ascribed salient features toward the gate control theory of pain.[20] These include the variable relationship of injury and pain, the possibility of pain being induced by non-noxious stimuli, the variable relationship between the location and the subjective experience of pain, the enduring nature of pain past its healing point, the multidimensional characterization of pain, and the lack of optimal pain treatments.[21] The neuromatrix theory of pain proposes that pain is a multidimensional experience that is produced by a characteristic of a widely distributed brain neural network called the body-self neuromatrix, which in turn incorporates cognitive-evaluative, sensory-discriminative, and motivational-affective components. This theory also posits that there is an engagement and interaction of the perceptual, behavioral, and homeostatic systems in response to chronic injury and stress. Therefore, the experience, expression, and management of pain in the LGBTQI+ community will likely be driven and influenced by other aspects or domains in the holistic or person-centered approach and not solely by a disease-centric paradigm.

Total Pain: Bringing Together the Biopsychosocial, Cultural, and Spiritual Dimensions

In the palliative care setting, Dame Cicely Saunders, who is considered the mother of the modern hospice movement, coined the term *total pain*, which illustrates clearly the biopsychosocial, cultural, and spiritual framework. Furthermore, this is linked to a person's personal narrative, ethnography, and all the suffering endured, thereby providing a foundation for this person-centered understanding of pain and suffering.[22] The subsequent domains explore more of their roles and contributions toward total pain experience for the LGBTQI+ community.

Psychosocial Domain

The health care disparities that members of the LGBTQI+ community face are not limited to physical health. One large study showed that half of the LGBTQI+ people and two-thirds of the transgender population have received disproportionate and suboptimal care in various medical settings.[23] There is clear robust evidence that the mental and psychological health outcomes resulting from long-standing oppressive and discriminatory practices are quite staggering.[6]

Experiences of victimization and abuse, such as physical attacks and hate crimes, are associated with negative mental health outcomes and more lifetime suicide attempts among LGBTQI+ adults.[24] Bisexual women and men showed more mental health distress compared to lesbian women and gay men, respectively. Moreover, bisexual and gay men reported higher levels of internalized homophobia, alcohol abuse, and suicidal ideation compared to bisexual and lesbian women.[24,25]

There are large studies underscoring the presence of diverse mood disorders such as anxiety, depression, and suicidal ideation. A 2011 study found that close to one-third of older LGBTQI+ adults reported symptoms of depression. Of the subgroups in the LGBTQI+ community, the transgender cohort reported the highest percentage of depression compared to their cisgender counterparts.[26] Another study found that older gay men who experienced internalized gay ageism in their lifetime had concurrent depression.[27] A subsequent study in 2013 examined suicidal ideation in this population and found that approximately 40% of LGBTQI+ participants seriously thought about committing suicide.[16] However, the patterns of suicidal behavior differed by age across the life span, with the majority of suicidal attempts (approximately 69%) occurred between ages 22 and 59 years. A small proportion (approximately 4%) occurred after age 60 years.[28]

Kenagy[29] found that in a sample of 182 transgender individuals, those who identified as male-to-female (i.e., transgender woman) were significantly more likely to be diagnosed with HIV, have attempted suicide, and experienced physical and/or sexual abuse than those who identified as female-to-male (transgender man). In 2015, a study of more than 27,000 transgender respondents in the United States revealed that 40% of them have attempted suicide in their lifetime,[24] which is approximately nine times the attempted suicide rate in the general population. This percentage did not differ significantly from that in a 2011 study in which 41% reported suicide attempts, which were largely associated with stressful causes such as unemployment; physical, verbal, and sexual harassment; poverty; and other types of assault.[26] Of note, transgender women of color are disproportionately at greater risk of victimization and violence.[30,31] Note that a major source of stigmatization in this population is the experience of going through conversion therapy, especially during adolescence, when the onset of structural gaps in SOGI disclosure realization comes to light.

Conversion therapy, also known as reparative therapy, pertains to interventions aimed at changing sexual orientation, gender identity, and gender expression. Common interventions include sexuality counseling, sexual reorientation efforts, and healing sexual brokenness. The net results include lowered self-esteem, self-hatred, depression, and suicidality. This practice has since been denounced by professional organizations and restricted in numerous U.S. states.[32] The negative consequences of reparative therapy include the rising prevalence of substance use disorder and risky sexual behavior and practices in the LGBTQI+ community. A few identifiable contributory factors leading to these problems include minority stressors, lack of social supports, internalized homophobia, internalized transphobia, peer pressure, and integration of clubs and bars into LGBTQI+ neighborhoods.[6,33] On the other hand, one study showed that LGBTQI+ persons were more likely to seek treatment compared to their heterosexual cohort (21% vs. 7%, respectively).[15]

The previously mentioned studies, however, showed overt gaps in cultural competency training for medical providers, leading to suboptimal care for the LGBTQI+ community but especially the transgender community.[24] Although the data on mental health outcomes are jarring, there are also a number of *buffering and redemptive factors* that cannot be overlooked. Examples include religiosity, spirituality, greater community connectedness, positive sense of sexual identity, higher perceived social support, self-efficacy especially in HIV+ men, and resiliency and robustness, among others.[34] In 2017, Monin et al.[35] examined mental health resiliency in sexual minority American veterans. They concluded that although older LGBTQI+ identified veterans were more resilient than their younger peers, they were also at higher risk of social isolation.

A core tenet in recognizing LGBTQI+ adults as people involves a lens of understanding of who they are through their *lived experiences*, including self-identification, proclamation, and revelation of their SOGI. The acceptance and celebration of their SOGI is a defining milestone in living authentically as they truly are. This process is often referred to as *coming out of the closet.* There are typically two phases: internal, during which individuals become aware of their SOGI; and external, during which they declare their SOGI to someone else. The timing and sequencing of these events are unique to the individual.[6] The coming out process varies from one individual to the next and is therefore unique to each individual. The trajectory could be met with acceptance and support from families and other networks. However, this could also be an incredibly stressful time for the individual, especially if met with rejection, ridicule, and ostracization by family and support networks. There is an intrinsic vulnerability in the lived experiences of the individuals, so much so that understanding their unique narratives can assist providers in cogently creating a space of compassion and deliberate consideration for a comprehensive management of their pain experience.

These narratives are embedded in the lived experiences of the LGBTQI+ community that in turn are shaped by two theories, namely life course theory and goal-oriented theory.[36] The former describes how adults change over time as influenced by transitions and choice points in the context of a larger sociocultural milieu. The latter pertains to further development of an adult whose goals are varied, including self-maintenance and balance. For transgender and gender diverse individuals, a significant part of coming out is another closely intertwined process called *transitioning*. This is a process that allows the individual to take steps to transition into the gender they truly identify as. These may or may not include medical and surgical treatments. It is also necessary to understand that there are generational challenges that older LGBTQI+ adults faced as they were coming out compared to millennials, for instance. This is best exemplified in the Caring and Aging study, which showed that more than 80% of older LGBTQI+ adults experienced at least one episode of victimization in their lifetime. The most common forms of victimization included verbal insults, threats of physical violence, being hassled or being ignored by police, damage to personal property, objects being thrown at them, and physical assault in all forms.[37]

The vulnerabilities persist across diverse clinical settings such as nursing home and rehabilitation facilities. There lies a real threat to returning to the closet and detransitioning for transgender and gender diverse individuals.[6] These are processes of retreating from their authentic selves, becoming invisible to the outside world while "blending in" toward a more cisgender and heteronormative archetype. Unfortunately, this concealment and nondisclosure of SOGI further puts this already marginalized population in extreme stress, thereby impacting the provision and access to necessary physical and mental health care. Ultimately, the decision to come out or remain out will largely depend on the safety of the environment (i.e., physical and social) that they are in.

An important element in understanding the psychosocial context in which LGBTQI+ adults exist is the presence or absence of support networks. It is rather common that members of this population have created their own networks of friends and families as a result of abandonment and/or rejection by their biological families and other blood relatives. *Chosen families*, also known as *lavender families*, are individuals whom LGBTQI+ adults have chosen to construct meaningful, familial, and relational ties with in place of their biological families. Examples of chosen family members include friends, roommates, neighbors, co-workers, distant relatives, partners, and children. This is in contradistinction to families of origin, whose kinship with LGBTQI+ adults is through blood or adoption.[38] LGBTQI+ individuals may or may not have good relationships with their families of origin. When they do have fractured relationships, these could be a source of great emotional distress and pain and could contribute to the physical manifestations of the pain experience. Often, chosen families and/or families of origin also serve as the caregivers for members of the LGBTQI+ community when they are faced with serious illness or when they advance in age. The converse is true in that LGBTQI+ people are more than likely to serve as caregivers for ailing family members. The 2006 MetLife survey showed that one in four LGBTQI+ adults serves as the caregiver for a family member as opposed to one in five for the cisgender heterosexual cohort.[39] The chosen families are not spared invisibility and prejudice, especially when LGBTQI+ adults approach the end of life. Without proper legal connections to the patients, they may not be recognized as salient support systems. Moreover, at the time of death, they are as much victims of disenfranchised grief as are the legal partners of LGBTQI+ patients. Kenneth Doka coined the term *disenfranchised grief* in 1989 to describe a pattern of grief that is not openly acknowledged, socially mourned, or publicly supported.[40] This is further rooted in the stigma associated with underrecognition and devaluation of chosen families as legitimate support networks for this community.

A few other key constructs (referenced in the preceding sections) that allow for a more expansive understanding of the textured psychosocial domains impacting LGBTQI+ people's experience of pain include internalized homophobia and transphobia and stigma-based rejection sensitivity. Whereas the former are described as the internalization of negative societal attitudes about one's sexual orientation or gender identity that are subsequently linked to unhealthy and risky behaviors, the latter is described as the psychological process through which some members of the minority groups are conditioned to be anxiously anticipating rejection due to prior experiences with prejudice and discrimination toward their group membership.[41,42]

Cultural Domain

Members of the LGBTQI+ community are cultural beings inasmuch as non-LGBTQI+ people are. They come from various backgrounds and diverse experiences. Culture influences the beliefs, values, and practices around the experience and response to various illnesses and associated symptoms, including pain. It is critical to understand that certain ethnic and racial groups express pain openly, whereas others are stoic about it.

No matter the manifestation, pain should be considered culturally acceptable.[43] The language to describe pain can be nuanced to specific racial and ethnic cultures. The LGBTQI+ community has a shared culture of being marginalized and oppressed, as evidenced by the minority stress model. Therefore, it is critical for providers to be cognizant of the inadvertent practice of *ethnocentrism*, which is the tendency to believe that one's own cultural norms are correct and evaluate other's beliefs in light of them. By this account, acknowledging the differences in pain expression and manifestation is a valid consideration in comprehensive pain assessment and management rather than ascribing judgment whether it is right or wrong. Furthermore, it is essential to be mindful of unique cultural practices such as underreporting of pain, reluctance to use pharmacotherapies, fear of further prejudice and discrimination, and fear of being unjustly labeled as drug-seekers or abusers, among others.

Religious and Spiritual Domain

The religious and spiritual domain or a lack thereof is an essential and interwoven aspect in the comprehensive management of pain by LGBTQI+ people. *Religion* is distinguished from *spirituality* in that the former is characterized by institutional beliefs and rituals, whereas the latter is an individualized journey influenced by experiential descriptors such as transcendence, connectedness, meaning, purpose, and energy.[44] Religion is often organized as a community but can also exist outside of an institution, and it may be practiced alone or in private. In contrast, spirituality has been much more broadly self-defined and can be anything a person wants it to mean. Spirituality may be deeply religious for some or not very religious for others. Secular humanism views human existence without reference to God, religion, the transcendent, and higher power.[45]

The experiences of LGBTQI+ people in relation to religion and spirituality is quite complex. Historically, health care systems affiliated with religious organizations have refused much needed medical care and ostracized this community. The discriminatory practices are rooted in traditions and beliefs that many monotheistic religions, such as Christianity and Islam, uphold. This has therefore caused tremendous emotional and spiritual pain for the LGBTQI+ community.[46] Moreover, in many of these religions that are non-LGBTQI+ affirming, the coming out process across ages could be fraught with fear of rejection, persecution, and exclusion from their spiritual and religious communities, resulting in dissociation and abandonment of their religion and spirituality and undesirable psychological outcomes such as anxiety, depression, poor self-esteem, and internalized homophobia and transphobia.[47] Regardless of sexuality, spiritual pain in the context of advanced or serious illness correlates with anxiety, depression, and lower quality of life. This is further defined as pain deep in one's soul that is not physical. Mako et al.[48] referred to three major components: intrapersonal (e.g., despair and isolation), interpersonal (e.g., isolation), and transpersonal (e.g., despair and anxiety).

Although there has been animosity between LGBTQI+ people and organized religions, there is also evidence that this population may ascribe to spiritual beliefs and practices as supported by a 2013 survey indicating that spirituality is a significant component of this population's sense of self, values, and worldviews.[49] Therefore, spirituality could act as a source of coping and support in this population. Spirituality has been described as acceptance and loving kindness.

Resilience, Robustness, and Crisis Competence

Due to long-standing oppression, discrimination, and abuse that members of the LGBTQI+ community have faced across time, they have collectively developed coping strategies in order to survive. Stress inoculation theories point to the fact that early exposure to various forms of stigma and marginalization have allowed an intersectional identity of resiliency to buffer that of the stressors associated with being a minority. Resilience is the ability to mitigate the adverse impact of stress and thrive in the face of adversity.[50] Moreover, coping is distinctive from resilience in that the former pertains to the effort put into adapting or responding to stress, whereas the latter is the result of a successful adaptation to stress in the hope of mitigating multiple stressors. Meyer categorizes resilience in two levels: personal or individual resilience and community resilience. *Individual resilience* describes a person's capability to cope with stress and triumph over adversity. Examples include spirituality, religiosity, support network, positive self-esteem, and exercise. *Community resilience* pertains to a community's capacity to empower marginalized members through the provision of both tangible and intangible resources. Examples include safe public spaces, protective policies, and other affirming services such as health care.[51] In 1978, Kimmel described the construct of *crisis competence* especially among adult and older adult gay men as patterns of survival strategies that have been utilized in response to managing a lifetime of minority stressors and adversities and would allow them to age successfully even if faced with a lack of social supports and financial resources, among others.[52,53] This was evidenced by the MetLife Survey in 2006, which showed that close to 40% of LGBTQI+ baby boomers believed that being a sexual and gender minority prepared them for the aging process (Figure 8.1).[54]

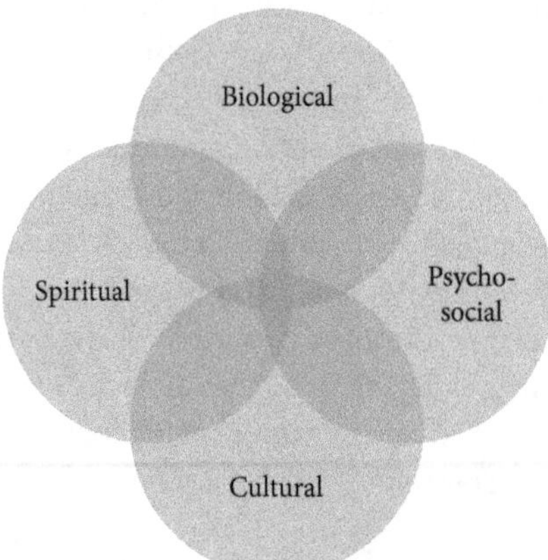

Figure 8.1 Proposed framework for pain assessment and management in the LGBTQ community: Biopsychosocial, cultural, and spiritual model of the pain experience.

Multidimensional Pain Assessment Tools

The tools used to assess and manage pain in non-LGBTQI+ individuals are the same ones used to assess and manage pain in the LGBTQI+ community. To my knowledge and based on a review of the literature, there are no existing studies to support that the perception, experience, and manifestation of pain between these two groups are different. Therefore, in the assessment of the severity of *physical pain*, we can utilize scales such as the numeric pain scale, the faces pain scale for those with cognitive impairment and very young patients, the visual analog scale, pain descriptor scales, and the combination of any of these, among others.[55] The older adult population might prefer pain terminologies such as discomfort, aches, pains, hurting, etc.; regardless of the scale used, it is essential to be consistent with its use to be able to track and monitor pain over time. An important multidimensional scale that can be utilized is the Brief Pain Inventory (BPI). This is a self-administered questionnaire that has been validated in both cancer and chronic non-cancer pain. It is available in a short form of 9 questions and a long form of 17 questions. The questionnaire typically consists of pain diagrams, pain intensity items, pain relief and treatments, and pain interference in day-to-day function.[56] In addition to these scales, we can further identify and expand on the quality, characteristics, and other descriptors of pain using the commonly used mnemonic PQRSTU, which stands for palliating and provoking factors (P), quality or nature of pain (Q), radiation and region of pain (R), severity and associated symptomatology (S), timing or temporality (T), and the overall effect on the quality of life and function (U).[57]

For the psychosocial assessment of pain, there are two well-known multidimensional scales that incorporate questions on psychological symptoms. The McGill Pain Questionnaire (MPQ) is a comprehensive measure that quantifies both neurophysiological and psychological domains of pain. Although extensively used in cancer populations, throughout the years this has gained popularity for use in those with chronic nonmalignant pain as well. This pain scale was developed based on the gate control theory. The MPQ includes four main measures: pain location, pain intensity, pain quality (that integrates sensory, affective, and cognitive dimensions), and pain pattern. A fifth additional measure evaluates alleviating and aggravating factors (i.e., behavioral dimension).[58] The second multidimensional scale is the Edmonton Symptom Assessment Scale, which is a self-reporting tool of symptom intensity that was developed in a palliative care unit in Canada. This has been validated in diverse diagnoses, including cancer and other serious illnesses such as heart failure. It consists of numerical rating scales among 10 commonly presenting symptoms: pain, nausea, tiredness, shortness of breath, drowsiness, appetite, sleep, psychological symptoms of depression and anxiety, and overall well-being.[59]

In performing a culturally humble approach to pain assessment and management, it is helpful for providers to understand the cultural background of the patient through a lens of curiosity and openness to be able to allow the patient to express how they feel and manifest pain. Moreover, it is helpful to understand nuances in interpretation and behaviors pertaining to the experience of pain because some pain assessment tools might be linguistically or culturally inappropriate. The explanatory model interview for pain assessment is a good template for a more open-ended approach to understanding the experience of pain of patients with diverse backgrounds and cultures.[60] The BPI and MPQ have both been translated and validated across cultural and linguistic groups.[43]

Regarding the spiritual assessment of pain, a tool that has been demonstrated to be effective in the palliative care literature is the FICA Spiritual History Tool. This instrument was created in 1996 by Christina Puchalski. FICA stands for faith (F), importance of faith (I), spiritual community (C), and interventions to address spiritual needs (A). This tool uses open-ended questions that can be incorporated into standard medical history by health care professionals.[61] Other spiritual assessment tools that might also be helpful are the Spiritual Injury Scale, the Functional Assessment of Chronic Illness Therapy—Spiritual Well-Being 12 Item Scale, and Spiritual Pain Screening Question. Schultz et al.'s[62] study on spiritual distress showed that among cancer patients followed over 12 months, the Spiritual Injury Scale had the best correlation with spiritual distress, although an imperfect one. Moreover, spiritual distress is not necessarily identical with spiritual pain, even though the latter showed a bivariate correlation with it.[62]

Remediation/Treatment

Sexual Orientation and Gender Identity Collection

One of the major pitfalls that leads to the perpetuation of these harsh realities is the lack of visibility, disclosure, and representation of LGBTQI+ people presenting in health care facilities due in large part to the health care system's failure to include sexual orientation and gender identity in electronic health records even though there is a significant LGBTQI+ population in mainstream society. The 2017 EQUALITY study highlighted the importance for medical providers to ask for the SOGI of their patients in the emergency room setting.[63] This exploratory, sequential, and mixed methods study found that only 10% of respondents (regardless of their actual SOGI) would refuse to provide their SOGI information. However, more than two-thirds of health care professionals assumed that their patients were not willing to disclose their SOGI information. In a parallel study of exclusively transgender individuals, the majority believed that gender identity was more important to report than sexual orientation; however, they also stated that if asked their SOGI, they were willing to disclose this as long as the environment was LGBTQI+ friendly and the information was relevant to their chief complaint.[64] Patient acceptance of SOGI disclosure on intake forms has also been demonstrated in the outpatient setting. A pragmatic randomized multisite trial conducted by Rullo et al.[65] showed that collection of SOGI as a part of the routine clinical patient intake process was not distressing to 97% of patients who were heterosexual, cisgender, and older than age 50 years. This finding was consistent with the findings from an earlier study by Cahill et al.[31] that most respondents (both heterosexual and LGBTQI+) in four diverse U.S. community health centers were willing to answer SOGI questions on intake forms and were supportive of its inclusion in these forms.

Interprofessional Approach to Care

The proposed biopsychosocial, cultural, and spiritual model of care grounds its approach in a multidimensional manner. Having a team-based approach including diverse health care professionals is integral to holistic care. The team members include, but are not limited to, physicians, nurses, mid-level providers, social workers, chaplains, pharmacists, rehabilitation therapists, psychologists, and nutritionists. The core tenets of this approach include ongoing education, training, collaboration, feedback, cooperation, and teamwork. A study by Damsgard et al.[66] in Norway highlights the importance of collaboration of trainees from various disciplines (i.e., nursing, physical therapy, pharmacy, and medical education) in developing a comprehensive pain management plan for older adults in a nursing home. Interprofessional collaboration fostered enthusiasm and a more holistic pain management approach. Moreover, the approach also assisted in mitigating presumptions about patients' pain experience.[66] These results are further supported by a 2020 study of pre-licensure health professional students utilizing an interprofessional learning module for cancer pain treatment.[67] Through close collaboration with diverse members from multiple disciplines, a patient-centered approach in pain management was achieved. The ultimate goal is to normalize and standardize the routine collection of SOGI on intake forms and electronic medical records so that members of the LGBTQI+ community will be recognized for who they are and will receive optimal health care based on their unique needs and concerns.

Multimodal Approach to Pain Management

Currently, there is no literature indicating that the use of various modalities of pain management is different for LGBTQI+ and non-LGBTQI+ individuals. Multimodal approaches for the management of acute and chronic pain include the use of pharmacotherapy such as nonsteroidal anti-inflammatory drugs and opioids, interventional pain strategies such as neuraxial blocks, rehabilitation therapies (e.g., physical therapy, occupational therapy, and speech–language pathology), and other methods of pain management such as integrative therapies. This approach is consistent with the biopsychosocial framework in managing patients with pain. After all, pain is a complex biopsychosocial disease that can affect many facets of life, including sleep, cognition, mood, ambulation, and other activities of daily living.[68] Physical pain and associated symptoms are the result of the dynamic interactions among the biological, psychological, and social factors.[69] Moreover, the psychosocial, cultural, and spiritual strategies to mitigate pain include the presence of social supports, mental health counseling, spirituality and religion, volunteerism, community activities (e.g., group exercises), and access to LGBTQI+ resources. The involvement of an interprofessional team is crucial to a successful multidimensional program for holistic pain management.[50,68] The benefits of a multimodal approach include improvement in pain control, reduction in the use of opioids, and increased patient satisfaction.[70,71]

Case Example: How the Model Works

A 59-year-old Native American woman of transgender experience with a history of HIV was seen as a new consultation in the hospital after she was admitted for weakness and failure to thrive. She is visibly observed to have lost weight and extremely malnourished. She was recently diagnosed with HIV/AIDS. Upon query, she endorsed widespread bodily aches and pains. She described the pain as sharp with a burning feature to it. Her pain is most pronounced in both of her legs. She only takes acetaminophen with minimal relief. Her pain experience has impacted her ability to sleep, think clearly, and walk for long periods of time. She shared that she no longer wanted to take her antiretroviral therapies. She expressed being fed up with taking too many pills and frequently seeing her medical providers. One day, she decided to stop them altogether. She further shared that there is no other purpose for her existence. She did not endorse any depression or loss of interest in her daily activities. She has not attempted suicide in the past. She is not using illicit substances from the street. She is resigned to dying with this disease. She did not identify any religious affiliations, although in the past she attended a Christian church. She is currently unemployed and living on disability. Her partner died a few years ago. She has no relationship with her mother, who at disapproved of her lifestyle and abandoned her (Figure 8.2).

A multimodal approach to pain management could include pharmacotherapy using opioids for her sharp pain and non-opioid medications such as gabapentinoids for her neuropathic pain; mental health and social support using

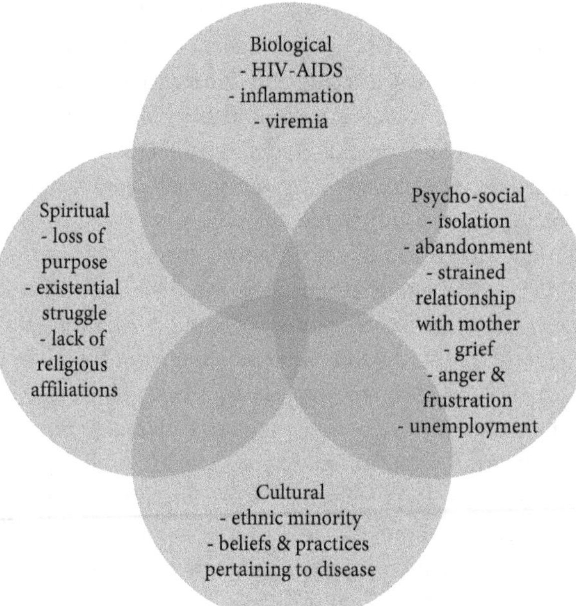

Figure 8.2 Conceptual framework: Biopsychosocial, cultural, and spiritual paradigm.

cognitive-behavioral therapy and counseling; chaplaincy support to explore existential crises using dignity therapy; and involvement of other members of the interprofessional team, such as rehabilitation specialists to assist with functionality. Moreover, if consistent with overall goals of care, she could benefit from palliative/hospice care support, especially because HIV/AIDS is a progressive disease without antiretroviral therapies.

Conclusion

The LGBTQI+ community is a marginalized population that continues to experience oppression and discrimination in various clinical settings. A multidimensional approach utilizing the biopsychosocial, cultural, and spiritual model of care is integral to understanding the pain experience of this population. Therefore, the strategies in addressing and managing the pain experience are multimodal, including pharmacologic and nonpharmacologic interventions. The active involvement of all the members of the interprofessional team from various disciplines is crucial to optimizing pain control in a holistic manner.

References

1. Jones JM. LGBT identification rises to 5.6% in latest U.S. estimate. February 24, 2017. https://news.gallup.com/poll/329708/lgbt-identification-rises-latest-estimate.aspx
2. Migdon B. US LGBT+ population hits 20 million. *The Hill.* December 14, 2021. https://thehill.com/changing-america/respect/diversity-inclusion/585711-us-lgbtq-population-hits-20-million
3. Institute of Medicine Committee on Lesbian, Gay, Bisexual, and Transgender Health Issues and Research Gaps and Opportunities. *The Health of Lesbian, Gay, Bisexual, and Transgender People: Building a Foundation for Better Understanding.* National Academies Press; 2011.
4. Pérez-Stable EJ. Director's message. October 6, 2016. https://www.nimhd.nih.gov/about/directors-corner/messages/message_10-06-16.html
5. Fredriksen-Goldsen KI, Kim HJ, Bryan AEB, Shiu C, Emlet CA. The cascading effects of marginalization and pathways of resilience in attaining good health among LGBT older adults. *Geronologist.* 2017;57(Suppl 1):S72–A83.
6. Yarns BC, Abrams JM, Meeks TW, Sewell DD. The mental health of older LGBT adults. *Curr Psychiatry Rep.* 2016;18(60):1–11.
7. GLAAD. *Accelerating Acceptance 2019: A survey of American acceptance and attitudes toward LGBTQ Americans.* GLAAD; 2019.
8. Gatchel RJ, Peng YB, Peters ML, Fuchs PN, Turk DC. The biopsychosocial approach to chronic pain: Scientific advances and future directions. *Psychol Bull.* 2007;133(4):581–624.
9. Meyer IH. Prejudice, social stress, and mental health in lesbian, gay, and bisexual populations: Conceptual issues and research evidence. *Psychol Bull.* 2003;129(5):674–697.
10. Guidi J, Lucente M, Sonino N, Fava GA. Allostatic load and its impact on health: A systematic review. *Psychother Psychosom.* 2021;90:11–27.
11. Meyer IH. Resilience in the study of minority stress and health of sexual and gender minorities. *Psychol Sex Orient Gender Divers.* 2015;2:209–213.
12. Witten TM. It's not all darkness: Robustness, resilience, and successful transgender aging. *LGBT Health.* 2014;1(1):24–33.

13. Seng J, Lopez W, Sperlich M, et al. Marginalized identities, discriminate burden and mental health: Empirical exploration of an interpersonal-level approach to modeling intersectionality. *Soc Sci Med*. 2012;75:2437–2445.
14. Foronda C, Baptiste DL, Reinholdt MM, Ousman K. Cultural humility: A concept analysis. *J Transcult Nurs*. 2016;27:210–217.
15. Wallace S, Cochran S, Durazo E, Ford C. The health of aging lesbian, gay, and bisexual adults in California. Policy Brief UCLA Cent Health Policy Res. 2011;(PB2011-2):1–8.
16. Fredriksen-Goldsen KI, Kim HJ, Barkan SE, Muraco A, Hoy-Ellis CP. Health disparities among lesbian, gay, and bisexual older adults: Results from a population-based study. *Am J Public Health*. 2013;103(10):1802–1809.
17. Fredriksen-Goldsen KI. Resilience and disparities among lesbian, gay, bisexual, and transgender older adults. *Public Policy Aging Rep*. 2011;21(3):3–7.
18. Grulich AE, Poynten IM, Machalek DA, Jin F, Templeton DJ, Hillman RJ. The epidemiology of anal cancer. *Sex Health*. 2012;9:504–508.
19. Palefsky JM, Giuliano AR, Goldstone S, et al. HPV vaccine against anal HPV infection and anal intraepithelial neoplasia. *N Eng. J Med*. 2011;365:1576–1585.
20. Moayedi M, Davis KD. Theories of pain: From specificity to gate control. *J Neurophysiol*. 2013;109(1):5–12.
21. Kusnanto H, Agustian D, Hilmanto D. Biopsychosocial model of illnesses in primary care: A hermeneutic literature review. *J Family Med Prim Care*. 2018;7(3):497–500.
22. Ong CK, Forbes D. Embracing Cicely Saunder's concept of total pain. *BMJ*. 2005;331(7516):576–577.
23. Lambda Legal. When health care isn't caring? Lambda Legal survey on LGBT people and people living with HIV. 2010. https://legacy.lambdalegal.org/publications/when-health-care-isnt-caring
24. James SE, Herman JL, Rankin S, et al. *The Report of the 2015 US Transgender Survey*. National Center for Transgender Equality; 2016.
25. Choi SK, Meyer IL. LGBT aging: A review of research findings, needs, and policy implications. The Williams Institute, UCLA School of Law. 2016. https://www.lgbtagingcenter.org/resources/pdfs/LGBT-Aging-A-Review.pdf
26. Grant JM, Mottet LA, Tanis J, et al. *Injustice at Every Turn: A Report of the National Transgender Discrimination Survey*. National Center for Transgender Equality and National Gay and Lesbian Task Force; 2011.
27. Carter PL, Reardon SF. Inequality matters. William T. Grant Foundation. 2014. Accessed June 14, 2022. https://wtgrantfoundation.org/wp-content/uploads/2015/09/Inequality-Matters.pdf
28. D'Augelli AR, Grossman AH, Hershberger SL, O'Connell TS. Aspects of mental health among older lesbian, gay, and bisexual adults. *Aging Ment Health*. 2001;5(2):149–158.
29. Kenagy GP. Transgender health: Findings from two needs assessment studies in Philadelphia. *Health Soc Work*. 2005;30(1):19–26.
30. Lombardi E, Wilchins R, Priesling D, Malouf D. Gender violence: Transgender experiences with violence and discrimination. *J Homosex*. 2002; 42(1):89–101.
31. Cahill S, Singal R, Grasso C, et al. Do ask, do tell: High levels of acceptability by patients of routine collection of sexual orientation and gender identity data in four diverse American community health centers. *PLoS One*. 2014;9(9):1–8.
32. Byne W. Regulations restrict practice of conversion therapy. *LGBT Health*. 2016;3(2):97–99.
33. Balsam KF, Molina Y, Beadnell B, Simoni J, Walters K. Measuring multiple minority stress: The LGBT people of color microaggressions scale. *Cult Divers Ethnic Minor Psychol*. 2011;17(2):163–174.
34. Fredriksen-Goldsen KI, Emlet CA, Kim HJ, et al. The physical and mental health of lesbian, gay male, and bisexual older adults: The role of key health indicators and risk and protective factors. *Gerontologist*. 2013;54(4):664–675.
35. Monin JK, Mota N, Levy B, Pachankis J, Pietrzak RH. Older age associated with mental health resiliency in sexual minority US veterans. *Am J Geriatr Psych*. 2017;25(1):81–90.

36. Aldwin CM, Igarashi H, Gilmer DF, Levenson MR. *Health, Illness, and Optimal Aging: Biological and Psychological Perspectives*. 2nd ed. Springer; 2013.
37. Fredriksen-Goldsen KI, Kim HJ, Shiu C, Goldsen J, Emlet CA. Successful aging among LGBT older adults: Physical and mental health-related quality of life by age group. *Gerontologist*. 2015;55(1):154–168.
38. Neville S, Henrickson M. The constitution of "lavender families": A LGB perspective. *J Clin Nurs*. 2009;18:849–856.
39. MetLife Mature Market Institute and American Society on Aging. Still out, Still Aging: The MetLife Study of lesbian, gay, bisexual, and transgender baby boomers. 2010. Accessed June 14, 2022. https://www.asaging.org/sites/default/files/files/mmi-still-out-still-aging.pdf
40. Cardoza K, Schneider CM. The importance of mourning losses (even when they seem small). NPR. 2021. Accessed June 14, 2022. https://www.npr.org/2021/06/02/1002446604/the-importance-of-mourning-losses-even-when-they-seem-small
41. Hatzenbuehler ML, Pachankis JE. Stigma and minority stress as social determinants of health among lesbian, gay, bisexual, and transgender youth. *Pediatr Clin North Am*. 2016;63:985–997.
42. Mendoza-Denton R, Downey G, Purdie VJ, et al. Sensitivity to status-based rejection: Implications for African American students' college experience. *J Pers Soc Psychol*. 2002;83(4):896–918.
43. Narayan MC. Culture's effects on pain assessment and management. *Am J Nurs*. 2010;110(4):38–47.
44. Pesut B, Fowler M, Taylor EJ, Reimer-Kirkham S, Sawatzky R. Conceptualising spirituality and religion for healthcare. *J Clin Nurs*. 2008;17:2803–2810.
45. Koenig HG. Religion, spirituality, and health: A review and update. *Adv Mind Body Med*. 2015;29(3):19–26.
46. Higgins A, Hynes G. Meeting the needs of people who identify as lesbian, gay, bisexual, transgender, and queer in palliative care settings. *J Hosp Palliat Nurs*. 2019;21(4):286–290.
47. Gibbs JJ, Goldbach J. Religious conflict, sexual identity, and suicidal behaviors among LGBT young adults. *Arch of Suicide Res*. 2015;19(4):472–488.
48. Mako C, Galek K, Poppito SR. Spiritual pain among patients with advanced cancer in palliative care. *J Palliat Med*. 2006;9:1106–1113.
49. Porter KE, Ronnenberg CR, Witten TM. Religious affiliation and successful aging among transgender older adults: Findings from the Trans MetLife Survey. *J Relig Spiritual Aging*. 2013;25:112–138.
50. Frost DM, Meyer IH. Measuring community connectedness among diverse sexual minority populations. *J Sex Res*. 2012;49:36–49.
51. McConnell EA, Janulis P, Phillips G II, Truong R, Birkett M. Multiple minority stress and LGBT community resilience among sexual minority men. *Psychol Sex Orientat Gend Divers*. 2018;5(1):1–12.
52. Kimmel DC. Adult development and aging: A gay perspective. *J Soc Issues*. 1978;34:113–130.
53. Brown MT, Grossman BR. Same-sex sexual relationships in the national social life, health, and aging project: Making a case for data collection. *J Gerontol Soc Work*. 2014;57(2–4):108–129.
54. MetLife Mature Market Institute, American Society on Aging, and Zogby International. Out and aging: The MetLife study of lesbian & gay baby boomers. 2006. Accessed June 14, 2022. https://www.lgbtagingcenter.org/resources/resource.cfm?r=31
55. Karcioglu O, Topacoglu H, Dikme O, Dikme O. A systematic review of the pain scales in adults: Which to use? *Am J Emerg Med*. 2018;36(4):707–714.
56. Poquet N, Lin C. The Brief Pain Inventory. *J Physiother*. 2016;62(1):52.
57. McPherson ML. *Demystifying Opioid Conversion Calculations*. American Society of Health System Pharmacists; 2010.
58. Ngamkam S, Vincent C, Finnegan L, et al. The McGill Pain Questionnaire as a multidimensional measure in people with cancer: An integrative review. *Pain Manag Nurs*. 2012;13(1):27–51.

59. Wong A, Tayjasanant S, Rodriguez-Nunez A, et al. Edmonton Symptom Assessment Scale time duration of self-completion versus assisted completion in patients with advanced cancer: A randomized comparison. *Oncologist.* 2021;26(2):165–171.
60. Lasch KE. Culture, pain, and culturally sensitive pain care. *Pain Manag Nurs.* 2000;1(3 Suppl 1):16–22.
61. Borneman T, Ferrell B, Puchalski C. Evaluation of the FICA tool for spiritual assessment. *J Pain Symptom Manage.* 2010;40(2):163–173.
62. Schultz M, Meged-Book T, Maschiach T, Bar-Sela G. Distinguishing between spiritual distress, general distress, spiritual well-being, and spiritual pain among cancer patients during oncology treatment. *J Pain Symptom Manage.* 2017;54(1):66–73.
63. Haider AH, Schneider EB, Kodadek LM, et al. Emergency department query for patient-centered approaches to sexual orientation and gender identity: The EQUALITY study. *JAMA Intern Med.* 2017;177(6):819–828.
64. Maragh-Bass AC, Torain M, Adler R, et al. Is it okay to ask: Transgender patient perspectives on sexual orientation and gender identity collection in healthcare. *Acad Emerg Med.* 2017;24(6):655–667.
65. Rullo JE, Foxen JL, Griffin JM, et al. Patient acceptance of sexual orientation and gender identity questions on intake forms in outpatient clinics: A pragmatic randomized multisite trial. *Health Serv Res.* 2018;53(5):3790–3808.
66. Damsgard E, Solgard H, Johannessen K, et al. Understanding pain and pain management in elderly nursing home patients applying an interprofessional learning activity in health care students: A Norwegian pilot study. *Pain Manag Nurs.* 2018;19(5):516–524.
67. Fishman SM, Copenhaver D, Mongoven JM, Lorenzen K, Schlingmann E, Young HE. Cancer pain treatment and management. *MedEdPORTAL.* 2020;16:10953.
68. Schwan J, Scalafani J, Tawfik VL. Chronic pain management in the elderly. *Anesthesiol Clin.* 2019;37(3):547–560.
69. Cohen SP, Vase L, Hooten WH. Chronic pain: An update on burden, best practices, and new advances. *Lancet.* 2021;397(10289):2082–2097.
70. Helander EM, Menard BL, Harmon CM, et al. Multimodal analgesia, current concepts, and acute pain considerations. *Curr Pain Headache Rep.* 2017;21(1): Article 3.
71. Slawek DE. People living with HIV and the emerging field of chronic pain: What is known about epidemiology, etiology, and management. *Curr HIV/AIDS Rep.* 2021;18(5):436–442.

9

Vulnerability to Pain-Related Disability Following Occupational Injury

A Diathesis–Stress Perspective

Raymond C. Tait

Introduction

In a book dedicated to the issue of vulnerability, some may question the inclusion of a chapter focused on people with pain (PwP) secondary to occupational injury. People who sustain work-related injuries do not lack access to treatment: Federal law mandates treatment of occupational injuries through state-based workers' compensation (WC) systems. Treatment is provided regardless of sociodemographic factors (e.g., race/ethnicity) known to occasion treatment disparities for PwP in the general population.[1] These elements separate PwP related to occupational injury from other vulnerable groups, who may lack access to treatment secondary to socioeconomic or other sociocultural factors.[2]

Because PwP following occupational injury benefit from WC-related protections, they fall outside dictionary definitions of vulnerability[3]: "Someone who is . . . weak and without protection, with the result that they are easily hurt." Similarly, the WC cohort does not meet bioethics definitions of vulnerability involving capacity to provide informed consent[4]: Aside from the choice of a treating physician (restricted in many states), injured workers provide consent prior to treatment. Instead, this chapter considers vulnerability from a risk perspective: A patient cohort is deemed vulnerable when it experiences greater risk for poor treatment/outcomes relative to other patient groups with comparable health conditions.

From a risk perspective, people who sustain occupational injuries that occasion persistent pain clearly are vulnerable: Outcomes are significantly poorer for workers with low back pain (LBP) and other musculoskeletal injuries treated through a WC system than for people with LBP treated outside WC systems.[5] A meta-analysis of surgical outcomes for people treated through WC versus non-WC systems found that the odds of a good recovery were almost four times worse for those treated through WC systems.[6] Indeed, relative to non-occupational injuries, work-related injuries occasion disproportionate levels of Social Security disability claims/enrollment.[7] Furthermore, despite WC requirements that workers with job-related injuries receive treatment, disparities within WC systems mirror those found more broadly: Minorities with LBP receive significantly less treatment than non-minorities,[8] undergo significantly fewer surgical interventions,[9] and demonstrate poorer treatment outcomes.[10,11] Moreover, socioeconomic status (SES) factors adversely impact long-term outcomes following WC treatment.[12]

Researchers have proposed that a diathesis–stress perspective be applied to chronic pain secondary to occupational injury,[13–15] arguing that multiple factors affect a patient's treatment response: individual vulnerabilities, pain-related stressors, and WC-specific stressors. Individual vulnerabilities, well studied in the clinical literature, include dysfunctional coping skills,[16] depression,[17] and other psychosocial factors.[18] Similarly, pain-specific stressors are well studied, such as inconsistencies between objective medical evidence and self-reported symptoms that occasion providers discounting the severity of pain.[19] Less attention has been paid to WC-specific effects.[20,21]

This chapter applies a diathesis–stress perspective to painful occupational injuries in WC settings. The following section describes the diathesis–stress model in more detail, including a brief history of its neuropsychiatric origins. It also outlines chronic pain-related factors related to that model: baseline stresses associated with chronic pain, WC system stresses, and patient-related vulnerabilities that interact poorly with WC system stresses. Sections that follow address each of these factors in greater detail. The chapter concludes with a discussion of strategies that may attenuate the adverse effects experienced by PwP who are engaged with WC systems.

The Diathesis–Stress Model

As noted above, the diathesis–stress model derives from a neuropsychiatric literature that attempted to explain the discontinuous development of schizophrenia[22] and then was extended to explain the development of major depressive disorders.[23] The premise underlying these models involved pre-existing genetic vulnerabilities: When stresses exceed their coping capacity, patients with these vulnerabilities experience changes in psychopathology beyond expected, additive effects. Empirical studies, enabled by recent technologic advances in genetic research, have supported the model. For example, depression research has shown that the levels of psychopathology exhibited by patients with genetic predispositions exceed what would be predicted by direct effects of stressors.[24]

Application to Chronic Pain Following Occupational Injury

The constructs of the diathesis–stress model—vulnerability and stress—have been adapted to chronic pain research, albeit without assumptions regarding genetic predispositions. Turk and Banks[13] have proposed that a diathesis–stress model could be used as a heuristic within which to consider "the interaction of predisposing factors with a trauma, setting in motion a cascade of interpretive cognitive processes . . . that maintain disability following the trauma" (p. 9). This formulation is supported by longitudinal studies of patients with low back injuries showing that disability 1 year after injury is more strongly associated with psychosocial factors than with injury-related biomedical factors.[18]

Turk and Banks'[13] focus on psychological factors fails to consider the role of system-related stressors in the development of pain-related disability, as well as system-related stressors that interact adversely with psychosocial vulnerabilities. Figure 9.1 extends the diathesis–stress model of chronic pain to the context of a WC system. It outlines three domains that may occasion disability: medical system stresses, WC system stresses, and psychosocial vulnerabilities.

The following medical system stresses have been shown to operate within WC systems[25]: (1) treatment complications associated with inconsistencies between confirmatory medical evidence and reported pain severity and pain-related dysfunction and (2) racial/ethnic disparities in pain-related treatment and outcomes. Secondary to the medicolegal underpinnings of WC systems, evidence of impairment is critical to disability determinations,[26] despite the frequent lack of association between such findings and ultimate occupational status.[27] Similarly, although less studied than the latter issue, there is evidence of significant racial/ethnic disparities in state WC systems.[25] Because of the substantial overlap between the WC literature and the general medical literature on these topics, however, the WC literature on these topics is not reviewed. Instead, system-related stresses more specific to WC are reviewed: (1) operational issues that disadvantage PwP, (2) WC-related patient–provider issues that undermine effective collaboration, and (3) WC conditions that promote litigation and undermine treatment.

The chapter also selectively reviews patient diatheses—the vulnerabilities/coping resources that WC claimants bring to the experience of persistent pain. As noted above, diatheses that can influence response to treatment and adjustment to pain include SES, coping strategies, mood disorders, and many others. Again, given the broad scope of

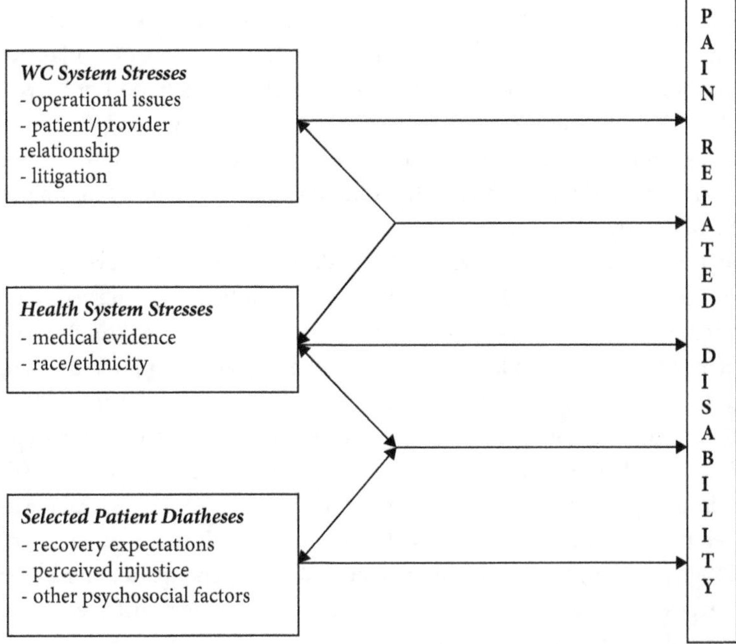

Figure 9.1 Diathesis–stress model: Pain-related disability with compensable injury. WC, workers' compensation.

this literature and its many commonalities with the broader chronic pain field, these diatheses are not reviewed here. Two other diatheses, however, that are clearly and directly relevant to WC systems are reviewed: recovery expectations linked to return to work (RTW) and perceived injustice, the perception of being treated unfairly. The following sections address these systemic stresses and patient diatheses in more detail.

Systemic Stresses in Workers' Compensation Programs

Operational Issues

Although this chapter largely treats WC systems as a unitary entity—a system common to all states—that perspective obscures differences. Indeed, the only truly common feature across state WC systems is that, since 1948, each state has one. Otherwise, systems diverge in numerous ways[25]: 30 states allow injured workers to choose their treating physicians, whereas 20 assign that function to the employer; 38 states use a schedule of impairments to determine PPD ratings, whereas 9 base PPD ratings on projected wage-loss consequences of an injury, and 3 do not consider disabilities as partial. States also diverge in their handling of injuries not on a benefit schedule (a common issue with pain): 19 states use a schedule that assigns a financial value to an impairment, 13 estimate the impact of an injury on future wage-earning, 10 base PPD on the difference between pre- and post-injury wages, and 8 use some combination of the above.

Although state WC programs represent a patchwork of different approaches, several issues are cross-cutting, with clear implications for managing pain-related disabilities. One issue involves delays in treatment by providers with experience in treating at-risk workers,[28] especially when treatment involves multidisciplinary care. Delays increase claim duration and increase the likelihood of chronicity[29,30]: 85% of workers with LBP return to work within 6 months of injury, after which the likelihood of RTW declines dramatically. Various factors contribute to delays: (1) determining that a worker is failing to respond to standard treatment; (2) obtaining additional approvals needed for further evaluation and treatment; and (3) initiating multidisciplinary care, a potentially successful but costly intervention.[31]

Delays run counter to the goals of "secondary prevention," preventing disability after a work-related injury.[32] Successful disability-mitigating interventions should be provided within 3 months of injury—further delays increase disability risk.[33] The Department of Labor and Industries in the state of Washington piloted a program in 2004 (the Centers of Occupational Health and Education [COHE]) aimed at delivering occupational medicine best practices within weeks of an injury[34]: (1) improved care coordination, (2) enhanced physician payment for delivering best practices, (3) training aimed at improving providers' ability to treat workplace injuries, (4) information systems developed to track patient progress, (5) support of health care leadership to reduce work disability, and (6) support of business and labor leadership. Relative to a standard care cohort, workers with LBP who participated in the pilot demonstrated a 30% reduction in long-term disability at a 2-year follow-up,[34] a pattern that was repeated 8 years post-injury.[35] These results have encouraged other states to consider similar secondary prevention practices.

Patient–Provider Relationship Issues

One differentiating feature across states involves the selection of a treating physician: 20 states assign that responsibility to the employer, whereas 30 assign it to an injured worker. WC providers, including those that workers choose, have responsibilities that differ from those associated with non-WC providers.[36] Whereas the primary responsibility of a non-WC provider is to treat painful symptoms, secondarily reducing pain-related disability, the primary responsibility of a WC provider is to the employer—to facilitate RTW. PwP are sensitive to these differences: WC patients referred to a pain clinic voiced significantly less confidence in their physicians than did patients referred through standard medical channels.[37]

Negative stereotypes regarding patients in compensation proceedings (e.g., compensation neurosis) also can influence patient–provider relationships, including the attribution of symptoms to psychological causes, especially when patients are distressed. Those patients are vulnerable to providers discounting the contribution of potential medical factors contributing to the pain condition,[38] even when neurologic findings are comparable to those of less distressed patients.[39]

Litigation-Related Issues

Secondary to its medicolegal underpinnings, injured workers are considered WC claimants, regardless of their legal representation. As noted above, claimants are viewed within the medical community with suspicion, making them vulnerable to negative stereotypes. Aside from stereotypes, data also show poorer outcomes for PwP who are involved in WC-related litigation.[5,6,40]

Litigation effects, however, may be more nuanced than previously thought. A study of PwP referred for pain treatment, controlling for legal representation (yes/no) and WC involvement (yes/no), showed that WC claimants with legal representation were less distressed than claimants without representation, whereas PwP with legal representation who were not involved in WC proceedings were more distressed than those without representation.[41] For the latter patients, the decision to retain legal representation likely reflected the cumulative burden of persistent pain, distress, and disability. WC patients, however, may have retained legal representation to cope with an adversarial system.

A study of WC claimants in the state of Missouri showed that the motivation behind the decision to retain legal representation also may be important.[21] Claimants who retained representation secondary to treatment dissatisfaction (54% of the sample) differed from those who retained representation for other reasons or who did not retain legal representation: The dissatisfied group was younger; less likely to have been diagnosed with a herniated disc; had a longer claim duration; had more economic difficulties; and reported more pain, distress, and disability. Seven years after claim settlement, the dissatisfied group still reported more disability and psychological distress than the other groups. Hence, although litigation had negative effects on treatment outcomes, the motivation to retain legal representation also was important.

Patient Pain-Related Diatheses

Many psychosocial issues have been identified that contribute to a poor adjustment to chronic pain. Some have spawned significant literatures, including depression,[42] anxiety,[43] catastrophizing,[42] fear-avoidance behaviors,[44] self-efficacy,[16] and pain-related coping.[16] Those issues also apply to WC claimants, including catastrophizing,[42] depression,[45] fear-avoidance behaviors,[46] and self-efficacy.[47] Because it is beyond the scope of this chapter to review the vast psychosocial literature reflecting vulnerabilities to pain-related disability, the chapter focuses on two issues directly relevant to WC: recovery expectations, especially those related to RTW, and perceived injustice. Each is included for two primary reasons: (1) evidence that each represents a vulnerability to pain-related disability following occupational injury; and (2) evidence that each can flag the presence of other psychosocial issues among at-risk injured workers, signaling the potential need for further assessment and/or treatment.[48]

Recovery Expectations

Support for significant, positive associations between recovery expectations and treatment outcomes spans a range of conditions[49]: cardiovascular disorders, psychiatric disorders, cancer, and various musculoskeletal disorders. Positive recovery expectations consistently predict successful functional and RTW outcomes among people experiencing acute and subacute musculoskeletal pain,[50] whereas negative expectations predict poor outcomes.[51] Recent studies of chronic pain have shown that recovery expectations also have predictive value in that cohort, despite its chronicity, for both clinical[52] and RTW outcomes.[53]

Although the above findings suggest reasonable agreement on the definition and measurement of recovery expectations, most studies have used single-item measures that assess expectations differently,[54] including the likelihood of RTW, estimating the number of days to RTW, etc. In fact, most measures have significant limitations (e.g., inconsistencies in terminology and lack of time references), and none have seen wide uptake.[54] Regardless of shortcomings in measurement, the critical outcome is RTW. Especially for pain in the acute and subacute stages, recovery expectations are highly predictive of a successful RTW (e.g., 80% accuracy at a 3-month post-injury assessment).[55] Although those expectations also predict RTW for workers with chronic pain, the rate of recovery is lower and more inconsistent.[55]

A recent study, however, suggests that workers' recovery expectations often are unrealistically optimistic.[56] Among workers with acute pain (<30 days), actual RTW often took twice the length of time that workers expected. Workers whose RTW estimates were greater than 60 days demonstrated much more variable rates of return (if they returned at all), and the recovery process was more likely to be complicated by psychological factors.[57]

Studies of workers with chronic pain are especially valuable relative to the identification of chronicity-related risks. Indeed, a key argument for examining recovery expectations after occupational injury involves the early identification of workers at risk of a failed recovery, enabling an early intervention that targets that subgroup. Research suggests that approximately 20% of injured workers fall into such a group, accounting for 80% of treatment, disability, and lost productivity costs.[58] Consistent with that formula, in a study of 1,068 workers with LBP, 196 (18.4%) received disability payments at 6-month follow-up,[46] a cohort that also reported higher baseline levels of pain and lower recovery expectations than workers who successfully returned to work.

A study of more than 3,000 PwP seen through multidisciplinary pain treatment centers examined variables potentially related to recovery expectations.[59] Two health-related variables emerged: (1) pain duration—longer duration was associated with lower expectations; and (2) general health status—better perceived health was associated with higher expectations. Several psychological variables also emerged, including depression and catastrophizing. Studies focused on RTW have yielded similar results: Among patients with whiplash-associated disorders, lower RTW expectancies were associated with lower SES, higher and more widespread pain, and depression.[60]

Although psychosocial factors remain a significant influence among WC claimants, contextual factors also play a role. For example, a study of WC claimants with acute LBP found that RTW within 3 months of injury showed that organizational support, among other factors, predicted RTW.[61] A study of workers with subacute pain implicated other contextual factors[62]: RTW expectations were adversely influenced when workers perceived a lack of control over the RTW process, received inadequate recognition of an injury's impact, feared reinjury, and lacked workplace accommodations for limited RTW. A study of workers with failed RTW identified another contributing factor[63]: They blamed the workplace for their pain conditions.

Despite the sprawling nature of research on recovery expectations, two patterns emerge: (1) Recovery expectations consistently predict RTW, especially with acute and subacute pain; and (2) psychosocial and cognitive factors contribute significantly to recovery expectations and to RTW. Thus, assessing recovery expectations early in treatment can help flag at-risk workers, for whom further evaluation of psychosocial and/or contextual factors may be indicated. If conducted early in treatment, an evaluation also can guide modifications. For many workers, treatment modifications may be minimal, although others may require more costly modifications. For example, multidisciplinary treatment can yield good outcomes,[64] but it must be employed selectively secondary to its costs. In short, recovery expectations tap an important dimension in the rehabilitation and RTW of PwP: positive expectations often predict RTW, and problematic expectations can signal the need for an early intervention, when a good recovery is more likely. Table 9.1 summarizes clinical correlates that have been associated with recovery expectations; a more detailed assessment of these correlates may be warranted for injured workers with problematic expectations.

Perceived Injustice

Perceived injustice (PI) is defined as "a dissatisfied state of mind: a felt discrepancy between what is perceived to be and what is perceived should be."[65(p272)] Perceptions of "what should be" are influenced by just world beliefs—that people generally get "what they deserve."[66] These beliefs are violated when people encounter health events perceived as undeserved and associated with the loss of important capacities. Injuries

Table 9.1 Recovery Expectations: Clinical Correlates

Clinical Domain	Correlated Factors	Association with Expectation (+/–)
Psychological factors	Catastrophizing	–
	Fear of pain/re-injury	–
	Emotional distress (depression, anxiety)	–
	Active coping	+
	Return-to-work confidence	+
	Blaming workplace/others	–
	Positive perception of general health	+
Injury factors	High pain severity/extent	–
	High pain interference	–
	Pain duration/longer recovery trajectory	–
Social/environmental factors	Job flexibility	+
	Supervisor/co-worker support	+
	Lower socioeconomic status	–
	Male gender	–
	Racial/ethnic minority status	–
	Younger age	–

are common triggers for PI when they occasion persistent adverse outcomes that generally are inconsistent with just world beliefs and often are associated with attributions of blame for the event and its sequelae.

Two scales have been developed to measure PI: the Injustice Experiences Questionnaire (IEQ)[67] and the Perceived Justice of the Compensation Process Scale (PJCPS).[68] The PJCPS was developed to assess PI associated with WC systems, and an initial validation study showed that higher scores were associated with such factors as the length of time between filing and having a claim validated, as well as perceptions of premature/forced RTW. Because the scale's content only applies to WC processes, it has seen restricted use.

The IEQ, however, is a 12-item questionnaire that has seen widespread use. Although it was designed with three subscales (severity of loss, irreparability of loss, and blame for loss), studies have supported two subscales[67]: severity/irreparability of loss and blame/unfairness. The IEQ has been shown to correlate with measures of pain severity and disability,[69] as well as adverse pain outcomes for such conditions as fibromyalgia[70] and osteoarthritis.[71] Furthermore, the IEQ is correlated with pain catastrophizing,[69,72] anxiety,[72] depression,[69,72] and disability,[69,73] as well as adverse RTW outcomes. The initial validation study showed that higher IEQ scores were linked to ongoing work-related absence.[67] More recent studies have shown that elevated IEQ scores were associated with higher levels of depression and anxiety; lower rates of RTW; and a higher likelihood of seeking legal counsel, blaming another for an injury, and experiencing financial worries.[74]

Given the associations between PI (as measured by the IEQ), psychosocial factors, and outcomes, the sources of PI are of interest, especially as they relate to the workplace. A study of PwP with workplace injuries[75] found that the most-cited sources of unjust

Table 9.2 Perceived Injustice: Clinical Correlates

Clinical Domain	Correlated Factors	Association with Perceived Injustice (+/–)
Psychological factors	Catastrophizing	+
	Fear of pain/re-injury	+
	Emotional distress (depression, anxiety, anger)	+
	Pain acceptance	–
	Blaming workplace/others	+
	Maladaptive coping (passive)	+
Injury factors	High pain severity/extent	+
	High pain interference	+
	Pain duration/length of recovery period	+
Social/environmental factors	Job flexibility	–
	Supervisor/co-worker support	–
	Shared decision-making with workplace	–

treatment included employers (84.8%), insurers (60.9%), and health care providers (52.2%). Another study of employer practices found that two factors influenced perceptions of fairness[76]: Early supportive contact was associated with perceived fairness, whereas negative supervisory responses were associated with perceived unfairness. Interestingly, the behavior of an insurance claim agent also may influence recovery: Higher levels of PI were associated with poor experiences with claim agents and with poorer mental health.[77] Table 9.2 summarizes clinical correlates that have been associated with PI; each may merit assessment when response to treatment is suboptimal.

Workplace interventions such as ergonomic adjustments, changes in the work environment, changes in work relationships (e.g., with supervisors), and case management activities appear to be the most direct approach to mitigate PI.[78] In fact, a meta-analysis examined such interventions in 14 randomized controlled trials (involving almost 2,000 participants) and showed that RTW was speedier, especially for workers with musculoskeletal injuries.[79] In combination with studies that have found value in case management,[58] especially for vulnerable workers,[48] the results suggest that individualized case management may reduce PI-related risk of disability.

Discussion

This chapter reviewed a literature that attests to the problematic effects of selected systemic and psychosocial factors on the risk for pain-related disability among PwP with occupational injuries. Some factors are common to both the broad health care and WC systems, whereas other factors are more specific to WC systems, including operational issues that can introduce delays in providing treatment and issues that can undermine patient–provider collaboration. The chapter also touched on dysfunctional recovery expectations and PI, psychosocial issues that may adversely influence outcomes.

Although each of the above can contribute to a worker's vulnerability to persistent disability, a focus on single stresses and/or diatheses underrepresents the actual vulnerability that workers incur when an occupational injury occasions persistent pain. The actual risk that workers incur is magnified when stresses and diatheses interact. Below are two scenarios depicting hypothetical clinical cases that illustrate toxic combinations that can eventuate from an occupational injury.

Case Examples

Insufficient medical evidence: It is common for medical diagnostic findings to inadequately explain levels of pain severity that patients report (a medical system stressor). For an injured worker with pessimistic recovery expectations secondary to a mild depressive disorder (a recovery expectation diathesis), the lack of an explanation may weaken those expectations and worsen the depression. Lacking trust in a company-designated physician and afraid that symptoms will be dismissed as psychosomatic (WC system stressors), the worker may fail to disclose depressive symptoms that impede treatment. This combination of stressors and diatheses, common among WC claimants, can undermine recovery if not addressed early in treatment.

Unrealistic recovery expectations: Another problematic combination of stressors and diatheses could involve a worker with unrealistically positive expectations for RTW following a back injury (a patient diathesis), expectations shared by a supervisor (an institutional stressor). When rehabilitation does not progress speedily, the supervisor attributes the slow recovery to a lack of motivation. The slow progress also triggers worker concerns about a possible missed diagnosis, but those concerns are dismissed because the physical findings fail to justify further diagnostic workup (a medical system stressor). The situation is made worse by a failure to educate the worker about rehabilitation of musculoskeletal pain. The supervisor's unrealistic RTW expectations and the physician's refusal to educate adequately, combined with unrealistic recover expectations, occasion increased anxiety and concerns about being treated unfairly, triggering a decision to seek legal counsel (another general system stressor). The attorney validates injustice perceptions and initiates litigation. These factors combine to cause a prolonged work absence and pain-related disability that persists after case closure. An application for Social Security Disability Insurance is denied and an appeal is required (and so on . . .).

These scenarios, although fictional, exemplify toxic interactions between stressors and diatheses that can attend work injuries that occasion persistent pain. In combination, they increase the likelihood of prolonged disability beyond the levels associated with individual stressors and diatheses described in the literature. Fortunately, the literature also suggests some approaches to the management of injured workers that have potential to reduce these disability risks.

Treatment Considerations

As noted previously, treatment delays can contribute to an increased likelihood of chronicity. Through its COHE initiative, the state of Washington made changes in its WC program that addressed operational inefficiencies and reduced lag times. Furthermore, it recruited and trained a cadre of physicians with expertise in managing pain so that patients were assigned to a qualified provider in a timely manner. Consequently, the Washington WC system is more responsive to patient needs and more effectively returns injured workers to employable levels of functioning, yielding a 30% reduction in disability applications and a comparable reduction in treatment costs.[35]

In addition to these quantifiable changes, the program may have yielded other benefits, including reductions in the burden that providers assume in treating this vulnerable cohort. The pain of burdensome patients is likely to be discounted and attributed to psychological causes,[38] a toxic combination that can undermine effective treatment collaboration. The Washington program has taken steps to reduce that burden: (1) Training physicians in the treatment of persistent pain facilitates collaborative decision-making, and (2) funding trained providers at enhanced rates offsets the time demands that collaboration might require and enhances the likelihood of successful treatment.[80]

The above comments have focused primarily on WC-related system stresses. However, some elements of the Washington program have more general implications. For example, improved efficiencies in treatment delivery enhance claimant satisfaction. Similarly, training in the proper interpretation of diagnostic test results in nonspecific, musculoskeletal pain addresses another common medical system stressor—the inconsistencies that often can arise between diagnostic test results and patient symptom reports.

Indeed, the primary medical system stressor that was not addressed in the COHE initiative involved racial/ethnic disparities. As noted previously, those disparities remain problematic across the health system. Although the resolution of this issue remains a major challenge, one recommendation would help frame the issue for study in WC settings: requiring that racial/ethnic identifiers be included in WC databases. In the Missouri system, in which such elements were not included, such information required direct contact with each WC claimant, a logistically challenging and costly alternative to a database.[25] The inclusion of such data would facilitate the study of this important topic in WC systems.

Box 9.1 summarizes system-level recommendations that derive from the literature. Some are relatively straightforward and could be instituted readily, such as the routine assessment of recovery expectations. Others are more challenging because they would require an investment of time and money (e.g., developing information technology systems to track/communicate information) or require commitments from outside entities (e.g., case management resources in the workplace). Synergies are likely to derive from the broad adoption of strategies, but even a piecemeal implementation of selected strategies is likely to improve RTW outcomes for WC systems.

Although the above strategies address systemic stressors that affect RTW outcomes, implementing strategies at the patient–provider level also could improve outcomes. For example, a strategy of potential value would target patient diatheses through mechanisms such as tracking recovery expectations. As noted previously, many workers underestimate the time required for recovery.[56] Workers who progress more slowly than they expect are vulnerable to frustration and discouragement, both of which may contribute to the high rates of depression that have been reported following workplace injury. Education about musculoskeletal pain and coaching about adaptive approaches to treatment could help workers adopt more realistic expectations and build trust. Because recovery expectations are influenced not only by the pace of recovery but also by factors such as self-efficacy (positively) and depression (negatively), problematic expectations also could signal the presence of psychosocial issues that could compromise recovery if not addressed in a timely manner.[46]

Box 9.2 lists recommendations that could be adopted at the clinical level. Unlike recommendations in Box 9.1, those in Box 9.2 do not require significant investments. For example, physicians can maintain regular communications with rehabilitation providers, not only for progress reports but also to coordinate medical and rehabilitative treatment. Clearly, this and other recommendations (e.g., routine tracking of recovery expectations) can be implemented independent of system-level initiatives.

Box 9.1 Recommendations for Workers' Compensation Systems

Providers
- Establish and train a cadre of physicians in the evaluation and treatment of common workplace injuries.
- Enhance physician reimbursement for best practices.

Health systems
- Develop information technology systems to track and communicate information regarding response to treatment.
- Conduct routine assessments of treatment response (e.g., functional changes and recovery expectation changes).
- Initiate timely interventions (e.g., enhanced assessment and specialist referral) when treatment response does not follow expectations.
- Implement stepped intervention program when worker response to standard care is inadequate (e.g., education > pain specialist referral > multidisciplinary treatment).
- Maintain racial/ethnic identifiers to identify and track potential disparities in treatment delivery/outcomes.

Workplace
- Provide case management and coordination for injured workers.
- Consider job modifications (e.g., ergonomic adjustments) to promote successful return to work.
- Monitor work relationships (e.g., supervisory and collegial) to promote successful return to work.

Box 9.2 Recommendations for Workers' Compensation Clinicians

Injured worker
- Evaluate recovery expectations and educate when expectations are unrealistic.
- Conduct routine (e.g., every 2 weeks) assessments of response to treatment (functional gains and recovery expectations).
- If response to treatment is poor and/or recovery expectations worsen, assess and/or refer for psychosocial complications (e.g., catastrophizing, fear avoidance, depression, and dissatisfaction with treatment).

Health and workers' compensation systems
- Establish regular communication with and feedback from physical/occupational therapists.
- Maintain regular contact with case manager (especially important when response to treatment is problematic).
- Maintain consistent documentation in information technology systems regarding treatment progress/problems.
- Make timely referrals (i.e., minimize time lag) if worker demonstrates inadequate response to treatment despite adjustments.

General
- Maintain training to ensure delivery of best practices (e.g., mechanisms and treatment of musculoskeletal pain).
- Guard against negative stereotypes that can adversely influence clinical judgments.

Conclusion

There is abundant evidence that injured workers with persistent pain are vulnerable to the development of chronic, pain-related disability when treated through WC systems. That vulnerability is secondary to health care system stresses that can interact with patient diatheses in a significant minority of injured workers. The most effective approach to disability risk reduction requires attention to both patient- and system-level factors. Absent an integrated approach, incremental, clinic-level initiatives also are likely to yield benefits, although to a lesser extent. Indeed, a diathesis–stress perspective argues for a combination of health care, research, and administrative actions, involving an ongoing commitment from industry, academic, health care, and governmental (federal and state) partners, to address the many factors that a comprehensive solution will require. At a time in the United States when the workforce has been eviscerated by a pandemic and a wave of retirements, it has never been more important (or timely) to take steps that will restore and retain the workforce.

References

1. Green CR, Anderson KO, Baker TA, et al. The unequal burden of pain: Confronting racial and ethnic disparities in pain. *Pain Med.* 2003;4:277–294.
2. Agency for Healthcare Research and Quality. 2021 National Healthcare Quality and Disparities report. 2021. Accessed January 14, 2022. https://www.ahrq.gov/research/findings/nhqrdr/nhqdr21/index.html
3. Vulnerable. In: *Collins English Dictionary*. n.d. Accessed April 25, 2022. https://www.collinsdictionary.com/dictionary/english/vulnerable
4. Murray B. Informed consent: What must a physician disclose to a patient? *AMA J Ethics.* 2012;14:563–566.
5. Murgatroyd DF, Casey PP, Cameron ID, Harris IA. The effect of financial compensation on health outcomes following musculoskeletal injury: Systematic review. *PLoS One.* 2015;10(2):e011759. doi:10.1371/journal.pone.0117597
6. Harris I, Mulford J, Solomon M, van Gelder JM, Young J. Associations between compensation status and outcome after surgery: A meta-analysis. JAMA 2005;293:1644–1652.
7. Buffie N, Baker D. Rising disability payments: Are cuts to workers' compensation part of the story? Center for Economic and Policy Research. 2015. Accessed April 26, 2022. https://cepr.net/report/rising-disability-payments-are-cuts-to-workers-compensation-part-of-the-story
8. Tait RC, Chibnall JT, Andresen EM, Hadler NM. Management of occupational back injuries: Differences among African Americans and Caucasians. *Pain.* 2004;112(3):389–396. PMID:15561395
9. Chibnall JT, Tait RC, Andresen EM, Hadler NM. Race differences in diagnosis and surgery for occupational low back injuries. *Spine.* 2006;31(11):1272–1275.
10. Chibnall JT, Tait RC, Andresen EM, Hadler NM. Race and socioeconomic differences in post-settlement outcomes for African American and Caucasian workers' compensation claimants with low back injuries. *Pain.* 2005;114(3):462–472. PMID:15777871
11. Tait RC, Chibnall JT. Legal sequelae of occupational back injuries: A longitudinal analysis of Missouri judicial records. *Spine.* 2011;36(17):1402–1409. PMID:21217454
12. Chibnall JT, Tait RC. Long-term adjustment to work-related low back pain: Associations with socio-demographics, claim processes, and post-settlement adjustment. *Pain Med.* 2009;10(8):1378–1388. PMID:20021598
13. Turk DC, Banks C. A diathesis–stress model of chronic pain and disability following traumatic injury. *Pain Res Manage.* 2002;7:9–19.
14. Tait RC. Compensation claims for chronic pain: Effects on evaluation and treatment. In: Dworkin RH, Breitbart WS, eds. *Psychosocial Aspects of Pain: A Handbook for Health Care Providers.* IASP Press; 2004:547–570.
15. Tait RC, Miller L. The multidisciplinary treatment of pain in vulnerable populations. In Schatman ME, Campbell A, eds. *Chronic Pain Management: A Guidebook for Multidisciplinary Program Development.* Informa Healthcare; 2007:129–150.
16. Edwards RR, Dworkin RH, Sullivan MD, Turk DC, Wasan AD. The role of psychosocial processes in the development and maintenance of chronic pain. *J Pain.* 2016;17(Suppl 2):T70–T92.
17. IsHak WW, Wen RY, Naghdechi L, et al. Pain and depression: A systematic review. *Harvard Rev Psychiatry.* 2018;26:352–363.
18. O'Donnell ML, Varker T, Holmes AC, et al. Disability after injury: The cumulative burden of physical and mental health. *J Clin Psychiatry.* 2013;74:e137–e143.
19. Tait RC, Chibnall JT, Kalauokalani DC. Provider judgments of patients in pain: Seeking symptom certainty. *Pain Med.* 2009;10:11–34.
20. Hadler NM. The illness of work incapacity. *Occup Med.* 2016;66:346–348.
21. Chibnall JT, Tait RC. Legal representation and dissatisfaction with workers' compensation: Implications for claimant adjustment. *Psychol Inj Law.* 2010;3:230–240.
22. Rosenthal D. A suggested conceptual framework. In: Rosenthal D, ed. *The Genain Quadruplets: A Case Study and Theoretical Analysis of Heredity and Environment in Schizophrenia.* Basic Books; 1963:505–511.

23. Robins CJ, Block P. Cognitive theories of depression viewed from a diathesis–stress perspective: Evaluations of the models of Beck and of Abramson, Seligman, and Teasdale. *Cognit Ther Res.* 1989;13:296–313.
24. Colodro-Conde L, Couvey-Duchesne B, Ahu G, et al. A direct test of the diathesis–stress model for depression. *Mol Psychiatry.* 2018;23:1590–1596.
25. Tait RC, Chibnall JT. Management of occupational low back pain: A case study of the Missouri workers' compensation system. *Psychol Inj Law.* 2016;9:298–312.
26. Rondinelli RD, Genovese E, Katz RT, Mayer TG, Mueller K, Ranavaya M, eds. *AMA Guides to the Evaluation of Permanent Impairment.* 6th ed. American Medical Association; 2008.
27. Tait RC, Chibnall JT, Andresen EM, Hadler NM. Disability determination: Validity with occupational low back pain. *J Pain.* 2006;7:951–957.
28. Schultz IZ, Crook JM, Berkowitiz J, Meloche GR, Prkachin KM, Chlebak CM. Early intervention with compensated lower back-injured workers at risk for work disability: Fixed versus flexible approach. *Psychol Inj Law.* 2013;6:258–276.
29. Besen E, Young A, Gaines B, Pransky G. Lag times in the work disability process: Differences across diagnoses in the length of disability following work-related injury. *Work.* 2018;60:635–648.
30. Wynne-Jones G, Cowen J, Jordan JL, et al. Absence from work and return to work in people with back pain: A systematic review and meta-analysis. *Occup Environ Med.* 2014;71:448–456.
31. Gallagher RM. Referral delay in back pain patients on worker's compensation: Costs and policy implications. *Psychosomatics.* 1996;37:270–284.
32. Frank JW, Kerr MS, Brooker AS, et al. Disability resulting from occupational low back pain: Part I. What do we know about primary prevention? A review of the scientific evidence on prevention before disability begins. *Spine.* 1996;21:2908–2917.
33. Frank JW, Brooker AS DeMaio SE, et al. Disability resulting from occupational low back pain: Part II. What do we know about secondary prevention? A review of the scientific evidence on prevention after disability begins. *Spine.* 1996;21:2918–2929.
34. Wickizer TM, Franklin G, Fulton-Kehoe D, et al. Improving quality, preventing disability and reducing costs in workers' compensation healthcare: A population-based intervention study. *Med Care.* 2011;49:1105–1111.
35. Wickizer TM, Franklin GM, Fulton-Kehoe D. Innovations in occupational health care delivery can prevent entry into permanent disability: 8-Year follow-up of the Washington State Centers for Occupational Health and Education. *Med Care.* 2018;56:1018–1023.
36. Hadler NM. Back pain and the vortex of disability determination. *Semin Spine Surg.* 1992;4:35–41.
37. Tait RC, Margolis RB, Krause SJ, Liebowitz E. Compensation status and symptoms reported by patients with chronic pain. *Arch Phys Med Rehabil.* 1988;69:1027–1029.
38. Chibnall JT, Tait RC, Gammack JK. Physician judgments and the burden of chronic pain. *Pain Med.* 2018;19:1961–1971.
39. Gallagher RM, Williams RA, Skelly J, et al. Workers' compensation and return-to-work in low back pain. *Pain.* 1995;61:299–307.
40. Cheriyan T, Harris B, Cheriyan J, et al. Association between compensation status and outcomes in spine surgery: A meta-analysis of 31 studies. *Spine J.* 2015;15:2564–2573.
41. Tait RC, Chibnall JT, Richardson WD. Litigation and employment status: Effects on patients with chronic pain. *Pain.* 1990;43:37–46.
42. Arnow BA, Blasey CM, Constantino MJ, et al. Catastrophizing, depression and pain-related disability. *Gen Hosp Psychiatry.* 2011;33:150–156.
43. Leman SF, Rudich Z, Brill S, Shalev H, Shahar G. Longitudinal associations between depression, anxiety, pain, and pain-related disability in chronic pain patients. *Psychosom Med.* 2015;77:333–341.
44. Leeuw M, Goossens ME, Linton SJ, Crombez G, Boersma K, Vlaeyen JWS. The fear avoidance model of musculoskeletal pain: Current state of scientific evidence. *J Behav Med.* 2007;30:77–94.

45. White MI, Wagner SL, Schultz IZ, et al. Non-modifiable worker and workplace risk factors contributing to workplace absence: A stakeholder-centred synthesis of systematic reviews. *Work.* 2015:52:353–373.
46. Turner JA, Franklin G, Fulton-Kehoe D, et al. Worker recovery expectations and fear-avoidance predict work disability in a population-based workers' compensation back pain sample. *Spine.* 2006;31:682–689.
47. Black O, Keegel T, Sim MR, Collie A, Smith P. The effect of self-efficacy on return-to-work outcomes for workers with psychological or upper-body musculoskeletal injuries: A review of the literature. *J Occup Rehabil.* 2018;28:16–27.
48. Kendall NAS, Linton SJ, Main CJ. *Guide to assessing psychosocial yellow flags in acute low back pain: Risk factors for long-term disability and work loss.* Accident Rehabilitation and Compensation Insurance Corporation of New Zealand and the National Health Committee; 1997.
49. Ebrahim S, Malachowski C, el Din MK, et al. Measures of patients' expectations about recovery: A systematic review. *J Occup Rehabil.* 2015;25:240–255.
50. Laisne F, Lecomte C, Corbiere M. Biopsychosocial predictors of prognosis in musculoskeletal disorders: A systematic review of the literature. *Disabil Rehabil.* 2012;34:355–382.
51. Cormier S, Levigne GL, Choiniere M, Rainville P. Expectations predict chronic pain treatment outcomes. *Pain.* 2016;157:329–338.
52. Iles RA, Davidson M, Taylor NF. Psychosocial predictors of failure to return to work in non-chronic non-specific low back pain: A systematic review. *Occup Environ Med.* 2008;63:507–517.
53. Opsommer E, Rivier G, Crombez G, Hilfiker R. The predictive value of subsets of the Orebro Musculoskeletal Pain Screening Questionnaire for return to work in chronic low back pain. *Eur J Phys Rehabil Med.* 2017;53:359–365.
54. Young AE, Besen E, Choi Y. The importance, measurement and practical implications of worker's expectations for return to work. *Disabil Rehabil.* 2015;37:1808–1816.
55. Schultz IZ, Crook J, Meloche GR, et al. Psychosocial factors predictive of occupational low back disability: Towards development of a return-to-work model. *Pain.* 2004:107(1–2):77–85.
56. Young AE, Besen E, Willetts J. Expectations for return to work after workplace injuries: The relationship between estimated time to return to work and estimate accuracy. *J Occup Rehabil.* 2018;28:711–720.
57. Carstens JK, Shaw W, Boersma K, Reme SE, Pransky G, Linton SJ. When the wind goes out of the sail: Declining recovery expectations in the first weeks of back pain. *Eur J Pain.* 2014;18:269–278.
58. Boone E. Changing the game in workers' compensation: Liberty Mutual's new predictive model takes claims management to the next level. December 2011. Accessed July 9, 2022. https://roughnotes.com/rnmagazine/2011/december2011/2011_12p078.htm
59. Cormier S, Levesque-Lacasse A. Biopsychosocial characteristics of patients with chronic pain expecting different levels of pain relief in the context of multidisciplinary treatments. *Clin J Pain.* 2021;37:11–19.
60. Ozegovic D, Carroll LF, Cassidy JD. What influences positive return to work expectation? Examining associated factors in a population-based cohort of whiplash-associated disorders. *Spine.* 2010;35:E708–E713.
61. Besen E, Young AE, Shaw WS. Returning to work following low back pain: Towards a model of individual psychosocial factors. *J Occup Rehabil.* 2015;25:25–37.
62. Stewart AM, Polak E, Young R, Schultz IZ. Injured workers' construction of expectations of return to work with sub-acute back pain: The role of perceived uncertainty. *J Occup Rehabil.* 2012;22:1–14.
63. Jensen OK, Stengaard-Pedersen K, Jensen C, Nielsen CV. Prediction model for unsuccessful return to work after hospital-based intervention in low back pain patients. *BMC Musculoskel Dis.* 2013;14: Article 140.
64. Kamper SJ, Apeldoorn AT, Chiarotto A, et al. Multidisciplinary biopsychosocial rehabilitation for chronic low back pain. Cochrane Database Syst Rev. 2014;2014(9):CD000963.

65. Adams JS. Inequity in social exchange. *Adv Exp Soc Psychol.* 1965;2:267–299.
66. Lerner MJ. The belief in a just world. In: *Belief in a Just World: A Fundamental Delusion.* Springer; 1980:9–30.
67. Sullivan MJL, Adams H, Horan S, Maher D, Boland D, Gross R. The role of perceived injustice in the experience of chronic pain and disability: Scale development and validation. *J Occup Rehabil.* 2008;18:249–261.
68. Franche RL, Severin CN, Lee H, et al. Perceived justice of compensation process for return-to-work: Development and validation of a scale. *Psychol Inj Law.* 2009;2:225–237.
69. Reme SE, Ljosaa TM, Stubhaug A, Granan LP, Falk RS, Jacobsen HB. Perceived injustice in patients with chronic pain: Prevalence, relevance, and associations with long-term recovery and deterioration. *J Pain.* 2022;23(7):1196–1207.
70. Rodero B, Luciano JV, Montero-Marin J, et al. Perceived injustice in fibromyalgia: Psychometric characteristics of the Injustice Experience Questionnaire and relationship with pain catastrophising and pain acceptance. *J Psychosom Res.* 2012;73:86–91.
71. Yakobov E, Scott W, Stanish W, Dunbar M, Richardson G, Sullivan M. The role of perceived injustice in the prediction of pain and function after total knee arthroplasty. *Pain.* 2014;155:2040–2046.
72. Martinez-Borba V, Ripoll-Server P, Yakobov E, Suso-Ribera C. Predicting the physical and mental health status of individuals with chronic musculoskeletal pain from a biopsychosocial perspective: A multivariate approach. *Clin J Pain.* 2021;37:211–218.
73. Carriere JS, Sturgeon JA, Yakobov E, Kao M-C, Mackey SC, Darnall BD. The impact of perceived injustice on pain-related outcomes: A combined model examining the mediating roles of pain acceptance and anger in a chronic pain sample. *Clin J Pain.* 2018;34:739–747.
74. Giummarra MJ, Cameron PA, Ponsford J, et al. Return to work after traumatic injury: Increased work-related disability in injured persons receiving financial compensation is mediated by perceived injustice. *J Occup Rehabil.* 2017;27:173–185.
75. Scott W, McEvoy A, Garland R, et al. Sources of injustice among individuals with persistent pain following musculoskeletal injury. *Psychol Inj Law.* 2016;9:6–15.
76. Hepburn CG, Kelloway EK, Franche R-L. Early employer response to workplace injury: What injured workers perceive as fair and why these perceptions matter. *J Occup Health Psychol.* 2010;15:409–420.
77. Orchard C, Carnide N, Smith P. How does perceived fairness in the workers' compensation claims process affect mental health following a workplace injury? *J Occup Rehabil.* 2020;30:40–48.
78. Iles RA, Sheehan LR, Gosling C McR. Assessment of a new tool to improve case manager identification of delayed return to work in the first two weeks of a workers' compensation claim. *Clin Rehabil.* 2020;34:656–666.
79. van Vilsteren M, van Oostrom SH, de Vet HCW, Franche R-L, Boot CRL, Anema JR. Workplace interventions to prevent work disability in workers on sick leave. *Cochrane Database Syst Rev.* 2015;2015(10):CD006955.
80. Frantsve LME, Kerns RD. Patient–provider interactions in the management of chronic pain: Current findings within the context of shared medical decision making. *Pain Med.* 2007;8:25–35.

10

Pain in Cognitive Impairment

Cynthia M. A. Geppert and Karen E. Cardon

> Neuroplasticity contributes to both the constrained and unconstrained aspects of our nature. It renders our brains not only more resourceful, but also more vulnerable to outside influences.
>
> —Norman Diodge[1(pxx)]

Introduction

There are likely no two greater sources of vulnerability in the human condition than cognitive impairment and pain. These vulnerabilities may adversely affect the most essential aspects of what makes life worth living. Cognitive impairment interferes with the ability of individuals to fully participate in close relationships; express their innermost thoughts and feelings; creatively pursue work, interests, and recreation; organize their time and efforts to manage daily affairs; and respond to challenges. Pain, particularly chronic pain, often prevents persons from exercising and enjoying the outdoors, being socially active and involved in the community, maintaining gainful employment, and even meeting their own hierarchy of needs. When a person suffers from both pain and cognitive impairment, their burden of misery is increased; the expanse of their life trajectory shrinks even further; and their vulnerability to dependency and exploitation, additional medical and psychiatric disorders, poverty, and loneliness is amplified and intensified.

This chapter traces the complex patterns of interaction between pain and cognitive impairment as a way of constructing a framework for the consideration of models of vulnerability in this patient population. Within the larger cohort of patients with comorbid pain and cognitive impairment, this chapter focuses on the growing populations of patients with dementia, and traumatic brain injury (TBI) and those with developmental delay. The specific vulnerabilities and unique challenges to accurate assessment of pain and its safe, efficacious, and holistic management for each of the three conditions are presented. The chapter concludes with a discussion of strategies to ameliorate the wider contextual features that frame pain in patients with cognitive impairment and sketch the therapeutic potential of a patient-centered approach to their care.

Discussion

Cognitive Impairment and Pain

The Centers for Disease Control and Prevention (CDC) offers a concise definition of this complicated problem: "Cognitive impairment is when a person has trouble remembering, learning new things, concentrating or making decisions that affect their everyday life."[2] Although cognitive impairment is often treated as synonymous with dementia, it is a broader category that includes stroke, TBI, and developmental delay. Many of the chief biomedical, environmental, genetic, and psychosocial risk factors for cognitive impairment are listed in Box 10.1. Given the variety of factors and the high prevalence of many of them, it is likely most of the public has at least one risk factor for cognitive impairment.

Whatever the cause(s) of cognitive impairment, the disorder shares a set of common symptoms, such as memory loss; impaired insight and judgment; agnosia; changes in mood and behavior; and deficits in executive function such as planning, set shifting, and problem-solving.

In 2020, the International Association for the Study of Pain (IASP) revised its often-cited definition of pain: "An unpleasant sensory and emotional experience associated with, or resembling that associated with, actual or potential tissue damage."[3(p1977)] Research into the bidirectional interaction of pain and cognitive impairment suggests chronicity of pain may contribute to cognitive impairment. For this reason, this chapter concentrates on chronic rather than acute pain. The Health and Retirement Study

Box 10.1 Risk Factors for Cognitive Impairment

- Family history of cognitive impairment
- Lower educational level
- Brain injuries
- Exposure to toxins and pesticides
- Physical inactivity
- Cardiac disease
- Diabetes
- Parkinson's disease
- Stroke
- Vitamin deficiencies
- Hypertension
- Hypercholesteremia
- Consuming alcohol
- Smoking
- Depression

assessed 8,515 adults older than age 65 years regarding the effect of pain persistence, intensity, and interference with daily activities on the development of cognitive impairment. The study adjusted for confounding factors such as demographics, depression, and medical comorbidities. Results showed that persistent interference of pain with daily activities of living, but not the intensity of pain, was associated with a 21% increase in the odds of developing cognitive impairment.[4]

Vulnerability Models in Dementia

Scientists have proposed illness models to explain how pain and cognitive impairment generate vulnerability in each of the three subgroups. The fifth edition of the American Psychiatric Association's *Diagnostic and Statistical Manual of Mental Disorders* does not use the diagnostic label dementia.[5] The syndrome is designated as either minor or major neurocognitive disorder. Dementia is the more broadly recognized term in public and professional parlance and so is used in this chapter. Researchers analyzed the relationship of pain and dementia with social vulnerability in a subset of participants in the Canadian Health and Aging Study. A cross-sectional study of 3,776 community-dwelling older Canadian adults identified an independent association of moderate to severe pain and cognitive impairment with higher scores on the Social Vulnerability Index. The index is a self-report measure of 39 different variables comprising an individual's social circumstances and how these impact involvement in the community.[6] Surprisingly, the interaction between the two variables of pain and cognitive impairment with social vulnerability did not reach statistical significance. Comorbidities such as depressed mood and functional impairment decreased the strength of the association for moderate and severe pain as a cause of social vulnerability, but the same effect was not found for cognitive impairment.[7]

Each of the two variables was also independently related to impairments in activities of daily living (ADLs) and instrumental activities of daily living (IADLs). Individuals with both cognitive impairment and pain were found to have more serious problems managing ADLs and IADLs. In turn, impairments in these crucial living skills would likely amplify social vulnerability, although this was not a hypothesis the study directly investigated.[8] Results from another secondary analysis of data from the Canadian Health and Aging Study showed that over a period of 5 years, participants with high social vulnerability scores had 36% higher odds of experiencing cognitive decline.[9] Although the cross-sectional nature of these studies did not allow for determination of causation, the authors suggest that improvement in the management of pain and increased attention to social vulnerability, especially in cognitively impaired older adults, may improve their quality of life.

Neuroscience Vulnerability Model

A growing body of basic and clinical neuroscience research literature is evincing a bidirectional relationship between pain and cognition. Research is ongoing to determine whether the nature of the relationship is associational or causational.[10] Studies of

Box 10.2 Cognitive Domain Deficits Associated with Pain

- Attention
- Processing speed
- Learning
- Language
- Concentration
- Psychomotor coordination
- Working memory
- Recall
- Recognition
- Spatial learning
- Reaction time
- Decision-making
- Executive function

common chronic pain–generating conditions such as fibromyalgia, migraine, osteoarthritis, and chronic lower back pain, among other disorders, have shown deficits in important areas of cognition, as summarized in Box 10.2.[11–13] Several of these conditions, such as arthritis, are more common in older individuals, who are already at higher risk of developing cognitive impairment.[14]

There are several proposed models of this pain-cognition vulnerability. It is well known that pain alters the hypothalamic–pituitary axis, raising cortisol, and resulting in inflammation and neuronal degeneration that are neurobiological pathways to cognitive decline.[15] A neuropsychological theory posits that coping with pain, especially chronic pain, appropriates and diverts psychological energy and focus, resulting in attentional and memory deficits.[16] Pain also interrupts sleep, which is neurobiologically necessary for memory consolidation. Both nociceptive and neuropathic pain conditions frequently restrict the ability to obtain mental and physical exercise that is a protective factor for cognitive impairment. Stress, distraction, and sleep deprivation adversely affect cognition even in young persons, but the deleterious effects are more serious and consequential in older adults, who do not have the cerebral reserve to compensate. Major impairments in cognition noted in persons with chronic pain are listed in Box 10.2.

Epidemiology of Pain and Dementia

Modern Western society has enjoyed the benefits of increased longevity and suffered the harms that accompany living longer, such as higher rates of dementia. Age is the single greatest risk factor for the development of dementia, and current demographic predictions of dementia prevalence are alarming. The Alzheimer's Association[17] estimates that by 2050, the number of persons older than age 65 years diagnosed with

Table 10.1 Pain in Subtypes of Dementia

Type of Dementia	Clinical Pathophysiology	Pain Features
Alzheimer's disease	Accumulation of β-amyloid plaques and τ tangles in temporal and parietal lobes leading to death of neurons.	Heightened reaction to pain stimulus
Cerebrovascular	Insufficient oxygen and nutrition to cerebral blood vessels leads to tissue damage and brain injuries (stroke).	Higher pain prevalence possibly due to white matter lesions causing central pain Similar pain intensity to that of patients without vascular dementia but more severe suffering
Frontotemporal	Abnormal proteins in neurons in temporal and frontal lobes lead to atrophy and abnormal tissue.	Increase in pain threshold and possible higher pain tolerance. Temperature dysregulation, hallucinations associated.
Lewy body dementia	Abnormal clumps of protein α-synuclein in the cortex.	Severe, may increase with age Poorly localized Associated with gastrointestinal disturbance, hallucinations.

Sources: References 17, 24, 64, and 65.

the disease will reach 1.7 million. This staggering figure in part reflects the fact that the population of individuals older than age 65 years will grow from 58 million in 2021 to 88 million in 2050.

Pain, especially in its chronic form, is also more prevalent in older populations. In 2019, the CDC[2] reported that the percentage of American adults older than age 65 years with high-impact pain was 11.8%, higher than in all younger cohorts. The percentage of persons with comorbid pain and dementia is not precisely known. Estimates are that more than half of community-dwelling elders are afflicted with both daily pain and dementia.[18] The statistic is even higher in nursing home populations, approaching 80% in some studies.[19] Patients with advanced dementia experience more severe pain than those with mild or moderate dementia.[20]

Although Alzheimer's disease is the most-diagnosed type of dementia, the rates of other subtypes are also rising exponentially. Other prevalent forms of dementia include cerebrovascular dementia, Lewy body dementia, and frontotemporal dementia, with the second most common type being mixed. Recent research shows that each of the major subtypes has its own pain profile, summarized in Table 10.1.

Assessment of Pain in Patients with Dementia

Three vulnerabilities seriously limit the accurate and consistent assessment of pain in persons with dementia, and indeed most forms of cognitive impairment. The first is the lack of clinical research in these populations, leaving health care professionals to extrapolate from similar groups (e.g., older persons without dementia) or to exercise their best clinical judgment based on experience, training, and expert consensus guidelines. A striking example of the detrimental effect of this paucity of data is earlier research that suggested persons with dementia, especially in more advanced stages, feel less pain.[21] Newer studies have demonstrated the opposite conclusion: Persons with dementia feel pain more intensely.[22]

Notes accompanying the revised IASP definition of pain emphasize its subjective and individualized nature: "Pain is always a personal experience that is influenced to varying degrees by biological, psychological, and social factors."[3(p1977)] The irreducible subjectivity of pain is the rationale for self-report being the objective criterion of pain assessment. The second vulnerability is that inherent in cognitive impairment are deficits in ability to reflect, remember, abstract, and communicate the experience of pain necessary for accurate self-report.[24] A prerequisite for efficacious and safe treatment of pain in patients with cognitive impairment is valid and reliable assessment of pain. Patients with mild cognitive impairment can frequently use basic verbal self-report tools. It is an ethical and clinical best practice for practitioners to make every feasible effort to facilitate a patient's participation in their own pain assessments. This must be balanced with the need to obtain an accurate register of the patient's pain and the recognition that patients with even moderate dementia may not be able to respond meaningfully to visual analog scales. They may do better with simple verbal or facial recognition instruments.[24]

In patients with advanced dementia or other severe forms of cognitive impairment who have lost the self-referential and linguistic capacities required for self-report, the locus of assessment must shift to the observations of caregivers. The internal states of patients with end-stage dementia are almost entirely manifest through observable behaviors such as body movements, posture, vocalizations, and facial expressions. Even when trained observers familiar with the patient assess their pain, the externalization of the assessment introduces added potential for misapprehension and misinterpretation of the internal experience of the patient. A salient contributor to these errors is the phenomenological and neurobiological overlap between physical pain and other forms of distress.[25] Confounding or confusing the behavioral and psychological symptoms of dementia (BPSD) with pain can lead to incorrect and ineffective treatment, often with antipsychotic medications that also carry their own risks. Although there is a relative lack of evidence for pain causing BPSD, it is likely a contributor, requiring more complex treatment regiments with increased potential for adverse events.[26]

The third vulnerability is that despite intensive efforts, researchers have not yet produced a valid and reliable tool to clinically evaluate pain in patients with dementia. A 2014 systematic review of pain assessment tools evaluated the psychometric profiles and clinical utility of 28 separate tools that had been used in different care sites. The authors concluded that "we cannot at present recommend any particular tool for use in any clinical setting, due to the lack of comprehensive evidence of the reliability, validity, feasibility or clinical utility of any particular tool."[27] Despite the inadequacy of these tools, there is evidence that if caregivers use them consistently, correctly, and compassionately, they can improve the identification of pain in persons with dementia compared to casual observation or care as usual.[28] For this reason, the use of various instruments is recommended in almost all expert guidelines.

Treatment of Pain in Persons with Dementia

The same intrinsic limitations that cognitive impairment imposes on pain assessment also restrict the use of current treatment modalities. Many persons with moderate or severe dementia lack the abilities needed to participate in therapies that are increasingly the mainstay of nonpharmacological chronic pain management. Cognitive–behavioral therapy (CBT) is among the treatment modalities with the strongest evidence base and is a recommended first-line treatment for most forms of chronic pain.[29] As its name implies, intact abilities to set goals, control impulses, problem-solve, abstract, remember, and learn are prerequisites for successful CBT.

The same vulnerability restricts the use of some pharmacological treatments, ironically in the wake of the opioid crisis, likely *not* rational pharmacotherapy with opioids. There has long been a presumption, reinforced by the opioid epidemic, that opioids would worsen cognition in persons with dementia. In fact, cognitive decline is more strongly associated with the use of nonsteroidal anti-inflammatory drugs.[30] There is clinical consensus that acetaminophen is likely the gold standard for non-acute, non-cancer patients with dementia, at least in the short term.[31] However, recently reviews have advised that there is a dearth of research to inform judgments about the relative safety of frequently prescribed agents.[32]

Consequently, the pain of persons with dementia is often undertreated or when treated done so ineffectually and inappropriately. There is emerging evidence that untreated pain at least accelerates, if it does not cause, cognitive decline and exacerbates behavioral and psychological disturbances of dementia.[33] This underscores the need for health care professionals to work with caregivers and patients to develop multimodal treatment plans that weigh the risks and benefits of various combinations of therapies for the individual patient in their particular care context and considering other medical and psychiatric comorbidities. Advance care planning offers an opportunity for patients to express their values and preferences regarding pain management before they lose capacity.[34]

Pain in Patients with Developmental Delay

The same vulnerabilities that lead to inadequate assessment and treatment of pain in patients with dementia even more seriously impede the care of persons with developmental delay. There is an even greater paucity of research and lack of reliable, valid, clinically useful assessment instruments for patients with intellectual and developmental disabilities (IDD) than for those with dementia. Thus, whatever clinical guidance is available is primarily generalized from other populations. What little is known about pain management in persons with developmental delay comes from studies in pediatric patients and is thus not discussed in this chapter on cognitive impairment in adults.

The literature on adults more frequently uses the terms intellectual and developmental disabilities (IDD) than developmental delay, the more common designation for these disorders in children: "Developmental disabilities are a group of conditions due to an impairment in physical, learning, language, or behavior areas. These conditions begin during the developmental period, may impact day-to-day functioning, and usually last throughout a person's lifetime."[35] Intellectual disabilities are a subset of this larger category: "Intellectual disability is a condition characterized by significant limitations in both intellectual functioning and adaptive behavior that begins before the age of 22."[36] The intellectual disabilities span conceptual, social, and practical skills, all integral to adaptive functioning. Examples of adult IDDs include autism, some cases of cerebral palsy, and Down's syndrome.

Model of Vulnerability in Developmental Disability

Adults with IDD are among the most vulnerable populations in a Western postmodern, highly technological, economically competitive, and socially fragmented society. Persons with developmental and intellectual disabilities are more likely than adults without them to suffer social victimization and exploitation.[37] Individuals with intellectual disabilities are often impoverished due to inability to find and maintain gainful employment, further compounding social isolation.[38] Compared to other populations, those with IDD have long suffered health care disparities, including the negative impact of social determinants of health, reduced access, lack of cultural competence among health care practitioners, and exclusion from public health initiatives.[39]

Assessment of Pain in Patients with Developmental Disabilities

Among the most troubling health care disparity is the poor quality of pain assessment and management in persons with IDD. Similar to patients with dementia, there was long an assumption that persons with developmental disabilities experience pain less frequently than persons without them. Research has now disproved that presumption, finding that persons with developmental disability experience acute and chronic pain at least as often as the general population.

This erroneous view of pain, as with dementia, can be traced to poor assessment of pain in this group due to the lack of standardized evidence-based tools. Although there has been progress in developing such instruments, there is little evidence so far that it has translated into improved evaluation and management of pain in patients with IDD. Part of the difficulty lies in the unconscious bias, ignorance, or insensitivity of the professional and informal caregivers who are the "proxy" reporters of pain, especially for nonverbal individuals and those with severe impairments in language skills.

Treatment of Pain in Patients with Intellectual and Developmental Disabilities

The result of flawed assessment is once more inadequate and often dangerous pain management practices, largely based on data from other populations, that may worsen pain when utilized in persons with developmental disabilities.[40] This is particularly unfortunate in persons with IDD, who are more likely to suffer medication-related side effects.[41]

Pain in Patients with Traumatic Brain Injury

Traumatic brain injuries are classified according to severity. Given that up to 90% of TBIs in both civilian and military cohorts are mild rather than moderate or severe, the focus of this section is on mild TBIs (mTBIs).[42] Because it is the persistent nature of the deficits from mTBIs that is the parameter of interest in this chapter on pain in cognitive impairment, acute management of mTBIs is not covered. The financial cost of mTBIs in the United States is estimated at $17 billion annually. The human cost in inability to return to work, lost productivity for those who can return to employment, and social stressors on families and communities are incalculable.

Multiple organizations have defined mTBIs in slightly different ways.[43] This lack of consistency in the use of terminology has compounded extant confusion among the public, and even nonspecialty health care professionals, about this complicated and often controversial topic.[44] A frequently cited definition is that of the American Congress of Rehabilitation Medicine. The definition first formulated in 1993 is in the process of being updated[45(pp86–87)]:

> A patient with a mTBI, also referred to as concussion, is a person who has had a traumatically induced physiologic disruption of brain function, as manifested by at least one of the following:
> 1. any period of loss of consciousness;
> 2. any loss of memory for events immediately before or after the accident;
> 3. any alteration in mental state at the time of the accident (e.g., feeling dazed, disoriented, or confused); and
> 4. focal neurological deficits that may or may not be transient; but when the severity of the injury does not exceed the following;
>   a. loss of consciousness for approximately 30 minutes or less;
>   b. after 30 minutes an initial Glasgow Coma Scale (CGS) of 13–15;
>   c. post-traumatic amnesia not greater than 24 hours.[46]

Initial psychophysical symptoms of mTBIs include dizziness, irritability, headache, fatigue, depression, and anxiety—a constellation often called post-concussive syndrome (PCS). Earlier studies estimated that only a small percentage of mTBI patients continue to exhibit PCS symptoms after the acute phase of injury. This is despite the documented pathophysiologic changes in the brain that could form the neuropsychiatric substratum of impaired cognition. Historically, this inconsistency has been the object of legal, political, clinical, and ethical debate regarding whether the etiology of PCS and the attendant cognitive impairment are primarily due to depression, chronic pain, or a result of primary neurobiological insult.[47] A 2017 scoping review of 45 studies suggests that the rate of PCS has been underestimated at approximately 15% and that up to half of individuals who suffer a single mTBI exhibit long-term cognitive impairment.[48] Premorbid

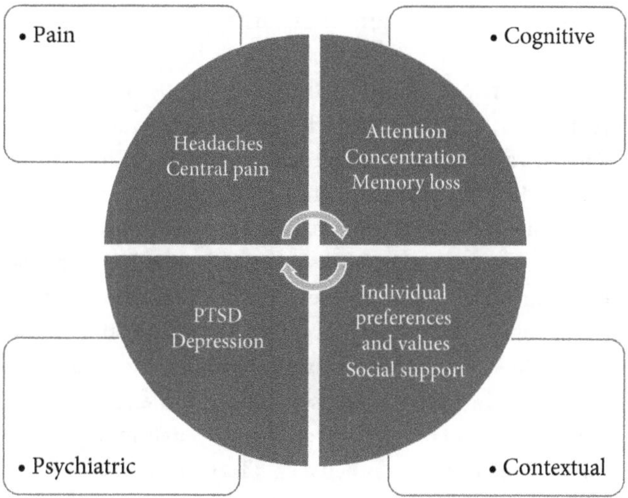

Figure 10.1 Complexity of TBI.

psychiatric history is associated with PCS at 3 months, emphasizing the importance of psychiatric assessment soon after the brain injury.[49] See Figure 10.1.

As the authors of one recent review state,

> Overall, there is an abundance of evidence that shows that both mTBI and chronic pain are complex problems that impact mood, cognitive function, and physical function. It is also clear that both problems have shared neurobiological CNS mechanisms that underlie and account for their complexity in symptom and functional impact. To date, it is not clear to what extent the problems encountered are comorbid rather than overlapping related conditions.[50]

A corollary of this complexity is that each mTBI patient will present with a unique profile of symptoms that warrants an equally individualized approach and will have a variable outcome even with optimal care.[51] The relationship of pain and cognitive impairment in mTBI is an exemplar of this complexity—and of the difficulty in ascertaining the distinct contribution of multiple interacting factors. The model of neuropsychiatric vulnerability proposed earlier in the chapter shows how pain, especially chronic pain, can amplify, and perhaps cause, cognitive impairment. Studies have shown that depression and post-traumatic stress disorder (PTSD), along with sleep disturbances, are frequently diagnosed, particularly in military patients and Veterans with mTBIs. The Traumatic Brain Injury Center of Excellence conducted a research review on the relationship between PTSD and mTBI and found that each condition can increase the severity of the other.[52] Persistent cognitive impairments in executive function, learning, and memory are associated with each disorder. Regarding the crucial question of whether each individual disorder can increase the incidence and severity of the other, the review determined that "the results are inconclusive."[52]

Assessment of Pain in Traumatic Brain Injury

The lacunae in psychometrically sound instruments that also have clinical utility for the assessment of pain in dementia and the lack of research in pain assessment in IDD are major obstacles to pain assessment in subgroups of persons with cognitive impairment. During the past few decades, the prevalence of TBI and its enormous financial and human costs, especially in military cohorts, has driven a large research enterprise. The gold standard of self-report is more valid and reliable in mTBI patients, although the same difficulties encountered in IDD and severe dementia arise in severe TBI patients.

The greatest challenge in assessing pain in mTBI is identical with the source of the condition's vulnerability—its complexity. Nampiaparampil's[53] 2008 systematic review is one of the most significant attempts to isolate the prevalence of chronic pain in TBI from the many other related factors that have contributed to its underdiagnosis. The review also examined the correlation between TBI severity and chronic pain, as well as the varying profiles of pain post-TBI in civilian and military populations. His analysis of 23 different studies found the prevalence of the most common pain complaint (chronic headache) to be 57.8%. The prevalence of chronic pain was higher in patients with mTBI than those with moderate or severe injuries and higher among civilian than military cohorts. The most significant finding from the perspective of complexity was that chronic pain "was independent of psychological disorders such as PTSD and depression."[53(p1977)]

Treatment of Mild Traumatic Brain Injury

As for persons with dementia and IDD, nonpharmacological treatments for chronic pain are first line. Unfortunately, systematic reviews and meta-analyses have found that even first-line treatments recommended in most expert guidelines for PCS have weak evidence.[54] These recommendations include education about diagnosis and course of mTBI, support for gradual return to activities, reassurance of likely good outcome (all provided as soon as possible after the injury), cognitive rehabilitation therapy, and cognitive–behavioral therapy.[55,56] Primarily psychological interventions for the frequent sleep difficulties that arise in mTBI are crucial to recovery.[57] Persons with mTBI have endorsed perceived injustice (the belief that one has been treated unfairly and disrespectfully), which makes their efforts and reintegration into society even more difficult.[58]

The pharmacological treatment of pain in patients with TBI aims to avoid medications that will exacerbate cognitive impairment, worsen comorbidities (e.g., lowering seizure threshold), or cause other harms, such as addiction. Agents should be chosen to target specific symptoms or disorders (e.g., depression) in accordance with established psychiatric standards of practice for those conditions. Before prescribing, practitioners will want to rule out other psychosocial etiologies that warrant nonpharmacological therapies. Although some mTBI patients may be more sensitive to side effects, toxicity, and drug interactions, they usually require therapeutic trials of dosing and duration to be effective.[59]

Given the neuropsychiatric linkage between pain and mental health conditions, effective treatment of pain would in theory improve cognitive impairment. However, the most-prescribed medication for post-traumatic headache (amitriptyline) has not conclusively shown benefit.[60] Pharmacological and psychological therapies that concurrently address both PTSD and cognitive impairment are under investigation, and efforts are underway to identify psychopharmacological agents or neuromodulation techniques that would target cognitive impairment.

Remediation of Vulnerability

It is unfortunate that the current state of medical science cannot offer persons with dementia and IDD a definitive cure or even a substantive therapy that can reverse or ameliorate their cognitive impairment. The prospects for the creation of higher quality pain assessment methods and the assembly of a fund of knowledge that can inform skilled pain management with lower risk and greater benefit for these vulnerable groups are much brighter. Currently, researchers are investigating automatic pain and facial recognition technology, machine learning algorithms, neuroimaging and neurophysiologic recording, among other cutting-edge methods of assessing pain that would greatly benefit nonverbal individuals.[61,62] The perfection of these techniques and their translation to clinical use will require the multi- and interdisciplinary collaboration that is the hallmark of the most successful treatments of pain in the cognitively impaired.

Similar innovation is occurring in the treatment of pain in persons with dementia and IDD, especially in the nonpharmacological realm. There is emerging evidence for music therapy, guided graded exercise and other movement-based therapies, massage and therapeutic touch, simple relaxation techniques, and the simplest yet most powerful intervention—human compassion and relationship.[63]

There is more hope for mTBI patients. The "VA/DoD Clinical Practice Guideline for the Management and Rehabilitation of Post-Acute Mild Traumatic Brain Injury"[59] describes multimodal therapies for the treatment of cognitive impairment associated with mTBI. It also recommends a comprehensive, holistic, patient-centered recovery program.

A consistent theme of this chapter has been the need for more research in the diagnosis and treatment of pain in the cognitively impaired. Yet if there is ever to be meaningful progress in the remediation of the conditions that make these groups among the most vulnerable, biomedical research is not enough. Generalizable, realizable improvement in the quality of life of individuals with dementia, IDD, and TBI will require change across multiple domains, as illustrated in Figure 10.2. The circle of concern must encompass the families and caregivers of these vulnerable persons, who need education; financial support; respite care; and competent, compassionate, accessible, integrated health care. Providing this level of assistance will necessitate stronger laws to protect the rights and safeguard the well-being of persons with cognitive impairment and pain. Intensive advocacy efforts must be launched to reduce the stigma, inequity, and social injustice that these cohorts continue to bear. Simultaneously, the many strengths of persons with dementia, IDD, and mTBI must be capitalized on and maximized so that

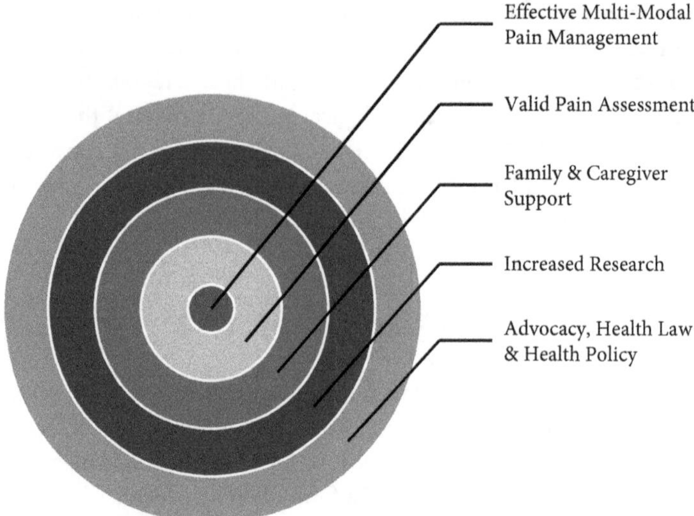

Figure 10.2 Encompassing better pain management in patients with cognitive impairment.

every individual can realize their personal potential to work, have relationships, and be part of the community.

Conclusion

This chapter has explored pain in patients with cognitive impairment. Three specific subgroups, each with its own unique profile for pain vulnerability, were examined: patients with dementia, intellectual disabilities, and mTBI. An illness model explicating the unique vulnerability of each cohort was proposed. Finally, remediation strategies for individual patients as well as patient-centered changes in the broader social context to promote the welfare and well-being of persons with pain and cognitive impairment were outlined.

References

1. Diodge N. *The Brain That Changes Itself: Stories from the Frontiers of Brain Science.* Penguin; 2007.
2. Centers for Disease Control and Prevention. Cognitive impairment: A call for action, now! 2011. https://www.cdc.gov/aging/pdf/cognitive_impairment/cogimp_poilicy_final.pdf
3. Raja SN, Carr DB, Cohen M, et al. The revised International Association for the Study of Pain definition of pain: Concepts, challenges, and compromises. *Pain.* 2020;161:1976–1982.
4. Bell T, Franz CE, Kremen WS. Persistence of pain and cognitive impairment in older adults. *J Am Geriatr Soc.* 2022;70:449–458.
5. American Psychiatric Association. *Diagnostics and Statistical Manual of Mental Disorders.* 5th ed. American Psychiatric Publishing; 2013.
6. Andrew MK, Mitnitski AB, Rockwood K. Social vulnerability, frailty and mortality in elderly people. *PLoS One.* 2008;3:e2232.

7. Shega JW, Andrew M, Hemmerich J, et al. The relationship of pain and cognitive impairment with social vulnerability: An analysis of the Canadian Study of Health and Aging. *Pain Med.* 2012;13:190–197.
8. Shega JW, Weiner DK, Paice JA, et al. The association between noncancer pain, cognitive impairment, and functional disability: An analysis of the Canadian Study of Health and Aging. *J Gerontol A Biol Sci Med Sci.* 2010;65:880–886.
9. Andrew MK, Rockwood K. Social vulnerability predicts cognitive decline in a prospective cohort of older Canadians. *Alzheimers Dement.* 2010;6:319–325.
10. Khera T, Rangasamy V. Cognition and pain: A review. *Front Psychol.* 2021;12:673962.
11. Innes KE, Sambamoorthi U. The potential contribution of chronic pain and common chronic pain conditions to subsequent cognitive decline, new onset cognitive impairment, and incident dementia: A systematic review and conceptual model for future research. *J Alzheimers Dis.* 2020;78:1177–1195.
12. Wu YL, Huang CJ, Fang SC, Ko LH, Tsai PS. Cognitive impairment in fibromyalgia: A meta-analysis of case–control studies. *Psychosom Med.* 2018;80:432–438.
13. Corti EJ, Gasson N, Loftus AM. Cognitive profile and mild cognitive impairment in people with chronic lower back pain. *Brain Cogn.* 2021;151:105737.
14. Shane Anderson A, Loeser RF. Why is osteoarthritis an age-related disease? *Best Pract Res Clin Rheumatol.* 2010;24:15–26.
15. Peavy GM, Salmon DP, Jacobson MW, et al. Effects of chronic stress on memory decline in cognitively normal and mildly impaired older adults. *Am J Psychiatry.* 2009;166:1384–1391.
16. Schoth DE, Nunes VD, Liossi C. Attentional bias towards pain-related information in chronic pain: A meta-analysis of visual-probe investigations. *Clin Psychol Rev.* 2012;32:13–25.
17. Alzheimer's Association. 2022 Alzheimer's disease facts and figures. 2022. https://www.alz.org/media/Documents/2022-Facts-and-Figures-Report_1.pdf
18. Barry HE, Parsons C, Passmore AP, Hughes CM. Exploring the prevalence of and factors associated with pain: A cross-sectional study of community-dwelling people with dementia. *Health Soc Care Community.* 2016;24:270–282.
19. Corbett A, Husebo B, Malcangio M, et al. Assessment and treatment of pain in people with dementia. *Nat Rev Neurol.* 2012;8:264–274.
20. Van Kooten J, Smalbrugge M, Van der Wouden JC, Stek ML, Hertogh C. Prevalence of pain in nursing home residents: The role of dementia stage and dementia subtypes. *J Am Med Dir Assoc.* 2017;18:522–527.
21. Scherder EJ, Sergeant JA, Swaab DF. Pain processing in dementia and its relation to neuropathology. *Lancet Neurol.* 2003;2:677–686.
22. Defrin R, Amanzio M, De Tommaso M, et al. Experimental pain processing in individuals with cognitive impairment: Current state of the science. *Pain.* 2015;156:1396–1408.
24. Achterberg W, Lautenbacher S, Husebo B, Erdal A, Herr K. Pain in dementia. *Pain Rep.* 2020;5:e803.
25. Van Dalen-Kok AH, Pieper MJ, De Waal MW, Lukas A, Husebo BS, Achterberg WP. Association between pain, neuropsychiatric symptoms, and physical function in dementia: A systematic review and meta-analysis. *BMC Geriatr.* 2015;15: Article 49.
26. Atee M, Morris T, Macfarlane S, Cunningham C. Pain in dementia: Prevalence and association with neuropsychiatric behaviors. *J Pain Symptom Manage.* 2021;61:1215–1226.
27. Lichtner V, Dowding D, Esterhuizen P, et al. Pain assessment for people with dementia: A systematic review of systematic reviews of pain assessment tools. *BMC Geriatr.* 2014;14: Article 138.
28. Rostad HM, Utne I, Grov EK, Smastuen MC, Puts M, Halvorsrud L. The impact of a pain assessment intervention on pain score and analgesic use in older nursing home residents with severe dementia: A cluster randomised controlled trial. *Int J Nurs Stud.* 2018;84:52–60.
29. McCracken LM, Turk DC. Behavioral and cognitive–behavioral treatment for chronic pain: Outcome, predictors of outcome, and treatment process. *Spine.* 2002;27:2564–2573.
30. Dublin S, Walker RL, Gray SL, et al. Prescription opioids and risk of dementia or cognitive decline: A prospective cohort study. *J Am Geriatr Soc.* 2015;63:1519–1526.

31. Husebo BS, Achterberg W, Flo E. Identifying and managing pain in people with Alzheimer's disease and other types of dementia: A systematic review. *CNS Drugs.* 2016;30:481–497.
32. Erdal A, Ballard C. Vahia IV, Husebo BS. Analgesic treatments in people with dementia: How safe are they? A systematic review. *Expert Opin Drug Saf.* 2019;18:511–522.
33. Nowak T, Neumann-Podczaska A, Deskur-Smielecka E, Styszynski A, Wieczorowska-Tobis K. Pain as a challenge in nursing home residents with behavioral and psychological symptoms of dementia. *Clin Interv Aging.* 2018;13:1045–1051.
34. Booker SS, Booker RD. Shifting paradigms: Advance care planning for pain management in older adults with dementia. *Gerontologist.* 2018;58:420–427.
35. Rubin IL, Crocker AC. *Developmental Disabilities: Delivery of Medical Care for Adults and Children.* Lea & Febiger; 1989.
36. American Association for Intellectual and Developmental Disabilities. Defining criteria for intellectual disability. 2022. Accessed May 28, 2022. https://www.aaidd.org/intellectual-disability/definition
37. Fisher MH, Moskowitz AL, Hodapp RM. Vulnerability and experiences related to social victimization among individuals with intellectual developmental disabilities. *J Ment Health Res Intellect Disabil.* 2012;5:32–48.
38. Emerson E. Poverty and people with intellectual disabilities. *Ment Retard Dev Disabil Res Rev.* 2007;13:107–113.
39. Anderson LL, Humphries K, McDermott S, Marks B, Sisirak J, Larson S. The state of the science of health and wellness for adults with intellectual and developmental disabilities. *Intellect Dev Disabil.* 2013;51:385–398.
40. Lonchampt S, Gerber F, Aubry JM, Desmeules J, Kosel M, Besson M. Pain interventions in adults with intellectual disability: A scoping review and pharmacological considerations. *Eur J Pain.* 2020;24:875–885.
41. Barney CC, Andersen RD, Defrin R, Genik LM, McGuire BE, Symons FJ. Challenges in pain assessment and management among individuals with intellectual and developmental disabilities. *Pain Rep.* 2020;5:e821.
42. Hoge CW, McGurk D, Thomas JL, Cox AL, Engel CC, Castro CA. Mild traumatic brain injury in U.S. soldiers returning from Iraq. *N Engl J Med.* 2008;358:453–463.
43. National Academies of Sciences, Engineering, and Medicine. *Evaluation of the Disability Determination Process for Traumatic Brain Injury in Veterans.* National Academies Press; 2019.
44. Lefevre-Dognin C, Cogne M, Perdrieau V, Granger A, Heslot C, Azouvi P. Definition and epidemiology of mild traumatic brain injury. *Neurochirurgie.* 2021;67:218–221.
45. Silverberg ND, Iverson GL; ACRM Mild TBI Definition Expert Consensus Group and the ACRM Brain Injury Special Interest Group Mild TBI Task Force. Expert panel survey to update the American Congress of Rehabilitation Medicine definition of mild traumatic brain injury. *Arch Phys Med Rehabil.* 2021;102:76–86.
46. Mild Traumatic Brain Injury Committee of the Brain Injury Interdisciplinary Special Interest Group of the American Congress of Rehabilitation Medicine. The definition of traumatic brain injury. *J Head Trauma Rehabil.* 1993;8:86–87.
47. Nicholson K. Pain, cognition and traumatic brain injury. *NeuroRehabilitation.* 2000;14:95–103.
48. McInnes K, Friesen CL, Mackenzie DE, Westwood DA, Boe SG. Mild traumatic brain injury (mTBI) and chronic cognitive impairment: A scoping review. *PLoS One.* 2017;12:e0174847.
49. Levin HS, Diaz-Arrastia RR. Diagnosis, prognosis, and clinical management of mild traumatic brain injury. *Lancet Neurol.* 2015;14:506–517.
50. Grandhi R, Tavakoli S, Ortega C, Simmonds MJ. A review of chronic pain and cognitive, mood, and motor dysfunction following mild traumatic brain injury: Complex, comorbid, and/or overlapping conditions? *Brain Sci.* 2017;7(12): Article 160.
51. Comper P, Bisschop SM, Carnide N, Tricco A. A systematic review of treatments for mild traumatic brain injury. *Brain Inj.* 2005;19:863–880.

52. Sloley S. Research review on mild traumatic brain injury and post-traumatic stress disorder. Traumatic Brain Injury Center of Excellence; 2020.
53. Nampiaparampil DE. Prevalence of chronic pain after traumatic brain injury: A systematic review. *JAMA*. 2008;300:711–719.
54. Rytter HM, Graff HJ, Henriksen HK, et al. Nonpharmacological treatment of persistent postconcussion symptoms in adults: A systematic review and meta-analysis and guideline recommendation. *JAMA Netw Open*. 2021;4:e2132221.
55. Comper P, Bisschop SM, Carnide N, Tricco A. A systematic review of treatments for mild traumatic brain injury. *Brain Injury*. 2005;19(11):863–880. doi:10.1080/02699050400025042
56. Snell DL, Surgenor LJ, Hay-Smith EJ, Siegert RJ. A systematic review of psychological treatments for mild traumatic brain injury: an update on the evidence. *J Clin Exp Neuropsychol*. 2009;31(1):20–38.
57. Pilon L, Frankenmolen N, Bertens D. Treatments for sleep disturbances in individuals with acquired brain injury: A systematic review. *Clin Rehabil*. 2021;35:1518–1529.
58. Iverson GL, Terry DP, Karr JE, Panenka WJ, Silverberg ND. Perceived injustice and its correlates after mild traumatic brain injury. *J Neurotrauma*. 2018;35:1156–1166.
59. U.S. Department of Veterans Affairs. VA/DoD clinical practice guideline for the management and rehabilitation of post-acute mild traumatic brain injury. 2021. https://www.healthquality.va.gov/guidelines/Rehab/mtbi/VADoDmTBICPGFinal508.pdf
60. Hurwitz M, Lucas S, Bell KR, Temkin N, Dikmen S, Hoffman J. Use of amitriptyline in the treatment of headache after traumatic brain injury: Lessons learned from a clinical trial. *Headache*. 2020;60:713–723.
61. Atee M, Hoti K, Chivers P, Hughes JD. Faces of pain in dementia: Learnings from a real-world study using a technology-enabled pain assessment tool. *Front Pain Res*. 2022;3:827551.
62. Kunz M, Seuss D, Hassan T, et al. Problems of video-based pain detection in patients with dementia: A road map to an interdisciplinary solution. *BMC Geriatr*. 2017;17: Article 33.
63. Pieper MJ, Van Dalen-Kok AH, Francke AL, et al. Interventions targeting pain or behaviour in dementia: A systematic review. *Ageing Res Rev*. 2013;12:1042–1055.
64. Binnekade TT, Van Kooten J, Lobbezoo F, et al. Pain experience in dementia subtypes: A systematic review. *Curr Alzheimer Res*. 2017;14:471–485.
65. Chang JY, Rukavina K, Lawn T, Chaudhuri KR. Pain in neurodegenerative diseases with atypical parkinsonism: A systematic review on prevalence, clinical presentation, and findings from experimental studies. *J Integr Neurosci*. 2021;20:1067–1078.

11
Pain in Military Personnel

Major Sara M. Wilson and Captain Taylor J. Byrne

Introduction

"Vulnerable" is a derivative of the Latin word meaning wounded.[1] Any given population or group of people can be "wounded" for numerous reasons. In the context of health care, Flaskerud and Winslow[2] defined vulnerable populations as social groups that experience limited resources and as a result have an increased risk for poor health outcomes, morbidity, and premature mortality. Social groups classically recognized as vulnerable include minorities; the lesbian, gay, bisexual, transgender, and queer (LGBTQ) community; immigrants; the elderly; and women and children.[2] However, additional vulnerable populations exist that society may overlook.[3] The military population, including active duty and veterans, is one such population that is not commonly recognized as vulnerable. However, due to the soldier experience, the state of being vulnerable is a common risk when defined as the "exposure to the possibility of being attacked or harmed, either physically or emotionally."[4] This chapter explores the vulnerability of the military population, the impact of chronic pain in this unique population, and both risk factors and protective factors for developing chronic pain. It also outlines many of the strategies and programs the U.S. Department of Defense has instituted to improve chronic pain measurement and outcomes.

What Makes Military Service Members More Vulnerable to Pain?

Military service members face unique stressors that contribute to their inclusion as a vulnerable population as well as increase their risk for chronic pain states. Military service members are defined in this chapter as active duty, National Guard, and Reserve members of the U.S. Army, Navy, Air Force, Marine Corps, or Coast Guard.

The military has been described as the most engrossing and demanding institution in American society.[5] Unique experiences of the service member include special training requirements, frequent relocations, geographic isolation from support structures, deployments and redeployments, integrating from the military to the civilian workforce, and financial stressors.[6] Additional contributors to vulnerability include a rigid command structure, a pervasive military culture, and predominance of force priorities over individual concerns.

In addition to vulnerability as a population due to the institutional nature of service, military-specific requirements and exposures increase service members' vulnerability to developing illness and injury at an increased rate compared to the general population. These unique exposures increase the rate of depression, post-traumatic stress disorder (PTSD), and traumatic brain injury (TBI) compared to the general civilian population.[7–9] The increased rates of these mental health disorders are important contributors to vulnerability. In recent years with the wars in Iraq [Operation Iraqi Freedom (OIF) and Operation New Dawn] and Afghanistan [Operation Enduring Freedom (OEF)], 6,783 service members were killed and more than 50,000 wounded in action.[10] This unprecedented survival rate and increased wounded-to-fatality ratio has led to increased medical, psychological, and social costs to service members, their families, and the Department of Defense and Veterans Affairs (VA) medical systems.[11] The medical system is challenged to provide complex care to these patients. In addition, patients are at risk of not receiving the services they need, especially when discharged from the military.

In contrast to active duty service members, the veteran population is more synchronous with vulnerability due to the plethora of social challenges they encounter as they transition from the military to the civilian population.[12] Social challenges experienced by veterans include limited access to care, disability, unemployment, homelessness, and social isolation.[13] Because the homeless population is commonly considered a vulnerable population, it is important to note that veterans make up 8% of the adult homeless population.[14] The obstacles faced by homeless veterans can significantly impact their ability to access care. These obstacles include lack of transportation, lack of continuity of care, distrust of health care providers, and poor social support.[15]

Discussion

One such medical condition that is highly prevalent within the veteran population is chronic pain. Approximately half of all veterans enrolled in the VA health care system experience chronic pain compared to just 30% of the civilian population.[13] Furthermore, compared to nonveterans, veterans with chronic pain suffer from more complex pain syndromes often associated with comorbid psychiatric conditions such as depression and PTSD.[13,16]

Chronic pain is defined as pain that is present for 3 months or more. Chronic pain affects more than 100 million U.S. adults.[17] This is more than the number of U.S. adults suffering from diabetes, cancer, and heart disease combined.[18] Pain is a universal phenomenon, and everyone is at risk of experiencing acute or chronic pain. However, some populations are at increased risk and thus are at increased risk of suffering its disabling effects.[17] The prevalence of chronic pain is even higher among U.S. military personnel. The prevalence of chronic pain among active duty service members is estimated to range from 31% to 44%.[19,20] In comparison to military rates in 2016, only 20–30% of U.S. nonmilitary service-connected adults were estimated to have chronic pain.[13,21] Furthermore, approximately half of all veterans enrolled in the VA health care system experience chronic pain compared to 30% of the U.S. population.[13] The difference between prevalence in the military and nonmilitary populations can be attributed to the high demands and risk factors that military service exposes its members to, including mental and physical demands; injuries sustained during deployment; a delay by service members to seek treatment due to the high job demands; lack of access; and a culture that praises selflessness, toughness, and willingness to accept pain.[22–25]

Managing chronic pain in the military population is of significant concern due to the impact within the military, the Department of Defense, and the general U.S. health care system. There are more than 1.3 million active duty personnel and more than 1 million Ready Reserve members, including the National Guard and Reserves.[26] Chronic pain imposes a significant burden on society and is the leading cause of medical discharge, resulting in a significant cost to the Department of Defense for disability payments.[27] The musculoskeletal system is the most commonly injured and is the leading cause of disability for the U.S. Armed Forces. The Department of Defense spends more than $1.5 billion per year paying disabled veterans, and musculoskeletal conditions are responsible for 40–50% of the total amount.[27–29] It can cost approximately $250,000 in lifetime disability costs, excluding health care costs, for the medical discharge of one active duty service member, discharged in their late twenties.[27] Furthermore, it can cost up to and exceed $1 million to retrain a replacement.[30]

Types of Pain

Potential risks for injury and hazard exposures for soldiers depend on the specific job performed during their military service. Research specific to the post–September 11, 2001, soldier depicts an abundance of unique hazards, including but not limited to combat smoke, burn pits, landmines, improvised explosive devices, rocket-propelled grenades, mortar and rocket fire, depleted uranium, and aircraft and artillery noise.[31–35] Depending on the specialty within the military, some soldiers are also required to routinely carry heavy equipment, including weapons, armor, and personal gear, that can weigh more than 100 pounds.[31] Not surprisingly, the musculoskeletal system is the most commonly injured system in the U.S. Armed Forces, and many of these musculoskeletal injuries occur during military training. A survey of U.S. Army trainees found that 50% of musculoskeletal injuries occurred gradually as opposed to being associated with a single specific event. These types of injuries are typically unintentional and result from acute or chronic overuse. This high prevalence of musculoskeletal injuries that begin during training, combined with the mental and physical challenges associated with military duties, places service members at increased risk for both acute and chronic pain issues.[22] In addition to training-related injuries, combat-related injuries are more prevalent than ever before. It is estimated that more than 90% of soldiers survive combat-related injuries. As such, increasingly high rates of chronic pain conditions related to combat injuries are being diagnosed in military combat personnel. These painful combat-related injuries are often comorbid with TBI and PTSD.[36]

A study by Reif et al.[22] found that 63% of soldiers had at least one pain diagnosis during fiscal year 2012. The most frequent primary diagnoses were back and neck pain (22%), nontraumatic joint disorders (28%), and other musculoskeletal pain (30%). Severe or moderate pain scores were reported by 55% of soldiers who carried a primary pain diagnosis. Of these categories, soldiers complaining of neck or back pain were the most common category to develop chronic pain (62%) during that fiscal year.[22] An earlier study investigating 359 OIF/OEF veterans found that the most common medical condition was chronic pain. This high prevalence of musculoskeletal injuries among service members has prompted injury risk reduction efforts by the U.S. Army.

In addition to the musculoskeletal injuries highlighted above, service members also have the potential to develop behavioral health conditions that predispose them to increased chronic pain states, including PTSD, depression, TBI, sleep disorders, smoking, and substance use disorder. The nature of military service also provides protective factors that can improve pain outcomes in the military population, including physical fitness requirements, weight parameters, a focus on nutrition, and educational and employment status opportunities.

Post-Traumatic Stress Disorder

Post-traumatic stress disorder occurs at an increased rate in the military population. In the United States, PTSD prevalence is estimated to be 6% in males and 12% in females, with an estimated lifetime prevalence of 7.8%.[37] In a comprehensive study on the effects of war on combatants, the National Vietnam Veterans Readjustment Study found a lifetime rate of patients with PTSD as high as 30% and a current rate of 15%.[38,39] Within a population diagnosed with PTSD, there is a high rate of chronic pain. In one study performed on veterans with PTSD, the results of a self-reported questionnaire showed that 80% of patients diagnosed with PTSD also reported the presence of a chronic pain condition.[40] Research shows that patients affected by PTSD and chronic pain in combination experience greater pain, distress, and disability than patients with either condition alone.[41] The co-prevalence of chronic pain and PTSD negatively impacts both disorders. There are proposed theoretical models to elucidate the link as well as proposed neurologic factors that may contribute to the co-prevalence of disease. Some theoretical models include the mutual maintenance model, the shared vulnerability model, the fear avoidance model, and the triple vulnerability model.[39,42–46] Although more research is needed, preliminary research indicates a shared pathophysiology between the neuroanatomic pathway of both chronic pain and PTSD—as well as the dysregulation of neurohormones, neurotransmitters, and inflammatory system factors (neuropeptide Y) and the GABAergic neuroactive steroid immune factors—and cellular second messenger systems.[41,47–51]

Depression

Depression is recognized as one of the leading causes of global disability, estimated to affect more than 264 million people worldwide.[52] One study suggests the prevalence of depression may be even higher in the military compared to civilian populations.[53] A survey of soldiers found as many as 38% reported clinically significant depressive symptoms after returning from 12-month OIF/OEF deployments.[54] Likewise, a study by Seal et al.[55] tracking the prevalence of mental health diagnoses in OEF/OIF veterans receiving health care at the VA documented a sevenfold increase in depression diagnoses from 2002 to 2008. This high prevalence of depression within the military population is often complicated by comorbid diagnoses. Pain, for example, may mask symptoms of depression, leading to underdiagnosis or delayed diagnosis.[56] Unfortunately, chronic pain and depression are commonly comorbid conditions, with up to 60% of chronic pain patients also presenting with symptoms of depression.[57]

The relationship between chronic pain and depression is complex. It is thought to be a reciprocal or bidirectional relationship, because having chronic pain increases the risk of developing depression and vice versa.[58,59] Pain, in particular, is associated with worse depression.[60] Although there is strong evidence for pain predicting depression onset and outcomes, there is weaker evidence for depression predicting pain intensity and outcomes.[59] Even so, another opinion argues that chronic pain is actually a type of depression.[61] In many cases, it can be difficult to determine whether pain caused depression or depression caused pain, but in most instances the two disease processes are clearly intertwined. Clinical studies show that pain often induces depression, and up to 85% of patients with chronic pain also suffer from depression.[61–63]

The current literature suggests the need to treat depression and chronic pain together in order to deliver effective care. This is especially true with emerging evidence showing neuroplasticity mechanism changes that are common to both chronic pain and depression. Recent studies have reviewed the shared structural foundations for the coexistence of pain and depression, including connections between the insular cortex, prefrontal cortex, anterior cingulate, thalamus, hippocampus, and amygdala.[61,64] Monoamine neurotransmitters have also been studied for their molecular mechanism involved in chronic pain and depression. Transmitters such as serotonin, dopamine, and norepinephrine have been studied as a molecular link between chronic pain and depression.[61] Other factors studied as potential links between depression and chronic pain include brain-derived neuropathic factor, inflammatory factors, and glutamate levels.[61] Failing to recognize the comorbid diseases may increase the likelihood of negative outcomes for the patient's overall health.[58]

Traumatic Brain Injury

Traumatic brain injury is defined as an injury to the brain, typically from an external force, that causes traumatic structural and physiologic disruption of normal brain function. Depending on the severity of a TBI, service members may experience a range of symptoms, including confusion, disorientation, loss of consciousness, memory loss, and neurologic deficits. TBIs are typically classified as mild, moderate, or severe based on clinical and radiographic criteria associated with the injury. The incidence of TBI has increased significantly in both the active duty and veteran population because of recent military and combat operations. TBI became so common during OEF and OIF that it would eventually be described as the "signature injury" of these conflicts.[65]

The number of service members reporting TBI symptoms after returning from recent conflicts is staggering. Approximately 22–97% of service members returning from OEF and OIF suffered from mild TBI.[66–69] Although many comorbid health issues occur because of TBI, pain is one of the most common. Clark and colleagues[70] found that returning service members and veterans report pain as the most common TBI-associated symptom, with pain affecting 30%–90% of service members following a deployment related TBI. A study by Taylor et al.[71] found that recent veterans with mild

TBI were 70% more likely to report head, neck, or back pain compared to veterans who had not sustained a TBI.

Sleep Disorders

Sleep disorders continue to occur at high rates within the military population. This is in large part attributed to deployment-related demands, which typically necessitate long shiftwork, irregular sleep schedules, and potentially unsafe sleep environments. These stressors, combined with the potential for psychological trauma, PTSD, and TBI, make military personnel highly susceptible to chronic sleep disturbances.[72] In a study by Troxel and colleagues,[73] nearly half of all military personnel reported poor sleep when using the Pittsburgh Sleep Quality Index. The high prevalence of sleep disorders within the U.S. military was further supported when Moore et al.[74] found that the incidence of obstructive sleep apnea and insomnia had increased enormously across all branches of the military since 2005.

As the incidences of chronic pain states and sleep disorders continue to rise among service members, research has begun to focus on the relationship between sleep and pain. The current literature supports a bidirectional relationship between pain and sleep, in which chronic pain conditions negatively impact sleep, and sleep disorders worsen chronic pain conditions.[75] A review by Andersen and colleagues[75] found that many sleep disorders, including sleep deprivation and insomnia, are associated with increased pain severity and frequency. This is further supported by Afolalu et al.,[76] who found that adults with reduced sleep duration and quality were at a three times greater risk of developing a chronic pain condition. This study also found that improvements in sleep quality and duration resulted in improved physical functioning.

Smoking

From a historical perspective, smoking has long been associated with military culture. In general, the military population is more likely to engage in cigarette smoking compared to civilian populations.[77] In a report by the Institute of Medicine in 2009,[78] cigarette smoking among military personnel was found to negatively affect readiness by impairing physical fitness and cognitive performance. In addition to negatively impacting physical and cognitive performance, the negative health impacts of smoking include cardiovascular disease, respiratory disease, periodontal disease, peptic ulcer disease, and increased risk for acute respiratory illness.[79] Cigarette smoking and its negative impacts have been estimated to cost the Department of Defense more than $1 billion per year.[80] Due to the negative effect smoking has within the military, several efforts have been made by the Department of Defense to mitigate this impact, including tobacco cessation counseling, increasing access to tobacco cessation products, and instituting tobacco-free areas.[81,82] Although these efforts were initially successful, the conflicts in Iraq and Afghanistan and the associated deployments resulted in an increase in smoking initiation and resumption.[83]

Cigarette smoking is known to cause multiorgan system dysfunction. Interestingly, cigarette smoking has also been shown to have a negative impact on chronic pain conditions. Because low back pain is one of the most common pain-related musculoskeletal diagnoses among service members, a focus on smoking cessation in this population may have a significant impact on patient outcomes with regard to pain management.

Substance Use Disorder

In addition to smoking, substance use and substance use disorders are common in the veteran population. Illicit substances including marijuana and cocaine are generally used less among veterans compared to nonveterans, whereas use of licit substances such as alcohol is higher among veteran than nonveterans.[84] Studies show that there is a high prevalence of heavy alcohol use among veterans. In a recent study assessing male participants aged 18–25 years, 17.6% reported heavy drinking compared to 12.2% of nonveterans.[85] Lan et al.[86] performed a systematic review of 72 studies examining more than 125,000 veterans and reported a 32% prevalence of alcohol use disorder and a 20% prevalence of drug use disorder. In addition to alcohol use, veterans also engage in higher rates of polysubstance use, including opioid use disorder. Mental health diagnoses increase the likelihood of receiving an opioid prescription, and patients with a diagnosis of PTSD also received higher doses of opioid medications and were more likely to receive an early refill.[84] The interplay between chronic pain, mental health disorders, and substance use requires subspecialty use services that some veterans do not engage in or have access to.[85] This leads to increased high-risk behaviors and adverse clinical outcomes and increases the complexity of pain and pain management.[31] Recent efforts to bring awareness to this issue within the Department of Defense showed encouraging improvements, with the prevalence of long-term opioid use among service members declining from a peak of 12.3% in 2007 to 3.9% in 2018.[87]

Protective Factors

Although occupation within the military and its unique requirements place service members at risk for developing chronic pain conditions, there are also aspects of service that may protect service members from developing chronic pain, including physical fitness requirements, weight parameters, a focus on nutrition, and educational and employment status opportunities.

A systematic review identified nine studies supporting physical activity for the prevention of chronic pain.[88] A more recent study by Fancourt and colleagues[89] found that vigorous weekly physical activity was protective against the development of chronic pain in older adults. In addition, they also found that psychosocial factors such as cultural engagement may be protective against the development of chronic pain. Because regular physical training and physical fitness tests are requirements across all military branches, this may serve to protect service members from developing chronic pain conditions if applied appropriately with proper training and rest periods. In addition to physical fitness requirements, all branches have height and weight requirements which could help attenuate chronic pain given that a high body mass index can be a predictor of chronic pain.[90]

Nutrition is an important lifestyle factor that can impact chronic pain states. Poor nutrition is considered a predicting, perpetuating, or underlying factor in chronic musculoskeletal pain.[91] Brain et al.[92] conducted a systematic review that showed nutritional interventions with altered diet and altered nutrition significantly reduced pain scores in patients with non-cancer pain. Most military bases provide a centralized subsidized dining facility with access to healthy food options. The military has also instituted a Go for Green campaign, sponsored by the Consortium for Health and Military Performance, that labels food in a manner that makes it easy to identify high-performance foods and drinks that will boost fitness, strength, and health.

Other protective factors include educational and employment opportunities. The educational landscape among military personnel varies between officer and enlisted. Military officers have higher levels of education, on average, than both enlisted personnel and the average U.S. nonmilitary adult. More than 80% of active duty officers have at least a bachelor's degree, and 42% hold an advanced degree and are four times as likely as the average adult to have completed a postgraduate degree.[93] The enlisted personnel education profile shows that 92% of enlisted personnel have completed high school or some college, compared to 60% of U.S. nonmilitary adults. Research also shows that only 7% of enlisted personnel have a bachelor's degree compared to 19% of all adults aged 18–44 years.[93] Although more research is needed to fully understand the link between chronic pain and education, some studies suggest that lower education levels may correlate with increased prevalence of chronic pain.[21,94] Given the higher education levels within the U.S. military, education status may be a protective factor for developing chronic pain. Similarly, employment status of the active duty population may be a protective factor against developing chronic pain. However, more research is needed.

Solutions to Chronic Pain in the Military

Due to the high prevalence of chronic pain within the military health system, aggressive efforts have been made to improve pain management care. In 2009, the Army Surgeon General chartered a Pain Management Task Force. This task force published a report outlining 109 recommendations to improve pain management care within the veteran and military health system. The recommendations focus on four areas: providing infrastructure to support research in pain management, utilizing evidenced-based best practices, maintaining a patient- and family-centered approach, and creating a culture of pain awareness and education. Some key strategies include standardizing pain management care, the use of an interdisciplinary and multimodal approach to pain management, as well as adopting the stepped-care approach utilized by the Veterans Health Administration.[95,96] The stepped-care model of pain management is a biopsychosocial approach focusing on the patient as a whole. It addresses physical, psychological, and social factors that contribute to chronic pain states. This model also provides a framework for escalating care of pain patients from primary to tertiary.[97] Following this report, the

Department of Defense developed a comprehensive pain management policy in 2011 to implement the above strategies.

In 2014, the Department of Defense issued a report to Congress outlining its progress. Several key changes were outlined that improved overall patient satisfaction with pain management. These include the implementation of a patient-centered medical home (PCMH) model within primary care clinics to increase access to pain care, an increase in the number of pain management specialists, and the development of new tools and training to improve pain management care.[98] The PCMH model places the primary care physician as the team leader of patient care, responsible for addressing pain conditions early and initiating timely referral to pain specialists when indicated.[98] The highest level of care involves treatment at an interdisciplinary pain management center (IPMC). These centers are sophisticated pain rehabilitation programs that use advanced diagnostic techniques, pain medicine, and functional rehabilitation to treat complex pain conditions. As such, in addition to increasing the number of pain specialists, the military continues to focus on the development of IPMCs at its major military treatment facilities.[95,98]

A more recent report to Congress in 2021 outlined additional progress in the ongoing implementation of a comprehensive pain management policy within the Department of Defense. In addition to continued efforts to improve the current PCMH, stepped-care models, and IPMCs, this report highlights progress with regard to the implementation of pain-related clinical practice guidelines; expansion of pain telehealth services; annual training in primary care and specialty care pain skills; as well as research efforts to examine complementary and alternative medicine treatment modalities for chronic pain syndromes, including physical therapy, occupational therapy, chiropractic treatment, acupuncture, and cognitive–behavioral therapy. These strategies were complemented by the development of the Pain Assessment Screening Tool and Outcomes Registry (PASTOR) to be used as a performance measure for the above implemented pain care strategies. PASTOR is a patient survey tool that produces a detailed and comprehensive report of a patient's chronic pain. As such, in addition to providing data and performance measures, PASTOR also serves as a pain registry and clinical decision-making tool for providers. In 2021, PASTOR was enabled at all military treatment facilities.

Conclusion

The Department of Defense and support organizations throughout the country continue to make concerted efforts to decrease the risk factors and effects of chronic pain in the military as well as enhance the protective factors.

Acknowledging the vulnerability of this unique population can also improve outcomes by promoting better understanding of the specific comorbid diseases, experiences of the service members, and inherent limitations to care. Given the broad burden of pain in this population, devoting resources to improve pain will have widespread effects on this special population as well as the Department of Defense and the U.S. population as a whole.

References

1. King TE, Wheeler MB. *Medical Management of Vulnerable and Underserved Patients: Principles, Practice, and Populations*. 2nd ed. McGraw Hill; 2016.
2. Flaskerud JH, Winslow BJ. Conceptualizing vulnerable populations health-related research. *Nurs Res*. 1998;47(2):69–78. doi:10.1097/00006199-199803000-00005
3. Waisel DB. Vulnerable populations in healthcare. *Curr Opin Anaesthesiol*. 2013;26(2):186–192. doi:10.1097/ACO.0b013e32835e8c17
4. Benzel E. On being vulnerable. *World Neurosurg*. 2020;142. doi:10.1016/j.wneu.2020.07.157
5. Moon Z. Pastoral care and counseling with military families. *J Pastoral Care Counsel*. 2016;70(2):128–135. doi:10.1177/1542305016633663
6. Ormeno MD, Roh Y, Heller M, et al. Special concerns in military families. *Curr Psychiatry Rep*. 2020;22(12): Article 82. doi:10.1007/s11920-020-01207-7
7. Blore JD, Sim MR, Forbes AB, Creamer MC, Kelsall HL. Depression in Gulf War veterans: A systematic review and meta-analysis. *Psychol Med*. 2015;45(8):1565–1580. doi:10.1017/s0033291714001913
8. Gates MA, Holowka DW, Vasterling JJ, Keane TM, Marx BP, Rosen RC. Posttraumatic stress disorder in veterans and military personnel: Epidemiology, screening, and case recognition. *Psychol Serv*. 2012;9(4):361–382. doi:10.1037/a0027649
9. Ommaya AK, Ommaya AK, Dannenberg AL, Salazar AM. Causation, incidence, and costs of traumatic brain injury in the U.S. military medical system. *J Trauma*. 1996;40(2):211–217. doi:10.1097/00005373-199602000-00007
10. U.S. Department of Defense. Immediate release casualty status 2022. n.d. https://www.defense.gov/casualty.pdf
11. Gibson CA. Review of posttraumatic stress disorder and chronic pain: The path to integrated care. *J Rehabil Rese Dev*. 2012;49(5):753–776. doi:10.1682/jrrd.2011.09.0158
12. Baria AM, Pangarkar S, Abrams G, Miaskowski C. Adaption of the biopsychosocial model of chronic noncancer pain in veterans. *Pain Med*. 2019;20(1):14–27. doi:10.1093/pm/pny058
13. Gallagher RM. Advancing the pain agenda in the veteran population. *Anesthesiol Clin*. 2016;34(2):357–378. doi:10.1016/j.anclin.2016.01.003
14. Henry M, de Sousa T, Tano C, et al. The 2021 Annual Homeless Assessment Report (AHAR) to Congress. U.S. Department of Housing and Urban Development, Office of Community Planning and Development; 2021.
15. O'Toole TP, Johnson EE, Aiello R, Kane V, Pape L. Tailoring care to vulnerable populations by incorporating social determinants of health: The Veterans Health Administration's "Homeless Patient Aligned Care Team" Program. *Prev Chronic Dis*. 2016;13:E44. doi:10.5888/pcd13.150567
16. Kerns RD, Otis J, Rosenberg R, Reid MC. Veterans' reports of pain and associations with ratings of health, health-risk behaviors, affective distress, and use of the healthcare system. *J Rehabil Res Dev*. 2003;40(5):371–379. doi:10.1682/jrrd.2003.09.0371
17. Institute of Medicine Committee on Advancing Pain Research, Care, and Education. *Relieving Pain in America: A Blueprint for Transforming Prevention, Care, Education, and Research*. National Academies Press; 2011.
18. Tsang A, Von Korff M, Lee S, et al. Common chronic pain conditions in developed and developing countries: Gender and age differences and comorbidity with depression-anxiety disorders. *J Pain*. 2008;9(10):883–891. doi:10.1016/j.jpain.2008.05.005
19. Toblin RL, Quartana PJ, Riviere LA, Walper KC, Hoge CW. Chronic pain and opioid use in US soldiers after combat deployment. *JAMA Intern Med*. 2014;174(8):1400–1401. doi:10.1001/jamainternmed.2014.2726
20. Sherry TB, Roth CP, Bhandarkar M, Hepner KA. *Chronic Pain Among Service Members: Using Administrative Data to Strengthen Research and Quality Improvement*. RAND Corporation; 2021.

21. Dahlhamer J, Lucas J, Zelaya C, et al. Prevalence of chronic pain and high-impact chronic pain among adults—United States, 2016. *MMWR Morb Mortal Wkly Rep*. 2018;67(36):1001–1006. doi:10.15585/mmwr.mm6736a2
22. Reif S, Adams RS, Ritter GA, Williams TV, Larson MJ. Prevalence of pain diagnoses and burden of pain among active duty soldiers, FY2012. *Mil Med*. 2018;183(9–10):e330–e337. doi:10.1093/milmed/usx200
23. Clark ME. Post-deployment pain: A need for rapid detection and intervention. *Pain Med*. 2004;5(4):333–334. doi:10.1111/j.1526-4637.2004.04059.x
24. Gironda RJ, Clark ME, Massengale JP, Walker RL. Pain among veterans of Operations Enduring Freedom and Iraqi Freedom. *Pain Med*. 2006;7(4):339–343. doi:10.1111/j.1526-4637.2006.00146.x
25. Office of the Army Surgeon General. Pain Management Task Force: Providing a standardized DoD and VHA vision and approach to pain management to optimize the care for warriors and their families. 2010. https://permanent.fdlp.gov/gpo60064/Pain-Management-Task-Force.pdf
26. U.S. Department of Defense, Office of the Deputy Assistant Secretary of Defense for Military Community and Family Policy. 2019 Demographics: Profile of the military community. 2019. https://download.militaryonesource.mil/12038/MOS/Reports/2019-demographics-report.pdf
27. Gatchel RJ, McGeary DD, Peterson A, et al. Preliminary findings of a randomized controlled trial of an interdisciplinary military pain program. *Mil Med*. 2009;174(3):270–277. doi:10.7205/milmed-d-03-1607
28. Berkowitz SM, Feuerstein M, Lopez MS, Peck CA Jr. Occupational back disability in U.S. Army personnel. *Mil Med*. 1999;164(6):412–418.
29. Huang GD, Feuerstein M, Berkowitz SM, Peck CA Jr. Occupational upper-extremity-related disability: Demographic, physical, and psychosocial factors. *Mil Med*. 1998;163(8):552–558.
30. Cohen SP, Griffith S, Larkin TM, Villena F, Larkin R. Presentation, diagnoses, mechanisms of injury, and treatment of soldiers injured in Operation Iraqi Freedom: An epidemiological study conducted at two military pain management centers. *Anesth Analg*. 2005;101(4):1098–1093. doi:10.1213/01.ane.0000169332.45209.cf
31. Waszak DL, Holmes AM. The unique health needs of post-9/11 U.S. veterans. *Workplace Health Saf*. 2017;65(9):430–444. doi:10.1177/2165079916682524
32. Falvo MJ, Osinubi OY, Sotolongo AM, Helmer DA. Airborne hazards exposure and respiratory health of Iraq and Afghanistan veterans. *Epidemiol Rev*. 2015;37:116–130. doi:10.1093/epirev/mxu009
33. Franklin M, Hintze W, Hornbostel M, et al. 2010 Wounded Warrior Project Survey. Wounded Warrior Project; 2010.
34. Gajewski D, Granville R. The United States Armed Forces Amputee Patient Care Program. *J Am Acad Orthop Surg*. 2006;14(10 Spec No.):S183–S187. doi:10.5435/00124635-200600001-00040
35. Kelly U, Boyd MA, Valente SM, Czekanski E. Trauma-informed care: Keeping mental health settings safe for veterans. *Issues Ment Health Nurs*. 2014;35(6):413–419. doi:10.3109/01612840.2014.881941
36. Casey K, Demers P, Deben S, Nelles ME, Weiss JS. Outcomes after long-term follow-up of combat-related extremity injuries in a multidisciplinary limb salvage clinic. *Ann Vasc Surg*. 2015;29(3):496–501. doi:10.1016/j.avsg.2014.09.035
37. Kessler RC, Sonnega A, Bromet E, Hughes M, Nelson CB. Posttraumatic stress disorder in the National Comorbidity Survey. *Arch Gen Psychiatry*. 1995;52(12):1048–1060. doi:10.1001/archpsyc.1995.03950240066012
38. Kulka RA, Schlenger WE, Fairbank JA, et al. *Trauma and the Vietnam War Generation: Report of Findings for the National Vietnam Veterans Readjustment Study*. Brunner/Mazel; 1990.

39. Otis JD, Keane TM, Kerns RD. An examination of the relationship between chronic pain and post-traumatic stress disorder. *J Rehabil Res Dev*. 2003;40(5):397–405. doi:10.1682/jrrd.2003.09.0397
40. Beckham JC, Crawford AL, Feldman ME, et al. Chronic posttraumatic stress disorder and chronic pain in Vietnam combat veterans. *J Psychosom Res*. 1997;43(4):379–389. doi:10.1016/s0022-3999(97)00129-3
41. Scioli-Salter ER, Forman DE, Otis JD, Gregor K, Valovski I, Rasmusson AM. The shared neuroanatomy and neurobiology of comorbid chronic pain and PTSD: Therapeutic implications. *Clin J Pain*. 2015;31(4):363–374. doi:10.1097/ajp.0000000000000115
42. Sharp TJ, Harvey AG. Chronic pain and posttraumatic stress disorder: Mutual maintenance? *Clin Psychol Rev*. 2001;21(6):857–877. doi:10.1016/s0272-7358(00)00071-4
43. Asmundson GJ, Coons MJ, Taylor S, Katz J. PTSD and the experience of pain: Research and clinical implications of shared vulnerability and mutual maintenance models. *Can J Psychiatry*. 2002;47(10):930–937. doi:10.1177/070674370204701004
44. Norton PJ, Asmundson GJ. Amending the fear-avoidance model of chronic pain: What is the role of physiological arousal? *Behav Ther*. 2003;34:17–30.
45. Vlaeyen JWS, Linton SJ. Fear-avoidance and its consequences in chronic musculoskeletal pain: A state of the art. *Pain*. 2000;85(3):317–332. doi:10.1016/s0304-3959(99)00242-0
46. Barlow DH, ed. *Anxiety and Its Disorders*. Guilford; 2002.
47. Morgan CA 3rd, Wang S, Southwick SM, et al. Plasma neuropeptide-Y concentrations in humans exposed to military survival training. *Biol Psychiatry*. 2000;47(10):902–909. doi:10.1016/s0006-3223(99)00239-5
48. Morgan CA 3rd, Rasmusson AM, Wang S, Hoyt G, Hauger RL, Hazlett G. Neuropeptide-Y, cortisol, and subjective distress in humans exposed to acute stress: Replication and extension of previous report. *Biol Psychiatry*. 2002;52(2):136–142. doi:10.1016/s0006-3223(02)01319-7
49. Rasmusson AM, Hauger RL, Morgan CA, Bremner JD, Charney DS, Southwick SM. Low baseline and yohimbine-stimulated plasma neuropeptide Y (NPY) levels in combat-related PTSD. *Biol Psychiatry*. 2000;47(6):526–539. doi:10.1016/s0006-3223(99)00185-7
50. Sah R, Ekhator NN, Strawn JR, et al. Low cerebrospinal fluid neuropeptide Y concentrations in posttraumatic stress disorder. *Biol Psychiatry*. 2009;66(7):705–707. doi:10.1016/j.biopsych.2009.04.037
51. Charlet A, Lasbennes F, Darbon P, Poisbeau P. Fast non-genomic effects of progesterone-derived neurosteroids on nociceptive thresholds and pain symptoms. *Pain*. 2008;139(3):603–609. doi:10.1016/j.pain.2008.06.016
52. GBD 2017 Disease and Injury Incidence and Prevalence Collaborators. Global, regional, and national incidence, prevalence, and years lived with disability for 354 diseases and injuries for 195 countries and territories, 1990–2017: A systematic analysis for the Global Burden of Disease Study 2017. *Lancet*. 2018;392(10159):1789–1858. doi:10.1016/s0140-6736(18)32279-7
53. Gadermann AM, Engel CC, Naifeh JA, et al. Prevalence of DSM-IV major depression among U.S. military personnel: Meta-analysis and simulation. *Mil Med*. 2012;177(8 Suppl):47–59. doi:10.7205/milmed-d-12-00103
54. Lapierre CB, Schwegler AF, Labauve BJ. Posttraumatic stress and depression symptoms in soldiers returning from combat operations in Iraq and Afghanistan. *J Trauma Stress*. 2007;20(6):933–943. doi:10.1002/jts.20278
55. Seal KH, Metzler TJ, Gima KS, Bertenthal D, Maguen S, Marmar CR. Trends and risk factors for mental health diagnoses among Iraq and Afghanistan veterans using Department of Veterans Affairs health care, 2002–2008. *Am J Public Health*. 2009;99(9):1651–1658. doi:10.2105/ajph.2008.150284
56. Jaracz J, Gattner K, Jaracz K, Górna K. Unexplained painful physical symptoms in patients with major depressive disorder: Prevalence, pathophysiology and management. *CNS Drugs*. 2016;30(4):293–304. doi:10.1007/s40263-016-0328-5

57. Hooten WM. Chronic pain and mental health disorders: Shared neural mechanisms, epidemiology, and treatment. *Mayo Clin Proc.* 2016;91(7):955–970. doi:10.1016/j.mayocp.2016.04.029
58. Antioch I, Ilie OD, Ciobica A, Doroftei B, Fornaro M. Preclinical considerations about affective disorders and pain: A broadly intertwined, yet often under-explored, relationship having major clinical implications. *Medicina.* 2020;56(10): Article 504. doi:10.3390/medicina56100504
59. Bondesson E, Larrosa Pardo F, Stigmar K, et al. Comorbidity between pain and mental illness: Evidence of a bidirectional relationship. *Eur J Pain.* 2018;22(7):1304–1311. doi:10.1002/ejp.1218
60. DeVeaugh-Geiss AM, West SL, Miller WC, Sleath B, Gaynes BN, Kroenke K. The adverse effects of comorbid pain on depression outcomes in primary care patients: Results from the ARTIST trial. *Pain Med.* 2010;11(5):732–741. doi:10.1111/j.1526-4637.2010.00830.x
61. Turk DC, Salovey P. "Chronic pain as a variant of depressive disease": A critical reappraisal. *J Nerv Ment Dis.* 1984;172(7):398–404. doi:10.1097/00005053-198407000-00004
62. Sheng J, Liu S, Wang Y, Cui R, Zhang X. The link between depression and chronic pain: Neural mechanisms in the brain. *Neural Plast.* 2017;2017:9724371. doi:10.1155/2017/9724371
63. Agüera-Ortiz L, Failde I, Mico JA, Cervilla J, López-Ibor JJ. Pain as a symptom of depression: Prevalence and clinical correlates in patients attending psychiatric clinics. *J Affect Disord.* 2011;130(1–2):106–112. doi:10.1016/j.jad.2010.10.022
64. Bair MJ, Robinson RL, Katon W, Kroenke K. Depression and pain comorbidity: A literature review. *Arch Intern Med.* 2003;163(20):2433–2445. doi:10.1001/archinte.163.20.2433
65. Meerwijk EL, Ford JM, Weiss SJ. Brain regions associated with psychological pain: Implications for a neural network and its relationship to physical pain. *Brain Imaging Behav.* 2013;7(1):1–14. doi:10.1007/s11682-012-9179-y
66. Management of Concussion/mTBI Working Group. VA/DoD clinical practice guideline for management of concussion/mild traumatic brain injury. *J Rehabil Res Dev.* 2009;46(6):CP1–CP68.
67. Hoge CW, McGurk D, Thomas JL, Cox AL, Engel CC, Castro CA. Mild traumatic brain injury in U.S. soldiers returning from Iraq. *N Engl J Med.* 2008;358(5):453–463. doi:10.1056/NEJMoa072972
68. Schwab KA, Ivins B, Cramer G, et al. Screening for traumatic brain injury in troops returning from deployment in Afghanistan and Iraq: Initial investigation of the usefulness of a short screening tool for traumatic brain injury. *J Head Trauma Rehabil.* 2007;22(6):377–389. doi:10.1097/01.Htr.0000300233.98242.87
69. Theeler BJ, Flynn FG, Erickson JC. Headaches after concussion in US soldiers returning from Iraq or Afghanistan. *Headache.* 2010;50(8):1262–1272. doi:10.1111/j.1526-4610.2010.01700.x
70. Clark ME, Bair MJ, Buckenmaier CC 3rd, Gironda RJ, Walker RL. Pain and combat injuries in soldiers returning from Operations Enduring Freedom and Iraqi Freedom: Implications for research and practice. *J Rehabil Res Dev.* 2007;44(2):179–194. doi:10.1682/jrrd.2006.05.0057
71. Taylor BC, Hagel EM, Carlson KF, et al. Prevalence and costs of co-occurring traumatic brain injury with and without psychiatric disturbance and pain among Afghanistan and Iraq War Veteran V.A. users. *Med Care.* 2012;50(4):342–346. doi:10.1097/MLR.0b013e318245a558
72. Bramoweth AD, Germain A. Deployment-related insomnia in military personnel and veterans. *Curr Psychiatry Rep.* 2013;15(10): Article 401. doi:10.1007/s11920-013-0401-4
73. Troxel WM, Shih RA, Pedersen ER, et al. Sleep in the military: Promoting healthy sleep among U.S. servicemembers. *Rand Health Q.* 2015;5(2): Article 19.
74. Moore BA, Tison LM, Palacios JG, Peterson AL, Mysliwiec V. Incidence of insomnia and obstructive sleep apnea in active duty United States military service members. *Sleep.* 2021;44(7):zsab024. doi:10.1093/sleep/zsab024
75. Andersen ML, Araujo P, Frange C, Tufik S. Sleep disturbance and pain: A tale of two common problems. *Chest.* 2018;154(5):1249–1259. doi:10.1016/j.chest.2018.07.019

76. Afolalu EF, Ramlee F, Tang NKY. Effects of sleep changes on pain-related health outcomes in the general population: A systematic review of longitudinal studies with exploratory meta-analysis. *Sleep Med Rev*. 2018;39:82–97. doi:10.1016/j.smrv.2017.08.001
77. Bray RM, Marsden ME, Peterson MR. Standardized comparisons of the use of alcohol, drugs, and cigarettes among military personnel and civilians. *Am J Public Health*. 1991;81(7):865–869. doi:10.2105/ajph.81.7.865
78. Institute of Medicine Committee on Smoking Cessation in Military and Veteran Populations; Bondurant S, Wedge R, eds. *Combating Tobacco Use in Military and Veteran Populations*. National Academies Press; 2009.
79. Office of the Surgeon General; Office on Smoking and Health. *The Health Consequences of Smoking: A Report of the Surgeon General*. Centers for Disease Control and Prevention; 2004.
80. Dall TM, Zhang Y, Chen YJ, et al. Cost associated with being overweight and with obesity, high alcohol consumption, and tobacco use within the military health system's TRICARE prime-enrolled population. *Am J Health Promot*. 2007;22(2):120–139. doi:10.4278/0890-1171-22.2.120
81. Jahnke SA, Hoffman KM, Haddock CK, et al. Military tobacco policies: The good, the bad, and the ugly. *Mil Med*. 2011;176(12):1382–1387. doi:10.7205/milmed-d-11-00164
82. National Center for Chronic Disease Prevention and Health Promotion Office on Smoking and Health. *The Health Consequences of Smoking—50 Years of Progress: A Report of the Surgeon General*. Centers for Disease Control and Prevention; 2014.
83. Smith B, Ryan MA, Wingard DL, Patterson TL, Slymen DJ, Macera CA. Cigarette smoking and military deployment: A prospective evaluation. *Am J Prev Med*. 2008;35(6):539–546. doi:10.1016/j.amepre.2008.07.009
84. Seal KH, Shi Y, Cohen G, et al. Association of mental health disorders with prescription opioids and high-risk opioid use in US veterans of Iraq and Afghanistan. *JAMA*. 2012;307(9):940–947. doi:10.1001/jama.2012.234
85. Agaku I, Odani S, Nelson JR. U.S. military veteran versus nonveteran use of licit and illicit substances. *Am J Prev Med*. 2020;59(5):733–741. doi:10.1016/j.amepre.2020.04.027
86. Lan CW, Fiellin DA, Barry DT, et al. The epidemiology of substance use disorders in US veterans: A systematic review and analysis of assessment methods. *Am J Addict*. 2016;25(1):7–24. doi:10.1111/ajad.12319
87. Office of the Secretary of Defense. The implementation of a comprehensive policy on pain management by the military health care system for fiscal year 2019. U.S. Department of Defense; 2019.
88. Steffens D, Maher CG, Pereira LS, et al. Prevention of low back pain: A systematic review and meta-analysis. *JAMA Intern Med*. 2016;176(2):199–208. doi:10.1001/jamainternmed.2015.7431
89. Fancourt D, Steptoe A. Physical and psychosocial factors in the prevention of chronic pain in older age. *J Pain*. 2018;19(12):1385–1391. doi:10.1016/j.jpain.2018.06.001
90. Webb R, Brammah T, Lunt M, Urwin M, Allison T, Symmons D. Prevalence and predictors of intense, chronic, and disabling neck and back pain in the UK general population. *Spine*. 2003;28(11):1195–1202. doi:10.1097/01.Brs.0000067430.49169.01
91. Elma Ö, Yilmaz ST, Deliens T, et al. Chronic musculoskeletal pain and nutrition: Where are we and where are we heading? *PM R*. 2020;12(12):1268–1278. doi:10.1002/pmrj.12346
92. Brain K, Burrows TL, Rollo ME, et al. A systematic review and meta-analysis of nutrition interventions for chronic noncancer pain. *J Hum Nutr Diet*. 2019;32(2):198–225. doi:10.1111/jhn.12601
93. Parker K, Cilluffo A, Stepler R. 6 facts about the U.S. military and its changing demographics: Pew Research Center; 2017. https://www.pewresearch.org/fact-tank/2017/04/13/6-facts-about-the-u-s-military-and-its-changing-demographics
94. Zajacova A, Rogers RG, Grodsky E, Grol-Prokopczyk H. The relationship between education and pain among adults aged 30–49 in the United States. *J Pain*. 2020;21(11–12):1270–1280. doi:10.1016/j.jpain.2020.03.005

95. Vallerand AH, Cosler P, Henningfield JE, Galassini P. Pain management strategies and lessons from the military: A narrative review. *Pain Res Manag.* 2015;20(5):261–268. doi:10.1155/2015/196025
96. Families. Office of the Army Surgeon General; 2010.
97. Veterans Health Administration. Pain management. VHA Directive 2009-053. Department of Veterans Affairs, Veterans Health Administration; 2009. https://www.va.gov/PAINMANAGEMENT/docs/VHA09PainDirective.pdf
98. Office of the Secretary of Defense. The implementation of a comprehensive policy on pain management by the military health care system. U.S. Department of Defense. 2014. Accessed June 7, 2022. https://health.mil/Reference-Center/Reports/2014/08/11/Implementation-of-a-Comprehensive-Policy-on-Pain-Management-by-the-Military-Health-System

12
Pain at the End of Life

Frey Gugsa, Lauren E. Berninger, Eric J. Wang, and Thomas J. Smith

Introduction

A vulnerable population comprises individuals at "greater risk for poor health status and healthcare access [and who] experience significant disparities in life expectancy [and] access to and use of healthcare services."[1] Individuals in need of pain care at the end of life represent a group at increased risk of vulnerability, often with a lower quality of life[2] and inadequate end-of-life pain management.[3] Although there is no standard definition of "end of life" or "terminal illness," in general, patients at end of life show evidence of "irreversible decline" in the setting of chronic and life-limiting disease(s).[2–5] Time-based definitions of end of life are highly variable, ranging from days to less than 2 years.[4,5] Several factors increase vulnerability at end of life, including culture, ethnicity, race, indigeneity, immigration, socioeconomic, gender, incarceration, intellectual capability, poverty, housing instability, lack of health insurance, limited English proficiency, age, cognitive impairment, and physical disability.[5–7] Foreseeably, geriatric patients may be among the most vulnerable adults, with factors such as frailty, cognitive impairment, lack of social support, and fear of loss of independence which can lead to high risk behaviors that may result in negative outcomes.[7]

What Makes Individuals at the End of Their Life More Vulnerable to Pain?

End of life is commonly described as the phase of life when a person is living with, and impaired by, an eventually fatal condition. Although there is currently no standardized time frame describing the end-of-life period, U.S. hospice eligibility criteria limit a patient's estimated prognosis to 6 months or less.[4,5]

Among vulnerable populations, there are two distinct but overlapping at-risk populations: (1) clinically at-risk individuals and (2) socially and structurally disadvantaged groups (Figure 12.1).[5,6] Clinically at-risk individuals are those who do not or cannot receive timely and high-quality health care, which predisposes them to poor medical outcomes.[6] For example, patients with inadequate end-of-life pain treatment are at greater risk of lower quality of life and greater functional impairment.[5] Socially disadvantaged groups whose social, economic, or geographic characteristics limit their ability to obtain high-quality care may not achieve desired health outcomes.[6] A higher vulnerability for inadequate end-of-life pain management is found to a greater degree

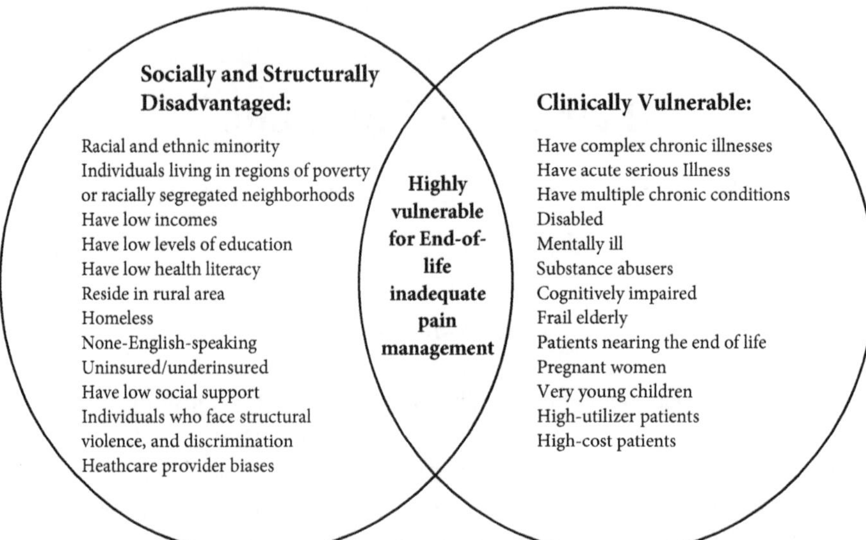

Figure 12.1 Socioeconomic, structural, and clinical factors contributing to end-of-life pain management vulnerability.
Source: Based on References 4–6.

between the intersection of the two distinct but overlapping categories of vulnerable populations (see Figure 12.1).[6]

Socially and structurally disadvantaged and clinically at-risk individuals (see Figure 12.1) are more likely to wait to receive care when sick, encounter delays in care, experience poorly coordinated care and lack of access to health care, and may encounter health care provider biases.[5,6,8] Those patients often suffer more severe end-of-life pain, pain-related disabilities, and have a lower quality of life.[2,7] A 2021 retrospective study of Medicare beneficiaries with disabilities found significant racial inequities in the receipt of prescription opioids.[9] In the study, Black patients on average received lower doses and smaller quantities in each filled prescription.[9]

Such differences in practice may be a result of clinicians' conscious and unconscious racial bias, including a mistaken belief that Black patients misuse prescription opioids more than do White patients.[9] Other factors, such as lack of effective patient–physician communication and systemic structural racism (e.g., racially segregated neighborhoods and a lower density of pharmacies in predominantly Black neighborhoods than in predominantly White neighborhoods), likely contribute to the disparity.[9]

In another study, low access to chronic pain care was independently associated with Hispanic ethnicity with limited English proficiency in a nationally representative sample of African Americans, Hispanics, and Caucasians.[10] The net effect of one's background and life experience, along with inequalities the individual may endure, can lead to undertreatment of pain at the end of life.

Using evidence-based practices, palliative care teams address pain and symptom management for patients at all stages of serious illness.[11] The World Health Organization (WHO)[12] defines the goal of palliative care as facilitating the "quality of life of patients and that of their families who are facing challenges associated with life-threatening illness, whether physical, psychological, social, or spiritual." Providing pain relief, comfort, and symptom management at the end of life is a critical component of high-quality, patient-centered, and culturally competent palliative care.[11] In addition, the care plan for patients with life-threatening illnesses should consider the complex interplay among the physical, cognitive, social, and spiritual experiences of a person's life.[12] Life-threatening illnesses can present with symptoms including, but not limited to, pain, shortness of breath, fatigue, nausea, and agitation.[12] Those symptoms affect an individual's quality of life, disrupt relationships, contribute to worsened mental health, and lead to social withdrawal.[3,11,13] Hence, palliative care teams aim to improve the quality of life for both patients and their families.[11] In this chapter, we (1) further define dimensions of pain at the end of life; (2) identify specific, evidence-based strategies to evaluate and provide end-of-life pain relief; and (3) review some of the challenges faced during end-of-life pain management. We also suggest best practices.

Dimensions of Pain at the End of Life

Background

Patients and families receiving end-of-life care have numerous physical, psychological, social, and spiritual needs.[13] Despite a rapid increase in hospice and palliative care services, many patients continue to experience unmet pain and symptom management.[13] Palliative care can be provided at the discretion of the physician and patient at any stage of illness, from initial diagnosis through end of life, whether disease is terminal or not.[13–15] This is not to be confused with hospice services, which provide comprehensive comfort-focused care and family support exclusively to patients with terminal illness with a life expectancy of fewer than 6 months.[14]

The ideal end-of-life care team is interdisciplinary and may include physicians, nurse practitioners, physician assistants, nurses, chaplains, pharmacists, social workers, and music and art therapists.[14,15] The aim of the interdisciplinary team is to address pain and symptom management and ensure the physical, psychological, social, and spiritual needs of patients and families are met.[15] This team also brings a unique and holistic perspective to address the needs of patients and their families.[14,15] It is essential to assess end-of-life pain through a multidimensional perspective that allows for the appreciation of all probable causes and influences.

Definitions of Pain

In the early 20th century, pain was theorized to be a physiological signal sent to the brain from noxious stimuli within the body.[16] Melzack and Wall's gate control theory (1965) emphasized that nervous stimuli could be inhibited at the level of the substantia gelatinosa in the dorsal horn of the spinal cord, prior to reaching the thalamus and cerebral cortex.[14] The gate control theory conceptualized pain as a primarily physiological event while acknowledging the potential for psychological factors to influence pain perception, such as past experiences and emotions.[16]

Other paradigms theorized an even broader definition of pain. For example, Dame Cicely Saunders articulated the theory of "total pain" to describe the sum of suffering (physical, spiritual, psychological, and social) experienced by patients with advanced disease and terminal illness.[17] The combination of these experiences is believed to result in a total pain experience that is personalized and specific to each patient.

The definition of pain by the International Association for the Study of Pain (IASP) also encompasses the physiological and emotional aspects of pain experience.[18] Pain is defined as "an unpleasant sensory and emotional experience associated with, or resembling that associated with, actual or potential tissue damage."[18] The idea that pain at the end of life involves physical, psychological, social, and spiritual aspects is widely acknowledged; however, clinical practice may only focus on the physical determinants. Without thorough assessments of other relevant factors that contribute to pain perception, it is difficult to obtain a comprehensive understanding of a patient's pain management needs and goals.

Pathophysiology of End-of-Life Pain

End-of-life pain is typically related to the underlying terminal disease process (e.g., cancer) and associated medical treatments as well as other comorbidities that commonly produce pain (e.g., osteoarthritis and diabetes).[19] Although pain can be either acute or chronic, there are three recognized mechanistic categories of pain: neuropathic, nociceptive (further subdivided into visceral and somatic), and nociplastic.[13,20] Understanding the etiology of a patient's pain helps inform treatment.

Acute and Chronic Pain

Acute and chronic pain have unique etiologies and treatments.[13,21] Acute pain can arise from inflammation, tissue damage, injury, illness, or recent surgery, and it usually lasts less than 1 or 2 weeks but may last up to 3 months.[21] Acute pain draws attention to the injury and usually resolves after the underlying cause is treated.[21] Although chronic pain (defined as pain lasting 3 months or more) can develop from acute pain, the mechanisms mediating the transition from acute to chronic pain remain poorly understood.[21,22] The literature on chronic pain acknowledges pain as a subjective experience that is a summation of sensory input, genetic composition, prior cognitive appraisal, mood states, expectations, and the sociocultural environment.[13,20,21] Chronic pain may persist for years.[13,21,22]

Neuropathic Pain

Neuropathic pain is caused by direct damage or injury to the somatosensory system and can be broadly organized into two basic categories: peripheral and central etiologies.[23,24] Common peripheral neuropathic conditions include chemotherapy-induced peripheral neuropathy, metabolic disorders (e.g., diabetic peripheral polyneuropathy), and radicular pain.[23,24] Radicular pain is a subset of neuropathic pain, arising from the compression or inflammation of a spinal nerve root, which may occur with osteoarthritis, lumbar disc herniation, or tumor invasion.[25] Central neuropathic conditions include multiple sclerosis, post-stroke pain, spinal cord injury–related pain, complex regional pain syndrome, and trigeminal neuralgia.[23,24] The clinical presentation of neuropathic pain includes abnormal hypersensitivity to noxious stimuli (hyperalgesia), pain with non-noxious stimuli (allodynia), and the perception of spontaneous aberrant sensations (dysesthesias).[23,24] Neuropathic pain is often perceived as spontaneous, manifesting in the absence of an identifiable stimulus.[24]

Nociceptive Pain (Visceral and Somatic)

Nociceptive pathways lead to the sensation of noxious stimuli in the body.[22,23] There are two main subcategories of nociceptive pain: somatic and visceral. Somatic pain is caused by the activation of nociceptors from a site of injury or inflammation, and it may be perceived as "deep" or "superficial," with pain being a response to inflammation of the skeletal structure, tendons, or muscles. It is often described as localized, "aching," "throbbing," or "squeezing."[23] Visceral pain emanates from the internal organs and is caused when nociceptors are activated from compression, obstruction, infiltration, ischemia, stretching, or inflammation.[23] Visceral pain is often described as vague in regional distribution rather than localized, and it may be perceived as "cramping," "spasmodic," or "stabbing" sensations.[23]

Nociplastic Pain

Nociplastic pain is pain that arises from the abnormal processing of afferent signals and is characterized by the lack of objective evidence of tissue or somatosensory system injury.[20] The term "nociplastic pain" was officially defined by the IASP in 2017,[26] although the clinical characteristics had previously been observed and described by terms such as "functional pain syndrome" or "primary pain syndrome."[26,27] Fibromyalgia and irritable bowel syndrome are examples of pain conditions primarily mediated via a nociplastic mechanism.[26] A characteristic of nociplastic pain conditions is the absence of identifiable lesions or biomarkers that can be directly correlated with the pain symptoms, and centrally directed therapies (e.g., cognitive-based therapy or antidepressants with analgesic effects) are more likely to be beneficial compared to peripherally acting medications (e.g., nonsteroidal anti-inflammatory drugs [NSAIDs]), surgeries, or injections.[20,27]

Recognition of Concomitant Disease Processes and Pain Mechanisms

Most patients with advanced stage or metastatic cancer experience some degree of pain, and the specific type of cancer is a poor predictor of pain prevalence or severity.[28] Severe nonmalignant organ dysfunction is also frequently associated with pain, such as in renal disease[29] and chronic obstructive pulmonary disease.[30] There are limited data suggesting that the prevalence of pain in end-stage organ dysfunction (e.g., cardiac, renal, and pulmonary) might be similar to that of cancer.[31] In addition, the specific categorical mechanisms (e.g., nociceptive, neuropathic, and nociplastic) leading to pain symptoms might vary widely between patients even in the context of similar disease processes. For example, cancer-associated bone pain likely involves nociceptive and neuropathic mechanisms,[32] but the proportion of each mechanism's contribution to a particular patient's symptoms likely varies according to individualized factors. It is therefore important to recognize that several concomitant disease processes and pain mechanisms might be co-prevalent and contributing to the totality of an individual patient's symptoms. Carefully identifying and addressing these different contributors to pain is essential for developing and revising comprehensive treatment plans that are tailored to a patient's clinical course.

Specific, Evidence-Based Strategies to Evaluate Pain and Provide Relief

End-of-Life Pain Evaluation and Treatment

History and Goals of Care Discussion

A comprehensive patient history is key and should be performed to outline the course of the disease and formulate an optimal end-of-life pain management plan.[19] Early discussions regarding prognosis and goals of care with patients and their caregivers can help facilitate advance care planning and decrease the use of possible inappropriate life-sustaining therapies.[19] Open-ended questions help ascertain the patient's expectations regarding care.[19] An interdisciplinary team should consider the patient's physical, spiritual, psychological, and social experiences to develop a holistic plan.[15,19] This collaborative approach to decision-making and power-sharing should aim to facilitate patient-centered care.[19]

Physical Examination

A comprehensive physical examination should include a head-to-toe assessment of physical factors that may contribute to pain.[19] For example, patients who have been in bed for prolonged periods of time may develop skin breaks or pressure ulcers.[19] Constipation or urinary retention can also lead to significant distress and can present abdominal fullness.[19] Other nonverbal physical signs of pain may include facial grimacing, restlessness, consolability, tachypnea, and tachycardia especially in patients who are unable to communicate for themselves.[19] In addition, a general assessment of hygiene and well-being of the patient is essential to maintain the patient's dignity.[19]

Evaluation of End-of-Life Pain

End-of-life pain evaluation follows the general pattern of pain assessment, which includes location, onset, quality, severity, and exacerbating and attenuating factors.[13, 19] The cornerstone of effective pain management includes routine pain assessment and re-evaluations, especially following interventional procedures.[13,19]

Several validated pain grading scales have been developed that help standardize care and provide an objective assessment. [13, 19] The Likert-type scale (or numeric rating scale) grades pain on a 0–10 scale, where 0 is defined as no pain at all and 10 is defined as the worst pain imaginable. [13, 19] The Wong–Baker FACES Pain Rating Scale has a series of six gender-neutral cartoon faces that range from depicting a neutral facial expression of "no pain/no hurt" to the "worst possible pain/hurt" depicting a crying face.[19] This scale provides superior assessment in children and adult patients who are unable to communicate verbally.[19] The Pain Assessment in Advanced Dementia (PAINAD) scale helps assess pain in patients with cognitive impairment and dementia.[19] The PAINAD scale assesses pain via five criteria: breathing, vocalization, facial expression, body language, and consolability that can be observed by caregivers and health care providers.[19]

For nonverbal adults who are unable to communicate, additional pain assessment tools include the Behavioral Pain Scale (BPS) and Behavioral Pain Scale–Non-Intubated (BPS-NI), both of which have been predominately studied in the critical care setting.[33] The BPS is formulated based on facial expressions, upper limb movement, and compliance with mechanical ventilation, whereas the BPS-NI substitutes mechanical ventilation compliance with vocalization for patients with delirium who are not intubated.[33] Additional pain scales include the Critical Care Pain Observational Tool; the Faces, Legs, Activity, Cry, Consolability pain tool; the Multidimensional Observational Pain Assessment Tool; and the Nonverbal Pain Scale.[33] Although these tools represent practical frameworks for assessing nonverbal indicators of pain in nonverbal, noncommunicative patients, research on the use of these tools in the general palliative care population is currently limited and further study is needed.

The appropriate scale(s) should be consistently used among physicians and health care providers for the same patient to maintain quality of care for the duration of pain management. As a patient's condition changes, often selection of a new tool may be required (e.g., if the patient develops delirium or becomes noncommunicative). There is minimal evidence to suggest the use of one tool over another in the palliative care setting, and the selection of tools is highly individualized to the patient's clinical condition and needs.

Treatment of End-of-Life Pain

Effective end-of-life pain management requires timely recognition, a comprehensive and interdisciplinary assessment, an appropriate treatment plan, and monitoring of treatment outcomes.[13, 19] The management of end-of-life pain includes nonpharmacological, pharmacological, and psychosocial measures.[13,19]

Pharmacological Management End-of-Life Pain

Categories of pharmacological pain medications that are used in end-of-life care include non-opioids, opioids, and adjuvants.[13,19,34] WHO devised a cancer pain ladder to guide physicians and caregivers in selecting pharmacological agents for managing pain.[19,34] The first step is to begin with a non-opioid medication and consider the use of an adjuvant medication (e.g., antiemetics, anxiolytics, antipyretic, antidepressants, anticonvulsants, and anti-inflammatory drugs). The non-opioid medications include acetaminophen and NSAIDs.[19,34] Opioid analgesics are used to treat moderate to severe pain.[19,34]

Non-Opioid Analgesics

Acetaminophen

Although acetaminophen is recommended as a first-line agent by WHO for the treatment of mild to moderate cancer pain,[34] it confers only modest analgesia for chronic nociceptive pain symptoms[35] and does not appear to be effective for chronic neuropathic pain symptoms.[36] There are only limited data via murine models regarding its efficacy for nociplastic pain symptoms.[37] However, acetaminophen might be a useful adjunct for acute pain because a large meta-analysis demonstrated at least a 50% reduction in acute postsurgical pain symptoms.[38]

Acetaminophen is recognized for its generally favorable safety profile and can be utilized in the setting of pre-existing renal, cardiovascular, or gastrointestinal disease. It also does not require dose reduction based on patient age.[39] Doses should not exceed 2 g within 24 h in the setting of severe or chronic liver dysfunction (e.g., cirrhosis), but in patients without significant liver disease, doses up to 4 g within 24 h are considered safe and unlikely to cause hepatotoxicity.[19,40]

Nonsteroidal Anti-Inflammatory Drugs

Nonsteroidal anti-inflammatory drugs are the most frequent initial pharmacological agents used to treat pain, fever, and other inflammatory processes.[19,34] Their mechanism of action is based on the inhibition of cyclooxygenase enzymes COX-1 and COX-2, with the COX-2 enzyme playing a key role in pain generation by inflammatory cells.[19,34] Some NSAIDs can also inhibit the lipoxygenase pathway and interfere with G protein-mediated signal transduction processes that mediate pain.[19]

Opioid Analgesics

Opioids are often used to treat acute or refractory end-of-life pain. Opioids mimic the actions of endogenous opioid peptides by interacting with μ-, δ-, or κ-opioid receptors to relieve pain.[19,34] It is key to understand the pharmacokinetics of different opioids (e.g., time to peak analgesic effect, duration of analgesia, and time to clearance) in order to provide appropriate dosing and to monitor possible side effects.[17] Common side effects of opioids include sedation, decreased respiratory rate, bradycardia, nausea, vomiting, constipation, and a reduction in gastric motility.[19,34] Hence, clinicians must monitor and perform constant assessments to detect and treat any adverse events.

Opioids can be administered through several routes, including oral, intravenous, subcutaneous, intramuscular, transmucosal, nasal, transdermal, and rectal.[19,34] In addition, patient-controlled analgesia (PCA) via an infusion pump is another modality that can be utilized when frequent or high doses of opioids are necessary or when the patient is unable to tolerate oral opioids.[19] Nurse-controlled analgesia pump (NCA) can also be used.[19] In NCA, a PCA pump is used to deliver nurse-initiated opioids for patients unable to press the PCA button because of age or physical or developmental disabilities.[41]

Special considerations may warrant the use of methadone and the partial μ-agonist buprenorphine in the management of end-of-life pain.[42,43] Opioid use disorder is common in the United States, and deaths related to opioid use are rising.[42,43] From 2019 to 2020, there was a 38% overall increase in deaths involving opioid use, and prescription opioid-involved death rates increased by 17% and synthetic opioid-related deaths rose by 56%.[43] These deaths did not involve palliative care patients.

Clinicians must be cognizant of the current state of the opioid epidemic in the United States and should screen for opioid use disorder in all patients, including patients at end of life.[43] It is equally important to individualize patient care and avoid adhering to a rigid application of opioid doses or limits for pain control.[44] Methadone and buprenorphine may be appropriate for managing opioid use disorder, and they can also be effective in the management of pain when used appropriately.[42,43] Methadone is a long-acting full opioid agonist medication with additional *N*-methyl-D-aspartate receptor antagonist activity that is commonly used in both substance use disorder and pain management.[45]

Beneficial features of methadone for patients with serious illness include that it is available in multiple forms (tablet, liquid, and intravenous), it can be used as a long-acting opioid, it is inexpensive, it has demonstrated success for complex pain refractory to other opioids, and it is safe in the treatment of renal failure.[45] For patients on daily methadone maintenance therapy for opioid use disorder, daily dosing is effective in managing cravings for as long as 36 h.[45]

When faced with serious illness (e.g., cancer), daily methadone dosing for opioid use disorder can be divided into three equal doses administered every 8 h, increased slowly to the desired analgesic effect with allowance of additional short-acting opioids as needed for breakthrough pain.[45] For patients with active substance use disorder not already on maintenance therapy or those at high risk for opioid misuse, methadone should be used with caution given the potential for overdose without close monitoring.[45]

Buprenorphine is a partial μ-opioid agonist with additional κ and δ receptor antagonist activity.[46] It has a high affinity for the μ-opioid receptor along with prolonged dissociation from the receptor.[46] Decreased opioid craving and antidepressant properties result from the drug's κ receptor antagonism and can be helpful in managing concomitant depression and anxiety.[46] Overall, buprenorphine has fewer adverse effects than full opioid agonists, with decreased risk of respiratory depression, misuse, and all-cause mortality following overdose.[46] For these reasons, it is considered a drug of choice in managing opioid use disorder.[46]

Furthermore, buprenorphine is an effective analgesic medication when used appropriately and should be considered as first line in patients with serious illness who have both pain and opioid use disorder as a safer alternative to full agonist opioid medications such as fentanyl, oxycodone, and morphine.[46] The drug has multiple formulations and can be used in patients for end-of-life care with dysphagia in transdermal, sublingual, or buccal formulations, and it may be used more safely in older adults and those with renal failure.[46] Although used infrequently in the general end-of-life population, there is evidence that buprenorphine has similar efficacy to morphine in the treatment of moderate to severe pain. Other advantages to the use of buprenorphine in patients at end of life include less risk of respiratory depression, less effect on cognition, and decreased constipation.[47] Further research is underway on the use of buprenorphine in this population.

Nonpharmacological Management of End-of-Life Pain

Nonpharmacological measures are an important modality of end-of-life pain management and quality of life. For example, the use of gel foam pads on skin-to-appliance interfaces and frequent repositioning and offloading of dependent areas of the body can help prevent decubitus ulcers.[19] In addition, proper head positioning and neck support can minimize neck pain.[19] Furthermore, oral care and proper hydration can prevent painful oral ulcers and dental decay.[19]

Counseling with family members regarding end-of-life decisions (e.g., financial and property-related decisions) and devising robust goals of care with the patient can help alleviate anxiety and improve interpersonal relationships.[19,48] Spiritual counseling and pastoral visits can support patients and families through the end-of-life and grieving process.[19,48] Alternative medicinal therapies such as acupuncture can be offered to support pharmacological measures in managing pain.[49]

Challenges Faced During End-of-Life Pain Management

Managing pain at the end of life in a manner that aligns with patients' expectations and beliefs can present a challenge for health professionals.[11] Practicing in an ethnically and culturally diverse society requires health care providers to understand, respect, and consider the cultures from which their patients come.[11] Health professionals who learn the nuances of their patients' cultures are more effective in understanding the contexts through which their patients experience pain.[11,50] Also, they are better able to help guide their patients' family and friends through the dying process.[11,50]

Cultural and Spiritual Considerations of End-of-Life Pain

Cultural and spiritual beliefs surrounding pain and death affect patients' attitudes and preferences in end-of-life care.[11,50] For example, some cultures do not accept or encourage the use of opioids and may discourage the use of services such as palliative care despite severe pain at the end of life.[11,50] A lack of understanding regarding the beliefs of patients and their families can potentially damage the patient–provider relationship.[11,17,50] Furthermore, this lack of trust can act as a significant barrier to appropriate pain management, including nonpharmacological and non-interventional modalities (e.g., pastoral care).[11,19,50] Open-ended questions and discussions are needed to ascertain patient's expectations of care, in addition to any relevant religious or cultural beliefs.[11,19,50]

At the end of life, individuals from all varieties of cultural and religious backgrounds tend to reflect over their lives and many may take a "spiritual inventory." [11,19,50] Dame Cicely Saunders explained in the theory of "total pain" that unresolved emotional and spiritual issues can amplify the pain of dying.[11,19,50] She called this "spiritual pain" and stated that it comes from "a desolate feeling of meaninglessness."[11,19,50] Therefore, finding meaning in suffering is a healthy process that can make pain and other uncomfortable symptoms more manageable.[11,19,50]

Racial and Ethnic Inequality in End-of-Life Pain and Symptom Management

According to the Declaration of Montreal, access to adequate pain treatment is a fundamental human right.[51] Yet, the experience of pain, especially at the end of life, varies across the global population.[52] For example, results from the 2000 Health and Retirement Study, a cross-sectional study of 13,777 persons aged 51 years or older, indicated similar pain prevalence rates across racial/ethnic groups, but among those reporting pain, African Americans and Hispanic Whites (27%) were more likely than non-Hispanic Whites (17%) to report severe pain.[52]

Racial and ethnic inequities in pain management have been well documented in peer-reviewed literature.[52] In the United States, racial and ethnic minorities and individuals with lower socioeconomic status face structural, health system, and interpersonal barriers to optimal health care, including palliative care.[53]

Palliative care and hospice services may disproportionately benefit White patients in the United States, but there is scant research dedicated to identifying differences in the benefits of palliative care received by ethnic and racial minorities and subsequently fewer studies suggesting potential methods to decrease these gaps.[54,55] Nonetheless, the limited data available suggest that minority groups experience poorer access to quality end-of-life care. Medicare data outlined by the National Hospice and Palliative Care Organization suggest continued disparities in hospice utilization at the end of life by minority Medicare beneficiaries in comparison to Caucasian Medicare beneficiaries.[56] Compared to 53.8% of Caucasian Medicare beneficiaries, 42.7% of Hispanic patients, 40.8% of Black patients, 39.8% of Asian American patients, and 38.5% of American Indian/Alaska Native patients utilized the Medicare hospice benefit.[56]

General mistrust of the medical system, poor previous experiences, or equating hospice with death or "giving up" all reflect reasons for underutilization of hospice services.

As documented in the congressionally mandated Institute of Medicine (IOM) report, *Unequal Treatment: Confronting Racial and Ethnic Disparities in Healthcare*, stark differences in health outcomes exist solely based on race, sex, age, socioeconomic status, or community characteristics.[57] For example, studies have shown that Black patients receive fewer pain assessments and are less appropriately managed for adverse effects (e.g., opioid-induced constipation) compared to their White peers over the course of serious illnesses.[58] Other studies have found that the odds of undertreatment for pain are twice as high for racial and ethnic minority patients.[59] In addition, it has been shown that White patients are more likely to receive prescription opioids, as well as higher doses.[60,61] Although physicians must balance the benefits of opioid prescribing against the potential harms of overdose and dependence, it is possible that misguided beliefs or biases regarding pain sensitivity, or population-level risks of opioid misuse, may be contributing to these discrepancies.[58–61]

An analysis of 1,117,086 individuals aged 12 years or older from the 1999–2018 National Survey on Drug Use and Health that compared the relative prevalence for prescription opioid misuse across six racial/ethnic groups revealed that relative to White individuals, adjusted prevalence estimates of prescription opioid misuse were lower among Black, Hispanic, and Asian individuals across all time periods.[62] The misuse of opioid peaked for White individuals at 5.7% (during 2007–2010); the corresponding peak rates were 3.9% among Black individuals (2011–2014), 3.8% among Hispanic individuals (2011–2014), and 2.5% among Asian individuals (2007–2010). In addition, heroin use among White individuals significantly surpassed that of all other groups in 2011–2015 and continued to increase, more than doubling from 1999–2002 (0.16%) to 2015–2018 (0.41%).[62] Opioid prescribing has historically been highest among non-Hispanic White individuals, which might have contributed to the higher risk for misusing prescription opioids among White individuals relative to other racial/ethnic groups.[62]

The existence of disparities in pain treatment among racial and ethnic minorities is a complex issue and involves an interplay among patient-specific factors (e.g., distrust of health care providers or medications), health care provider behaviors and practices (e.g., unconscious biases), and variations among health care systems (e.g., access to adequate supplies of pain medication).[58–61] IOM identifies two specific sources of disparities: (1) health care systems and the legal and regulatory climates in which they operate and (2) discrimination such as biases and stereotyping in clinical communication and decision-making.[57]

Implicit biases decrease the quality of treatment recommendations and hinder effective communication, leading to poorer outcomes.[63] Policies aimed at improving culturally appropriate care and diversifying the medical workforce and improving education regarding health inequities felt by specific populations could potentially help address health disparities and racial biases in health care.[58,64] There is a need for raising public and provider awareness of racial/ethnic disparities across all levels of health care, expanding health insurance coverage, improving the resources and number of providers in underserved communities, and improving educational training for health care providers.[65] In addition, a comprehensive pain research agenda is necessary to decrease future pain disparities among racial and ethnic minorities.[58] Finally, there is a need to develop culturally competent strategies that optimize physician–patient communication and facilitate an understanding of patients' pain management goals.[11,50]

Terminal Illness/End-of-Life Pain Management in Vulnerable Populations

Terminal illness or life-limiting disease often refers to an illness or disease process that cannot be cured or adequately treated and that will worsen and is expected to result in the death of the patient.[66] Patients with a terminal illness may live for days, weeks, months, or years.[4,66] The estimation of time to death from the terminal illness varies significantly and can be more predictable based on illness with somewhat anticipated trajectories, such as cancer.[66] In contrast, other common life-limiting illnesses, such as organ system failure (e.g., chronic kidney disease, congestive heart failure, and liver failure), lung disease, Alzheimer's disease, and AIDS may exhibit much less predictable disease trajectories and may not result in death for months or years, and many patients diagnosed with such conditions may die from another cause.[66]

Terminally ill patients commonly experience substantial pain and are at increased risk of vulnerability and inadequate end-of-life pain care.[2,66] The following factors further increase their vulnerability: poor mental health; social isolation; homelessness;

immigration; social, cultural, and economic barriers; and intellectual and developmental disability.[2,66] Unresolved pain in terminally ill patients has been cited as evidence that end-of-life care is of poor quality.[66] To better illustrate the challenges and potential opportunities for improving the experience of end-of-life care in terminally ill patients, we provide two case studies.

Case Example: Dalia

Dalia is a 45-year-old woman with advanced ovarian cancer complicated by worsening malignant ascites for which she is admitted to the inpatient oncology unit. Her disease has progressed through multiple lines of treatment. The palliative medicine team is consulted for pain management and adjusting to life-limiting illness. Her overall functional status is poor (Eastern Cooperative Oncology Group Performance Status score is 4), and she is no longer a candidate for further disease-directed treatment. She reports 8/10 pain in her abdomen described as pressure-like pain or "fullness" that is sharp at times. At home, she was taking 650 mg of acetaminophen per os (P.O.) every 6 h in addition to tramadol 50 mg twice a day without relief. She had been hesitant to further escalate her pain regimen due to the concern that the effects of opioid medications could compromise her ability to care for her three young children at home. Pain is partially relieved (pain decreased from 8/10 to 5/10) by 1 mg of intravenous hydromorphone, which she is taking every 3 h around the clock. Any movement or Valsalva worsens her pain, and she is mostly confined to a bed or chair throughout the day. She believes a pain level of 3/10 would be tolerable and would like to work toward that goal. The thought of uncontrolled pain has led to increased anxiety levels and depressed mood. Recently, she has developed nausea and vomiting. Her appetite has been poor, and she has been tolerating only small bites and sips throughout the day.

A "goals of care" meeting is held, and a prognosis of weeks to months is given. Dalia is agreeable to comfort-focused care and would like to go home but worries about increasing needs with minimal social and financial support to facilitate a home care plan. She also worries about the logistics of returning to the hospital for frequent paracentesis and/or pain crises given her debilitated state and family's lack of personal vehicle for transportation. She admits to increasing spiritual distress and difficulty coping with the thought of leaving her family members behind. She is Catholic and welcomes the support of the palliative chaplain in her care.

Following in-depth discussions, a decision is made to send Dalia home and place a peritoneal catheter for management of her ascites as well as olanzapine 5 mg P.O. at bedtime for her nausea. Given her need for around-the-clock medications with inadequate pain relief and difficulty taking oral medications, she is given a hydromorphone PCA pump. In addition, she has started on a daily pharmacologic bowel regimen for opioid-induced constipation, which could contribute to her pain.

Dalia opts for home hospice services to provide an extra layer of support and symptom management as her disease progresses. Palliative social work explores resources with Dalia's husband, and they determine a plan for time off work without significant additional financial strain. In addition, further support systems are explored, and a schedule is created between Dalia's mother and sister to provide care when her husband is unavailable.

Anticipatory guidance on the dying process is provided, and legacy work is begun. Dalia is assured that bereavement services will be available for her family members through their local hospice agency for 1 year after her death. Dalia was discharged to home hospice and passes away at home several weeks later.

Case Example: Martin

Martin is a 62-year-old man with a history of amyotrophic lateral sclerosis (ALS). Four months ago, he became wheelchair bound due to progressive weakness and now resides in a long-term care facility. He is experiencing recurrent bouts of aspiration pneumonia along with worsening fatigue. He verbalized to physicians and other health care providers that he does not want a tracheostomy for mechanical ventilation nor a feeding tube. He understands he has a terminal illness and does not want to prolong his dying process.

During the past months, Martin developed a stage IV sacral decubitus ulcer with associated sharp, sometimes stinging, pain that is made worse by lying in the same position. Offloading the area sometimes provides relief. He also reports occasional pain in his bilateral shoulders and upper back described as "stiffness" and "tightness." He does not take pain medications, stating that he "deals with it and does not like to cause trouble."

Martin is estranged from his family following a conviction of armed robbery at the age of 45 years and was imprisoned until age 58 years. He avoided the health care system most of his life due to poor prior experiences while imprisoned and a feeling that "no one really cares." He finds comfort in watching television and listening to jazz. He describes himself as a private person who prefers keeping to himself. Supportive listening is provided, allowing Martin to express his hesitations with speaking to health care providers and mistrust of the medical system, which has been a barrier to improving his quality of life and symptom control.

Following a discussion of Martin's prognosis and anticipated disease trajectory, Martin decided to enroll in hospice services at his long-term care facility. He is provided with meticulous wound care for his decubitus ulcer and more frequent positional changes and passive range-of-motion exercises to assist with his pain. Martin works closely with the hospice social worker on coping skills and adjusting to illness. He decides he would like to have his body donated to science with the hope that this will help others in the future dealing with ALS. For his pain regimen, Martin is given scheduled liquid acetaminophen, lidocaine patches for musculoskeletal pain, and low-dose sublingual morphine as needed for pain. He is monitored closely for nonverbal indicators of pain and discomfort as his disease progresses. He is eventually transferred to an inpatient hospice unit for subcutaneous administration of opioids and benzodiazepines for signs of increased dyspnea, terminal agitation, and pain as he approaches end of life in the setting of his progressing ALS. He passed away comfortably several days after admission to inpatient hospice and appropriate administration of comfort-focused medications.

Conclusion

Pain at the end of life is influenced by a complex interplay of a person's physical, psychological, social, and spiritual experiences. Individuals in need of end-of-life pain care are more vulnerable, have a lower quality of life, and have greater functional impairment. Disparities in end-of-life pain care may stem from health care provider biases; gaps in knowledge; racial, cultural, and/or structural barriers; and policies that may exclude or stigmatize different populations. Involving an interdisciplinary team of health care professionals and palliative care services is essential for optimizing outcomes and assessing the multifaceted nature of pain. Inclusive and accessible end-of-life pain management can be achieved through further expanding existing strengths in palliative care and eliminating barriers to access.

References

1. Vulnerable populations: Who are they? *Am J Manag Care*. 2006;12(13 Suppl):S348–S352.
2. Hagarty AM, Bush SH, Talarico R, Lapenskie J, Tanuseputro P. Severe pain at the end of life: A population-level observational study. *BMC Palliat Care*. 2020;19(1): Article 60. doi:10.1186/s12904-020-00569-2
3. Phipps EJ. What's end of life got to do with it? Research ethics with populations at life's end. *Gerontologist*. 2002;42(Spec No. 3):104–108. doi:10.1093/geront/42.suppl_3.104
4. Hui D, Nooruddin Z, Didwaniya N, et al. Concepts and definitions for "actively dying," "end of life," "terminally ill," "terminal care," and "transition of care": A systematic review. *J Pain Symptom Manage*. 2014;47(1):77–89. doi:10.1016/j.jpainsymman.2013.02.021
5. Craig KD, Holmes C, Hudspith M, et al. Pain in persons who are marginalized by social conditions. *Pain*. 2020;161(2):261–265. doi:10.1097/j.pain.0000000000001719
6. Lewis VA, Larson BK, McClurg AB, Boswell RG, Fisher ES. The promise and peril of accountable care for vulnerable populations: A framework for overcoming obstacles. *Health Aff*. 2012;31(8):1777–1785. doi:10.1377/hlthaff.2012.0490
7. Ward H, Finucane TE, Schuchman M. Challenges related to safety and independence. *Med Clin North Am*. 2020;104(5):909–917. doi:10.1016/j.mcna.2020.06.006
8. Meghani SH, Polomano RC, Tait RC, Vallerand AH, Anderson KO, Gallagher RM. Advancing a national agenda to eliminate disparities in pain care: Directions for health policy, education, practice, and research. *Pain Med*. 2012;13(1):5–28. doi:10.1111/j.1526-4637.2011.01289.x
9. Morden NE, Chyn D, Wood A, Meara E. Racial inequality in prescription opioid receipt: Role of individual health systems. *N Engl J Med*. 2021;385(4):342–351. doi:10.1056/NEJMsa2034159
10. Nguyen M, Ugarte C, Fuller I, Haas G, Portenoy RK. Access to care for chronic pain: Racial and ethnic differences. *J Pain*. 2005;6(5):301–314. doi:10.1016/j.jpain.2004.12.008
11. Givler A, Bhatt H, Maani-Fogelman PA. The importance of cultural competence in pain and palliative care. In: *StatPearls*. StatPearls Publishing; May 23, 2022.

12. World Health Organization. Palliative care. 2020. Accessed August 31, 2022. https://www.who.int/news-room/fact-sheets/detail/palliative-care
13. Goebel JR, Doering LV, Lorenz KA, Maliski SL, Nyamathi AM, Evangelista LS. Caring for special populations: Total pain theory in advanced heart failure: Applications to research and practice. *Nurs Forum*. 2009;44(3):175–185. doi:10.1111/j.1744-6198.2009.00140.x
14. Shalev A, Phongtankuel V, Kozlov E, Shen MJ, Adelman RD, Reid MC. Awareness and misperceptions of hospice and palliative care: A population-based survey study. *Am J Hosp Palliat Care*. 2018;35(3):431–439. doi:10.1177/1049909117715215
15. Wittenberg-Lyles E, Parker Oliver D, Demiris G, Regehr K. Interdisciplinary collaboration in hospice team meetings. *J Interprof Care*. 2010;24(3):264–273. doi:10.3109/13561820903163421
16. Trachsel LA, Munakomi S, Cascella M. Pain theory. In: *StatPearls*. StatPearls Publishing; April 20, 2022.
17. Clark D. "Total pain," disciplinary power and the body in the work of Cicely Saunders, 1958–1967. *Soc Sci Med*. 1999;49(6):727–736. doi:10.1016/s0277-9536(99)00098-2
18. Raja SN, Carr DB, Cohen M, et al. The revised International Association for the Study of Pain definition of pain: Concepts, challenges, and compromises. *Pain*. 2020;161(9):1976–1982. doi:10.1097/j.pain.0000000000001939
19. Sinha A, Deshwal H, Vashisht R. End of life evaluation and management of pain. In: *StatPearls*. StatPearls Publishing; April 4, 2022.
20. Fitzcharles MA, Cohen SP, Clauw DJ, Littlejohn G, Usui C, Häuser W. Nociplastic pain: Towards an understanding of prevalent pain conditions. *Lancet*. 2021;397(10289):2098–2110. doi:10.1016/S0140-6736(21)00392-5
21. Gupta A, Kaur K, Sharma S, Goyal S, Arora S, Murthy RS. Clinical aspects of acute post-operative pain management & its assessment. *J Adv Pharm Technol Res*. 2010;1(2):97–108.
22. Katz J, Seltzer Z. Transition from acute to chronic postsurgical pain: Risk factors and protective factors. *Expert Rev Neurother*. 2009;9(5):723–744. doi:10.1586/ern.09.20
23. Omoigui S. The biochemical origin of pain: The origin of all pain is inflammation and the inflammatory response. Part 2 of 3—Inflammatory profile of pain syndromes. *Med Hypotheses*. 2007;69(6):1169–1178. doi:10.1016/j.mehy.2007.06.033
24. Mitsikostas DD, Moka E, Orrillo E, et al. Neuropathic pain in neurologic disorders: A narrative review. *Cureus*. 2022;14(2):e22419. doi:10.7759/cureus.22419
25. Dydyk AM, Khan MZ, Singh P. Radicular back pain. In: *StatPearls*. StatPearls Publishing; November 2, 2021
26. International Association for the Study of Pain. IASP terminology. 2017. Accessed November 8, 2022. https://www.iasp-pain.org/terminology
27. Nijs J, Lahousse A, Kapreli E, et al. Nociplastic pain criteria or recognition of central sensitization? Pain phenotyping in the past, present and future. *J Clin Med*. 2021;10(15):3203. doi:10.3390/jcm10153203
28. Van den Beuken-van Everdingen MH, de Rijke JM, Kessels AG, Schouten HC, van Kleef M, Patijn J. Prevalence of pain in patients with cancer: A systematic review of the past 40 years. *Ann Oncol*. 2007;18(9):1437–1449. doi:10.1093/annonc/mdm056
29. Murtagh FE, Addington-Hall J, Higginson IJ. The prevalence of symptoms in end-stage renal disease: A systematic review. *Adv Chronic Kidney Dis*. 2007;14(1):82–99. doi:10.1053/j.ackd.2006.10.001
30. Lee AL, Harrison SL, Goldstein RS, Brooks D. Pain and its clinical associations in individuals with COPD: A systematic review. *Chest*. 2015;147(5):1246–1258. doi:10.1378/chest.14-2690
31. Solano JP, Gomes B, Higginson IJ. A comparison of symptom prevalence in far advanced cancer, AIDS, heart disease, chronic obstructive pulmonary disease and renal disease. *J Pain Symptom Manage*. 2006;31(1):58–69. doi:10.1016/j.jpainsymman.2005.06.007
32. Falk S, Dickenson AH. Pain and nociception: Mechanisms of cancer-induced bone pain. *J Clin Oncol*. 2014 Jun 1;32(16):1647–1654. doi:10.1200/JCO.2013.51.7219
33. McGuire DB, Kaiser KS, Haisfield-Wolfe ME, Iyamu F. Pain assessment in noncommunicative adult palliative care patients. *Nurs Clin North Am*. 2016 Sep;51(3):397–431. doi:10.1016/j.cnur.2016.05.009

34. Anekar AA, Cascella M. WHO analgesic ladder. In: *StatPearls*. StatPearls Publishing; May 15, 2022.
35. Dowell D, Haegerich TM, Chou R. CDC guideline for prescribing opioids for chronic pain—United States, 2016. *MMWR Recomm Rep*. 2016;65(No. RR-1):1–49. http://dx.doi.org/10.15585/mmwr.rr6501e1er
36. Chaparro LE, Wiffen PJ, Moore RA, Gilron I. Combination pharmacotherapy for the treatment of neuropathic pain in adults. *Cochrane Database Syst Rev*. 2012;2012(7):CD008943.
37. Yajima M, Sugimoto M, Sugimura YK, Takahashi Y, Kato F. Acetaminophen and pregabalin attenuate central sensitization in rodent models of nociplastic widespread pain. *Neuropharmacology*. 2022;210:109029.
38. Toms L, McQuay HJ, Derry S, Moore RA. Single dose oral paracetamol (acetaminophen) for postoperative pain in adults. *Cochrane Database Syst Rev*. 2008;2008(4):CD004602.
39. Alchin J, Dhar A, Siddiqui K, Christo PJ. Why paracetamol (acetaminophen) is a suitable first choice for treating mild to moderate acute pain in adults with liver, kidney or cardiovascular disease, gastrointestinal disorders, asthma, or who are older. *Curr Med Res Opin*. 2022;38(5):811–825. doi:10.1080/03007995.2022.2049551
40. Chandok N, Watt KD. Pain management in the cirrhotic patient: The clinical challenge. *Mayo Clin Proc*. 2010;85(5):451–458. doi:10.4065/mcp.2009.0534
41. Donado C, Solodiuk J, Rangel SJ, et al. Patient- and nurse-controlled analgesia: 22-year experience in a pediatric hospital. *Hosp Pediatr*. 2019;9(2):129–133. doi:10.1542/hpeds.2018-0179
42. Centers for Disease Control and Prevention. Understanding the opioid overdose epidemic. 2022. Accessed November 10, 2022. https://www.cdc.gov/opioids/basics/epidemic.html#print
43. Gabbard J, Jordan A, Mitchell J, Corbett M, White P, Childers J. Dying on hospice in the midst of an opioid crisis: What should we do now? *Am J Hosp Palliat Care*. 2019;36(4):273–281. doi:10.1177/1049909118806664
44. Dowell D, Ragan KR, Jones CM, Baldwin GT, Chou R. CDC clinical practice guideline for prescribing opioids for pain—United States, 2022. *MMWR Recomm Rep*. 2022;71(3):1–95. doi:10.15585/mmwr.rr7103a1
45. McPherson ML, Walker KA, Davis MP, et al. Safe and appropriate use of methadone in hospice and palliative care: Expert consensus white paper. *J Pain Symptom Manage*. 2019;57(3):635–645. doi:10.1016/j.jpainsymman.2018.12.001
46. Neale KJ, Weimer MB, Davis MP, et al. Top ten tips palliative care clinicians should know about buprenorphine [published online ahead of print, 2022 Sep 6]. *J Palliat Med*. 2023;26(1):120–130. doi:10.1089/jpm.2022.0399
47. Kral L, Ku J, Kematick BS, Fudin J. Pearls for opioid use in seriously ill patients. *J Pain Palliat Care Pharmacother*. 2019;33(1–2):54–58. doi:10.1080/15360288.2019.1650870
48. Committee on Family Caregiving for Older Adults; Board on Health Care Services; Health and Medicine Division; National Academies of Sciences, Engineering, and Medicine; Schulz R, Eden J, eds. *Families Caring for an Aging America*. National Academies Press; 2016.
49. Singh P, Chaturvedi A. Complementary and alternative medicine in cancer pain management: A systematic review. *Indian J Palliat Care*. 2015;21(1):105–115. doi:10.4103/0973-1075.150202
50. Martin EM, Barkley TW Jr. Improving cultural competence in end-of-life pain management. *Nursing*. 2016;46(1):32–42. doi:10.1097/01.NURSE.0000475480.75266.9a
51. International Pain Summit of the International Association for the Study of Pain. Declaration of Montréal: Declaration that access to pain management is a fundamental human right. *J Pain Palliat Care Pharmacother*. 2011;25(1):29–31. doi:10.3109/15360288.2010.547560
52. Mossey JM. Defining racial and ethnic disparities in pain management. *Clin Orthop Relat Res*. 2011;469(7):1859–1870. doi:10.1007/s11999-011-1770-9
53. Griggs JJ. Disparities in palliative care in patients with cancer. *J Clin Oncol*. 2020;38(9):974–979. doi:10.1200/JCO.19.02108

54. Lee KT, George M, Lowry S, Ashing KT. A review and considerations on palliative care improvements for African Americans with cancer. *Am J Hosp Palliat Care*. 2021;38(6):671–677. doi:10.1177/1049909120930205
55. Johnson KS. Racial and ethnic disparities in palliative care. *J Palliat Med*. 2013;16(11):1329–1334. doi:10.1089/jpm.2013.9468
56. National Hospice and Palliative Care Organization. Hospice facts & figures. January 13, 2022. Accessed November 10, 2022. https://www.nhpco.org/hospice-care-overview/hospice-facts-figures
57. Institute of Medicine Committee on Understanding and Eliminating Racial and Ethnic Disparities in Health Care; Smedley BD, Stith AY, Nelson AR, eds. Unequal Treatment: Confronting Racial and Ethnic Disparities in Health Care. National Academies Press; 2003.
58. Green CR. Racial and ethnic disparities in the quality of pain care: The anesthesiologist's call to action. *J Am Soc Anesthesiologists*. 2007;106(1):6–8.
59. Booker SQ, Herr KA, Wilson Garvan C. Racial differences in pain management for patients receiving hospice care. *Oncol Nurs Forum*. 2020;47(2):228–240. doi:10.1188/20.ONF.228-240
60. Green CR, Anderson KO, Baker TA, et al. The unequal burden of pain: Confronting racial and ethnic disparities in pain [published correction appears in Pain Med. 2005 Jan–Feb;6(1):99. Kaloukalani, Donna A [corrected to Kalauokalani, Donna A]]. *Pain Med*. 2003;4(3):277–294. doi:10.1046/j.1526-4637.2003.03034.x
61. Tamayo-Sarver JH, Hinze SW, Cydulka RK, Baker DW. Racial and ethnic disparities in emergency department analgesic prescription. *Am J Public Health*. 2003;93(12):2067–2073. doi:10.2105/ajph.93.12.2067
62. Schuler MS, Schell TL, Wong EC. Racial/ethnic differences in prescription opioid misuse and heroin use among a national sample, 1999–2018. *Drug Alcohol Depend*. 2021;221:108588. doi:10.1016/j.drugalcdep.2021.108588
63. FitzGerald C, Hurst S. Implicit bias in healthcare professionals: A systematic review. *BMC Med Ethics*. 2017;18(1):19. doi:10.1186/s12910-017-0179-8
64. Togioka BM, Duvivier D, Young E. Diversity and discrimination In healthcare. In: *StatPearls*. StatPearls Publishing; May 3, 2022.
65. Betancourt JR. Eliminating racial and ethnic disparities in health care: What is the role of academic medicine? *Acad Med*. 2006;81(9):788–792.
66. Murray SA, Kendall M, Boyd K, Sheikh A. Illness trajectories and palliative care. *BMJ*. 2005;330(7498):1007–1011. doi:10.1136/bmj.330.7498.1007

13
Pain and Adverse Childhood Experiences

William G. Katzman and Anilla Del Fabbro

Introduction

Trauma has long been linked to the development of pain. Although pain can develop due to the experience of degenerative changes that occur in the body, it can also come about through the experiencing of traumatic events, such as through the terror associated with death, threatened death, serious injury, or sexual violence. These frightening experiences frequently lead to the development of psychological distress that can be classified by the acute stress disorder and post-traumatic stress disorder (PTSD) diagnoses, and they often simultaneously lead to the development of physical pain. Specifically, psychological trauma has widely been shown to be related to both functional somatic syndromes (fibromyalgia, chronic widespread pain, chronic fatigue syndrome, and many gastrointestinal syndromes)[1] and other chronic pain conditions.[2,3] Furthermore, the overlap between physical and psychological pain related to traumatic experiences has been thoroughly noted, and theories related to the development of both forms of pain have been discussed in the literature. Some argue for a mutual maintenance hypothesis stating that the cognitive, affective, and behavioral components of pain may contribute to the experience of psychological distress, whereas the physiologic, affective, and avoidance components of psychological distress contribute to the experience of chronic pain.[4,5] However, others argue for a vulnerability model stating that factors such as catastrophizing or anxiety sensitivity are required prerequisites for the experience of both physical and psychological pain following traumas.[2,6]

Adverse Childhood Experiences: Definition and Current Literature

Although the relationship between physical and psychological pain is still under investigation, it is clear that traumatic experiences lead to the development of various forms of pain. Specifically, adverse childhood experiences (ACEs) are one form of trauma that researchers and medical health providers have begun to consider. ACEs are traumatic experiences of abuse or household dysfunction that occur before age 18 years which have been shown to have lasting impacts on mental, physical, and behavioral health (Table 13.1). Between 1995 and 1997, researchers at Kaiser Permanente collaborated in a landmark study to examine more closely how early childhood adversity can negatively impact health throughout the life span.[7] More than 17,000 members from the health

Table 13.1 Adverse Childhood Experiences Questions Based on Abuse and Household Dysfunction Category

Abuse by Category
Psychological
(Did a parent or other adult in the household . . .)
Often or very often swear at, insult, or put you down?
Often or very often act in a way that made you afraid that you would potentially be physically hurt?
Physical
(Did a parent or other adult in the household . . .)
Often or very often push, grab, shove, or slap you?
Often or very often hit you so hard that you had marks or were injured?
Sexual
(Did an adult or person at least 5 years or older ever . . .)
Touch or fondle you in a sexual way?
Have you touch their body in a sexual way?
Attempt oral, anal, or vaginal intercourse with you?
Actually have oral, anal, or vaginal intercourse with you?
Substance Abuse
Live with someone who was a problem drinker or alcoholic?
Live with someone who used street drugs?
Mental Illness
Was a household member depressed or mentally ill?
Did a household member attempt suicide?
Mother Treated Violently
Was your mother (or step mother)
Sometimes, often, or very often pushed, grabbed, slapped, or had something thrown at her?
Sometimes, often, or very often kicked, bitten, hit with a fist, or hit with something hard?
Ever repeatedly hit over at least a few minutes?
Ever threatened with, or hurt by, a knife or gun?
Criminal Behavior in Household
Did a household member go to prison?

Source: Felitti et al.[7]

maintenance organization completed confidential surveys regarding their ACEs and current health status and behaviors. The number of ACE questions endorsed was then compared to measures of adult risk behavior, health status, and disease: 61% of adults endorsed at least one question, and 16% endorsed four or more types of ACEs. It was found that the higher the number of ACEs experienced, the greater the likelihood and severity of chronic health conditions and premature death. The original ACEs study has been replicated internationally, and as a result, ACEs have now been associated with many neurological chronic pain conditions (see Table 13.1).

What Makes People Exposed to ACEs More Vulnerable to Pain?

The documentation of ACEs has led to the development of numerous conceptual frameworks to better understand how ACEs lead to subsequent medical, behavioral, and mental health problems. Both animal and human studies suggest that fetal exposure to maternal stress can influence later stress sensitivity. In addition, ACEs have been shown to increase a child's allostatic load and negatively impact their developing brain due to excessive activation of the stress response system.[8] Furthermore, the negative impact of ACEs has been shown to be dependent on whether ACEs occur during a stress-sensitive period of the brain's development.[9] Considering the type and timing of ACEs improves understanding of vulnerability and should inform diagnostics of pain conditions. There are sensitive periods in early development, and without the protection of a safe environment, long-term disruptions in brain development and immune, hormonal, and metabolic systems can occur.

Social Determinants of Health—Another Predictor of Pain Vulnerability

Although ACEs have been shown to be predictive of later health consequences, it is important to note that these childhood experiences only capture a subset of the adverse experiences that are related to negative sequelae. Specifically, the documentation of ACEs can be considered as a life course approach for understanding social determinants influencing health because its focus is on the examination of the early sensitive period of development as a predictor of later health.[10] However, other social determinant approaches focus on the effects of social disadvantages such as neighborhood conditions; work environments; and sociodemographic factors, including class, gender, and race. These social determinants have been correlated with a plethora of later negative health outcomes, such as infant mortality and the development of an activity-limiting chronic medical condition, and it has been widely established that lower income, fewer years of education, and belonging to an ethnic minority increase one's chances of dealing with health-related consequences.[11,12]

Not surprisingly, a strong relationship exists between ACEs and these additional social determinants of health. For example, adults who report having experienced homelessness in childhood also report significantly greater exposure to higher numbers and types of ACEs than adults reporting no childhood homelessness.[13] Furthermore, when ACEs are examined alongside other social determinants of health, such as socioeconomic status, peer rejection, peer victimization, community violence exposure, and school performance, the predictive power of later mental and physical health symptoms is significantly improved.[14–16] Despite the strong overlap between ACEs and other social determinants of health, it appears that some individuals in diverse samples report primarily experiencing social determinants not measured by traditional ACE questions.[14] These additional social determinants have also been shown to be uniquely predictive of later outcomes such as seeking behavioral health services.[17] Given these findings, researchers have begun to propose and develop expanded assessments of ACEs to include questions that ask about community-wide adverse experiences along with socioeconomic status. Despite these attempts, many studies continue to report on early adverse experiences that occur only within the home. Regardless, it appears likely that individuals who endorse experiences such as abuse and neglect likely have also faced challenges in their wider communities that further contribute to their later health detriments.

Discussion

Relationship of Psychological Pain and Adverse Childhood Experiences

The early stages of human development are of critical importance for cognitive and emotional adaptations later in life.[18] In addition, these early milestones are marked by rapid physical changes while children are simultaneously attending to their environments in order to learn about their own and others' mental states.[19] Thus, experiencing ACEs not only impacts the biological processes of the developing child but also can prohibit the development of psychological capacities allowing a child to gain a proper understanding of the world around them. These consequences have been widely shown to manifest in a variety of psychological experiences of pain. Specifically, experiences of sexual abuse, physical abuse, and violence in the home throughout childhood have been related to greater mental health symptoms and risk-taking behaviors later in life.[20] Of note, the increased number of ACEs results in a dose–response in which the accumulation of ACEs leads to poorer mental health outcomes.[7,21] Research investigations have uncovered the many ways in which ACEs can manifest as psychological experiences of pain and have argued for the large contribution that ACEs play in the development of psychopathology. For women, it has been estimated that 22–32% of mental disorders can be attributed to ACEs, and for men this percentage ranges from 20% to 24%.[22]

It has been observed that the effects of ACEs can manifest in affective and anxiety disorders. In line with the dose–response theory, the greater number of reported ACEs has been shown to increase the probability of a recent or lifetime depressive disorder (major depression or dysthymia) among both men and women.[23,24] Furthermore, women who have experienced childhood sexual abuse are more likely to report later depressive, anxiety, and other interpersonal sensitivity.[25] In addition, the experiencing of early emotional abuse has been found to have a strong relationship with the development of affective disorders.[24] Notably, the presence of a depressed mood occurring as early as young adulthood has been linked to the occurrence of ACEs.[26]

The probability of suicidality at a later age also increases based on the number of reported ACEs.[24,27] Specifically, among women, suicidality has been significantly correlated with childhood physical abuse and sexual abuse; among men, it has been significantly correlated with childhood physical abuse and witnessing domestic violence.[22] Furthermore, depressed mood, alcohol abuse, and illicit drug use have been found to mediate the relationship between ACEs and suicidality.[27]

There also exists a clear relationship between ACEs and substance use. Notably, it has been argued that ACEs may account for one-half to two-thirds of serious problems with drug use.[28] It has been shown that household drug use, household mental illness, and emotional abuse during childhood are strong predictors of drug use, drug addiction, parental drug use, and heavy drinking during adulthood.[24,28] It has also been illustrated that a greater number of reported ACEs leads to an earlier age in which one begins their drug use. Furthermore, ACEs have been shown to lead to additional problematic health behaviors such as smoking and thus subsequent increased risk of lung cancer.[29]

Although ACEs are in themselves traumatic, they can lead to the increased likelihood that traumatic experiences later in life will cause PTSD. For example, in a sample of individuals in the military, those who reported ACEs were more likely to be diagnosed with post-deployment PTSD than those who did not endorse any ACEs.[30] It seems probable that the influence of ACEs likely leads to limited psychological capacities and biological vulnerabilities, which in turn leave individuals less able to cope with future terrors. Although those who experience a high degree of ACEs may be more vulnerable in the face of future traumatic events, individuals who experience ACEs have been found to have greater general traumatic stress, which points to the likely continued impact of the stress related to the original ACEs.[31]

ACEs are often seen in individuals who are diagnosed with a personality disorder. Specifically, in a clinical sample of individuals diagnosed with a personality disorder, 73% of the individuals reported experiencing abuse and 82% reported experiencing neglect.[32] The relationship between ACEs and personality disorders has also been investigated in nonclinical samples, and it has been found that ACEs are most consistently associated with schizotypal, antisocial, borderline, and narcissistic personality disorders.[33] Furthermore, compared to other personality disorders, borderline personality disorder is most commonly associated with childhood abuse and neglect.[34] Given the high correlation between borderline personality disorder and ACEs, some have argued that borderline personality disorder should be considered a trauma spectrum disorder.[32]

Although the relationship between ACEs and psychological experiences of pain is consistently identified, further research has begun to hypothesize and uncover factors that may mediate this relationship. One common framework for understanding these factors comes from a biopsychosocial approach, which views biological, psychological, and social factors as interrelated and continually influencing one another over the course of development.[35] Using this model as a guide, research findings are beginning to highlight specific elements of each aspect of the biopsychosocial model that have direct impacts on psychological pain when ACEs are present.[36]

With regard to the biological processes that are affected by the presence of ACEs, one way in which ACEs have been shown to have detriments on health is through neurophysiological changes occurring in the body.[37] Specifically, sensitized corticoamygdala neural circuitry has been found in those who have experienced ACEs. It is thought that this then leads to heightened reactivity to future stressors and a subsequent activation of the sympathetic nervous system and the hypothalamic–pituitary–adrenocortical axis. In addition, abnormal changes in both oxytocin and serotonin, along with deficient opioid receptors in the brain, have been found in individuals who have disrupted relationships with their caregivers, and these chemical processes have been found to play important roles in the development of mental disorders.[38]

ACEs have also been shown to impact how individuals choose to respond and interact with their environments.[36] Specifically, individuals who have experienced a greater number of ACEs are more likely to perceive their surroundings as threatening and thus subsequently more likely to engage in avoidant coping strategies.[28] These strategies often are characterized by drug and alcohol use, negative eating patterns, and avoidance of stressful environments and relationships. Although avoidance can be understood as an adaptive form of coping when abuse or neglect is present during childhood, the continued use of avoidant coping strategies later in life often manifests in these problematic ways. As would be expected, given the heightened use of avoidant coping strategies within this population, those who have experienced ACEs are less likely to use adaptive coping skills such as actively engaging, planning, and reframing their emotional experiences.[39] Furthermore, ACEs been correlated with self-regulatory deficits, poorer attention, decreased inhibition, difficulties in delaying gratification, and less reward sensitivity, all of which likely contribute to high-risk behaviors later in life.[36]

Although ACEs impact biological and behavioral processes, these early experiences also have a significant impact on the psychological capacities of the developing individual. Specifically, from a cognitive perspective, ACEs have been shown to lead to an increased use of negative cognitive styles and negative self-schemas.[40,41] A negative cognitive style describes the process of making negative interpretations regarding stressful life events as these moments are attributed to stable and global factors. In addition, a negative self-concept leaves individuals prone to self-criticism and doubt. Ultimately, this way of understanding oneself and the environment has been shown to manifest in disorders such as depression.[42]

The emotional experience of individuals with ACEs is also significantly affected. Specifically, the process of emotion regulation, defined as an individual's ability to recognize, monitor, express, and modify their emotions in a manner that facilitates adaptive functioning, has been found to contribute to the relationship between ACEs and mental health outcomes such as depression and PTSD.[43,44] Furthermore, although problems with emotion regulation are central to the development of psychopathology,[45] emotional difficulties are often also correlated with aggression and impulsivity, both of which have also been shown to increase in the presence of ACEs.[38]

The relationship between ACEs and psychological pain can also be understood as stemming from problematic parent–child attachment relationships that form when children are exposed to a high number of ACEs. A secure attachment relationship develops when children can readily rely on their attachment figures to function as a secure base, which is understood as a presence that will provide the growing child with comfort and security during moments of distress.[46] However, when children perceive their caregivers as threatening due to ACE experiences such as abuse or neglect, this often leads to the development of a disorganized attachment relationship in which the children desire connection but fear that this proximity may bring them harm.[19] Adults who experienced a greater number of ACEs and less emotional support in childhood have been shown to be more likely to have a disorganized mental representation of their early attachment experiences.[47] Disorganized attachment later in life limits one's capacity to function optimally in adult relationships because these individuals often assume that their friends or romantic partners may similarly be the rejecting, abusive, or neglecting others that they experienced in childhood.[48] Thus, disorganized attachment has been correlated with psychopathology such as borderline personality disorder.[49]

While the development of a secure attachment relationship is affected by the presence of ACEs, a child's developing capacity to mentalize is simultaneously impaired. Mentalization describes the ability to understand the mental states that underlie the behavior of both the self and others.[19] This capacity develops when children's mental states are adequately understood by caring, attentive, and nonthreatening attachment figures. This is an important developmental process because mentalizing deficits have been shown to be related to emotional and interpersonal difficulties later in life.[50] Furthermore, deficient mentalization capacities have been observed in a wide range of mental disorders.[51] Whereas the capacity to mentalize develops under optimal conditions, the experience of ACEs can affect the development of a child's mentalization capacity because abusive parents often fail to acknowledge the intentionality of their developing child. It is also thought that when children experience abuse by their caregivers, this presents children with an emotional disincentive to understand the intentions of others given the real threat of the abuse. Multiple studies have not only documented the effect of ACEs on individuals' capacity to mentalize but also shown how these individuals with deficient mentalization capacities are more likely to develop disorganized attachment relationships with their own children.[52] This highlights an important mechanism underlying the intergenerational transition of ACEs.

Relationship of Physical Pain and Adverse Childhood Experiences

Adverse childhood experiences have been associated with physical pain in youth and adulthood.[53] Early studies have identified heart disease, cancer, rheumatologic syndromes, and many types of chronic pain as some of the conditions associated with a history of ACEs.[54] In the original ACE study, researchers noted a dose–response between the number of ACEs and the severity of a particular health outcome or chronic pain condition.[7] Other studies have confirmed a similar relationship between the number of ACEs and the development of certain chronic pain conditions, such as headaches, fibromyalgia, and abdominal pain.[54,55] It is not yet well understood which ACEs, or which combination of ACEs, place a child at most risk for developing long-term chronic pain or other deleterious health outcomes.

Both chronic pain and anxiety have been found to be associated with childhood trauma (emotional abuse, emotional neglect, and physical neglect).[56] Many investigators have thus argued that psychological symptoms, particularly anxiety in youth, are a strong mediator in the development of chronic pain both in childhood and in adulthood).[26,57] However, it has also been noted that being given a chronic pain diagnosis can result in increased anxiety, so the timeline of developing both physical and psychological pain in the presence of ACEs is not always clear.[58,59] Some of the most common physical symptoms and syndromes associated with ACES include fibromyalgia; headaches; and gastrointestinal, pelvic, and bladder pain.[60]

Fibromyalgia

Fibromyalgia has commonly been associated with injuries and medical procedures.[61] Symptoms of fibromyalgia include chronic widespread pain, sleep-related disorder, anxiety and/or depression, and cognitive difficulties. However, the relationship between ACEs, other precipitating events, and the development of fibromyalgia is not universally accepted. Unfortunately, many early studies proved inconclusive due to poor quality of research design. Nonetheless, the vast majority of research in this field does point to some association between ACEs and chronic widespread pain or fibromyalgia, which is thought to be caused by a heightened, centralized pain state.

Specifically, research has noted an increased risk of fibromyalgia in individuals whose family had financial stress, family conflict, divorce, serious illness, and/or alcohol problems.[62] In other studies examining adults with fibromyalgia, risk factors included poor emotional relationship with parents, financial stress, alcohol misuse in the mother, and parental discord and/or separation occurring before the participants were aged 7 years.[63] In addition, compared to healthy adults without fibromyalgia, those with fibromyalgia have more often experienced physical and emotional neglect and abuse, as well as sexual abuse.[64]

Headaches

Headaches, especially migraines, are increasingly recognized as associated with stress and ACEs.[65] Migraine headaches usually begin in childhood and can transform to a chronic pattern of pain by central sensitization.[66] Results from large-scale cohort studies have concluded that a lack of parental warmth, paternal alcoholism, suicide attempt of a family member, and living in an unsafe neighborhood increase the likelihood of headaches.[67] Other researchers have identified that emotional abuse, neglect, and/or sexual abuse can transform an episodic migraine pattern into a chronic condition.[68] A study conducted by the National Survey of Children's Health found that children with three ACEs were 3.40 times more likely to report headaches compared to those without any ACEs. Interestingly, no particular ACE was more independently associated with headaches except for financial stress, at 2.46 times higher.[69]

Abdominal Pain

Abdominal pain associated with ACEs is most commonly seen in irritable bowel syndrome (IBS). The pathophysiology of IBS is complex and may include "altered gastrointestinal motility, visceral and food hypersensitivities, brain–gut interactions, alteration in fecal and micro flora, bacterial overgrowth," etc.[70] ACEs were found to be associated with IBS in females, with an odds ratio of 2.20, but no association was found in males.[71] In a separate case–control study of 148 patients with IBS, a greater number of ACEs increased the odds of having IBS. The three most significant predictors were family member with mental illness, emotional abuse, and incarceration of a family member.[72]

Pelvic Pain

Pelvic pain is usually seen in women, and many studies suggest an association with ACEs. There are many neuropathophysiological mechanisms of chronic pelvic pain, including neuropathic and non-neuropathic, depending on the origin of the pain.[73] A meta-analysis found that sexual abuse and PTSD were associated with pelvic pain, in addition to dysmenorrhea and dyspareunia.[74] In another study, women with and without pelvic pain were surveyed. The researchers concluded that 57% of those suffering chronic pelvic pain had four or more ACEs compared to 27% of women without chronic pelvic pain. Physical, sexual, and emotional abuse were also significantly more common in women with chronic pelvic pain.[75]

Interstitial Cystitis

Interstitial cystitis and overactive bladder, which are painful conditions in the pelvis, have also been associated with early childhood trauma. Researchers have surveyed women with and without interstitial cystitis and overactive bladder. Compared to controls, women with interstitial cystitis and overactive bladder had significantly increased likelihood of physical, sexual, or emotional abuse and/or having witnessed domestic violence.[76] A recent study suggests that depression may mediate the pain intensity in both men and women with chronic pelvic pain syndrome who have suffered from ACEs.[77] Similarly, researchers have studied patients with urologic chronic pelvic pain syndrome and found that patients suffering pelvic pain symptoms had a high degree of ACEs, along with frequent catastrophizing, anxiety, depression, perceived stress, and total somatic complaints.[78]

The recent literature suggests that early childhood trauma is associated with the development of certain chronic pain conditions. Family discord, parental alcohol misuse, physical/emotional neglect, and/or financial instability may be particularly associated with fibromyalgia, whereas physical/emotional/sexual abuse may be more commonly associated with pelvic pain. In addition, the higher the number of ACEs suffered during early childhood, the higher the risk for the development of chronic pain and poor health outcomes.

Treatment

Given that ACEs frequently lead to long-term associations with adolescent and adult health risk behaviors and resultant diseases, it is imperative that increased attention be paid to primary, secondary, and tertiary prevention strategies. These strategies include prevention of the occurrence of ACEs, preventing high-risk health behaviors as responses to ACEs during childhood and adolescence, and helping change the high-risk behaviors among adults whose health problems may represent long-term consequences of ACEs.

Primary intervention strategies that aim to prevent ACEs are ideal but challenging to achieve. The Centers for Disease Control and Prevention has provided specific strategies regarding the prevention of ACEs and strategies for mitigating the negative, potentially harmful effects of ACEs.[79] Research has indicated that ACEs can be prevented by bolstering financial support for families, teaching skills to help parents and their children better handle stress and regulate emotions, and connect children and adolescents to caring adults and health-promoting activities. As a further primary intervention strategy, it is valuable to implement high-quality home visiting programs such as the Nurse–Family Partnership. These programs can improve outcomes for children and families, particularly those facing added challenges such as teen or single parenthood, maternal depression, and lack of social and financial supports.[80]

Secondary prevention opportunities that may be leveraged after an individual has experienced a traumatic event include the development of skill-building, the promotion of resilience, and fostering supportive communities. This may also include interventions such as providing education about ACEs to high-risk populations, including teen parents, parents with substance use issues, or parents facing significant financial issues or homelessness. Education regarding the long-term sequelae and how to moderate the effects of ACEs has been shown to be a valuable point of intervention. In addition, child–parent psychotherapy[81] and the Circle of Security–Intensive model[82] are two attachment-based therapeutic strategies that help young children and families build resilience and interact more harmoniously with each other and thereby improve the frequency to which a child's experience is mentalized within the family environment.

Tertiary interventions for adults who are dealing with sequelae of childhood adversity may include approaches that account for the low frustration tolerance and emotional dysregulation that are often seen in people who have endured a high degree of trauma. A trauma-focused approach (specific PTSD/trauma) and a trauma-informed approach have merit. Specifically, trauma-informed care and trauma- and violence-informed care (TVIC) are considered valuable approaches for this population.[83,84] TVIC includes five components that are well worth integrating with any patient and especially with individuals who have experienced ACEs. Primarily, this treatment approaches care with "safety first" as an improved feeling of safety, and trustworthiness is a key component of change. Additional components include trauma awareness, cultural and individual deference, a focus on strengths and skill-building, as well as providing a combination of collaboration and individual choice and control. Treatment approaches that focus on improving outcomes for individuals who have experienced ACEs, especially with subsequent pain symptomatology, may include augmenting traditional pain-focused cognitive–behavioral therapy with specific trauma-focused cognitive–behavioral therapy.[55]

In addition to these specific interventions, combining conventional or traditional treatments with complementary or holistic approaches can be helpful for improving mental health, as well as physical health. Research has demonstrated the beneficial effects of repetitive transcranial magnetic stimulation, acupuncture, hypnotherapy, meditation, and visualization for PTSD symptoms.[85] More study is warranted to explore potential benefits of other mind–body strategies such as yoga, biofeedback, mindfulness, meditation, and neuromuscular relaxation training. In addition, improving sleep, ensuring exercise, and enhancing relaxation techniques, as well as pain-coping skills, may address some of the modifiable manifestations of childhood adversity. Last, interventions targeted at regulating stress physiology and helping reduce stigmatization of patients include routine physical activity, implementing anti-inflammatory diets, improving and strengthening nurturing relationships, addressing insomnia, and starting mindfulness practices.[86]

Conclusion

Adverse childhood experiences and social determinants of health can increase the risk of developing pain later in life. There are now many efficacious and multimodal treatments for pain, including those most commonly diagnosed in patients who suffer from multiple adverse childhood experiences. Primary prevention of ACEs, however, may certainly decrease the prevalence of certain psychological and physical sequelae.

References

1. Afari N, Ahumada SM, Wright LJ, et al. Psychological trauma and functional somatic syndromes: A systematic review and meta-analysis. *Psychosom Med.* 2014;76(1):2–11.
2. Kind S, Otis JD The interaction between chronic pain and PTSD. *Curr Pain Headache Rep.* 2019;23(12):1–7.
3. Otis JD, Keane TM, Kerns RD. An examination of the relationship between chronic pain and post-traumatic stress disorder. *J Rehabil Res Dev.* 2003;40(5–6):397–406.
4. Sharp TJ. The prevalence of post-traumatic stress disorder in chronic pain patients. *Curr Pain Headache Rep.* 2004;8(2):111–115.
5. Sharp TJ, Harvey AG. Chronic pain and posttraumatic stress disorder: Mutual maintenance? *Clin Psychol Rev.* 2001;21(6):857–877.
6. Asmundson GJ, Coons MJ, Taylor S, Katz J. PTSD and the experience of pain: Research and clinical implications of shared vulnerability and mutual maintenance models. *Can J Psychiatry.* 2002;47(10):930–937.
7. Felitti VJ, Anda RF, Nordenberg D, et al. Relationship of childhood abuse and household dysfunction to many of the leading causes of death in adults: The Adverse Childhood Experiences (ACE) study. *Am J Prev Med.* 1998;14(4):245–258.
8. Shonkoff JP, Garner AS; Committee on Psychosocial Aspects of Child and Family Health; Committee on Early Childhood, Adoption, and Dependent Care; and Section on Developmental and Behavioral Pediatrics. The lifelong effects of early childhood adversity and toxic stress. *Pediatrics.* 2012;129(1):e232–e246.
9. Schalinski I, Teicher MH, Nischk D, Hinderer E, Müller O, Rockstroh B. Type and timing of adverse childhood experiences differentially affect severity of PTSD, dissociative and depressive symptoms in adult inpatients. *BMC Psychiatry.* 2016;16(1):1–15.
10. Bharmal N, Derose KP, Felician M, Weden MM. Understanding the upstream social determinants of health. Working paper No. WR-1096-RC. RAND Corporation; 2015.
11. Braveman P, Barclay C. Health disparities beginning in childhood: A life-course perspective. *Pediatrics.* 2009;124(Suppl 3):S163–S175.
12. Braveman P, Gottlieb L. The social determinants of health: It's time to consider the causes of the causes. *Public Health Rep.* 2014;129(1 Suppl 2):19–31.
13. Radcliff E, Crouch E, Strompolis M, Srivastav A. Homelessness in childhood and adverse childhood experiences (ACEs). *Matern Child Health J.* 2019;23(6):811–820.
14. Cronholm PF, Forke CM, Wade R, et al. Adverse childhood experiences: Expanding the concept of adversity. *Am J Prev Med.* 2015;49(3):354–361.
15. Finkelhor D, Shattuck A, Turner H, Hamby S. Improving the Adverse Childhood Experiences Study Scale. *JAMA Pediatr.* 2013;167(1):70–75.
16. Finkelhor D, Shattuck A, Turner H, Hamby S. A revised inventory of adverse childhood experiences. *Child Abuse Neglect.* 2015;48:13–21.
17. Lee E, Larkin H, Esaki N. Exposure to community violence as a new adverse childhood experience category: Promising results and future considerations. *Fam Soc.* 2017;98(1):69–78.
18. Chapman DP, Dube SR, Anda RF. Adverse childhood events as risk factors for negative mental health outcomes. *Psychiatr Ann.* 2007;37(5):359–364.
19. Fonagy P, Target M. Fonagy and Target's model of mentalization. In: *Psychoanalytic Theories: Perspectives from Developmental Psychopathology.* Brunner-Routledge; 2003:270–282.
20. Edwards VJ, Holden GW, Felitti VJ, Anda RF. Relationship between multiple forms of childhood maltreatment and adult mental health in community respondents: Results from the Adverse Childhood Experiences Study. *Am J Psychiatry.* 2003;160(8):1453–1460.

21. Mullen PE, Martin JL, Anderson JC, Romans SE, Herbison GP. The long-term impact of the physical, emotional, and sexual abuse of children: A community study. *Child Abuse Neglect.* 1996;20(1):7–21.
22. Afifi TO, Enns MW, Cox BJ, Asmundson GJ, Stein MB, Sareen J. Population attributable fractions of psychiatric disorders and suicide ideation and attempts associated with adverse childhood experiences. *Am J Public Health.* 2008;98(5):946–952.
23. Chapman DP, Whitfield CL, Felitti VJ, Dube SR, Edwards VJ, Anda RF. Adverse childhood experiences and the risk of depressive disorders in adulthood. *J Affect Disord.* 2004;82(2):217–225.
24. Merrick MT, Ports KA, Ford DC, Afifi TO, Gershoff ET, Grogan-Kaylor A. Unpacking the impact of adverse childhood experiences on adult mental health. *Child Abuse Neglect.* 2017;69:10–19.
25. McCauley J, Kern DE, Kolodner K, et al. Clinical characteristics of women with a history of childhood abuse: Unhealed wounds. *JAMA.* 1997;277(17):1362–1368.
26. Schilling EA, Aseltine RH, Gore S. Adverse childhood experiences and mental health in young adults: A longitudinal survey. *BMC Public Health.* 2007;7(1):1–10.
27. Dube SR, Anda RF, Felitti VJ, Chapman DP, Williamson DF, Giles WH. Childhood abuse, household dysfunction, and the risk of attempted suicide throughout the life span: Findings from the Adverse Childhood Experiences Study. *JAMA.* 2001;286(24):3089–3096.
28. Dube SR, Felitti VJ, Dong M, Chapman DP, Giles WH, Anda RF. Childhood abuse, neglect, and household dysfunction and the risk of illicit drug use: The Adverse Childhood Experiences Study. *Pediatrics.* 2003;111(3):564–572.
29. Kalmakis KA, Chandler GE. Health consequences of adverse childhood experiences: A systematic review. *J Am Assoc Nurse Pract.* 2015;27(8):457–465.
30. LeardMann CA, Smith B, Ryan MA. Do adverse childhood experiences increase the risk of postdeployment posttraumatic stress disorder in US Marines? *BMC Public Health.* 2010;10(1):1–8.
31. Wu NS, Schairer LC, Dellor E, Grella C. Childhood trauma and health outcomes in adults with comorbid substance abuse and mental health disorders. *Addict Behav.* 2010;35(1):68–71.
32. Battle CL, Shea MT, Johnson DM, et al. Childhood maltreatment associated with adult personality disorders: Findings from the Collaborative Longitudinal Personality Disorders Study. *J Pers Disord.* 2004;18(2):193–211.
33. Afifi TO, Mather A, Boman J, et al. Childhood adversity and personality disorders: Results from a nationally representative population-based study. *J Psychiatr Res.* 2011;45(6):814–822.
34 Gunderson JG, Chu JA. Treatment implications of past trauma in borderline personality disorder. *Harv Rev Psychiatry.* 1993;1(2):75–81.
35. Borrell-Carrió F, Suchman AL, Epstein RM. The biopsychosocial model 25 years later: Principles, practice, and scientific inquiry. *Ann Fam Med.* 2004;2(6):576–582.
36. Sheffler JL, Stanley I, Sachs-Ericsson N. ACEs and mental health outcomes. In: Asmundson GJG, Afifi TO, eds. *Adverse Childhood Experiences: Using Evidence to Advance Research, Practice, Policy, and Prevention.* Academic Press; 2020:47–69.
37. Nusslock R, Miller GE. Early-life adversity and physical and emotional health across the lifespan: A neuroimmune network hypothesis. *Biol Psychiatry.* 2016;80(1):23–32.
38. Brodsky BS, Stanley B. Adverse childhood experiences and suicidal behavior. *Psychiatr Clin North Am.* 2008;31(2):223–235.
39. Helitzer D, Graeber D, LaNoue M, Newbill S. Don't step on the tiger's tail: A mixed methods study of the relationship between adult impact of childhood adversity and use of coping strategies. *Community Ment Health J.* 2015;51(7), 768–774.
40. Liu RT, Choi JY, Boland EM, Mastin BM, Alloy LB. Childhood abuse and stress generation: The mediational effect of depressogenic cognitive styles. *Psychiatry Res.* 2013;206(2–3):217–222.
41. Sachs-Ericsson N, Verona E, Joiner T, Preacher KJ. Parental verbal abuse and the mediating role of self-criticism in adult internalizing disorders. *J Affect Disord.* 2006;93(1–3):71–78.
42. Sachs-Ericsson N, Joiner TE, Cougle JR, Stanley IH, Sheffler JL. Combat exposure in early adulthood interacts with recent stressors to predict PTSD in aging male veterans. *Gerontologist.* 2015;56(1):82–91.

43. Cloitre M, Khan C, Mackintosh MA, et al. Emotion regulation mediates the relationship between ACES and physical and mental health. *Psychol Trauma*. 2019;11(1):82–89.
44. Gratz KL, Roemer L. Multidimensional assessment of emotion regulation and dysregulation: Development, factor structure, and initial validation of the difficulties in emotion regulation scale. *J Psychopathol Behav Assess*. 2004;26:41–54.
45. Sheppes G, Suri G, Gross JJ. Emotion regulation and psychopathology. *Annu Rev Clin Psychol*. 2015;11:379–405.
46. Bowlby J. *A Secure Base: Clinical Applications of Attachment Theory*. Routledge; 1988.
47. Murphy A, Steele M, Dube SR, et al. Adverse childhood experiences (ACEs) questionnaire and Adult Attachment Interview (AAI): Implications for parent child relationships. *Child Abuse Neglect*. 2014;38(2):224–233.
48. Levy KN, Meehan KB, Weber M, Reynoso J, Clarkin JF. Attachment and borderline personality disorder: Implications for psychotherapy. *Psychopathology*. 2005;38(2):64–74.
49. Fonagy P. Attachment and borderline personality disorder. *J Am Psychoanal Assoc*. 2000;48(4):1129–1146.
50. Fonagy P, Allison E. The role of mentalizing and epistemic trust in the therapeutic relationship. *Psychotherapy*. 2014;51(3):372–380.
51. Bateman AW, & Fonagy PE. *Handbook of Mentalizing in Mental Health Practice*. American Psychiatric Publishing; 2012.
52. Ensink K, Berthelot N, Bernazzani O, Normandin L, Fonagy P. Another step closer to measuring the ghosts in the nursery: Preliminary validation of the Trauma Reflective Functioning Scale. *Front Psychol*. 2014;5:1471.
53. Nelson SM, Cunningham NR, Kashikar-Zuck S. A conceptual framework for understanding the role of adverse childhood experiences in pediatric chronic pain. *Clin J Pain*. 2017;33(3):264–270.
54. Kerker BD, Zhang J, Nadeem E, et al. Adverse childhood experiences and mental health, chronic medical conditions, and development in young children. *Acad Pediatr*. 2015;15(5):510–517.
55. Groenewald CB, Murray CB, Palermo TM. Adverse childhood experiences and chronic pain among children and adolescents in the United States. *Pain Rep*. 2020;5(5):e839.
56. Kascakova N, Furstova J, Hasto J, Madarasova Geckova A, Tavel P. The unholy trinity: Childhood trauma, adulthood anxiety, and long-term pain. *Int J Environ Res Public Health*. 2020;17(2): Article 414.
57. Battaglia, M., Garon-Carrier, G., Brendgen, M., Feng, B., Dionne, G., Vitaro, F., Tremblay, R.E. and Boivin, M., 2020. Trajectories of pain and anxiety in a longitudinal cohort of adolescent twins. *Depression and anxiety*, 37(5), pp.475–484.
58. Campo JV, Di Lorenzo C, Chiappetta L, et al. Adult outcomes of pediatric recurrent abdominal pain: Do they just grow out of it? *Pediatrics*. 2001;108(1):e1.
59. Quartana PJ, Campbell CM, Edwards RR. Pain catastrophizing: A critical review. *Expert Rev Neurother*. 2009;9(5):745–758.
60. Dobson K, Pusch D, Allan L, Gonzalez S, Poole J, Mar G. The long shadow of adverse childhood events: 2. Physical health outcomes in an adult community sample. *Am J Prev Med Public Health*. 2020;6(2):39–49.
61. Clauw DJ. Fibromyalgia: A clinical review. *JAMA*. 2014;311(15):1547–1555.
62. Eich M, Hartmann A, Müller H, Fischer W. The role of psychosocial factors in fibromyalgia syndrome. *Scand J Rheumatol*. 2000;29(109):30–31.
63. Imbierowicz K, Egle UT. Childhood adversities in patients with fibromyalgia and somatoform pain disorder. *Eur J Pain*. 2003;7(2):113–119.
64. Olivieri P, Solitar B, Dubois M. Childhood risk factors for developing fibromyalgia. *Open Access Rheumatol*. 2012;4:109–114.
65. Tietjen GE, Brandes JL, Peterlin BL, et al. Childhood maltreatment and migraine (Part I). Prevalence and adult revictimization: A multicenter headache clinic survey. *Headache*. 2010;50(1):20–31.

66. Torres-Ferrús M, Ursitti F, Alpuente A, et al. From transformation to chronification of migraine: Pathophysiological and clinical aspects. *J Headache Pain.* 2020;21(1):1–12.
67. Anto M, Jaffee S, Tietjen G, Mendizabal A, Szperka C. Adverse childhood experiences and frequent headache by adolescent self-report. *Pediatr Neurol.* 2021;121:51–55.
68. Tietjen GE, Brandes JL, Peterlin BL, et al. Childhood maltreatment and migraine (Part II). Emotional abuse as a risk factor for headache chronification. *Headache.* 2010;50(1):32–41.
69. Mansuri F, Nash MC, Bakour C, Kip K. Adverse childhood experiences (ACEs) and headaches among children: A cross-sectional analysis. *Headache.* 2020;60(4):735–744.
70. Saha L. Irritable bowel syndrome: Pathogenesis, diagnosis, treatment, and evidence-based medicine. *World J Gastroenterol.* 2014;20(22):6759–6773.
71. Joshee S, Lim L, Wybrecht A, Berriesford R, Riddle M. Meta-analysis and systematic review of the association between adverse childhood events and irritable bowel syndrome. *J Investig Med.* 2022;70(6):1342–1351.
72. Park SH, Videlock EJ, Shih W, Presson AP, Mayer EA, Chang L. Adverse childhood experiences are associated with irritable bowel syndrome and gastrointestinal symptom severity. *Neurogastroenterol Motil.* 2016;28(8):1252–1260.
73. Vercellini P, Somigliana E, Viganò P, Abbiati A, Barbara G, Fedele L. Chronic pelvic pain in women: Etiology, pathogenesis and diagnostic approach. *Gynecol Endocrinol.* 2009;25(3):149–158.
74. Moussaoui, D. and Grover, S.R., 2022. The association between childhood adversity and risk of dysmenorrhea, pelvic pain, and dyspareunia in adolescents and young adults: a systematic review. *Journal of Pediatric and Adolescent Gynecology*, 35(5), pp.567–574.
75. Krantz TE, Andrews N, Petersen TR, et al. Adverse childhood experiences among gynecology patients with chronic pelvic pain. *Obstet Gynecol.* 2019;134(5):1087–1095.
76. Komesu YM, Petersen TR, Krantz TE, et al. Adverse childhood experiences in women with overactive bladder or interstitial cystitis/bladder pain syndrome. *Female Pelvic Med Reconstr Surg.* 2021;27(1):e208–e214.
77. Piontek K, Apfelbacher C, Ketels G, Brünahl C, Löwe B. Depression partially mediates the association of adverse childhood experiences with pain intensity in patients with chronic pelvic pain syndrome: Results from a cross-sectional patient survey. *Pain Med.* 2021;22(5):1174–1184.
78. Schrepf A, Naliboff B, Williams DA, et al.; MAPP Research Network. Adverse childhood experiences and symptoms of urologic chronic pelvic pain syndrome: A multidisciplinary approach to the study of chronic pelvic pain research network study. *Ann Behav Med.* 2018;52(10):865–877.
79. Centers for Disease Control and Prevention. *Preventing Adverse Childhood Experiences: Leveraging the Best Available Evidence.* National Center for Injury Prevention and Control, Centers for Disease Control and Prevention; 2019.
80. Olds DL, Eckenrode J, Henderson CR Jr, et al. Long-term effects of home visitation on maternal life course and child abuse and neglect: Fifteen-year follow-up of a randomized trial. *JAMA.* 1997;278(8):637–643.
81. Lieberman A, Ippen C, Horn P. Child–parent psychotherapy: 6-month follow-up of a randomized controlled trial. *J Am Acad Child Adolesc Psychiatry.* 2006;45:913–918.
82. Hoffman K, Marvin R, Cooper G, Powell B. Changing toddlers' and preschoolers' attachment classifications: The Circle of Security Intervention. *J Consult Clin Psychol.* 2006;74:1017–1026.
83. Purkey, E., Davison, C., MacKenzie, M. et al. Experience of emergency department use among persons with a history of adverse childhood experiences. *BMC Health Serv Res* **20**, 455 (2020). https://doi.org/10.1186/s12913-020-05291-6.
84. Ranjbar N, Erb M. Adverse childhood experiences and trauma-informed care in rehabilitation clinical practice. *Arch Rehabil Res Clin Transl.* 2019;1(1–2):100003.
85. Wahbeh, H., Senders, A., Neuendorf, R., & Cayton, J. (2018). Complementary and alternative medicine for posttraumatic stress disorder symptoms: A systematic review. *Focus*, 16(1), 98–112.
86. Ortiz R, Gilgoff R, Harris NB. Adverse childhood experiences, toxic stress, and trauma-informed neurology. *JAMA Neurol.* 2022;79(6):539–540.

14
Vulnerable Populations
Disparate Pain Care

Jana M. Mossey and Emily A. Haozous

Introduction

For the past several decades, countless resources have been invested exploring differences in how people respond to pain. It is now well established that culture, race, and ethnicity are closely woven into how individuals experience and react to pain.[1,2] More recently, attention has been directed to the examination of how pain care is delivered. Since 1993 when Todd et al.[3] reported Hispanic males seen in the emergency department (ED) with a long bone fracture received substandard pain care compared to non-Hispanic White (NHW) males, a large number of publications have reported evidence that unequal assessment and management of all types of pain continue. The research reports are uncomfortably predictable: Patients who have limited resources or are any population other than NHW are less likely to have their pain consistently and accurately assessed, are offered fewer options for treatment, and are prescribed fewer medications or at inadequate doses.[4] Clearly, there is a tolerance for the suffering of others within health care where pain is concerned. At this point in history, while further exploring the tacit acceptance of this disparity despite the mountain of evidence, we must pivot and (1) refine our understanding of the meaning and etiologies of "vulnerability" to inequitable pain care; and (2) identify, implement, and evaluate actions designed to diminish pain care disparities and to achieve equity in pain care delivery to all individuals and "population groups."

Consistent with the work of Mathur et al.[5] regarding the experience of pain, we view disparate pain care, vulnerability to receipt of such care, and lack of optimal treatment outcomes from an "injustice perspective," where "injustice" is defined as "unfairness, violations of equity and/or the rights of individuals or population groups."[5(p999),6] In Figure 1 in their paper,[5(p1001)] Mathur et al. present a multilevel hierarchy that specifies cultural, institutional, and interpersonal injustices that impact each lower category. The fourth segment of Figure 1 specifies pain-specific intrapersonal processes (cognitive, emotional, behavioral, and biological) that reflect an individual's responses to the different levels of experienced injustice. Implicit in taking this approach is the recognition that injustices from each hierarchical level perpetrated on minoritized individuals and groups are the primary contributors to the observed disparities in their disease risk; health status disparities; and inequitable preventive, diagnostic, and treatment health services. This represents a paradigm shift because, historically, large segments of the general population, including many health care providers, have attributed the poorer health status and health care disparities experienced by minoritized group members to their supposed inadequacies, indifference, deceit, and/or stupidity. In acknowledging the fundamental etiologic importance of cultural, institutional, and interpersonal injustices, pain care providers must recognize that the achievement of health status and health care equity across all population groups will require the cessation of injustices at each level.

Reflecting the importance of the injustice perspective from which to address disparities in pain, the remainder of this chapter is presented in three sections: The background section identifies the most vulnerable and/or minoritized population groups and provides a summary of findings pertinent to pain care disparities, the next section characterizes multilevel sources of injustices and intrapersonal consequences of such injustices, and the third section identifies issues pertinent to the development and implementation of anti-racial educational programs.

Background

Historically, a population group has been considered "vulnerable" as a function of age, maternity status, physical disability, disease, and/or prolonged poverty. Other population groups become vulnerable when they uniquely experience high-risk negative events or when members of the dominant, powerful group identify them as unequal, deficient, unworthy, or inadequate. Not all vulnerable groups become "minoritized,"[7] an imposed lesser status characterized by disenfranchisement and deprivation of amenities, services, social acceptance, wealth, etc. Phenotype (e.g., skin color, hair texture, and other easily observable physical characteristics), differences in cultural behaviors (e.g., familial organization, societal role assignments, and religious beliefs), and/or the absence of mastered skills such as reading, writing, and fluency in the language of those in power have been used to devalue multigenerational populations. In the United States, descendants of dark-skinned Africans, purchased as slaves and, until emancipation, treated as property, continue to be thought of, by many, as "lesser." Whether due to fear of losing their long-standing power, complacency, or ignorance, many NHW Americans remain hostile and suspicious toward darker skinned individuals. Through laws, policies, and behaviors, NHW appear to continually strive to keep "others" marginalized. Regrettably, children, elders, pregnant women, and disabled or infirm individuals whose skin color is darker (e.g., non-Hispanic Black [NHB], Hispanic [HISP], American Indians and Alaska Natives [AI/AN], and Native Hawaiian/ Pacific Islander [NHPI]) appear particularly vulnerable to receipt of substandard pain care compared to that provided NHW.[8] Other population subgroups that have experienced pain care disparities include individuals of all backgrounds who are poor[9]; active drug abusers[10]; LGBTQ individuals[11]; persons not fluent in English[12]; and women of all racial/ethnic groups, including NHW females.[13]

As mentioned previously, a large literature exists concerning disparities in pain care, and several recent comprehensive literature reviews are available.[8,14–19] Rather than provide yet another lengthy summary of the evidence pertinent to disparate pain care, in Table 14.1 the findings of previous reviews are summarized. As seen here, compared to NHW patients, the pain levels of minoritized individuals (NHB, AI/AN, and HISP),

Table 14.1 Summary: Identified Published Evidence of Disparities in Pain Care

Disparity Evidence: Compared to Non-Hispanic Whites	Racial/Ethnic, Age, Sex, Groups Impacted[a]
Pain Assessment	
Pain level not assessed by treating provider (EMT, ED)	NHB, HISP, AN/AI (C&A, M&F)
Provider pain assessment lower than patient's report (ED)	NHB, HISP (C&A, M&F)
Provider told patient she/he was lying about pain or said pain was "imaginary" or due to emotions (PCP office)	NHB, HISP, NHW, AN/AI (A mainly F)
Excessive time delay from ED arrival to initial pain assessment	NHB, HISP (C&A, M&F)
Provision Opioid Analgesic	
In transit to ED, opioid analgesic not prescribed or prescribed at dose insufficient for pain level	NHB, HISP (C&A, M&F)
Within ED, opioid analgesic not prescribed or at insufficient dose or less effective analgesic prescribed (e.g., NSAID)	NHB, HISP, AN/AI (C&A,M&F)
At ED discharge, opioid analgesic not prescribed or at insufficient dose or less effective analgesic prescribed	NHB, HISP, AI/AN (C&A, M&F)
During pre-/post-op surgical pain care, opioid analgesic not given or given at a lower dose	NHB, HISP (C,M&F)
Post cesarean section, prescribed opioid analgesic lower than for equivalent reported pain level	NHB (A, F)
At hospital discharge, opioid analgesic not prescribed or at lower dose or less effective analgesic prescribed	NHB, HISP (C&A, M&F)
Cancer patients prescribed lower opioid analgesic dose (annual prescriptions filled in morphine milligram equivalents)	NHB (A, M&F)
At PCP office, patients given lower dose opioid analgesic prescription at end of visit	NHB (A, M&F)
At PCP office, patients given opioid prescription are required to return for monitoring more frequently	NHB (A, M&F)
PCP refuses to "call in" an opioid analgesic prescription refill to the patient's pharmacy	NHB, HISP (A, M&F)
Other Evidence of Disparities	
At ED, patient discharged without complete assessment by physician	NHB (A, M&F)
Patient returns, within 30 days, to ED with same presenting pain complaint	NHB, AN/AI (A, M&F)
In PCP office, patient shown disrespect; provider scheduled shorter appointment time or cuts appointment short, ridicules patient, calls patient a liar	NHB, HISP, AN/AI (A, M&F)
Nursing home pain management inadequate; higher pain prevalence	NHB (A, M&F)

[a]All ethnic/racial groups for which published evidence has been identified are shown. Ethnic/racial groups not identified as impacted by the disparity may have experienced it, but evidence had not been found.

A, adults; AI, American Indian; AN, American Native; C, children; ED, emergency department; EMT, emergency medical technician; F, female; HISP, Hispanic; M, male; NHB, non-Hispanic Black; NHW, non-Hispanic White; NSAID, nonsteroidal anti-inflammatory drug; PCP, primary care physician.

including male and female, children and adults, consistently were less often assessed and less accurately determined by pain practitioners.

Without an accurate patient pain assessment, quality, appropriate care plans simply cannot be developed. During the past three decades, the failure to prescribe similarly effective opioid analgesics to NHB, AI/AN, and HISP by emergency medical technicians (EMTs) and in ED, hospital, and physician office settings relative to the NHW experiences consistently has been documented. Short- and long-term adverse impacts on the patient can be extensive. As Mossey[8] noted, prolonged acute pain due to long ED waits before receiving any analgesia can evoke anxiety, fear, desperation, or panic. Discharge from the ED or hospital without an effective analgesic prescription can prolong physical suffering and result in distrust, anger, and helplessness. Work or school absenteeism and delayed accomplishment of age-appropriate milestones may result in depression, anxiety, and low quality of life. In addition, long-term rates of chronic pain and postsurgical chronic pain have been observed for affected children and adults; increased pain severity and serious high-impact pain have been reported. Such consequences of past pain care disparities represent significant "injustices."

Multilevel Sources and Examples of Injustice Experienced by Minoritized Individuals

Reflecting the hierarchical classification of injustices perpetrated on minoritized individuals that was developed by Mathur et al.,[5] Box 14.1 identifies injustices and descriptive examples.

Reaction of Minoritized/Oppressed Individuals to Multiple Levels of Injustice

Regrettably, but not unexpected, members of minoritized groups often come to believe the pejorative, dismissive, demeaning messages they receive. "Internalized racism" can result in a passive acceptance of discriminatory messages and behaviors. Clinical depression, feeling worthless, can compound poorly treated pain. Coupled with persistent injustices of inadequate living circumstances (crowding, violence, poor schools, food insecurity, etc.), minoritized individuals endure chronic exposures to noxious stimuli. As noted in Chapter 4, such chronic exposure can evoke neurophysiological stress response system overload that may negatively impact central nervous system pain processing; increase depression risk; and alter the functioning of autonomic nervous, endocrine, and immune systems. Such neurophysiological changes increase risk of idiopathic chronic pain conditions.

The interpersonal injustices shown in Box 14.1, expose minoritized individuals to additional unfavorable circumstances. When a pain care provider displays ambivalent, dismissive, or indifferent reactions and behaviors toward patients, implicitly or explicitly, considered inadequate or unworthy, poorly treated patients withdraw their trust. The mutually positive doctor–patient relationship, crucial to effective communication regarding the occurrence and nature of self-reported pain, does not exist. Patients

Box 14.1 Categories and Examples of Injustices Experienced by Minoritized Groups

Cultural Injustices

- Beliefs that status and success are based on an individual's talent and effort (e.g., a meritocracy). A meritocracy can only be equitable if the playing field is level and every group has comparable access to resources (e.g., safe environments, quality education, accessible health care, and wealth). Minoritized population groups, especially, NHB, AI/AN, and HISP, do not have the same access to resources as NHW. White power-holders have intentionally limited their access and have often selectively punished those whose accomplishments were deemed threatening (e.g., creating targeted ineligibility rules, refusing promotions, withholding higher education opportunities, and threatening violence).
- Beliefs that multigenerational histories of slavery, denigration, submission, violence, etc. have no impact on younger descendants and can be disregarded. Such beliefs lay blame for lower achievement levels or transgressions on the minoritized individual so those in power can legitimately avoid reparations, affirmative action policies, or provision of compensatory resources such as excellent schools and mental health services.
- Beliefs that decisions regarding resource allocation or acceptances (e.g., promotions and school entrance) should be made "colorblind." The impact of this worldview is comparable to dismissing multigenerational histories and denies affirmative actions, selectively greater resource allocations, etc., and it serves to maintain the existing NHW power structure.
- Advocating that slavery protected "genetically lesser" NHB represents a pathetic and distorted justification for past transgressions.
- Reflecting their belief that NHB were "lesser," initiating and then hiding abusive medical experimentation on NHB (e.g., the Tuskegee Syphilis Study). The perpetrated abuse represents an extreme injustice and continues to diminish trust.
- Misinformed but persistently held "beliefs" that NHB and AN/AI males are genetically inferior and have violent natures have provided "righteous justification" for exerting harsh proactive punishments. Contemporarily this is manifest in beating and killing unarmed NHB by law officers and citizens.
- Ascribing to an individual characteristics of a group that are false but spread by those who are more powerful (e.g., NHB feel less pain than NHW; NHB are more likely to abuse opioid analgesics than NHW; immigrants are "rapists and criminals"; and women are "needy" and exaggerate). The individual becomes invisible.
- The enduring believe by dominant group members of their "right" to hold power because they are better and more worthy justifies "whatever it takes" to maintain their status, including violence.

Institutional Injustices

- Development and enforcement of laws designed to disenfranchise minoritized groups and deny them resources and opportunities (e.g., access to voting, well-funded school, and quality, funded health care). Despite civil rights and voting laws enacted during the 1960s, efforts currently are underway to reverse the gains toward equity by passing restrictive voting laws, reducing funding for public schools, etc.
- Tolerance of discrepancies between the written and enacted laws that allow stricter enforcement for NHB and Hispanic individuals (e.g., NHB and Hispanic individuals [especially males] are more likely than NHW to undergo "stop and frisk," be searched, receive physical abuse by police, be stopped by police while driving, be incarcerated pretrial due to inability to pay "cash bail," and receive longer sentences and disproportionate incarceration on death row).
- Legislative attempts to diminish government-funded health care and/or health insurance. This reduces already limited access to health care and further jeopardizes opportunities for preventive health care, early intervention, and appropriate management of chronic conditions.
- Persistent, subtle continuation of "redlining" policies to sustain neighborhood segregation. Residence in high concentrations of disadvantaged individuals increases exposure to noxious stressors such as violence, food and housing insecurity, etc.
- Preferential placement of toxic, polluting, undesirable structures and businesses near segregated neighborhoods selectively exposes minoritized individuals to dangerous chemical substances and noxious experiences.

Interpersonal Injustice

- Failure of a pain provider to address their own implicit and explicit biases. Such failure is irresponsible and exposes the patient to unpleasantness and potential danger through delivery of inferior pain care.
- Active displays of discriminatory and prejudicial behaviors (e.g., not greeting the patient pleasantly and/or inappropriately referring to an adult by their first name, calling the patient a liar, scheduling shorter appointment sessions, withholding information, and refusing to refer a patient to a relevant specialist).
- Treating individuals in discriminatory, demeaning, stereotypic ways due to failure to address, for example, one's racial or homophobic implicit biases (e.g., not making eye contact with the patient, not listening to what the patient says, and treating the patient with indifference or rudeness).
- Perpetrating subtle forms of discrimination through microaggressions (e.g., complementing an African American but, instead, indirectly denigrating the individual; the sentence, "You are great; you don't think like a Black person" is an example).
- Attributing to the patient false beliefs/stereotypes associated with their sex or presumed "racial/ethnic" background (e.g., believing NHB exaggerate their pain severity and not prescribing an adequate analgesic, withholding an opioid analgesic prescription because "the meds will be sold," and telling a woman complaining of widespread pain it is in her head because women exaggerate).

experience feelings of betrayal, distrust, powerlessness, etc., and providers tend to become frustrated and angry. Treatment success is compromised. Studies indicate that distrust with their physician, other pain care providers, and the health care system is prevalent among NHB, HISP, AI/AN, and other minoritized groups, including many women.[20]

Critical to the occurrence and persistence of pain care disparities, cultural and structural forms of racism and associated injustices have long and deeply rooted histories in the United States and elsewhere. Interpersonal injustices reflect culturally embedded values and laws/policies established long ago by NHW individuals. Such laws and policies are maintained at huge expense to minoritized individuals. Given strong cultural and structural influences on belief formation, it is not surprising that pain care providers have explicitly and implicitly adopted attitudes and behaviors modeled by those in power. Without numerous, strong anti-racist role models or a committed sense that equity/justice are essential values, delivery of disparate pain care is easy to imagine. Some have argued that the for-profit health care system perpetuated in the United States is responsible for most disparate care because physicians are expected to maximize the number of patients they see daily. Such pressure can impact practitioner equilibrium; however, the observation that minoritized patients, but not all patients, are adversely affected discredits this explanation. Irrespective of which explanations are most credible, substantial progress toward achieving equitable pain care should be possible if the negative, false, and dismissive attitudes and beliefs of pain care providers toward currently minoritized population groups were to accurately reflect the truth. It is clear that the delivery of universal, sustainable, equitable pain care is unlikely until the "upstream" cultural and systemic injustices have been eradicated. The next section focuses on issues important for the development of educational programs purposed to bring about sustainable changes in the beliefs, attitudes, and behaviors of existing and future pain care providers.

Moving Forward: Eliminating Ethnic/Racial and Gender Pain Care Disparities

As noted in the Introduction, the injustices due to disparate pain care have been documented in the scientific literature for more than three decades. Although changing current pain care practices is expected to require enormous effort and substantial time, years perhaps, continuation of inequitable pain care is untenable and unethical. Below, suggestions are presented pertinent to designing formal academic anti-racist educational programs and informal self-taught learning when anti-racist educational programs are unavailable.

Anti-Racist Academic Education Programs

Within the health care system, existing health care practitioners require re-education, and comprehensive anti-racist curricula are needed to accomplish this. Some anti-racist educational programs already had been established in health profession educational institutions, residency, and graduate programs prior to the Black Lives Matter movement in 2020; unfortunately, quality and effectiveness evaluations have reported discouraging results.[21] Examination of more recent program reviews and scientific articles indicates that antiracist education "best practice" guidelines suitable for use in the training of health care providers have not been established. Best practice guidelines should reflect the following:

- Comprehensive anti-racist education programs require a very long duration with periotic refresher sessions. The lengthy and repeated nature of the programs reflects the recognition that most target audiences are adults. Consequently, the first curriculum units will need to focus on unlearning held values and neutralizing past bad experiences. The second curricular components will need to focus on relearning new values and opinions. In the guidelines for learning a new skill, Adams[22] suggests, "[For each] skill we decide to learn, there are four learning stages . . . 1 Unconsciously unskilled . . . 2 Consciously unskilled . . . 3 Consciously skilled . . . 4 Unconsciously skilled." The author also notes, "Being aware of these stages helps us better accept that learning can be a slow and frequently uncomfortable process."[22]
- An important missing ingredient of many programs is "time." Acknowledgment and reversal of implicit biases so they do not "leak out" as microaggressions, or other injustices, require repetitive, mentored book and experiential learning and interactions with individuals from minoritized groups. Considerable time each year during undergraduate and graduate training should be allocated to allow for reflection, accumulative learning, and personal exploration. Ideally, students should enter anti-racist educational programs as soon as possible. Multiyear academic curricula could begin on entrance to college and continue through the individual's highest level graduation (e.g., advanced academic or professional degree).
- Unwavering commitment by administration and faculty, substantial focused and sustained personnel and financial resources, and extensive dedicated time are essential for the success of the educational program development, implementation, and evaluation. Recent reviews of anti-racism programs in medical education settings have observed many nascent programs with administrative "buy-in" but tenuous commitments for allocation of financial resources. Faculty appear interested, but an absence of qualified faculty for program planning, curriculum development, and student mentoring was seen in approximately 50% of the investigated sites.[23]
- The educational planning and teaching team should be composed of faculty with expertise in the relevant content and concept areas, such as culture and history of slavery; racism; White supremacy; intercultural relationships; the creation and persistence of minoritized populations; psychological, social, emotional, and health experiences of such populations; equity; justice and injustice; and health disparities. Faculty, students, and community members from diverse sociocultural backgrounds—including NHB, NHW, AI/AN, HISP, LGBTQ, racially mixed, etc.—need to be actively involved in planning, implementation, and evaluation. To facilitate unlearning and relearning, multiple program formats are required—for example, content lectures; seminars including students, faculty, and community

members to facilitate dialog, sharing, and interpretation; and experiential learning (e.g., short, intense experiences; periods embedded in an unfamiliar community; multicultural retreats; and regularly scheduled follow-up and refresher sessions).

Anti-Racist Education Activities When Institutional Academic Programs Are Unavailable

Although urgently needed, not all academic institutions can support a time-intensive, multiyear anti-racist educational program. When such programs are not supportable, students, administrative personnel, and practicing pain providers are encouraged to initiate their own anti-racist education activities, including the following:

- Self-education: Read scholarly and opinion materials; and attend lectures and classes addressing slavery, racism, the motives of those who marginalize others, the lived experiences of minoritized individuals, etc.
- Engage with others from diverse backgrounds; ask for help in identifying and addressing your implicit biases. Learn how others have overcome explicit, implicit, and false biases.
- Become familiar with important cultural histories and health-related norms held by NHN, AI/AN, HISP, and other groups, such as Asians and LGBTQ individuals.
- Daily observe the environment; watch for racist comments, interactions, policies, and laws; step up and advocate for equity, equal human rights, and justice rather than injustice.

Conclusion

This chapter began with the observations that knowledge of pain care disparities harming minoritized individuals has existed for decades, little progress has been made to diminish or eliminate inequitable care, and continuation of the past practices is untenable. In summarizing specific evidence of disparate care, an injustice framework has been used. From this approach, disparate care is not just poor pain care delivered to selective "minoritized" segments of the population; rather, it is an injustice perpetrated by individual providers and health care systems. Although many cultural and structural factors beyond the control of health care systems influence the status quo, pain care administrators, educators, and practitioners must take responsibility for their contributions to the existing injustices. It is essential that these groups speedily initiate the corrective changes necessary to provide pain care characterized by equity, quality, and compassion.

References

1. Mills SE, Nicolson KP, Smith BH. Chronic pain: A review of its epidemiology and associated factors in population-based studies. *Br J Anaesth*. 2019;123(2):e273–e283.

2. Macfarlane GJ. The epidemiology of chronic pain. *Pain*. 2016;157(10):2158–2159.
3. Todd KH, Samaroo N, Hoffman JR. Ethnicity as a risk factor for inadequate emergency department analgesia. *JAMA*. 1993;269(12):1537–1539.
4. Janevic MR, McLaughlin SJ, Heapy AA, et al. Racial and socioeconomic disparities in disabling chronic pain: Findings from the health and retirement study. *J Pain*. 2017;18(12):1459–1467.
5. Mathur VA, Trost Z, Ezenwa MO, et al. Mechanisms of injustice: What we (do not) know about racialized disparities in pain. *Pain*. 2022;163(6): Article 999.
6. Merriam-Webster. Equity. In: *Merriam-Webster.com Dictionary*. n.d. Accessed December 28, 2022. https://www.merriam-webster.com/dictionary/equity
7. Smith IE. Minority vs minoritized: Why the noun just doesn't cut it. *Odessey, Politics and Activism*. 2016. Accessed January 10, 2023. https://www.theodysseyonline.com/minority-vs-minoritize
8. Mossey JM. Disparities in pain care: Descriptive epidemiology-potential for primary prevention. In: Benzon HM, Rathmell JP, Wu CL, et al., eds. *Practical Management of Pain E-Book*. Elsevier; 2022.
9. Anastas TM, Miller MM, Hollingshead NA, et al. The unique and interactive effects of patient race, patient socioeconomic status, and provider attitudes on chronic pain care decisions. *Ann Behav Med*. 2020;54(10):771–782.
10. Dassieu L, Kaboré JL, Choinière M, et al. Chronic pain management among people who use drugs: A health policy challenge in the context of the opioid crisis. *Int J Drug Policy*. 2019;71:150–156.
11. Abd-Elsayed A, Heyer AM, Schatman ME. Disparities in the treatment of the LGBTQ population in chronic pain management. *J Pain Res*. 2021; 30:3623–3625.
12. Lor M, Koleck TA, Lee C, Moua Z, et al. Documentation of pain care and treatment for limited English proficiency minority patients with moderate-to-severe pain in primary care. *WMJ*. 2022;1:86–93.
13. Lloyd EP, Paganini GA, ten Brinke L. Gender stereotypes explain disparities in pain care and inform equitable policies. *Policy Insights Behav Brain Sci*. 2020;7(2):198–204.
14. Eze B, Kumar S, Yang Y, et al. Bias in musculoskeletal pain management and bias-targeted interventions to improve pain outcomes: A scoping review. *Orthop Nurs*. 2022;41(2):137–145.
15. Farcas AM, Joiner AP, Rudman JS, et al. Disparities in emergency medical services care delivery in the United States: A scoping review. *Prehosp Emerg Care*. 2022;14:1–4.
16. Morales ME, Yong RJ. Racial and ethnic disparities in the treatment of chronic pain. *Pain Med*. 2021;22(1):75–90.
17. Meghani SH, Byun E, Gallagher RM. Time to take stock: A meta-analysis and systematic review of analgesic treatment disparities for pain in the United States. *Pain Med*. 2012;13(2):150–1574.
18. Mossey JM. Defining racial and ethnic disparities in pain management. *Clin Orthop Relat R*. 2011;469:1859–1870.
19. Institute of Medicine. *Relieving Pain in America: A Blueprint for Transforming Prevention, Care, Education, and Research*. National Academies Press; 2011.
20. Sewell AA. Disaggregating ethnoracial disparities in physician trust. *Soc Sci Res*. 2015;54:1–20.
21. Hassen N, Lofters A, Michael S, et al. Implementing anti-racism interventions in healthcare settings: A scoping review. *Int J Environ Res Public Health*. 2021;18(6):2993.
22. Adams L. Learning a new skill is easier said than done. Gordon Training International. n.d. Accessed January 21, 2023. https://www.gordontraining.com/free-workplace-articles/learning-a-new-skill-is-easier-said-than-done
23. Fatahi G, Racic M, Roche-Miranda MI, et al. The current state of antiracism curricula in undergraduate and graduate medical education: A qualitative study of US academic health centers. *Ann Fam Med*. 2023;21(Suppl 2):S14–S21.

15
Pain in Patients Living in Congregant Settings
Incarceration and Nursing Homes

Donna Kalauokalani and Nitin Budhwar

The Patient Population in Prisons

Consideration for managing pain in prison settings begins with understanding the patient population. Although it might seem reasonable to think of this population as a microcosm of local communities, incarceration has not affected all communities equally. Approximately 2 million people are in prisons and jails in the United States, despite evidence that large-scale incarceration is not effective in achieving public safety.[1] There have been increasing trends of incarceration related to the war on drugs and changes in sentencing laws and policy, not related to crime rates. In fact, people incarcerated on drug-related convictions comprise the majority of the prison population.[2]

In terms of socioeconomic status, people in prison and jail are disproportionately poor compared to the overall U.S. population. Because of the high price of money bail, people with low incomes are more likely to face the harms of pretrial detention.[3] Poverty is not only a predictor of incarceration but also frequently the outcome because a criminal record and time spent in prison destroy wealth, create debt, and reduce job opportunities. People of color, who face much greater rates of poverty, are overrepresented in prisons and jails. Racial disparities are pronounced because Black Americans make up 38% of the incarcerated population despite representing only 12% of U.S. residents. Black men are six times as likely to be incarcerated as White men, and Latinos are 2.5 times as likely. For Black men in their 30s, approximately 1 in every 12 is in prison or jail on any given day.[4]

The overall health of people in prisons and jails is characterized by a high prevalence of chronic health problems, including diabetes, high blood pressure, and HIV, as well as substance use disorders, related infectious disease complications, and mental health problems. The likelihood of adverse childhood experiences (ACEs) is exceedingly high. Incarcerated people are 33% more likely to have one or more ACEs in their past compared to the general population. Nearly all incarcerated people have at least one ACE. There is also the aspect of incarceration that is traumatic. Prisons are traumatic places that dehumanize in the name of security and control. Incarcerated people navigate constant surveillance, social isolation, limited personal care services, ongoing harassment, and threats of violence and abuse. These experiences can accentuate trauma for those who have experienced victimization and abuse before their involvement with the justice system.[5]

Distrust of the health care system is common among the incarcerated. Many have not had a relationship with a physician or health care provider, either because previous exposures were characterized by rejection and discrimination or because of their selective avoidance of being judged by seeking assistance by health care. Therefore, interactions with doctors can be strained by not only the lack of control but also due to an underdeveloped ability for self-advocacy, which can have health implications. Despite this, incarcerated individuals have high utilization of medical services because of physical trauma and the risk of orthopedic problems and because they have a high rate of chronic pain. The addition of high psychological trauma and the increased burden of other chronic illnesses commensurate with the general population make assessing pain in this population very challenging. Because incarcerated individuals are at high risk of death after release from prison, largely due to drug overdose, interventions that mitigate risk must be considered for those preparing to transition back to their community.[6]

Pain Assessment

Assessment and documentation of pain should be done in a systematic and consistent manner. A complete history should be taken that includes comorbid conditions such as diabetes, cancer, hepatitis, renal disease, heart disease, and others, including any mental health history and treatment. The management of patients with chronic pain requires ongoing knowledge of any substance abuse and mental health issues. Pain cannot be properly managed without addressing both of these. Psychological factors may influence the experience, report, and display of pain. Identification and management of comorbid psychological disorders (especially anxiety and/or depression) will facilitate appropriate care because unrecognized and unmanaged comorbid mental health and other conditions may interfere with the patient's ability to meaningfully participate in a collaborative plan of care and likely diminish treatment effectiveness. Table 15.1 summarizes several useful instruments that help inform pain assessment.

Understanding the impact of pain on overall function and quality of life (e.g., ability to function at work, relationships, recreational activities, effects on sleep, changes in mood, and levels of stress) is essential because improvement in these domains may be a goal of pain treatment and a measure of the efficacy of interventions. In the correctional setting, functional assessment questions should elicit the impact of pain on ability to participate in prison programs, work, or education; ability to get in and out of their bunk bed; any effect on relationships with others; sleep disturbances; ability to get to meals, participate in outdoor yard time, get down on the ground for alarms, and stand for counts; and ability to engage in self-care behaviors such as showering, dressing, grooming, toileting, and daily exercise. The patient should be advised that the focus of treatment will be on improving their function.[10]

Treating Pain in Prison Using a Stepwise Approach

Managing pain in the vulnerable incarcerated population requires socioeconomic, cultural, and religious sensitivity. Therefore, the method in which care is delivered is

Table 15.1 Recommended Instruments and Their Scoring for Assessing Comorbid Substance Use and Mental Health Status[a]

Instrument	Used For	Completed By	No. of Items	Scoring
Patient Health Questionnaire-9 (PHQ-9)[7]	All patients with chronic pain given high rates of comorbid depression	Patient	9	Range: 0–27 (higher=worsedepression) 0–4 = None 5–9 = Mild 10–14 = Moderate 15–19 = Moderately severe 20–27 = Severe
Tobacco, Alcohol, Prescription Medication, and Other Substance Use Tool, Part 1 (TAPS-1)[8]	Screen for tobacco, alcohol, illicit drugs, and nonmedical use of prescription drugs	Patient or provider	4	Identifies the specific substance(s) use and risk level, ranging in severity from "problem use" to the more severe substance use disorder
TAPS-2	If TAPS-1 response is anything other than "never"; additional substance-specific assessment questions guide determining risk level for that substance	Provider	Up to 8	0 = No use in past 3 months 1 = Problem use 2+ = Higher risk
Clinical Opiate Withdrawal Scale (COWS)[9]	Characterizing misuse once opioid treatments begin	Provider	11	5–12 = Mild 13–24 = Moderate 25–36 = Moderate–severe >36 = Severe withdrawal

[a]Pain cannot be properly managed without adequately addressing both these concerns.

equally as important as the care itself.[11] When properly performed, patient-centered care may decrease patient anxiety, increase trust in physicians and other health care providers, and improve treatment adherence. As part of the patient-centered care approach, clinicians should review the patient's history, including previous treatments, their results, and overall progress. Clinicians should ask the patient about their interest in a referral to a substance use disorder program or mental health expert, when appropriate. In general, nonpharmacologic therapies and non-opioid therapies are preferred for managing chronic, non-cancer pain.[12]

Although some therapeutic modalities are limited in prison, such as the ability to offer the application of heat or ice, a biopsychosocial model and multimodal approach are recommended. In the biopsychosocial model, the experience of pain is sculpted by biological, psychological, and social influences. Each of these factors can independently influence pain; however, the complex interactions among these factors results in a unique mosaic of individual differences contributing to the individual's pain. The focus on management, therefore, must be holistic and recognize the long-term functional restoration as the treatment goal that is reliant on adaptive behaviors and choices. Each patient has different needs, and it is essential they play an active role in their own pain management program. A stepwise, graduated progression creates an individualized patient program.

Step 1: Self-Management

Self-management is recommended as first-line treatment for patients with chronic pain, and a host of tools and techniques are available that can be used to assist patients with the management of their chronic pain. Patients are much more likely to embrace self-management strategies if they are taught how to do things rather than being told "You need to learn to live with it."

Introducing concepts such as the mind–body connection, the importance of physical activity, sleep hygiene, healthy eating, relaxation techniques, as well as a host of coping strategies promotes a whole-person care approach to improving quality of life and increasing function.

Because patient beliefs and expectations about pain and its treatment are major determinants of treatment outcomes, patient education and engagement are essential in the treatment process and emphasize the patient's role in the care team.

Promoting a healthy lifestyle is just as important in managing chronic pain as it is for other chronic conditions. Patients should be encouraged to eat healthy, exercise, and maintain an ideal weight. Good sleep hygiene is important in pain management. Simple solutions such as using ear plugs or practicing meditation and relaxation exercises may improve a patient's sleep.

Mindfulness and meditation are among a host of self-management techniques that can be helpful to introduce and utilize for a variety of stressors, including physical and psychological pain. Because what patients think can affect their perception of pain, it is important to develop insight about the mind–body connection, and understanding how to use this to one's own advantage goes a long way in managing suffering. Patients can identify activities that distract them from their symptoms, such as leisure time activities, reading, drawing, watching television, listening to or playing music, or playing cards. With practice, intentional attention diversion can help reduce autonomic arousal.

Relaxation techniques aimed at reducing anxiety and pain also expand the patient repertoire of coping strategies for managing pain. Specific examples of techniques for patient self-management are shown in Table 15.2.

Table 15.2 Self-Management Techniques

Technique	Instructions
Deep-breathing exercises	Breathe in slowly and deeply through the nose to a count of 5. Hold the air in the lungs for a count of 5 and then breathe out slowly through the mouth to a count of 10. Repeat 5–10 times, several times each day, to trigger the body's normal relaxation response.
Progressive muscle relaxation	Tighten and then relax body parts one at a time, starting at either the head or the feet and progressing directionally toward the other.
Meditation	Focus on a single object or repeat a particular sound to help quiet the mind and relax the muscles.
Visualization/ imagery	Imagine a pleasant or relaxing scene, such as lying in the sun.

Peer/Other Support Groups

Peer support groups, if available, can be helpful in providing hope, modeling positive behaviors, and promoting a strong foundation of self-management. The availability of peer support groups varies greatly across institutions, and they may not be available. When they are available, however, there is little substitute for connecting with the support of a peer with lived experience.

Step 2: Nonpharmacologic Therapies

Many patients with chronic pain are able to manage adequately without medications and can function at a near-normal level. For patients who need more help managing their pain beyond self-management techniques, nonpharmacologic physical therapies and behavioral therapies can be added.[12]

Exercise

No one type of exercise has been shown to be more effective than another in the management of chronic pain. Exercise choices need to be individually tailored to each patient. Studies have shown flexion exercises, extension exercises, isokinetic muscle strengthening, and low-impact aerobic exercises to be beneficial. There is no significant difference in outcomes when comparing relatively inexpensive group aerobics/stretching to more traditional physiotherapy and muscle conditioning; thus, suggesting low-cost alternatives may be effective. Whereas patients with acute pain are often encouraged to rest to promote healing, patients with chronic pain often do worse with prolonged decreased activity, which leads to subsequent deconditioning. General activity should be encouraged and progressively increased where possible. Work classifications in prison may need to be modified in order to avoid specific activities that can exacerbate pain, such as heavy lifting or strenuous activity. Specific limitations need to be conveyed to custodial staff so that job assignments are modified as necessary. Similarly, sports and gym and other athletic activities should be assessed for continued or limited participation. Activities such as walking, stretching, and strength and balance exercises are encouraged as indicated.

Physical Therapy

Consultation with a physical therapist may be beneficial for patients who need help setting specific goals to restore function and/or for incorporating specific modalities into a rehabilitative program. General components of a physical therapy program include a gradually progressive therapeutic exercise program that includes goal-setting and interval progress reports; focused therapies designed to improve range of motion, gait, and mobilization of joints (including the spine) and soft tissues; supplemental modalities such as transcutaneous electrical nerve stimulation and traction; tips on how to complete assigned exercises (homework) between PT visits; and assessments for mobility assistive equipment.

Psychological Therapies

General counseling (i.e., education to promote wellness) can be accomplished and facilitated by a consistent primary care team that provides support of realistic goals and reinforcement of the patient's role in their improvement. Some patients may benefit from more formal psychotherapy sessions.

Cognitive–behavioral therapy (CBT) focuses on building skills to effectively control the tendency toward maladaptive thinking. CBT provides understanding and insight into the connection between one's thoughts and behaviors. Phases of CBT for pain management include reconceptualization of chronic pain as a chronic disease (i.e., pain as manageable and controllable); skills acquisition with emphasis on self-management, behavioral activation, and coping skills; and maintenance and relapse prevention with emphasis on problem-solving. Because CBT teaches self-monitoring for early recognition of triggering situations, and assists in developing strategies for coping with these, the skills acquired can be applied to many areas other than pain management.[13]

Dialectical behavioral therapy is a form of CBT that combines standard CBT techniques for emotion regulation and reality-testing with concepts of distress tolerance, acceptance, and mindful awareness. Originally designed to help people suffering from borderline personality disorder, the technique has had success in treating a broader selection of conditions, including substance use disorders, post-traumatic stress disorder, traumatic brain injuries, binge-eating disorder, and mood disorders.[14]

Motivational enhancement therapy (MET) is a technique that focuses on the treatment of substance use disorders. The goal of the therapy is not to guide the patient through the recovery process but, rather, to invoke inwardly motivated change, develop a plan for change, and improve coping strategies.[15] MET consists of five key components:

1. Express empathy—acknowledge (validate) the patient's pain, and establish trust and a sense of working together.
2. Develop discrepancy—establish goals and note the distance needed to travel to achieve those goals.
3. Avoid argument—skilled positive responses rather than negative ones.
4. Rolling with resistance—encourages the patient to recognize that there will be resistance at times and to "roll with" it.
5. Support self-efficacy—encourages the patient to realize they are capable of achieving the goals they set.

Step 3: Non-Opioid Pharmacologic Therapy

For patients who continue to have intolerable pain despite using nonpharmacologic approaches, select non-opioid therapy based on the type of pain and patient-specific comorbidities. The expectation is that the patient will maintain engagement in nonpharmacologic and self-care strategies, if possible, initiated as Steps 1 and 2. Selection of pharmacotherapy should be based on assessment of the underlying pain mechanism—that is, neuropathic versus somatic. Distinct from agents typically used to treat somatic pain, neuropathic analgesics generally exert their pain-relieving properties by gradually changing the patient's chemistry, thereby reducing neural responsiveness. As such, trials for neuropathic treatments tend to require several weeks to several months to adequately assess overall responsiveness. Attaining no response or intolerable side effects warrants taper/discontinuation and consideration for an alternative agent. Partial response, even with titration to maximal dosing, may warrant consideration for adding another agent with a different mechanism of action.

In the incarcerated setting, gabapentin and pregabalin may be abused and diverted, and so these should be avoided in lieu of other therapeutic agents such as tricyclic antidepressants and serotonin–norepinephrine reuptake inhibitors (SNRIs). Other anti-epileptic drugs (AEDs) also have limited roles. Carbamazepine is first-line agent for trigeminal neuralgia, but otherwise it should be rarely used due to its side effect profile. Oxcarbazepine may be used as an alternative to carbamazepine for trigeminal neuralgia; however, it has no utility in any other neuropathic pain condition and should rarely be used for pain management in general. Slow titration of AEDs is recommended to find the lowest effective dosage while avoiding adverse effects. A slow taper is recommended when discontinuing therapy. Monitoring is essential for worsening of depression, suicidal thoughts/behavior, and/or any other unusual changes in mood or behavior. Rare adverse effects include hepatitis and hematologic abnormalities.

Formularies tend to be limited in prison. Medications are often used as trade commodities, and if there is not a compelling indication, they can pose risk to the patient and/or the incarcerated population. Administration strategies are employed such that many medications utilized for analgesia are delivered daily at a medication station staffed by nurses rather than dispensing a supply that can be used discretionally. Because of the high rates of other chronic medical conditions, caution should be taken against prolonged regular use of medications such as anti-inflammatories because of the increased risk of adverse effects, including gastritis, gastrointestinal bleeding, edema, hypertension, cardiotoxicity, renal toxicity, central nervous system effects, and coagulopathy.

Step 4: Procedures/Interventions

Interventional techniques ranging from trigger point injections to intra-articular injections, spinal interventions, and surgery may be considered in select cases based on clinical findings and differential diagnosis.

Surgery

In the absence of neurological complications, it is typical to try at least several months of nonsurgical treatments, such as physical therapy and medications, before proceeding to surgery. Unless there is a discrete identifiable cause of pain, it is generally not recommended to treat chronic pain with surgery. There are significant risks associated with surgery, including no improvement and/or worsened pain. Postoperative care is particularly challenging in the carceral environment, and risk for postoperative infection and other complications is high.[16]

Opioid Therapy

Opioids are not the preferred treatment for chronic pain. In the carceral environment, select patients may be considered for opioid therapy in combination with nonpharmacologic treatments and non-opioid medication, using caution to prescribe the lowest effective dose and provide ongoing monitoring with urine drug testing and weighing risks versus benefits. In this population, medications are a commodity, and the risks of opioid misuse or diversion are high.

Careful screening of patients prior to treatment can ensure patients have access to safe, effective chronic pain treatment while reducing opioid-related morbidity and mortality. Clinical discretion remains an essential component to reducing misuse and diversion, and physicians must assess a range of external information, including patient drug utilization, drug screens, and information provided by the patient or others.

Invariably, there will be a need to restrict opioid therapy. A conversation is challenging when you are denying opioids to a patient who specifically requests them or informing a patient that their long-term opioid medication must be tapered and discontinued because risks of opioid therapy are outweighing benefits. It may be difficult to inform a patient that their urine drug screen shows illicit drugs and their opioid prescription will be tapered and discontinued because the risks of opioid therapy are outweighing benefits.

Maintaining a therapeutic relationship in the context of difficult conversations can be extremely challenging, especially when there is underlying pathology such as substance use disorder and/or borderline personality disorder. For example, the wild shift between idealization and devaluation, typically found in borderline personality disorder, is known as splitting, which signifies a disturbance in both thinking and emotion regulation. Idealization, devaluation, and splitting are considered to be subconscious defense mechanisms by which people view others, events, or even themselves as a way to protect themselves from perceived stress. When such defense mechanisms are consistent, distorted, and accompanied by other symptoms/behaviors, such as acting out, denial, and passive aggression, a mental health colleague should be consulted.

Although there are no easy answers for how best to deal with behaviors that manifest from subconscious defense mechanisms (e.g., splitting or devaluation), the following are some guiding principles:

Cultivate empathy. Devaluating is part of the disorder. Although certain actions may seem intentional and manipulative, these are simply defense mechanisms.

Manage your response. Control your tone and temper. Yelling or engaging in hostility will only serve to make the situation worse.

Remind your patient that you care. Knowing that someone cares often helps reduce the devaluating behavior because it lessens the fear of being rejected or abandoned.

Maintain lines of communication. Discuss isolated situations as they happen. Failure to communicate only serves to fuel rejection anxiety.

Set boundaries. Use the principles of an opioid agreement (even if you are not prescribing opioids) to establish expectations for behaviors. If a boundary is crossed, explain why you are proceeding as you are and try to do so dispassionately. Setting boundaries helps preserve the relationship rather than challenging it.

Encourage and support treatment. Consider and encourage alternate treatments, including medications and behavioral therapies (both cognitive and dialectical).

Take care of yourself. Engage with your peers and others for support. This is difficult work and you are not alone.

Comorbid Substance Use Disorders

Patients with coexisting chronic pain and opioid use disorders are particularly challenging to manage, in terms of both pharmacotherapy and other behavioral therapies.

Multidimensional biopsychosocial assessment developed by the American Society of Addiction Medicine can be useful to determine a level of care that is used for treatment planning.[17] Motivational interviewing techniques may assist with moving a patient along in the stages of change. Comprehensive treatment generally utilizes behavioral, pharmacologic, and/or housing modalities to stabilize an individual. These treatment modalities may be utilized individually or in combination based on patient need and consent. It is important for the patient to accept that they are responsible for their own recovery. The treatment team should work to provide all the evidence-based approaches that increase their chance at success. Behavioral treatment begins with motivational interviewing techniques and a therapeutic relationship with one's care team, and it may include cognitive–behavioral intervention, CBT, and peer support. Medication-assisted treatment (MAT) is available for patients with opioid use disorder or alcohol use disorder.[18] If considered a candidate for MAT based on assessment findings, the patient will be started on MAT after a signed informed consent. Follow-up appointments for patients on MAT are scheduled according to medication and duration of stability. Follow-up appointments for patients with substance use disorder are essential to monitor the disease, even if a patient is not on MAT. Urine drug screens are used to monitor MAT adherence and performed randomly at defined intervals.

If patients require surgery, advanced planning for patients on MAT who are scheduled for elective procedures is best. Treatment of acute postoperative pain in patients on buprenorphine maintenance includes continuing the patients' baseline dosing to avoid increased pain and/or withdrawal.[19] Total daily doses of buprenorphine may have to be increased postoperatively for no longer than 7 days for pain control and may be split to optimize analgesia (e.g., 24 mg/day changed to 8 mg every 8 h). If further pain control is needed, utilize multimodal pain management with non-opioids. Consider use of local and regional anesthesia as needed. If opioids are needed for breakthrough pain, standard dosing protocols should initially be utilized with careful monitoring and the understanding that patients with a history of opioid use disorder may require higher than usual doses due to cross-tolerance and increased pain sensitivity. Patient-controlled analgesia (PCA) without a basal component may be considered in addition to a patient's buprenorphine if pain is not adequately captured. If a PCA is utilized, oral PRN opioids should be discontinued. Coordination with the prescriber of MAT medication and others involved with patient care is essential. The patient should be scheduled to be seen by their physician or buprenorphine/naloxone prescriber within 1 week post-procedure. In order to overcome the pharmacologic blockade on extended-release injectable naltrexone or buprenorphine, extremely high doses of opioids are required to achieve adequate analgesia. This could lead to accidental overdose, respiratory depression, and death. Non-opioid analgesics are recommended whenever possible. Regional nerve blocks and dissociative analgesics such as ketamine may be considered. Generally, transfer to a higher level of care may be necessary to manage the patient in a setting that offers a full range of cardiopulmonary monitoring and ventilator support, if necessary.

Pain Management in Nursing Homes

As population demographics in the United States change, we are witnessing a shift in the settings where older patients spend their last years of life. Whereas the proportion of older patients residing in nursing homes has declined, there is an increase in the proportion of older patients in assisted living facilities and other similar long-term residential homes. All these long-term care settings offer additional challenges when trying to ensure the delivery of appropriate care. Most notable are systemic challenges that typically include staffing shortages, lack of standardized protocols, increasing cost of care, corporate priorities, and the interpretation and enforcement of rules and regulations. Compounding these challenges tied to long-term care settings are the unique medical risks of older patients, including an increased susceptibility to acute injury resulting in pain and having a higher prevalence of chronic illness that can result in a delay of recovery time, all of which can have far-reaching consequences on their overall well-being and independence. The following list provides the demographic makeup of U.S. nursing homes for 2021:[20]

Average age: 50% are aged 85 years or older.
Gender: 70% are women, and almost 70% of them have no spouse (widowed, divorced, or never married).
Activities of daily living (ADLs): More than 80% need help with at least three ADLs, including 90% who can walk but need assistance.
Incidence of dementia: 50–70% have some degree of impairment.[21]
Average length of stay: 2 years.

What Makes Older Adults Living in Long-Term Care Settings More Vulnerable?

The aging process brings with it numerous challenges. There is a general decline in physical abilities and physiological tolerances, which makes a person more susceptible to disease processes, injury, and a slower recovery time. This becomes more noticeable after one's sixth decade. The older adult is also at higher risk for conditions that are a direct cause for pain—that is, degenerative joint disease, osteoporotic fracture, muscle atrophy, etc.

Socioeconomic challenges potentially affecting populations living in nursing homes and group living facilities include limited financial assets to support ongoing care and the problem of outliving one's resources. In assisted living facilities, these financial constraints may pose significant challenges, especially when residents are responsible for services beyond what is part of the basic accommodation package, which is typically limited to covering accommodation, meals, housekeeping, and laundry. In contrast, nursing homes cover most of a patient's cost of living, including medications. Thus, the rising cost of medications and the need for additional medication can impact a patient's desire to voice complaints to avoid incurring additional expenses.

In this vulnerable group of patients, it is critical for patients or their advocates to clearly communicate their needs. Increased isolation from family or a support network is an ongoing problem, which was exacerbated during the COVID-19 pandemic. With aging, one's social network starts to diminish. Older patients in nursing homes have often lost their spouse (70%),[22,23] and family visits may not be as frequent as desired.

Not only does this have negative psychological effects for older patients but also there is a loss of advocacy for the patients, which can compound issues in their care.

Elder abuse is a concern that the clinician must keep in mind when noting physical findings that are overlooked by staff or dismissed by the patient for fear of retribution. Neurocognitive impairment (dementia) can be especially challenging as a comorbid condition because it impacts the foundation and reliability of expression and communication. In a congregant setting, conditions that impair the clear communication of needs must be considered.

Challenges in the Nursing Home Setting

There are several challenges for pain treatment specific to the nursing home setting that should be considered. Pain assessments and pain control have not been adequately studied or tracked in the nursing home setting, especially in the last 6 months of life. Studies suggest that up to 60% of patients without severe cognitive impairment experience consistent low back pain, and up to 34% report moderate to severe musculoskeletal pain, with only 5% or 6% experiencing improvements in their pain.[24]

Pain trajectories are noted to be worse in those who are severely impaired both physically and cognitively. Cognitive impairment can reduce care for pain. Patients with cognitive impairment have fewer regular pain assessments and reassessments with resultant prescribing or deprescribing in comparison to non-cognitively impaired patients. Older adults in nursing homes may view pain as part of normal aging, which limits their willingness to report it. Furthermore, there is also the fear or stigma of becoming addicted to controlled substances or becoming dependent on medications, both of which can reduce the desire to seek help for pain.[25]

There are systemic challenges in the nursing home setting as well. Staffing shortages and high staff turnover at long-term care facilities complicate the implementation of treatment plans. Studies and models have shown that when adequate staffing and low turnover can be achieved, patients receive better care, with lower admission and readmission rates.[26,27] Facilities may lack a formal or standardized approach to assessing and reassessing for pain, and even if such protocols exist, their routine use may be lacking. A long-term relationship with a patient, such as that seen in nursing home settings, has been shown to potentially influence pain assessments in a way that leads to underappreciation of pain because firsthand knowledge of prior behaviors can cause a confirmation bias in the evaluator assessment.

Improvements in Nursing Home Vulnerability

Recognition of a problem is the first step toward remediating it. A significant challenge in long-term care is the care of patients with cognitive impairment. Comprehensive pain assessment protocols have limitations when used in the cognitively impaired. Evaluations using tools such as the Minimum Data Set are required to be completed within 14 days of admission and thereafter every quarter or if there is a change in a patient's status.[28] There may be little incentive to perform more than the needed number of assessments, which may result in delays in assessing and treating pain.

Use of appropriate screening and monitoring tools in patients with cognitive impairment has been a subject of debate and study. Tools such as the Discomfort Scale for Dementia of Alzheimer Type[29] and Behavioral Pathology in Alzheimer's Disease[30] have been shown to significantly reduce discomfort and result in more frequent return to behavioral baselines. Facilities could consider adopting these tools into their pain management protocols.

Studies have shown that using a quality improvement process approach with a strong educational component led by nursing home staff can result in significant improvements in pain assessments and management.[31] Engaging the patient and the family is perhaps the most important aspect of any clinical care improvement process. Ensuring that patients are given a safe place to express their desires and concerns as well as engage in a dialog with all their health care team members can improve satisfaction and lead to realistic goal setting.

Staff education should draw attention to better recognition of pain, use of assessment tools, and the appropriate use of both pharmacological and nonpharmacological treatments. These interventions can be team-focused and include the physician as well as other providers, such as pharmacy, physical therapy, and behavioral health.

Management

Physiological Changes with Aging

Older adults present with differences in physiology. There are four key points to remember when using medications[32]:

1. In older adults, there is a relative increase in the body's percentage of fat and a decrease in muscle mass and water. Thus, water-soluble drugs become more concentrated and fat-soluble ones have a prolonged half-life.
2. Anatomically, the liver is functionally smaller with fewer hepatocytes and less blood flow, which can affect the clearance of medications and impact drug–drug interactions.
3. The renal system also changes with aging. Creatinine clearance can decline significantly, even when measured serum creatinine is in the normal range. This frequently requires dose adjustments and at times results in a relative contraindication for the use of certain classes of medications such as nonsteroidal anti-inflammatory drugs (NSAIDs).
4. Changes in the nervous system, such as a decrease in the number of pain receptors in the skin, and changes in the way nerve conduction occurs have been noted; however, this seems to have little influence on pain tolerance and pain perception.

Polypharmacy is a significant risk for adverse drug events (ADEs). Although the definition of polypharmacy is controversial, it is accepted that a patient taking more than five or six medications or nine or more doses a day is at risk of ADEs. Changes in the metabolism of drugs may result from the use of multiple medications that use the cytochrome P450 system and also from alternations in the anatomical and physiological systems associated with older adulthood. This effect can be compounded with the addition of supplements that increase an older adult's risk for ADEs.

Treatment

Acute pain generally has a prescribed treatment course. Chronic pain, however, is far more complicated to treat given its impact on multiple domains of a patient's life and the interplay on the success of chronic pain management. The treatment plan must address the psychological and social impacts of chronic pain, including depression, anxiety, stress, avoidance, social isolation, fear of movement, substance misuse, and impact on relationships. Medical complications arising from comorbid states such as weight gain, lack of sleep/insomnia, and pressure sores must also be considered in the plan.

An appropriate assessment and frequent reassessments are the cornerstone for any pain management plan. You must consider long-term plans, consequences, and realistic expectations.[33]

Nonpharmacological treatment options should always be considered as part of a treatment plan for pain.[34] Often, they are underutilized because they can be resource- and time-intensive. Examples of such modalities include physical therapy, massage therapy, movement-based therapies such as yoga and tai chi, and other structured exercise activities.

Involvement of other specialists, such as pain medicine specialists, physical therapists, and occupational therapists, can be considered. Behavioral health interventions such as CBT may help patients better cope with their pain. Interventional pain physicians can help with procedures that target specific pain sources. Complimentary modalities such as acupuncture should be considered as well because they have limited adverse effects or toxicities. Accessing some of these specialists may require leaving the facility, especially for more procedural-based interventions. The value of such treatments is variable and subject to availability, which can often be sparse and costly outside of large population centers.[34]

Pharmacological treatments may need adjustments based on age, comorbidity, potential drug interactions, and declining organ function.[35] Some agents may be contraindicated, and others often need dose adjustments. The geriatric prescribing principle of *start low–go slow* should be applied to the initiation of any medication, especially if it will have a systemic effect.

Topical agents are a reasonable first choice. These include topical NSAIDs; lidocaine-based creams/gels/patches; and capsaicin-, menthol-, and camphor-based creams/patches. These are widely available over-the-counter and include lower strengths and higher strengths as prescriptions. With topical NSAID creams, there is a small degree of systemic absorption. This is variable and will need to be considered in terms of the patient's underlying disease burden when prescribing.

Systemic agents can be considered next in treatment. They encompass six categories of medications: NSAIDs, acetaminophen, anticonvulsants, antidepressants, tramadol, and opioids. These agents are available in oral pill, oral liquid, intravenous, intramuscular, patch, or sublingual formulations, as well as in combination with each other. For instance, a frequent combination includes an NSAID or acetaminophen in combination with an opioid or tramadol. Some of these medications are described as follows:

Acetaminophen[36]: This is a widely used medication and can be reasonably effective and safe for joint, muscular, and back pain, as well as headaches. For healthy older adults, 4 g or less is appropriate, but a dose of 3 g per day is recommended for those with substantial risk factors for hepatotoxicity. It typically does not cause gastropathy, but it can be hepatotoxic in doses that exceed the recommended daily maximum. Renal damage is unlikely at prescribed doses. Common reactions may include nausea and headaches.

NSAIDs: They have well-known adverse effects on the stomach and bleeding (platelet inhibition). They can all worsen heart failure, renal impairment, and hypertension. Given the high prevalence of these conditions in the elderly, they are relatively contraindicated when taken systemically. Data on the use of topical NSAIDs such as diclofenac gel and their systemic safety are not definitive.[37,38] Although a degree of the topical drug is absorbed, the serum levels versus its oral dose will vary depending on the concentration and amount used. Therefore, the same cautions apply as when using oral NSAIDs.

Anticonvulsants: Their main use has been in the treatment of migraine and neuropathic pain. Some more widely prescribed medicines in this category in the United States include carbamazepine, valproic acid, topiramate, gabapentin, and pregabalin. (See Table 15.3 for indications and starting doses.)

Gabapentinoids (gabapentin and pregabalin): These are usually the first to be used for neuropathic pain, whereas valproic acid, carbamazepine, and topiramate may be incorporated for headache and facial pain conditions. Side effects need to be closely monitored because they may occur at lower doses in older adults. Drowsiness, fatigue, and cognitive disturbances may be more common. The physician should also be aware of specific adverse events related to the medication chosen that may require additional monitoring. In the older population, starting these medications at half or even less than half of the recommended starting dose is recommended, with a slow increase in dose and attention to possible adverse effects. When discontinuing medications in this category, it is current practice to taper them slowly over weeks, especially if the patient is taking a dose in the middle to higher range.[39,40] In non-epileptic patients, this is done to lessen withdrawal symptoms—for example, decreasing the dose by one-fourth per week.

Antidepressants: SNRIs have been shown to reduce chronic pain in the absence of depression. In the United States, these include duloxetine, venlafaxine, and desvenlafaxine. As a group, they are indicated for fibromyalgia,[41] neuropathic pain, and chronic musculoskeletal pain. Duloxetine may be better tolerated in older adults. Venlafaxine is also indicated in the use of migraine headache prophylaxis. As with anticonvulsants, one should be familiar with the monitoring requirements. Hyponatremia is a concern with both selective serotonin reuptake inhibitors (SSRIs) and SNRIs; it usually, but not always, occurs within the first 2 weeks.

Table 15.3 Indications and Starting Doses for Anticonvulsants and Antidepressants

Medication	U.S. Food and Drug Administration–Approved Pain Control Indication	General Starting Dose in the Elderly ± Renal or Hepatic Adjustment
Gabapentin	Post-herpetic neuralgia	Start at 100 mg QHS Renal adjustment: Yes Liver adjustment: No
Pregabalin	Diabetic neuropathy, spinal cord injury–associated neuropathy, post-herpetic neuralgia, fibromyalgia[1]	Start at 25 mg BID Renal adjustment: Yes Liver adjustment: No
Carbamazepine	Trigeminal neuralgia	Start at 100 mg BID Renal adjustment: Yes Liver adjustment: No
Valproic acid	Migraine headache prophylaxis	Start at 250 mg BID Renal adjustment: No Severe liver disease: Do not use
Topiramate	Migraine headache prophylaxis	Start at 25 mg at night with weekly titration if needed Renal adjustment: Yes Liver impairment: Caution
Venlafaxine	Migraine headache prophylaxis, diabetic neuropathy	Start at 37.5 mg ER QD Renal adjustment: Yes Liver adjustment: Yes
Duloxetine	Diabetic neuropathy, fibromyalgia, chronic musculoskeletal pain	Start at 20–30 mg QD Renal adjustment: Yes Liver adjustment: Yes
Desvenlafaxine	Diabetic neuropathy	Start at 50 mg QD Renal adjustment: Yes Liver adjustment: Yes

Tramadol

Low-dose tramadol (25–50 mg every 8 h) including in combination with acetaminophen can provide reasonably effective pain control for mild to moderate chronic pain. There may be a lower risk of falls and incidence of constipation in older patients. However, chronic use has been associated with a higher rate of all-cause mortality compared to Cox-2 inhibitors and NSAIDs, but not opioids such as codeine.[42] There is also an increased risk of serotonin syndrome and seizure activity when taken along with SSRIs and SNRIs.

Opioids (Non-Cancer Pain)

Patients can benefit from opioid therapy, but opioids are the subject of much debate and policy regulation. They pose several risks for older patients, such as cognitive decline, falls, worsening of sleep apnea, and constipation, and they are subject to misuse, overuse, and dependence with an escalating need for effect. For nonmalignant pain, they can be a reasonable and therapeutic option given a patient's other clinical morbidities that may preclude the use of other classes of medications. Given their inherent risk, physicians need to adhere to regulatory best practices, such as opioid agreements, goal setting and expectations, frequent monitoring for side effects, use of the lowest effective dose and shortest duration, and monitoring for misuse and use of other potentially harmful substances such as alcohol or marijuana. As with other medications in older adults, clinicians should start at low doses and make gradual increases. Long-acting opioids such as methadone should be used with caution given methadone's variable half-life (days), numerous drug interactions, and risk of arrythmia.[43] Other long-acting opioids or sustained-release opioids also carry an increased risk of unintended overdose,[44] but they may be considered with close monitoring if patients do not experience meaningful relief from short-acting agents.

Although this chapter highlights some of the better known concerns about the use of systemic agents, it is the physician's or provider's responsibility to be familiar with the side effects, drug interactions, and dose adjustments that may be necessary. Most patients residing in a long-term care setting have their medications regulated, but it is still possible for friends or family members to supply them with medications. Therefore, confirming all sources of medication is of significant value to ensure safe consumption. Moreover, consulting with an on-call pharmacologist, who is generally available to all long-term care facilities, can be helpful.

Complimentary Supplements

There has been an expansion in the sale and use of supplements. Although this chapter focuses on standard medical practice, both clinicians and patients may incorporate complimentary herbal/supplemental modalities based on their comfort and availability.[45] Some notable mentions include turmeric, glucosamine-chondroitin, S-adenosyl-L-methionine, cannabidiol extracts, and topical arnica. The National Center for Complementary and Integrative Health can be a useful resource for the practicing clinician to become familiar with some of these supplements, including their risks and potential benefits.[46,47]

Conclusion

Patients in the carceral environment pose management challenges because of chronic pain, substance use disorders, and adverse traumatic experiences that drive maladaptive behaviors, ill-formed coping strategies, and maladaptive social skills.

Clinicians should be well aware of the physiological and disease-related nuances that affect older and often cognitively impaired adults with pain in the long-term care setting. Medications in this group must be adjusted for physiological changes of aging, including renal and liver dysfunction. Reassessments of care plans should be performed on a frequent basis.

In both settings, a multimodal team approach can assist in providing thorough evaluations and treatments. System shortcomings in both the carceral environment and the long-term care system may impact the quality of care that physicians and other clinicians deliver. In addition, many patients in long-term care will spend their last years of life in such institutions; therefore, affording them a good quality of life should be a high priority.

References

1. National Academies of Sciences, Engineering, and Medicine. *The Effects of Incarceration and Reentry on Community Health and Well-Being: Proceedings of a Workshop*. National Academies Press; 2020. https://doi.org/10.17226/25471
2. Cohen A, Vakharia SP, Netherland J, Frederique K. How the war on drugs impacts social determinants of health beyond the criminal legal system. *Ann Med*. 2022;54(1):2024–2038.
3. Csete J, Kamarulzaman A, Kazatchkine M, et al. Public health and international drug policy. *Lancet*. 2016;387(10026):1427–1480.
4. MacDonald J, Arkes J, Nicosia N, Pacula RL. Decomposing racial disparities in prison and drug treatment commitments for criminal offenders in California. *J Legal Stud*. 2014;43(1):155–187.
5. Roos LE, Afifi TO, Martin CG, Pietrzak RH, Tsai J, Sareen J. Linking typologies of childhood adversity to adult incarceration: Findings from a nationally representative sample. *Am J Orthopsychiatry*. 2016;86(5):584–593.
6. Binswanger IA, Stern MF, Deyo RA, et al. Release from prison—A high risk of death for former inmates [published correction appears in N Engl J Med. 2007 Feb 1;356(5):536]. *N Engl J Med*. 2007;356(2):157–165.
7. Kroenke K, Spitzer RL, Williams JB. The PHQ-9: Validity of a brief depression severity measure. *J Gen Intern Med*. 2001;16(9):606–613.
8. McNeely J, Wu LT, Subramaniam G, et al. Performance of the Tobacco, Alcohol, Prescription Medication, and Other Substance Use (TAPS) Tool for substance use screening in primary care patients. *Ann Intern Med*. 2016;165(10):690–699.
9. Wesson DR, Ling W. The Clinical Opiate Withdrawal Scale (COWS). *J Psychoactive Drugs*. 2003;35(2):253–259.
10. Handtke V, Wolff H, Williams BA. The pains of imprisonment: Challenging aspects of pain management in correctional settings. *Pain Manag*. 2016;6(2):133–136.
11. Gil T, Metts J, Ugwueze G. The evaluation and management of chronic pain in the correctional setting. *J Correct Health Care*. 2019;25(4):382–393.
12. Skelly AC, Chou R, Dettori JR, et al. *Noninvasive Nonpharmacological Treatment for Chronic Pain: A Systematic Review Update*. Agency for Healthcare Research and Quality; 2020.
13. Ehde DM, Dillworth TM, Turner JA. Cognitive-behavioral therapy for individuals with chronic pain: Efficacy, innovations, and directions for research. *Am Psychol*. 2014;69(2):153–166.
14. Peprah K, Argáez C. *Dialectical Behavioral Therapy for Adults with Mental Illness: A Review of Clinical Effectiveness and Guidelines*. Canadian Agency for Drugs and Technologies in Health; 2017.
15. Center for Substance Abuse Treatment. Motivational interviewing as a counseling style. In: *Enhancing Motivation for Change in Substance Abuse Treatment*. Substance Abuse and Mental Health Services Administration; 1999. https://www.ncbi.nlm.nih.gov/books/NBK64964
16. Bryant MK, Tatebe LC, Siva NR, et al. Outcomes after emergency general surgery and trauma care in incarcerated individuals: An EAST multicenter study. *J Trauma Acute Care Surg*. 2022;93(1):75–83.
17. Graham AW. *Principles of Addiction Medicine*. 3rd ed., American Society of Addiction Medicine; 2003.
18. Substance Abuse and Mental Health Services Administration. *Use of Medication-Assisted Treatment for Opioid Use Disorder in Criminal Justice Settings*. HHS Publication No.

PEP19-MATUSECJS. National Mental Health and Substance Use Policy Laboratory, Substance Abuse and Mental Health Services Administration; 2019.
19. Kohan L, Potru S, Barreveld AM, et al. Buprenorphine management in the perioperative period: Educational review and recommendations from a multisociety expert panel. *Reg Anesth Pain Med.* 2021;46(10):840–859.
20. Healthy Aging. [Home page]. 2021. https://www.healthyaging.org
21. Centers for Disease Control and Prevention. Alzheimer's disease and healthy aging. 2021. https://www.cdc.gov/aging/index.html
22. Alzheimer's Association. Alzheimer's disease facts and figures. 2021. https://www.alz.org/alzheimers-dementia/facts-figures
23. Population Reference Bureau. [Home page]. 2021. https://www.prb.org
24. Farless LB, Ritchie CS. Challenges of pain management in long term care. *Annals of Long Term Care.* May 2012:2–8.
25. Wagatsuma S, Yamaguchi T, Berge LI, et al. How, why and where it hurts—Breaking down pain syndrome among nursing home patients with dementia: A cross-sectional analysis of the COSMOS trial. *Pain Manag Nurse.* 2021;22(3):319–326.
26. Sheikh F, Brandt N, Vinh D, Elon RD. Management of chronic pain in nursing homes: Navigating challenges to improve person-centered care. *J Am Med Dir Assoc.* 2021;22(6):1199–1205.
27. Zimmerman S, Bowers BJ, Cohen LW, et al. New evidence on the Green House model of nursing home care: Synthesis of findings and implications for policy, practice, and research. *Health Serv Res.* 2016;51(Suppl 1):475–496.
28. U.S. Centers for Medicare & Medicaid Services. MDS 3.0 Item Set. 2022. https://www.cms.gov/files/document/finalmds-30-rai-manual-v1181october2023.pdf
29. Van der Steen JT, Ooms ME, van der Wal G, Ribble MW. Measuring discomfort in patients with dementia: Validity of a Dutch version of the Discomfort Scale–Dementia of Alzheimer Type (DS-DAT). *Tijdschr Gerontol Geriatr.* 2002;33(6):257–263.
30. Reisberg B, Borenstein J, Salob SP, Ferris SH, Franssen E, Georgotas A. Behavioral symptoms in Alzheimer's disease: Phenomenology and treatment. *J Clin Psychiatry.* 1987;48(Suppl):9–15.
31. Swafford KL, Miller LL, Tsai PF, Herr KA, Ersek M. Improving the process of pain care in nursing homes: A literature synthesis. *J Am Geriatr Soc.* 2009;57(6):1080–1087.
32. American Medical Directors Association. *Pain Management in the Long-Term Care Setting.* American Medical Directors Association; 2009.
33. Cohen-Mansfield J, Lipson S. Pain in cognitively impaired nursing home residents: How well are physicians diagnosing it? *J Am Geriatric Soc.* 2002;50(6):1039–1044.
34. Robeck I. Chronic pain in the elderly: Special challenges. *Practice in Pain Management.* 2012;12(2).
35. 2019 American Geriatrics Society Beers Criteria Update Expert Panel. American Geriatrics Society 2019 updated Beers Criteria for potentially inappropriate medication use in older adults. *J Am Geriatric Soc.* 2019;67(4):674–694. https://doi.org/10.1111/jgs.15767
36. Alchin J, Dhar A, Siddiqui K, Christo PJ. Why paracetamol (acetaminophen) is a suitable first choice for treating mild to moderate acute pain in adults with liver, kidney or cardiovascular disease, gastrointestinal disorders, asthma, or who are older. *Curr Med Res Opin.* 2022;8(5):811–825.
37. Yoakum P, Kasen J, Hindahl S, Herndon C. Topical nonsteroidal anti-inflammatory drugs and nephrotoxicity: Is there a safer option? *Pract Pain Manag.* 2017;17(7).
38. Kim M, Laumbach S, Amico J. Are topical NSAIDs safer than oral NSAIDs when treating musculoskeletal pain? *Evidence-Based Pract.* 2021;24(1):43.
39. American Addiction Centers. Gabapentin withdrawal symptoms, signs & side effects. 2022. https://americanaddictioncenters.org/neurontin-abuse/gabapentin-cause-withdrawal-symptoms
40. American Addiction Centers. Lyrica withdrawal symptoms, timeline & treatment. 2022. https://americanaddictioncenters.org/prescription-drugs/lyrica-withdrawal-symptoms

41. National Center for Biotechnology Information. Treatments for fibromyalgia in adult subgroups. 2015. https://www.ncbi.nlm.nih.gov/books/NBK274463
42. Zen C, Dubreuil M, LaRochelle MR, et al. Association of tramadol with all-cause mortality among patients with osteoarthritis: *JAMA*. 2019;321(10):969–982. doi:10.1001/jama.2019.1347
43. Klein MG, Krantz MJ, Fatima N, et al. Methadone blockade of cardiac inward rectifier K^+ current augments membrane instability and amplifies U waves on surface ECGs: A translational study. *J Am Heart Assoc*. 2022;11(11):e023482.
44. Ray WA, Chung CP, Murray KT, Hall K, Stein CM. Prescription of long-acting opioids and mortality in patients with non-cancer pain. JAMA. 2016;315(22):2415–2423.
45. Anderson AR, Deng J, Anthony RS, Atalla SA, Monroe TB. Using complementary and alternative medicine to treat pain and agitation in dementia: A review of randomized controlled trials from long-term care with potential use in critical care. *Crit Care Nurs Clin North Am*. 2017;29(4):519–537.
46. National Center for Complementary and Integrative Health. [Home page]. 2022. https://www.nccih.nih.gov
47. National Center for Complementary and Integrative Health. Herbs at a glance. n.d. https://www.nccih.nih.gov/health/herbsataglance

16

Pain and Torture

War's Civilian Survivors and Refugees

Ramin Asgary and Amanda C. de C. Williams

Torture Survivors and Vulnerability

Modern humanitarian work perhaps started during the Battle of Solferino, between Franco-Sardinian and Austrian armies, where Henry Dunant started his work leading to the creation of the International Committee of the Red Cross. The events of World War II, particularly the Holocaust, led to organized humanitarian initiatives, exemplified by the 1948 Declaration of Human Rights and, later, through Refugee Law, International Humanitarian Law, and Conventions against Torture and Maltreatment. These human rights were intended to be supranational, but they were not enforceable. Early refugees during the Cold War were selectively represented as strong and politically oppressed heroes.[1] However, current asylum seekers are perhaps portrayed as politically neutral but individually victimized and traumatized. This helps elicit compassion and allows for an individualized approach within legal or health care systems, but it may lose the broader political and collective context and meaning of what was suffered and the reasons for fleeing their homes. In recognition of their autonomy, the term "survivor" is increasingly used rather than "victim," which is often used for the many who die.

Vulnerability is a characteristic assigned to an individual or group of people. In relation to survivors, the notion of vulnerability is often invoked as a political argument for scarce resources to be provided. Although within health care it indicates unmet needs and justifies interventions on humanitarian grounds,[2] it may inadvertently underrepresent the assets and strengths that individuals bring to that intersection and their individual or community-level coping abilities. The term "vulnerable" may imply inability to manage the demands of daily life because of some deficit or disability,[3] thus rendering the wrong done to survivors of torture and war an individual problem, often framed as poor mental health. In effect, vulnerability has both negative and positive connotations depending on the perspectives used and the audience. If it describes increased risk for specific conditions in clinical settings, it simply identifies the need for special attention and appropriate level of care. If it is presented as a sociopolitical background, it may represent a liability or burden. The balance and emphasis may have to be placed on transparency, clarification, the interface, and ultimately the outcomes of actions and the results.

Three aspects of health care for torture survivors who are refugees have been of particular interest: entitlement in law or policy, moral judgments of deservingness, and practical aspects of access.[4] Although there are accountability processes to provide social and health care resources to citizens, regulations and laws often require adjustment to include services for vulnerable populations irrespective of their legal status or available accountability mechanisms. Health care is established in some countries' constitutions as a basic human right, but its use may be restricted by bureaucratic complexities of claiming entitlement; misapplication of restrictions by health care staff; internalization of stigma; and often a situation in which accommodation, safety, jobs, and finances are precarious.[5,6] Restricted entitlement is countered by arguments about refugees' potential (and actual) value as workers and the risks to the wider society of neglecting health care, particularly of communicable diseases, and of children born in the host country.[7] Few of these initiatives seek the views of the refugees concerned, who may actively contest the frameworks that legitimize or delegitimize them.[8] Vulnerability summarizes the extent and complexity of problems, but it may risk an excessive individual focus on survivors' problems and detach them from past and present social and political contexts, and from the rights to rehabilitation and reparation.

Survivors presenting with pain, not least as part of their account of torture for their asylum claim, may be labeled as doubly illegitimate when there are no physical signs to "match" the pain they feel. Although pain is only very weakly related to evidence of tissue damage or pathology,[9] it entitles survivors to health care that may not be forthcoming for symptoms alone. On the other hand, symptoms may be more promptly referred to psychological services, which can be helpful in managing pain. In the end, survivors who present as patients with pain symptoms need to be evaluated considering their individual and group risks and associated factors; specific shortcomings in assessment of pain, especially chronic pain; and the individual, community, sociocultural, and political contexts. Recognition of different aspects of vulnerability and specific support systems needed is essential to effectively address pain in survivors.

Roles, Responsibilities, and Accountability Within Social and Health Care Systems and Psychosocial Burdens Among Refugees

Background

The number of refugees, internally displaced persons, and asylum seekers has doubled worldwide since 2010, mostly from countries with civil unrest or war and where human rights abuses have been commonly inflicted on civilians.[10] The international community has failed to address the fundamental causes of these conflicts or to adequately support civilians in the midst of brutal wars that recognize no rules. Consequently, populations living in danger zones have fled their countries to potential safe havens and countries[11] that, ironically, may be the key United Nations Security Council members.

Refugees, internally displaced persons, and asylum seekers are persons who have been forced to leave their homes or places of habitual residence, in particular as a result of or in order to avoid the effect of armed conflicts, situations of generalized violence, violation of human rights, or natural or man-made disasters, and who have or have not crossed an international border.[10] Refugees are recognized under the 1951 Convention relating to the Status of Refugees: "Asylum seekers are individuals who have sought international protection and whose claims for refugee status have not yet been determined."[10] In the United States, asylum seekers are individuals meeting the definition of refugee who are outside their country of nationality and are unable or unwilling to return to the home country because of persecution or a well-founded fear of persecution based on race, religion, nationality, membership in a particular social group, or political opinion. They need to already be in the United States or seeking admission at a port of entry.[12] Because the underlying characteristics and risk factors for poor access to health care for refugees in general and the subgroup of asylum seekers are closely related and often identical, the broad terminology of "refugees and asylum seekers" (also known as "asylees" in the United States) is used throughout this section.

A history of human rights abuse and torture is prevalent among refugees and asylum seekers.[13–18] They often demonstrate significant long- and short-term consequences from abuses, including post-traumatic stress disorder (PTSD), major depressive disorder, chronic pain syndromes, and physical limitations from physical trauma.[14,15,19–23] Asylum seekers in particular encounter numerous barriers to health care access, including emotional problems, discrimination, significant challenges of resettlement, constant fear of deportation, and barriers to social assimilation and language.[24–33] Therefore, most refugees and asylum seekers are either unable or afraid to seek health care services.[30,34]

In this section, we briefly review health care and social systems challenges and shed light on the related duties of providers and health systems in general, the social responsibilities of host societies, and the potential roles of health care organizations and professional associations. We introduce overarching themes to confer responsibility and accountability implications with a discussion and way forward.

Population and System Characteristics

Isolation, Guilt, Separation from Family, and Poor Social Network

Variations in disease presentation and effects of poor social networks with subsequent social isolation complicate management of psychological illness. Before arrival in host countries, refugees and asylum seekers are often held in custody or in a besieged state, are self-isolated, or flee to a neighboring country for temporary safety.[13,24] Usually, their physical injuries, including those from forced labor and beatings, go untreated. They commonly believe that their lives will never be normal.[13,24] After arrival, they often lack employment or steady housing, have no social and family support, and spend most of their time in isolation.[24] Many express guilt, particularly for leaving loved ones behind, being unable to provide for their families, or inadvertently causing them harm by association. They may assume guilt for their comrades or cellmates because they could not help them during their collective plight or journey.[13,24] Many meet multiple criteria for PTSD and depression, but the nuances of their unique situations complicate diagnostic practices. Social isolation is considered a symptom of depression, but it has a special context for survivors. Isolating themselves in their home countries or during their plight flight to safety was rational and intentional, given the dangers of active threats when hiding from perpetrators. This self-imposed social isolation continues in the host country due to a combination of predisposing and complicating social factors, which further limits refugees' social assimilation and hampers their participation in social activities, connection to the community, or semblance of normalcy. Both physical and psychological conditions are frequently left unaddressed due to poor access and limited cultural competence of providers.

Health Care and Social System Challenges

Current literature commonly groups together all refugees without attention to the unique challenges faced by the subgroups due to their legal status and experience of torture, and subsequent effects on their mental health and coping mechanisms, which makes it challenging to differentiate barriers and approaches.[13,18,27,30,35–39] Refugee and asylum seekers have unmet subsistence needs and continuously suffer from unemployment/underemployment, fragile legal status, lack of medical insurance, poor housing, and food insecurity.[13,35,39] Routine and efficient diagnostic and therapeutic modalities for psychosocial burdens are lacking. Health systems in host countries suffer from overall structural constraints, including inadequate training in cultural competence for providers.[40] Among health care providers, there is a perception of difficulty in addressing refugees' sociocultural problems and other medical priorities within constraints of the typical medical visit. Refugees and asylum seekers rarely receive help navigating the complex new health systems, especially for mental health services.

Basic logistics pose further barriers to deciphering appropriate psychosocial diagnoses. Language barriers are significant factors. Through the sieve of translation, nuances that are particularly necessary for understanding feelings are omitted from the patient–provider interaction.[25,41] Furthermore, some refugees or asylum seekers may not have previously encountered a physician or medical provider asking how they feel, if they feel sad, or enquiring about psychological symptoms. The Western model of psychiatric services in home countries is infrequently available,[13] and most people rely heavily on community coping strategies and approaches.[42] Allopathic mental health services alone are not commonplace in many original countries, and patients often have their own specific interpretations of mental health and are not prepared to reflect on their emotional states with a provider.[13,24,42] Prior to their arrival, some refugees may have had access to traditional care and community support that is more familiar and culturally appropriate, which often does not exist in host countries.[13,18,35] Refugee patients have often survived tremendous hardship and do not readily offer important details about their mental and emotional state in an environment that is so foreign and detached from what they know. They may internalize their trauma experiences because of lack of social and community support. This reticence, exacerbated by poor mental health, may result in masking of their symptoms when approached by physicians and other providers.[37]

Refugees often carry sustained distrust and fear of any government and its agents (and, by association, legal or medical personnel) due to their history of abuse and being discriminated against. Refugee patients who do not entirely fit the criteria for a specific disorder may nonetheless exhibit important and significant somatic and psychological symptoms,[35,39,43] and practitioners are challenged to characterize this mental anguish.[18,44] Once providers arrive at a mental health diagnosis, they need to recommend therapies. In addition, available therapies are regularly not accessed by or culturally adapted to these patients.[30]

In some host countries, refugees recognized by the United Nations High Commissioner for Refugees (UNHCR) may be connected with some type of formalized refugee services and are theoretically afforded some assistance in housing, health care, and employment upon arrival.[45] In practice, however, most refugees live in limbo or transitional states until their status is accepted, which takes a heavy toll and hinders any treatment and a productive, connected life. The imposed social isolation is particularly insidious, and it increases after arrival in the transitional or host country and puts them at risk for additional health problems.[39,46] Their status contributes to their isolation, in part due to limitations on engaging with their environment while in limbo legal status or due to restriction in employment and practical access to social services.[39]

Responsibility and Accountability

To effectively change the previously discussed dynamic, more needs to be done, beyond accepting refugees into the host societies, to facilitate some form of well-being and a dignified livelihood. Both social and health systems responses are needed to help integrate refugees into the existing health care and social systems and to navigate the divide between sociocultural backgrounds and experiences and practices and regulations regarding their care.

Professional Responsibilities

Health professionals' interest in social responsibility and the concepts of rights to health has been more pronounced with an increased appreciation of social determinants of health and the sociopolitical context of patients' illnesses. As resourceful members of their communities, they should not overlook the opportunity to improve the plight of refugees and could assume the role of advocate[47] and shed light on both medical and public health implications of inadequate treatment of refugees and the fundamental sociopolitical context that affect their health status. General practitioners and public health service members are often the first to come in contact with asylum seekers and can facilitate their individual and community well-being. They can help refugees in their documentation or asylum processes and secure a stable and legal status in some host countries.[13,24,43,44] Practitioners could help connect them with community organizations, community mental health providers, fellow refugee/asylum seekers, and other available social and medical services. Accordingly, at both the medical and public health levels, professional guidelines and targeted training in health care and ethics of working with asylum seekers need to be offered through respective professional societies, involving social scientists, bioethicists, and representatives of refugee communities, providers, and governmental agencies. Appropriate training for health care providers would prepare them to facilitate better communication and to identify and address the unique problems faced by this vulnerable population.[18,27,38] Simultaneously, public health and social service agencies have a critical role in providing and an obligation to ensure appropriate services by devising and maintaining culturally competent community-level interventions with active outreach and robust training for all service providers and comprehensive support centers. Psychosocial services and psychiatric treatment require tailoring to individual or community needs. Therefore, the health care system as a whole must consider it a professional responsibility to facilitate supportive modalities or adaption of refugees' local community coping strategies, and it must research their feasibility through community-based participatory approaches to fill in for the lack of access to, and validity and efficacy of, current Western therapeutic approaches to psychological illness.[30] This requires close collaboration between direct service providers, such as physicians, social workers, psychiatrists, and psychologists, and the public health system, social service agencies, and legal entities.

Health professionals, however, can only practice in a culture that supports this spirit, while the culture of medicine and its ethics and responsibilities continues to evolve toward a better and more rigorous discourse. A bottom-up approach is more likely to be effective by incorporating character building in the education of health professionals at their respective schools,[48–51] along with public advocate entities that could not only provide guidelines and adjust as we move forward in multicultural societies with new challenges and opportunities to our moral discourse but also redress and address diversions of sound and responsible health care practices.

Societal Responsibility and Accountability

Access to appropriate health care among refugees depends on the characteristics of the social and health systems and service accessibility in the host countries, which fundamentally relate to underlying accountability processes, expectations, views, and commitment to the rights of vulnerable populations. Developed countries welcome hundreds of thousands of refugees and asylum seekers annually. This welcome can be further supported by expanding cultural understanding and addressing psychosocial factors affecting their health, which requires a holistic approach in close collaboration between community organizations, government agencies, and service providers.[52–55] From a social responsibility perspective, structural support through government and not-for-profit sectors is not only an act of solidarity but also a just and sound measure. Minimum standards for access to care and social services have been devised in some U.S. states,[30,56–58] but they could be extended to meaningfully address important social factors such as appropriate housing, food security, vocational training, employment opportunities, cultural and linguistic immersion programs, and appropriate health insurance access. From a societal perspective, providing refugees with formal international and national recognition and adequate legal status would help alleviate structural barriers.[13,34] Awareness-raising and community education and networks of grassroots community organizations are likely to be effective in alleviating health inequalities and barriers to resources and helping refugees navigate complex social and health systems.[24]

Moving Forward

Social and health care government agencies have distinct accountability processes devised under the law and consistent with resources, characteristics, views, values, and expectations of the host societies, and they need to justify expansion of their services or accountability platforms. This will only be possible to realistically implement if the public at large is involved in these important societal decisions and expanding roles. The not-for-profit sector and scientific community could help generate proper evidence on the extent and nature of refugees' needs, the potential for public good from addressing their needs, and the impact on the broader interest of the public. This process must be transparent, away from political or charged views, with clear understanding of and communications about the advantages and disadvantages of proposed social and health care interventions. Government agencies could more systematically evaluate current interventions and provide public platforms to seek input from the public at large and create momentum and consensus regarding specific limits or expansion of potential resources. Passionate advocacy from advocacy-oriented organizations is helpful to raise awareness, but it requires transparency and evidence-based approaches, balancing advantages and disadvantages of the feasibility and effectiveness of interventions, and providing clear ways forward. Temporary programs might have to be implemented; however, more integrated and holistic interventions require a comprehensive, fair, balanced, humane, and accountable approach.

Pain Assessment and Treatment Among Torture Survivors and Asylum Seekers

Assessment

Conditions for Assessment

The prevalence of torture survivors among refugee and migrant populations is variable, but it is often estimated at between 30% and 50%; a recent U.S. estimate was 44%.[59] Torture survivors may be encountered anywhere in the health care system and in any specialist service, but they will not necessarily be identifiable as torture survivors, nor can it be assumed that they will disclose this to health care staff unless asked.[60] Their presentation of pain is often complicated by multiple factors: distrust in general or particularly of medical staff or anyone in state employment; lack of fluency in the language of the host country; lack of knowledge of anatomical terms appropriate for medical settings; fear of incurring health care costs; and multiple social problems, such as uncertain civil status, inadequate income, unstable accommodations, and lack of social support. Furthermore, the association of pain with the experience of torture may make survivors reluctant to discuss it, particularly when they have symptoms of post-traumatic stress.[13,24,26,44] To some extent, health care services can mitigate some of these difficulties by making interpreting services available, providing clear information on possible charges for health care and exemptions to those charges, communicating respect for confidentiality, and recognizing that trust may take time to establish and that several sessions may be required to obtain information useful for a complete assessment.[24,44,61] Interpretation by trained professionals should be offered, even when the patient has some host language skills, to make the assessment easier for the patient. The patient's need for a particular language or dialect, sex or ethnicity of interpreter, and a preference for phone or in-person interpretation should be met as much as possible. Interpreters who are not familiar with torture should be briefed and debriefed, and the importance of confidentiality should be emphasized.

Asking About Torture

Medical staff should be prepared to ask about torture if there are any grounds to suspect it has occurred, such as being a refugee from one of the many countries where it is practiced (by reference to information such as from Amnesty International, Human Rights Watch, or World Health Organization websites). Due to many missed opportunities in primary health care encounters in the United States, it is recommended that foreign-born patients should be routinely asked about torture.[14,15] The grounds for torture may be due to the individual's ethnicity, religion, sexuality, place of work or residence, membership in specific social groups, misidentification of the individual, or entirely random. Some survivors may have been well aware of the risks they took; others could have been tortured as a warning to a group or population.[62] However, most health care staff are reluctant to ask about torture, especially because they fear causing additional distress to the patient, and they have little confidence in being able to provide adequate medical or psychological support if torture is disclosed.[44] Knowing how to proceed if torture is disclosed requires training and support, but asking about torture is important, even if little can be offered immediately. The question can be prefaced by inquiries about detention, conflict, and ill-treatment in the patient's home country or during their journey to the host country, demonstrating to the patient that the staff member is inclined to recognize their account, in contrast to the disbelief and challenge that torture survivors routinely encounter when claiming asylum.[63,64] The expectation of being heard helps build trust, even if patients do not disclose their experience straightaway.[44]

Assessing Pain

Here, we discuss assessment for pain care and for medicolegal assessment to support the survivor's asylum claim, which is a specialized skill requiring training, system support, and knowledge of legal frameworks for understanding medical evidence.[43,44,51] One of the major challenges for the pain clinician can be unfamiliarity of the typical multiple injuries and assaults to which the body has been subjected, and presentation of the sequelae years (rarely months) later. The injuries are usually inflicted on people stressed by poor conditions and without any access to health care. In some countries, there is an effort not to leave visible signs on the body, thereby undermining the individual's claim to asylum on the grounds of torture. Many soft tissue injuries leave no obvious marks (e.g., most blunt traumas and some electrical torture) and require advanced knowledge and skills to identify. The same form of torture, such as beating the soles of the feet (falanga), can result in a range of different pain phenomena, at rest and/or on weight-bearing.[65–67] Severe strain on joints, prolonged forced positions, and plexopathies can be produced by hyperextension of limbs from which the survivor is hung.[68]

Accounts of injuries and abuse provided by survivors are often partial. Survivors may have been unconscious or drugged some of the time and not know what was done to them. There may be memory loss from head injuries, and recounting the torture can feel shameful and humiliating, particularly when rape and sexual torture have occurred.[44] It is therefore unclear to what extent a full account of physical torture is available for pain assessment. It might be helpful to focus on symptoms and to develop hypotheses about likely pain mechanisms that may be accessible to treatment, always bearing in mind to check for malunited fractures; shrapnel and other foreign bodies; experimental surgeries and pharmacological interventions; and acquired diseases, parasites, and nutritional deficiencies. Assessing chronic pain in general requires a nuanced approach with detailed history-taking over time, appropriate psychosocial history that could describe the psychological modulation of the pain experience, and perhaps trials of different therapeutic modalities based on potential hypotheses about specific mechanisms of pain. This is hampered in the case of persons who survive torture or maltreatment. There are no available tools to help diagnosis, and the Istanbul Protocol[69] that guides medicolegal examination is less helpful in identifying chronic pain than is the short-form Brief Pain Inventory[70,71] with which it has been compared.[72] Creating a therapeutic relationship based on trust, and allowing for and welcoming patients' participation in understanding and evaluating the origin and pattern of pain, is critical. Communicating hypotheses and findings with patients as assessment proceeds can be particularly useful in reducing anxieties and building a trusting relationship.

Types of Pain

There are no systematic studies of the prevalence and types of pain in torture survivors, and types of pain may vary with country of origin and at the time when torture was inflicted. Prevalence estimates are available from select populations, each with different biases, but most are very high considering the average age of the survivor population: often more than 80% of torture survivors.[73,74] Headache, musculoskeletal, and joint pain are very common,[75,76] as is widespread pain.[77] Foot or hand pain, and associated pain in the calf or forearm after beating on the soles of the feet or palm of hands, may have a predominantly neuropathic quality, a gait that avoids full weight on the sole, and pain that can be worse at rest.[65,66,77,78] A common type of torture that may leave no physical signs is suspension by the arms behind the back, leading to shoulder, arm, and neck pain and often associated with partial trauma to the brachial plexus, causing arm weakness and sensations of heaviness.[67] In general, most forced positions will cause significant chronic pain with varying degree of severity over time. Torture in the form of sexual assault can produce pelvic, genital, and anal pain and also urological and gynecological problems.[20,67,74,79] Sexual assaults in men are significantly underreported, and it is difficult to obtain information about their prevalence, severity, or associated factors due to pervasive stigma.[26]

The types of torture, even if survivors can give a full account, do not necessarily indicate the etiology of current pain problems. Whatever the local tissue injury, the overall conditions of risk, fear, and lack of hygiene, medical care, and even nutrition are likely to amplify central pain processing and undermine normal healing processes. Head injury can also be associated with the development of chronic pain,[80] and particular attention should be paid to the possibility of peripheral and central neuropathic pain processes.[67,75,81,82] Survivors are often exposed to further trauma during their flight to safety, thus complicating evaluation; therefore, exploration of additional traumas and the impact on pain presentation may be needed. In addition, pain presentation and its ethology may have significant cultural or social components that are not well known or recognized, with unfamiliar descriptions of some psychological problems in somatic terms. Physicians and other health care providers need to be vigilant and explore psychosocial issues in relation to pain.

Treatment

Establishing Shared Understanding

As with all chronic pain, establishing a shared understanding of the pain and of putative mechanisms helps lay the groundwork for discussion of medical and psychological interventions. Asking patients what they believe to be the cause of the pain may elicit culturally specific models that are unknown to clinicians or that may be familiar in terms of lay mechanistic beliefs about the body and about the meaning of pain. Torture survivors may feel irreparably damaged by torture.[26,67,68,76] Although some survivors show clear signs compatible with their account of pain and other persistent symptoms, an explanation of the body's healing capacity can still be helpful. Where investigation and examination find no signs, pain can be reformulated in terms of nervous system changes associated with persistent pain. Unfortunately, patient-friendly explanations of pain are scarce even in common languages, and perhaps absent in many languages and dialects spoken by survivors. This puts the onus on the clinician to describe the pain and its origin, using the survivor's own experience or those of others from the same sociocultural background as examples. Helping patients assist practitioners to better understand these nuances may require community collaboration and the use of informational materials.

Psychologically Informed Understanding of Pain

A further gap between clinicians and patients can arise with survivors' suspicion of the introduction of psychological terms into descriptions of how pain works. Psychological and psychiatric disorders may be seriously stigmatized in cultures with few psychiatrists or psychologists, who deal only with severely mentally ill patients whose needs have exhausted the resources of their extended families. For example, everyday distresses are often managed within the family network in many societies and are considered irrelevant or improper to share in medical settings. Depression and post-traumatic stress symptoms and disorders are common in survivors.[26,83] One large systematic review estimated approximately 30% prevalence for both depression and post-traumatic stress in refugee populations,[84] and this is likely higher among torture survivors[13,44,85] and even higher among those detained by immigration authorities.[86] There appears to be some mutual maintenance process, still poorly described, between pain and post-traumatic stress share threat, negative predictions, and avoidance, and this is described as "mutual maintenance" as they interact.[87–89] Post-arrival conditions, such as access to or lack of employment opportunities, adequate non-institutional accommodation, and current social support, are also important in mitigating or worsening refugees' mental health.[35,90] Ideally, health care providers working with survivors should liaise with social and welfare services to coordinate efforts to improve the overall health of survivors.[91]

The predominance of psychological therapies in not-for-profit and international aid sectors for torture survivors has not in general fostered good understanding or even recognition of pain problems. Rather, physical symptoms (usually without medical assessment or in the absence of obvious physical signs) have been conceptualized as somatic expression of distress and expected to resolve with treatment of distress.

Although reducing distress is likely to make pain itself somewhat easier to manage, the model of purely "psychosomatic" pain is inappropriate and lacks evidence. Pain is relatively rarely assessed in the treatment of post-traumatic stress or depression in torture survivors, and a systematic review reported that treatment effects were disappointingly small and short term,[92] although other narrative reviews are more optimistic.[93,94] Using purely Western psychiatric nosology to formulate psychological effects of torture and intervene accordingly will overlook important sociopolitical contexts of survivors' distress; interventions need to consider the broader context.[95–97]

Interventions for Chronic Pain

A systematic review and meta-analysis of any type of pain treatment offered to torture survivors found only three randomized controlled trials, very small (88 participants in total) and restricted to cognitive–behavioral therapy with biofeedback used in two trials and manual therapy in one trial.[98] Decrease in pain, disability, and distress was disappointingly small, with low confidence in estimates of effects and a high risk of bias. Grouping torture survivors together as the sole treated population may make little sense when treatment is surgical or pharmacological, and when it is physiotherapy- or psychology-based, aimed at rehabilitation, it is not clear whether torture survivors are better treated as an exclusive group or mixed with other patients. Arrangements may be based on practical rather than clinical considerations.[99] More recent controlled and uncontrolled accounts of multidisciplinary pain management have shown very modest outcomes, lower than those for a largely nontraumatized population. A systematic review of 15 controlled and uncontrolled studies of psychologically based interventions for torture survivors with PTSD and chronic pain demonstrated small benefit and some harms, which should not be overlooked, even though the majority of these studies did not intervene specifically for pain.[100]

Formulating the best plan of care to address pain requires liaising with psychologists and engaging the patient, building a trusting relationship, and ensuring that procedures are clearly explained so that unexpected flashbacks (e.g., from being naked or injected) are avoided. Physiotherapy is often a culturally acceptable intervention, and it can help the survivor adjust to being touched without undue fear arousal.[101] Rehabilitative approaches, such as pain management offered individually or in a group, are one of the more widely offered interventions because they do not require expensive medical equipment or personnel. However, they are often rather narrow in scope. Broader rehabilitative approaches for the mental health of refugees (rather than only torture survivors), which are rarely described in trials, engage with what participants themselves identify as their needs. These approaches may involve many components not usually seen within health care systems, including education, language classes, training in employment skills, and provision of childcare, offered alongside psychological interventions for individuals, groups, or families.[95,97] Pain self-management, where it is identified as a need, could also be considered in such programs.

The many uncertainties in torture survivors' lives, including whether they can remain in the host country, unsatisfactory and often temporary accommodation, restrictions on legal employment options, often insufficient financial resources to afford both a meal and a phone call to family left behind or travel to a medical appointment, and potential distrust and suspicion in the host country from the host or other refugee populations, can lead to nonadherence to health care recommendations and clinical and social service appointments. This in turn is discouraging for the health care team and can lead to a perception of survivors as unmotivated or ungrateful rather than struggling. There are obligations under human rights law to provide asylum, reparation, and rehabilitation to torture survivors,[102] which are rarely upheld. Many professional bodies that regulate the practice of health care personnel recognize the obligations to provide health care for torture survivors but provide little guidance or support for doing so, while some national organizations have failed to act against providers who developed and promoted techniques for maltreatment.[103]

Clinical care of torture survivors takes place in statutory health care systems, but it is also provided by charitable and not-for-profit organizations in poorly resourced settings without availability of trained medical staff. Pain expertise with knowledge of evidence for efficacy and harm of potential interventions may be lacking in deciding on appropriate and effective treatment, and untested or ineffective therapies may sometimes be promoted. Resource constraints in such settings, including a lack of trained practitioners, may lead to suboptimal plans of care and unrealistic expectations that cannot be met.

Health Care Beyond Direct Treatment

There are many opportunities to be considered beyond providing direct clinical care. Collaborations with charities and grassroots and nongovernmental organizations that provide social services to torture survivors could help provide better explanations and understanding of pain, and these organization could consult survivors regarding pain management. Such collaborations could improve services for survivors and help health care systems operate more effectively. Relevant clinical vignettes could be prepared and shared as educational materials for a wider audience in health care and/or published in single-person trials.[104,105] Key elements to consider in diagnosing and addressing pain relate to multiple factors, including the difficulty in establishing the origin of pain due to factors discussed above, important and pervasive psychosocial and sociocultural components, lack of training and support among the providers, limited evidence in diagnosis or treatment modalities, and competing social needs and requirements that significantly hamper survivors' engagement and their experience. However, there is opportunity to work collaboratively within academia and with community organizations, train health care providers, collect data and generate evidence, and support clinicians in a conducive and accommodating environment with the involvement of governmental and nongovernmental social service agencies. In the end, this field of study and practice has been significantly overlooked by the scientific community and requires further study and better collaboration between physicians, service providers, and academic institutions.

Screening for Torture, Provider Training, and Support Systems in Primary Care Settings

Background

Considering the mass influx of refugees from war-torn areas such as Syria, Afghanistan and Iraq, North Africa, and, most recently, Central and South America, appropriate public health and population-based strategies are needed to better address the health care of survivors of war trauma and human rights abuses. Torture and human rights abuses are reported in more than 150 countries, and they are commonly practiced in many. In the United States, approximately 12.5% of the population is foreign-born,[106] there are more than 11 million undocumented immigrants (mostly from developing regions),[107] and there are tens of thousands of refugees arriving in the country annually who are at higher risk for a history of human rights abuses. Although it is difficult to estimate the actual number of torture survivors worldwide, among foreign-born patients in urban primary care clinics in the United States, the prevalence of torture is estimated to be 7–11%,[14] with higher rates among certain subgroups. Prevalence is much higher among asylum seekers and refugees, and approximately 4% of torture survivors are children.

Medical and Social Challenges

Long-term and short-term physical and psychological consequences of torture are significant and interfere with survivors' social functioning. They include PTSD, major depressive disorder, chronic pain, and functional limitations from physical torture.[14,15,18–23] Foreign-born survivors face multiple barriers to health care access. These include existing mental illness, discrimination, fear of deportation, language barriers, unemployment, poor housing, food insecurity, barriers in social assimilation, and compounding factors such as providers' lack of cultural competencies and vigilance about mental illness that negatively affect their health.[24,27–29,31–33] Survivors often carry their burdens for many years without having the opportunity or awareness to discuss these issues with their physicians or other providers.

Role of Physicians and Health Care Providers

Because they have the pivotal role of addressing health care needs, primary care providers are often the gatekeepers for survivors' entry into the health care and legal systems. In addition to addressing the unique medical and psychiatric needs of these patients, primary care providers also have the opportunity to document the physical and mental scars of torture for the purpose of survivors being able to gain asylum.[43,48–50] Legal representation coupled with medical affidavits prepared by trained clinicians significantly increase asylum approval rates up to three times.[13,43,108]

Despite the ethical and professional obligation to train health professionals in the identification and treatment of survivors of torture, as set forth by the Convention Against Torture and adopted by the American College of Physicians,[102,109] there are very few such training opportunities. Less than 10% of all medical students receive an hour or more of formal training regarding torture,[110] and less than 20% of all medical schools have any formal international human rights curricula.[111] Health professional postgraduate training regarding care for survivors of torture is similarly uncommon, with just a few programs that offer formal curricula.[13,43,48–50]

With the many access barriers and constraints that torture survivors face, along with existing health and social system gaps and bureaucracy, contact with any medical professional would be an unmatched opportunity to screen for torture and direct them to proper medical and social services. However, screening for torture or human rights abuses has not been introduced into guidelines in the primary care setting, despite the high numbers of potential survivors.

Screening Could Create Opportunities

Considering the lack of social resources, higher occurrence of psychiatric illnesses, and issues with access, early detection and evaluation of torture among foreign-born and higher risk patients might help better address their specific needs. Screening could improve early access to mental health and social or legal services, especially for the nondocumented and uninsured. It might also help decrease individual, community, and societal costs. In addition, physicians and other providers can play the role of advocate and agent of social change by helping connect survivors to available resources. By providing documentation of torture, they not only give relief from risk of deportation and improve rates of asylum approval but also help survivors in their healing process. The introduction of screening among high-risk groups in the primary care setting also provides an opportunity to teach cultural competencies.[43,48–50] Not only does this introduce medical students and residents to the concept of cross-cultural medicine but also it introduces them to global sociopolitical issues and helps them connect with their patients more effectively and with better rapport. Similarly, this population is significantly understudied and there are limited evidence-based data to support therapeutic, social service, or advocacy efforts on behalf of survivors. Screening through identifying and shedding light on the lives of survivors provides further opportunities for researching and evaluating their needs, ultimately benefiting the community of survivors with tangible results, as well as society as a whole, and providing sound service through responsible participatory research.

There are examples of successful targeted screening for other forms of abuse, such as domestic or child abuse, well studied and introduced into practice in emergency rooms and primary care settings. These can therefore inform proper policy, system, and practice strategies for screening for torture. We recommend targeted screening for high-risk groups such as nondocumented and documented immigrants from developing regions or countries where torture and abuse are common; individuals who arrive with refugee status through the UNHCR; asylum seekers; immigrants from countries in which torture is commonly practiced; individual immigrants with a history of political activism; members of special social groups or ethnicities; and refugees with chronic pain, PTSD, or depression.[112] A criterion-based structured interview or questionnaire has been evaluated for its reliability and consistency with high sensitivity and specificity among specific subgroups of refugees.[113] In a refugee and immigrant clinic, a simple direct question regarding history of torture and abuse was introduced; if the answer was positive, this was followed by focused questions.[50] We emphasize the simplicity and ease of this screening question.

The Way Forward

Screening alone is obviously not enough. From a societal perspective, provision of care and services to torture survivors is not only a medical and professional issue but also a socioeconomic and political one. Changes are needed at multiple levels of health and social systems, in terms of both policies and services. These include providing affordable, culturally appropriate, and accessible health care to identified survivors, which necessitates a comprehensive and systematic approach in collaboration with social and community organizations. Further rollout and implementation of affordable health insurance through states or other entities could help improve opportunities for access to health care. At the provider level, professional and ethical guidelines must be developed with the involvement of physicians and other health care providers, public health professionals, social scientists, bioethicists, and health and human rights advocates, and perhaps drawing on other nations' experience. By updating continuous medical education programs, they could not only serve as a forum to provide skills in identifying and caring for survivors but also increase sensitivity and help generate critical self-evaluation among physicians and other health care providers. There may be a further need for development of standard and validated diagnostic and treatment guidelines. There are, however, multiple torture survivor clinics and centers in the United States that provide some services for physical and psychological sequelae of torture with promising results.[13,43,72,114]

References

1. Pupavac V. Refugees in the "sick role": Stereotyping refugees and eroding refugee rights. Research paper No. 128. United Nations High Commissioner for Refugees. 2006. https://www.unhcr.org/en-in/44e198712.pdf
2. Clark B, Preto N. Exploring the concept of vulnerability in health care. *Can Med Assoc J.* 2018;190(11):E308–E309.
3. Brown K. "Vulnerability": Handle with care. *Ethics Soc Welfare.* 2011;5(3):313–321.
4. Willen SS. Migration, "illegality," and health: Mapping embodied vulnerability and debating health-related deservingness. *Soc Sci Med.* 2012;74(6):805–811.
5. Larchanché S. Intangible obstacles: Health implications of stigmatization, structural violence and fear among undocumented immigrants in France. *Soc Sci Med.* 2012;74(6):858–863.
6. Quesada J. Special Issue Part II: Illegalization and embodied vulnerability in health. *Soc Sci Med.* 2012;74(6):894–896.
7. Viladrich A. Beyond welfare reform: Reframing undocumented immigrants' entitlement to health care in the United States, a critical review. *Soc Sci Med.* 2012;74(6):822–829.
8. Williams ACC. Are you working? *Br Med J.* 2009;338:a859.
9. Davis KD, Aghaeepour N, Ahn AH, et al. Discovery and validation of biomarkers to aid the development of safe and effective pain therapeutics: Challenges and opportunities. *Nat Rev Neurol.* 2020;16(7):381–400.
10. United Nations High Commissioner for Refugees. Mid-year trends 2015. 2015. https://data.unhcr.org/en/documents/details/48932. Accessed 12.27.22.
11. International Organization for Migration. Irregular migrants, refugee arrivals in Europe Top One Million in 2015. 2015. https://www.iom.int/news/irregular-migrant-refugee-arrivals-europe-top-one-million-2015-iom. Accessed 12.27.22.
12. U.S. Department of Homeland Security. U.S. Citizenship and Immigration Services. 2013. http://www.uscis.gov/portal/site/uscis. Accessed 12.27.22.

13. Asgary R, Charpentier B, Burnett DC. Socio-medical challenges of asylum seekers prior and after coming to the US. *J Immigr Minor Health*. 2013;15(5):961–968.
14. Crosby SS, Norredam M, Paasche-Orlow MK, Piwowarczyk L, Heeren T, Grodin MA. Prevalence of torture survivors among foreign-born patients presenting to an urban ambulatory care practice. *J Gen Intern Med*. 2006;21(7):764–768.
15. Eisenman DP, Keller AS, Kim G. Survivors of torture in a general medical setting: How often have patients been tortured, and how often is it missed? *West J Med*. 2000;172(5):301–304.
16. Marshall GN, Schell TL, Elliott MN, et al. Mental health of Cambodian refugees 2 decades after resettlement in the United States. *JAMA*. 2005;294(5):571–579.
17. Mollica RF, Caridad KR, Massagli MP. Longitudinal study of posttraumatic stress disorder, depression, and changes in traumatic memories over time in Bosnian refugees. *J Nerv Ment Dis*. 2007;195(7):572–579.
18. Silove D, Steel Z, Watters C. Policies of deterrence and the mental health of asylum seekers. JAMA, 2000;284(5):604–611.
19. Carinci AJ, Mehta P, Christo PJ. Chronic pain in torture victims. *Curr Pain Headache Rep*. 2010;14(2):73–79.
20. Norredam M, Crosby S, Munarriz R, Piwowarczyk L, Grodin M. Urologic complications of sexual trauma among male survivors of torture. *J Urol*. 2005;65(1):28–32.
21. Vorbrüggen M, Baer HU. Humiliation: The lasting effect of torture. *Mil Med*. 2007;172(12 Suppl):29–33.
22. Wenzel T. Torture. *Curr Opin Psychiatry*. 2007;20(5):491–496.
23. Wenzel T, Griengl H, Stompe T, et al. Psychological disorders in survivors of torture: Exhaustion, impairment and depression. *Psychopathology*. 2000;33(6):292–296.
24. Asgary R, Segar N. Barrier to healthcare access among refugee asylum seekers. *J Health Care Poor Underserved*. 2011;22(2):506–522.
25. Bischoff A, Bovier PA, Rrustemi I, et al. Language barriers between nurses and asylum seekers: Their impact on symptom reporting and referral. *Soc Sci Med*. 2003;57(3):503–512.
26. Burnett A, Peel M. Asylum seekers and refugees in Britain: The health of survivors of torture and organised violence. *Br Med J*. 2001;322(7286):606–609.
27. Hadgkiss E, Renzaho A. The physical health status, service utilization and barriers to accessing care for asylum seekers residing in the community: A systematic review of the literature. *Aus Health Rev*. 2014;38(2):142–159.
28. Ngo-Metzger Q, Massagli MP, Clarridge BR, et al. Linguistic and cultural barriers to care. *J Gen Intern Med*. 2003;18(1):44–52.
29. Piwowarczyk L, Keane TM, Lincoln A. Hunger: The silent epidemic among asylum seekers and resettled refugees. *Int Migration*. 2008;46(1):59–77.
30. Renner W, Bänninger-Hube E, Peltzer K. Culture-Sensitive and Resource Oriented Peer (CROP)-Groups as a community based intervention for trauma survivors: A randomized controlled pilot study with refugees and asylum seekers from Chechnya. *Aust J Dis Trauma Stud*. 2011;2011(1):1–13.
31. Weine S, Kulauzovic Y, Klebic A, et al. Evaluating a multiple-family group access intervention for refugees with PTSD. *J Marital Fam Ther*. 2008;34(2):149–164.
32. Wissink L, Jones-Webb R, DuBois D, et al. Improving health care provision to Somali refugee women. *Minn Med*. 2005;88(2):36–40.
33. Wong EC, Marshall GN, Schell TL, et al. Barriers to mental health care utilization for U.S. Cambodian refugees. *J Consult Clin Psychol*. 2005;74(6):1116–1120.
34. Heeren M, Whittmann L, Ehler U, et al. Psychopathology and resident status: Comparing asylum seekers, refugees, illegal migrants, labor migrants, and residents. *Compr Psychology*. 2014;56(4):818–825.
35. Gorst-Unsworth C, Goldenberg E. Psychological sequelae of torture and organised violence suffered by refugees from Iraq: Trauma-related factors compared to social factors in exile. *Br J Psychiatry*. 1998;172:90–94.
36. Harris M, Zwar N. Refugee health. *Aust Fam Physician*. 2005;34(10):825–829.

37. Mazur VM, Chahraoui K, Bissler L. Psychopathology of asylum seekers in Europe, trauma and defensive functioning. *Encephale.* 2015;41(3):221–228.
38. Slobodin O, de Jong JT. Mental health interventions for traumatized asylum seekers and refugees: What do we know about their efficacy? *Int J Soc Psychiatry.* 2015;61(1):17–26.
39. Warfa N, Curtis S, Watters C, et al. Migration experiences, employment status and psychological distress among Somali immigrants: A mixed-method international study. *BMC Public Health.* 2012;12: Article 749.
40. Savin D, Seymour DJ, Littleford LN, et al. Findings from mental health screening of newly arrived refugees in Colorado. *Public Health Rep.* 2005;120(3):224–229.
41. Bischoff A, Denhaerynck K. What do language barriers cost? An exploratory study among asylum seekers in Switzerland. *BMC Health Serv Res.* 2010;10: Article 248.
42. Cohen S, Asgary R. Community coping strategies in response to hardship and human rights abuses among Burmese refugees and migrants at the Thai–Burmese border: A qualitative approach. *Fam Community Health.* 2016;39(2):75–81.
43. Asgary R, Metalios EE, Smith CL, Paccione GA. Evaluating asylum seekers/torture survivors in urban primary care: A collaborative approach at the Bronx Human Rights Clinic. *Health Hum Rights.* 2006;9(2):164–179.
44. Asgary R, Smith CL. Ethical and professional considerations providing evaluation and care to refugee asylum seekers. *Am J Bioeth.* 2013;13(7):3–12.
45. Martin DC, Yankay YE. Annual flow report: Refugees and asylees: 2012. Department of Homeland Security, Office of Immigration Statistics. 2013. https://www.dhs.gov/sites/default/files/publications/Refugees_Asylees_2012.pdf. Accessed 12.27.22.
46. Pantell M, Rehkopf D, Jutte D, et al. Social isolation: A predictor of mortality comparable to traditional clinical risk factors. *Am J Public Health.* 2013;103(11):2056–2062.
47. Brown T, Fee E. Rudolf Carl Virchow. *Am J Public Health.* 2006;96(12):2104–2105.
48. Asgary R. Graduate public health training in healthcare of refugee asylum seekers and clinical human rights. *Int J Public Health.* 2016;61(3):279–287.
49. Asgary R, Saenger P, Jophlin L, Burnett D. Domestic global health: A curriculum teaching medical students to evaluate refugee asylum seekers and torture survivors. *Teach Learn Med.* 2013;25(4):348–357.
50. Asgary R, Smith CL, Sckell B, Paccione G. Teaching immigrant and refugee health to residents: Domestic global health. *Teach Learn Med.* 2013;25(3):1–8.
51. Metalios EE, Asgary R, Cooperman N, et al. Teaching residents to work with torture survivors: Experiences from the Bronx Human Rights Clinic. *J Gen Intern Med.* 2008;23(7):1038–1042.
52. Agger I, Ansari F, Suresh S, Pulikuthiyil G. Justice as a healing factor: Psycho-legal counseling for torture survivors in an Indian context. *Peace Conflict.* 2008;14(3):315–333.
53. Bodenmann P, Madrid C, Vannotti M, Rossi I, Ruiz J. Migration without borders, but . . . barriers of meaning. *Rev Med Suisse.* 2007;3(135):2710–2712, 2714–2717.
54. Gangsei D, Deutsch AC. Psychological evaluation of asylum seekers as a therapeutic process. *Torture.* 2007;17:79–87.
55. Germain R, Velez LE. Legal services: Best, promising, and emerging practices. *Torture.* 2011;21(1):56–60.
56. Department of Health. Introduction to the National Health Service. 2013. https://webarchive.nationalarchives.gov.uk/ukgwa/20130104183334/http://www.dh.gov.uk/en/Publicationsandstatistics/Publications/PublicationsPolicyAndGuidance/DH_4122587. Accessed 12.27.22.
57. Maier T, Schmidt M, Mueller J. Mental health and healthcare utilization in adult asylum seekers. *Swiss Med Wkly.* 2012;140:w13110. doi:10.4414/smw.2010.13110
58. Taylor K. Asylum seekers, refugees, and the politics of access to health care: A UK perspective. *Br J Gen Pract.* 2009;59(567):765–772.
59. Higson-Smith C. Updating the estimate of refugees resettled in the United States who have suffered torture. 2015. Accessed July 14, 2022.https://www.cvt.org/sites/default/files/SurvivorNumberMetaAnalysis_Sept2015_0.pdf

60. Crosby SS. Primary care management of non-English-speaking refugees who have experienced trauma: A clinical review. *JAMA*. 2013;310(5):519–528.
61. Haoussou K. When your patient is a survivor of torture. *Br Med J*. 2016;355:i5019. https://doi.org/10.1136/bmj.i5019
62. Turner S, Gorst-Unsworth C. Psychological sequelae of torture: A descriptive model. *Br J Psychiatry*. 1990;157(4):475–480.
63. Affolter L. Trained to disbelieve: The normalisation of suspicion in a Swiss asylum administration office. *Geopolitics*. 2022;27(4):1069–1092.
64. Herlihy J, Turner SW. The psychology of seeking protection. *Int J Refugee Law*. 2009;21(2):171–192.
65. Amris K, Torp-Pedersen S, Rasmussen OV. Long-term consequences of falanga torture: What do we know and what do we need to know? *Torture*. 2009;19:33–40.
66. Prip K, Persson AL. Clinical findings in men with chronic pain after falanga torture. *Clin J Pain*. 2008;24(2):135–141.
67. Rasmussen O, Amris S, Blaauw M, Danielsen L. Medical physical examination in connection with torture: Section II. *Torture*. 2005;15(1):37–45.
68. Kaur G. Chronic pain in refugee torture survivors. *J Global Health*. 2017;7(2):010303. doi:10.7189/jogh.07.020303
69. United Nations Office of the High Commissioner for Human Rights. *Istanbul Protocol: Manual on the Effective Investigation and Documentation of Torture and Other Cruel, Inhuman or Degrading Treatment or Punishment*. United Nations; 2001. https://www.ohchr.org/sites/default/files/documents/publications/training8rev1en.pdf
70. Daut RL, Cleeland CS, Flaner RC. Development of the Wisconsin Brief Pain Questionnaire to assess pain in cancer and other diseases. *Pain*. 1983;17(2):197–210.
71. Tan G, Jensen MP, Thornby JI, Shanti BF. Validation of the Brief Pain Inventory for chronic nonmalignant pain. *J Pain*. 2004;5(2):133–137.
72. Kaur G, Weinberg R, Milewski AR, et al. Chronic pain diagnosis in refugee torture survivors: A prospective, blinded diagnostic accuracy study. *PLoS Med*. 2020;17(6):e1003108.
73. Olsen D, Montgomery E, Bøjholm S, Foldspang S. Prevalent musculoskeletal pain as a correlate of previous exposure to torture. *Scand J Public Health*. 2006;34(5):496–503.
74. Williams AC, Peña CR, Rice AS. Persistent pain in survivors of torture: A cohort study. *J Pain Symptom Manag*. 2010;40(5):715–722.
75. Amris K, Williams A. Chronic pain in survivors of torture. *Pain: Clinical Updates*. 2007;15:1–4.
76. Rasmussen OV. Medical aspects of torture. *Dan Med Bull*. 1990;37(Suppl 1):1–88.
77. Edston E. The epidemiology of falanga: Incidence among Swedish asylum seekers. *Torture*. 2009;19(1):27–32.
78. Prip K, Persson AL, Sjolund BH. Self-reported activity in tortured refugees with long-term sequelae including pain and the impact of foot pain from falanga: A cross-sectional study. *Disabil Rehabil*. 2011;33(7):569–578.
79. Musisi S, Kinyanda E, Liebling H, Mayengo-Kiziri R. Post-traumatic torture disorders in Uganda. *Torture*. 2000;10(3):81–87.
80. Nampiaparampil DE. Prevalence of chronic pain after traumatic brain injury. *JAMA*. 2008;300(6):711–719.
81. Moreno A, Grodin M. Torture and its neurological sequelae. *Spinal Cord*. 2002;40(5):213–223.
82. Thomsen A, Eriksen J, Schmidt-Nielsen K. Chronic pain in torture survivors. *Forensic Sci Int*. 2000;108(3):155–163.
83. Watters C. Emerging paradigms in the mental health care of refugees. *Soc Sci Med*. 2001;52(11):1709–1718.
84. Steel Z, Chey T, Silove D, Marnane C, Bryant RA, van Ommeren M. Association of torture and other potentially traumatic events with mental health outcomes among populations exposed to mass conflict and displacement: A systematic review and meta-analysis. *JAMA*. 2009;302(5):537–549.

85. Song SJ, Subica A, Kaplan C, Tol W, de Jong J. Predicting the mental health and functioning of torture survivors. *J Nerv Ment Dis.* 2018;206(1):33–39.
86. Steel Z, Silove D, Brooks R, Momartin S, Alzuhairi B, Susjlik I. Impact of immigration detention and temporary protection on the mental health of refugees. *Br J Psychiatry.* 2006;188:58–64.
87. Liedl A, O'Donnell M, Creamer M, et al. Support for the mutual maintenance of pain and post-traumatic stress disorder symptoms. *Psychol Med.* 2010;40(7):1215–1223.
88. Nordin L, Perrin S. Pain and post-traumatic stress disorder in refugees who survived torture: The role of pain catastrophizing and trauma-related beliefs. *Eur J Pain.* 2019;23(8):1497–1506.
89. Otis JD, Keane TM, Kerns RD. An examination of the relationship between chronic pain and post-traumatic stress disorder. *J Rehabil Res Dev.* 2003;40(5):397–406.
90. Porter M, Haslam N. Predisplacement and postdisplacement factors associated with mental health of refugees and internally displaced persons: A meta-analysis. *JAMA.* 2005;294(5):602–612.
91. Esala JJ, Vukovich MM, Hanbury A, Kashyap S, Joscelyne A. Collaborative care for refugees and torture survivors: Key findings from the literature. *Traumatology.* 2018;24(3):168–185.
92. Hamid A, Patel N, Williams ACC. Psychological, social and welfare interventions for torture survivors: A systematic review and meta-analysis of randomised controlled trials. *PLoS Med.* 2019;16(9):e1002919.
93. McFarlane C, Kaplan I. Evidence-based psychological interventions for adult survivors of torture and trauma: A 30-year review. *Transcult Psychiatry.* 2012;49(3–4):539–567.
94. Nickerson A, Bryant RA, Silove D, Steel Z. A critical review of psychological treatments of posttraumatic stress disorder in refugees. *Clin Psychol Rev.* 2011;31(3):399–417.
95. Salo CD, Bray EM. Empirically tested interventions for torture survivors: A systematic review through an ecological lens. *Transl Issues Psychol Sci.* 2016;2(4):449–463.
96. Patel N, Kellezi B, Williams ACC. Reviewing outcomes of psychological interventions with torture survivors: Conceptual, methodological and ethical issues. *Torture.* 2016;21(1):2–16.
97. Van Wyk S, Schweitzer RD. A systematic review of naturalistic interventions in refugee populations. *J Immigr Minor Health.* 2014;16(5):968–977.
98. Baird E, Williams ACC, Hearn L, Amris K. Interventions for treating persistent pain in survivors of torture. *Cochrane Database Syst Rev.* 2017;8(8):CD012051.
99. Kuehler B, Childs S. One-stop multidisciplinary pain clinic for survivors of torture. *Pain Manag.* 2016;6(5):415–419.
100. Rometsch-Ogioun El Sount C, Windthorst P, Denkinger J, et al. Chronic pain in refugees with post-traumatic stress disorder (PTSD): A systematic review on patients' characteristics and interventions. *J Psychosom Res.* 2019;118:83–97.
101. Franklin C. Physiotherapy with torture survivors. *Physiotherapy.* 2001;87(7):374–377.
102. United Nations General Assembly. Conventions against torture and other cruel, inhuman or degrading treatment or punishment. 1984. https://www.ohchr.org/en/instruments-mechanisms/instruments/convention-against-torture-and-other-cruel-inhuman-or-degrading. Accessed 12.27.22.
103. American Psychological Association. Position on ethics and interrogation. 2009. Accessed July 11, 2022. https://www.apa.org/ethics/programs/position
104. McDonald S, Nikles J. N-of-1 trials in healthcare. *Healthcare.* 2021;9(3):330.
105. Morley SJ. *Single Case Methods in Clinical Psychology: A Practical Guide.* Routledge; 2018.
106. United States Census Bureau. QuickFacts. Foreign born persons, percent, 2017-2021. https://www.census.gov/quickfacts/fact/table/US/PST045222. Accessed 10.24.2023.
107. Passel JS, Cohn DV. Unauthorized immigrant population: National and state trends, 2010. Pew Research Center. 2011. http://pewhispanic.org/reports/report.php?ReportID=133. Accessed 12.27.22.
108. Lustig SL, Kureshi S, Delucchi KL, Iacopino V, Morse SC. Asylum grant rates following medical evaluations of maltreatment among political asylum applicants in the United States. *J Immigr Minor Health.* 2008;10:7–15.

109. American College of Physicians. The role of the physician and the medical profession in the prevention of international torture and in the treatment of its survivors. *Ann Intern Med.* 1995;122(8):607–613.
110. Boyd JW, Himmelstein D, Lasser K, et al. U.S. medical students' knowledge about the military draft, the Geneva Convention, and military medical ethics. *Int J Health Serv.* 2007;37:643–650.
111. Sofair AN, Lurie PG. Military medicine and human rights. *Lancet.* 2004;364(9448):1851.
112. Miles SH, Garcia-Peltoniemi RE. Torture survivors: What to ask, how to document. *J Fam Pract.* 2012;61(4):E1–E5.
113. Montgomery E, Foldspang A. Criterion-related validity of screening for exposure to torture. *Dan Med Bull.* 1994;41(5):588–591.
114. New York City Office of Immigrant Affairs. Asylum seeker response. n.d.https://www.nyc.gov/site/immigrants/help/asylum-seekers/asylum-seekers-help.page. Accessed 12.27.22.

17

Pain in Extreme Situations

The Battlefield and Disasters

Harold J. Gelfand, Erin A. Tracy, and Austin G. Bell

Introduction

Armed conflict and natural disaster both involve the imposition of a traumatic event onto an unprepared and unsuspecting population. This disruption can cause losses in human life, disrupt economic productivity, and create negative environmental impacts.[1] Even when the scope of the immediate disaster may be localized, the fallout will test the capacity of the affected community's resources, and victims often require additional assistance from the national or international community. This chapter examines the factors that predispose both battlefield and natural disaster victims to pain, with a particular focus on the battlefield and military populations.

Pain and Extreme Environments

Sociomedical factors can greatly impact pain outcomes. Increased preoperative anxiety and catastrophizing are known risk factors for the development of persistent post-surgical pain.[2] The presence of pre-existing pain in surgical patients is a known predictor of severe postoperative pain and the development of chronic post-surgical pain.[3] Multisystem injuries from natural disasters or the battlefield often present with both nociceptive and neuropathic pain. Victims suffering blast injuries have high rates of polytrauma and traumatic brain injury (TBI), complicating pain management.[4] Unfortunately, insufficient pain management is common in acute care. With the addition of disaster-caused disruption in services and paucity of resources, inadequate pain control becomes a greater issue.[5] An examination of injury patterns and treatment modalities utilized to treat American and coalition casualties provides a structure for treatment of populations affected by natural disasters.

Natural Disasters

Natural disasters have impacted humanity throughout history. However, the frequency and impact of such events have been on the rise. Compared to 1960, the worldwide incidence of natural disasters in 2019 increased by an order of magnitude—from 39 to 396, respectively.[6] The United Nations Office for Disaster Risk Reduction's 2022 "Global

Assessment Report" cautioned that human behavior was contributing to increased disasters and projected a rate of 1.5 disasters per day by 2030.[1] These trends are driven by several factors. First, the global population has more than doubled during the past 60 years (3 billion in 1960 to 8 billion in 2022), with the resultant increase in infrastructure required to support this growth.[7,8] The current global census and areas of growth are concentrated mostly in coastal areas, increasing humanity's exposure to hurricanes, tidal waves, and flooding. This confluence of growth and exposure alone would increase humanity's exposure to natural disasters; however, abundant evidence points to destabilizing climactic changes on a global scale.[9]

As global warming increases, both governmental and nongovernmental agencies throughout the world warn that increased natural disaster occurrence will continue at its current pace, if not worsen. In 2021, the Intergovernmental Panel on Climate Change reported that anthropogenic climate change is driving an increase in sea level rise and intensification of the water cycle, increasing the risk of flooding, landslides, and extreme weather events.[10] The injuries caused by these disasters frequently include blunt trauma, crush injury, drowning, and mental health issues. Because most people affected by natural disasters do not perish initially, timely intervention can have a significant impact on the number of overall casualties and the long-term harm experienced by those casualties.[11]

The preponderance of data on injuries from natural disasters derives from earthquakes. Among geophysical disasters, earthquakes have both the highest mortality rates and the largest burden of injuries, with lower extremity injuries being most common.[12] A retrospective analysis of injuries in victims of a 2016 Taiwan earthquake catalogued specific injury intensities and locations. Contusions and abrasions were the most common, present in 93% of victims. This was closely followed by crush injury, laceration, and fracture, which were present in approximately one-fourth of all injured, with compartment syndrome observed in 7% of victims. Injuries to the lower extremities were most frequent, followed by upper extremities, with head and neck, thorax, face, abdominal, and spine injuries occurring in the minority of victims.[13] Earthquake victims in less-developed countries can be expected to have worse mortality and morbidity outcomes, with less access to medical care, evacuation, or other humanitarian aid. Nonetheless, it seems general injury patterns remain consistent. A 2013 review of 31 articles on 15 major earthquakes found the leading injury was traumatic limb injury with an incidence of 68.0%.[14]

Terrorism

Like natural disasters, terrorist attacks vary widely in structure and sequence of events. They also tend to affect a group of unprepared victims from across the spectrum of age, gender, and physical fitness. Terrorist attacks typically produce injuries resembling those of the battlefield, yet civilian targets lack the protection that body armor or an organized system of medical evacuation confers. Furthermore, casualties in military conflicts are typically young with few pre-existing comorbidities, whereas civilian terror victims represent every level of society. A brief review of recent European terror attacks reveals significant heterogeneity in the scope and manner of attack. Some involve detonation of an improvised explosive device (IED) in a solitary location, whereas others involve several locations and a combination of bombings and shootings. Although all present medical and logistical challenges rarely seen in a civilian setting, the increasing complexity and number of victims magnify these challenges.[15] Those injured in a terrorist attack often benefit from early prioritization of pain treatment and control.

Disasters and the Development of Acute and Chronic Pain

Because both disasters and their victims vary greatly, it is difficult to ascertain any overarching protective factors against the development of acute or chronic pain. Psychosocial factors may predispose populations in general, and disaster victims specifically, to pain. Post-traumatic stress disorder (PTSD) following traumatic injury is known to aggravate pain symptoms and complicate pain treatment.[2] One factor that does seem to confer a benefit against the development of PTSD or PTSD symptoms is the existence of a social support network. Several studies examining the occurrence of PTSD symptoms and PTSD in earthquake victims have found that social factors play a vital role in the trauma recovery process, with high perceived social support decreasing the occurrence of acute and delayed post-traumatic stress symptoms.[16, 17]

Military Conflict

Injury Type and Distribution

The majority of modern battlefield wounds result from weapons that can be grouped into either explosive munitions or small arms. As weapons and tactics change, the etiology of injuries also evolves. Over the course of the 20th and 21st centuries, the predominant source of injury evolved from bullet and mortar fire to IEDs, as shown in Tables 17.1 and 17.2.[18,19]

Projectile Injury

Typically, projectile injury refers to wounds caused by kinetic objects such as bullets and fragmentation from explosions. As bullets travel through human tissue, they create both a permanent and temporary cavity. The permanent cavity is the tract whose width is roughly that of the projectile as it passes through tissue causing crush injury. Bullets often "tumble" in tissue, rapidly decelerate, and create nonlinear permanent cavities and greater damage. The temporary cavity is the transient displacement or disruption of tissues due to the round's kinetic, sonic, and thermal energy. It often causes extensive injury out of proportion to the size of the round and results in a primary wound tract that is surrounded by an area of damaged tissue.[20]

Since World War II, improving technology has led to the development of weapons that can be fired with increased accuracy, speed, and lethality. Concurrently, defensive tactics have also shifted from trench warfare to open or urban combat with close air support. Improved body armor and the adoption of aggressive tourniquet use have also greatly reduced the overall projectile mortality rate in recent conflicts.

Table 17.1 Causes of selected battle injuries in US casualties from WWII, Vietnam and operations from 2007-2017. Data adapted from (Cubano, 2018) and DODTR.

Causes of Battle Injury in US Casualties: Bougainville Campaign (WWII), Vietnam, and Military Operations 2007-2017			
Weapon	**Bougainville (%)**	**Vietnam (%)**	**Military Operations 2007-2017 (%)**
Bullet	33	30	19.2
Mortar/Rocket/Artillery	50	22	7.8
Grenade	12	11	4.6
RPG	N/A	12	4.5
Booby trap/IED	2	17	60.4
Other	3	8	3.5

Blast Injury

Explosive ordinance (rocket-propelled grenades, mortars, artillery, etc.) can inflict significant damage by creating a rapid exothermic reaction that transfers large amounts of energy to their surrounding environment.[21] Explosives can be subdivided based on their mechanism of detonation and subsequent energy release. Low-order explosives typically involve rapid conflagration of an ignitable fuel, whereas high-order explosives

Table 17.2 Distribution of injuries and mortality percentages from military conflicts over the past century. Data adapted from (Khorram-Manesh, Goniewicz, Burkle, & Robinson, 2021).

	Head and neck (%)	**Thorax (%)**	**Abdomen (%)**	**Pelvis (%)**	**Limbs (%)**	**Total mortality (%)**
WWI	17	4	2	-	70	21
WWII	4	8	4	-	75	30
Korean War	17	7	7	-	67	4-25
Vietnam War	14-21	5-7	5-18	-	56-74	3-24
Borneo	12	12	20	-	58	2-3
North Ireland	20	15	15	-	50	5
Falkland Islands	14-16	7-15	10-11.5	-	59-75	<1
Persian Gulf Wars	6-11	8-12	7-11	-	44-71	24
Afghanistan and Iraq	12-31	8.9-27	11-22	3.8	39-87	3.9-10
Chechnya	24-24.4	8.6-9	2.3-4	1.6	31-63.1	>20
Somalia	20	8	5	-	65	-
Pakistan	19.2	8.9	-	-	71.9	12.4
East DRC Conflict	8	16	13	-	60	-

create extreme heat, pressure, and are associated with a "blast wave" of transferred energy.

Land mines are explosive devices that are placed under or on the ground and when triggered damage their targets by either a primary explosion or secondary fragments. Most of the force is directed to the lower extremity and pelvis. Unfortunately, after conflicts end, land mines remain a threat to civilians, with noncombatants accounting for the majority of the estimated 5,000–7,000 victims injured or killed each year. [22]

Artillery makes use of large gun-type weapons utilizing a propellant charge to fire a projectile or explosive along an unpowered trajectory. All have a caliber greater than that of standard infantry weapons. [23] The size of the explosion is designed to cause significant destruction to personnel, vehicles, or other infrastructure.

IED attacks involve the use of a "homemade" bomb. [24] They can range from a small pipe bomb to a sophisticated device causing extensive destruction. IEDs are often packed with additional materials (nails, glass, ball bearings, etc.) to enhance the damage they inflict on their targets. Although IEDs have been utilized intermittently by domestic terrorists, their use increased exponentially during the Iraq and Afghanistan conflicts.

Wartime Injury Patterns

Over the course of its existence, the United States has seen vastly improved survivability from battlefield injuries. A soldier in the Revolutionary War had a 58% chance of surviving their injuries, and a soldier injured in the Civil War did not fare much better.[25] In the 20th century, modern medicine and organized casualty care improved survivability to approximately 80% by World War II and Vietnam.[25, 26] In Iraq and Afghanistan, U.S. and coalition forces witnessed a 90% survival rate among wounded,[26] the lowest wartime casualty rate in the modern era.[27] Advances in personal protective equipment, improved training of medics, and a deployed trauma system contributed to this improvement in survival.[26, 27] In addition, the increased use of air evacuation allowed the injured to reach stabilizing and definitive surgical care more expediently than in the past.[26] Short-term survival begets longer term survival, and as soldiers with increasingly severe injuries survive, there are significant ramifications for the long-term treatment and management of their pain.

An overarching theme in military and disaster injury is that patients frequently suffer multiple sites of injury. Polytrauma remains clinically challenging as multiple organ systems and priorities compete for treatment in resource-constrained environments. Patients may suffer from pulmonary, orthopedic, neurologic, or hemorrhagic injuries. Crush injuries from falling debris or overturned vehicles can lead to ischemic wounds with potentially prolonged recovery and chronic neuropathic pain. Burns and inhalational injury are a significant concern in war zones given numerous fuel and ignition sources. Although these injury patterns are common to combat and disasters, polytrauma can also easily occur in the setting of motor vehicle accidents, training mishaps, or friendly fire incidents.

Despite improvements in survivability, blast injuries are still associated with significant morbidity. IED injuries accounted for greater than 50% of the casualties suffered by U.S. military personnel in Iraq and Afghanistan, most commonly affecting the extremities. [28] The prompt application of tourniquets has significantly improved mortality by reducing blood loss and improving hemodynamics during initial treatment, but it may also contribute to the rate of subsequent fasciotomies.[29,30] Blasts create "dirty" injuries, introducing bacteria and fungi residing in soil and other surfaces directly into wounds. Resultant wound infections necessitate frequent washout and debridement surgeries following the initial injury. [31]

TBI impacts the disaster and blast injured. The lasting effects of TBI on the development of neurologic dysfunction or chronic pain are still being evaluated and not fully understood. In a study of veterans who suffered blast injuries, researchers found that exposure to a blast was later associated with higher levels of admission and discharge opioid analgesics, reduced improvement in pain intensity, and much higher rates of PTSD and other psychiatric diagnoses. [2]

During military conflicts and disasters, both soldiers and civilians are uniquely vulnerable to the increased threat of violence and the significantly enhanced hazards of their environment. Their treatment and survival are contingent on the available resources and ability to expeditiously transport them away from the battlefield to secure areas for definitive care.

Evolution of Casualty Movement and Evacuation

The ability to evacuate casualties safely and rapidly from the battlefield has always been understood by military commanders as the key to improving soldiers' survival. The Holy Roman Emperor Maximilian I is credited with structured triage, but it was not until the Napoleonic era that a formalized method of sorting battlefield injuries by severity and urgency was described. Baron Dominique Jean Larrey is often credited as the first modern military surgeon who adapted artillery carriages to create his *ambulance volantes* (flying ambulances) during the Battle of Metz in 1793. Furthermore, Larrey increased the organization of forward field hospitals, creating a framework for the casualty movement and tactical care that is still utilized by global militaries today. [32]

In the modern era, the U.S. military utilizes a system of tiered health care "roles" to treat its wounded from the point of injury on the battlefield to a military treatment facility in the continental United States (Figure 17.1). At each role, the patient is triaged and sorted based on injury severity and their need for further treatment. Patients may experience a prolonged stay at a specific role for geographical, security, or logistical reasons. Recent U.S. conflicts in the Middle East during the 21st century have maintained mostly open lanes of evacuation because of air superiority and an imbalance in military and technological prowess. As a result, casualties expeditiously received the appropriate care, which has been credited with the impressively low mortality and morbidity rates for U.S. soldiers during these conflicts. In contrast, during peer versus peer or near-peer conflicts, there may not be open lanes of evacuation by air or land and, more frequently, lower roles are required to establish prolonged casualty care.

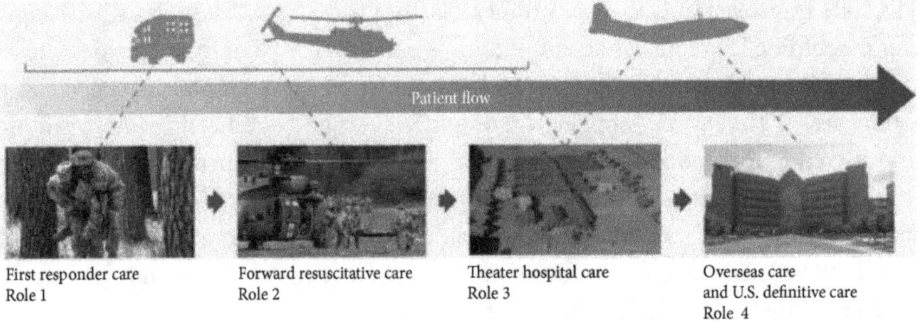

Figure 17.1 Roles of Operational Military Medical Care Provided by the Department of Defense's Medical Forces

Battlefield Assessment and Coordination of Pain Management

The Joint Trauma System (JTS) is a U.S. Department of Defense organization that addresses medical care in the deployed environment. It has established numerous evidence-based clinical practice guidelines that address in-theater management of combat casualties. These guidelines start with Tactical Combat Casualty Care (TCCC) [32] conducted at the point of injury and Role 1 facilities and progress through higher echelons of care with associated increased capabilities. Fundamental to the JTS model is ongoing assessment and management of pain throughout the continuum of casualty care.[33] All combat casualties are expected to experience pain associated with their injuries. At the point of injury and Role 1, seriously injured non-intubated patients are assessed for pain using the Defense and Veterans Pain Rating Scale every 1–4 h depending on the severity of pain and the treatments provided. For intubated patients, adequate analgesia and sedation are assessed using physiologic parameters. Sedation and anxiety are assessed using the Richmond Agitation Sedation Scale, and delirium is assessed using the Confusion Assessment Method.

At higher levels of care, a team-based approach is used to coordinate care.[33] Pain management is facilitated through a dedicated acute pain service (APS) with the resources to provide advanced interventions and consult on the care of pain for all patients in the facility on a 24-h basis. This service is staffed by personnel organic to the combat support hospital and consists of a consultant physician with extensive knowledge and skills in pain management, a dedicated chief pain nurse, and ward pain management nurse champions. The physician consultant develops a pain management plan in conjunction with the primary and consulting surgical services, performs advanced analgesic techniques (e.g., continuous peripheral nerve blocks), and is the primary provider managing analgesic care. The chief pain nurse assists in the performance of advanced regional interventions, oversees execution of pain management plans, and provides education and guidance to ward nurses. Ward pain management champions have additional training on equipment and agents used by the APS, are the first point of contact for ward nurses regarding questions on pain management, and serve as liaison between ward nurses and the chief acute pain nurse. The APS rounds on the patients daily either as integrated with trauma rounds or as an independent consulting service. Typically, the

APS will take direct and sole responsibility for directing and overseeing the execution of the pain management plan to avoid confusion and minimize the potential for errors.[34]

Tactical Combat Casualty Care and Role 1

Tactical Combat Casualty Care provides guidance on management of patients at the lowest echelon of casualty care, occurring at the point of injury through the Role 1 or field aid/triage station.[32] This is the most resource-limited level of care with respect to supplies, equipment, and available personnel. This level of care is typically provided by nonmedical first responders and trained medics with physician assistants or primary care physicians. If actively engaged in combat, casualties are expected to continue to support the mission to the extent possible. Casualties reposition themselves or are moved to cover, where self or buddy aid can be provided, with relocation of casualties to safe positions when more advanced care is required. When not engaged in combat or following conclusion of the engagement, definitive care is provided at the lowest echelon possible to permit return to active status. Where injuries prohibit return to duty, the casualty is advanced through the role system with eventual evacuation from theater.

Analgesia is available at all levels of care. At the point of injury, nonmedical responders (self-aid, buddy-aid, and Combat Life Savers) administer medications from combat wound medication packs. Combat medics and corpsmen and combat paramedics and providers (CPPs) are the first level of clinical staff who treat combat casualties and are equipped to escalate care. The basic analgesic options are provided as per the TCCC guidelines (Table 17.3).

Battlefield acupuncture (BFA; Figure 17.2) is used at this level of care to treat mild to moderate pain.[35] This integrative approach is minimally invasive, easy to teach and perform, and requires only acupuncture semipermanent needles.[36,37] The evidence supporting this modality, however, is mixed. A meta-analysis by Jan et al.[38] found benefit to the modality, whereas that by Yang et al.[39] found no significant difference compared to controls. Observational studies have suggested patient benefit from BFA.[36,40]

The TCCC guidelines for prehospital care have had a tangible effect on the attention given to and the analgesic treatments used to treat pain. A prospective multicenter observational study of prehospital analgesic administration to casualties in Afghanistan since adoption of the TCCC guidelines found that although there was inconsistent administration of pain medications at point of injury, by the time of their arrival to a Role 2, 100% of patients had received pain meds.[41] A systematic review covering the period before implementation of the 2012 TCCC guidelines and after found that the use of ketamine increased from less than 4% to nearly 20% of casualties, with more recent studies showing up to 50% of patients received ketamine, a 26% decrease in opioid use, and an overall 19% decrease in nausea.[42]

Prolonged Casualty Care

Prolonged casualty care (PCC) provides follow-on battlefield care guidance to point of injury and Role 1 providers when TCCC options are exhausted or the casualty cannot immediately be evacuated to the next echelon of care.[43] It represents a contingency care plan, not a substitute for evacuation to the next level of care or as a primary medical support resource, and is highly constrained by resources and personnel. Because priority is

Table 17.3 Roles of Care and analgesic capability (Gelfand, Kent, & Buckenmaier III, 2017).

ANALGESIC CAPABILITIES AT THE ROLES OF CARE			
Role	**Medical Capability**	**Time Until Transport to Higher Level of Care**	**Analgesic Capability**
1: Immediate first aid delivered at the scene	Basic first aid via medic or fellow soldier (tourniquet, bandage, splint, etc.)	Minutes to hours	"Pill Packs" (meloxicam + acetaminophen) Medic administered transmucosal fentanyl citrate 800 mcg and ketamine IV/IO/IN/IM
2: Forward surgical care	Forward surgical care (damage control resuscitation/surgery, blood product administration)	Within 24-48 h	Similar to role 1 with addition to general anesthesia, additional narcotics, single injection regional anesthesia
3: Combat support hospital	Highest level of care within theater (major surgical specialties, full anesthesia capability, intensive care, diagnostic imaging, laboratory, blood services)	Days	Advanced analgesic capabilities: Continuous peripheral/neuraxial techniques, patient controlled analgesia, analgesic infusions (ketamine, opioid, etc . . .)
4 and 5: Medical centers outside the theater of war	Full-service military hospitals	No limit	Manning capable of acute pain service, full capability of comprehensive pain care.

IN – Intranasal, IV – Intravenous, IO – Intraosseous, IM - Intramuscular

given to resuscitative efforts, analgesic options that maintain hemodynamic stability are preferred. PCC requires a slower, more deliberate approach to titration using lower doses of medication due to shock and low blood volume states.[44] Furthermore, prolonged administration of medications compounds the potential side effects, often necessitating the use of adjuncts to address symptoms such as nausea or agitation. Treatment may be needed to address both basal and breakthrough pain. These guidelines recognize that sedation may play a greater role in the context of prolonged in-place care, particularly in the agitated, anxious, combative, or intubated patient. Analgesia and sedation may need to extend to the point of amnestic anesthesia for painful procedures or if needed to continue the mission. PCC analgesic options are presented in Table 17.3.

Regional anesthetic (RA) techniques have been incorporated for casualty care across all military services.[45] Certain CPPs, particularly those assigned to Special Forces units, have the ability to perform a limited number of RA interventions[44] for extremity

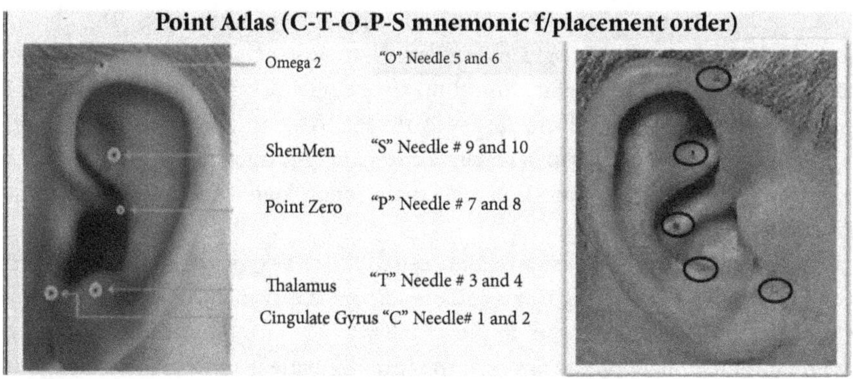

Figure 17.2 Battlefield Acupuncture Ear Points (Gurney, Onifer, & Pamplin, 2021)

analgesia (Table 17.4). RA provides superior analgesia compared to oral or intravenous medications.[25] RA carries a significantly lower risk of sedation, nausea, hypotension, and respiratory depression.[46] Although additional resources and training are required (e.g., needles, imaging equipment, lipid emulsion, etc.), RA provides extended analgesia that does not require the same level of monitoring and repeated medication dosing needed for other analgesics. However, a minimum of 20 min of physiologic monitoring (pulse oximetry) is required following the performance of a nerve block. Ultrasonography is the preferred nerve identification modality, but nerve stimulation or anatomic landmark-based techniques are acceptable alternatives for some blocks. Risks of RA include nerve injury, obscuring the diagnosis of compartment syndrome or pressure injury in insensate limbs, and local anesthetic toxicity. Providers skilled in

Table 17.4 Basic peripheral nerve blocks for use in combat casualties from the Joint Trauma System CPG 61 (Pamplin, Fisher, & Penny, 2017)

	Regional Anesthetic Technique
Upper Extremity	
Supraclavicular	Ultrasound guided only
Axillary	Ultrasound guided preferred, otherwise landmark
Wrist	Anatomic landmark based, +/- ultrasound guided
Digital	Anatomic landmark based
Lower Extremity	
Femoral	Ultrasound guided
Saphenous	Anatomic landmark based, +/- ultrasound guided
Subgluteal Sciatic	Ultrasound guided
Popliteal	Ultrasound guided
Ankle	Anatomic landmark based, +/- ultrasound guided
Digital	Anatomic landmark based

this modality may not be available at the majority of Role 1 care sites. The preferred local anesthetic is ropivacaine given its efficacy, duration of action, and improved cardiovascular risk profile. Current clinical practice guidelines discourage the use of RA by the untrained provider, if the patient is unable to communicate, or if the patient refuses. Potential contraindications include coexisting site infection or trauma, ongoing coagulopathy or anticoagulation use, pre-existing neurologic injury, or extremes of age (infants and the elderly).

The PCC guidelines also recognize the need to address expectant casualties and end-of-life care.[44] There are going to be clinical scenarios in which the severity of injury or resource limitations will result in the inability to adequately treat or resuscitate the patient. It is incumbent on the provider to minimize patient suffering and turn to palliative measures even if they further respiratory or hemodynamic compromise. Opioid analgesics and benzodiazepines are the first-line agents to address pain and anxiety. These are titrated until the patient reports relief or in the obtunded patient until respiratory rate falls to below 20 breaths per minute. The patient is positioned as comfortably as possible, with attention to pressure points. Attendants are to honor all patient comfort requests to the extent possible, such as cigarettes, water, food, talking, and physical contact. This is often the most traumatic level of care to the provider; debrief and counseling should be provided as soon as possible.

Role 2 Care

Role 2 is the first echelon of care where damage control surgery is performed and specialized providers with advanced analgesic/sedation training are routinely available. These include trauma surgeons, emergency medicine, and anesthesia providers.[33] Nonetheless, there remains variability in the resources available to manage casualties. Austere Role 2 sites may have a single operating room (OR) and intensive care unit (ICU) bed and be limited to the same supplies and equipment provided in the TCCC and PCC guidelines. Robust Role 2 facilities may have two or more ORs with several ICU capable beds, multiple specialty providers, and extended patient-holding capabilities; these are likely to have infusion pumps, ultrasound, machines, and staffing to manage infusions and patient-controlled analgesic (PCAs).

Role 2 is the point of care where it is likely that basic, single-injection RA techniques can be performed. The goal of these modalities is to decrease the patient transport burden by providing extended analgesia that requires a minimum amount of intervention on the part of the en route care provider.

Role 3 Care

Role 3 is the most robust echelon of casualty care within the theater of combat operations and is comparable to a civilian urban trauma center. It is staffed and equipped to provide advanced specialized surgical, medical, and ancillary care and services. It is the first echelon of care able to provide an APS team [33] capable of performing and handling advanced pain management techniques such as continuous peripheral nerve block and patient-controlled epidural anesthesia infusions, PCA infusions, other analgesic medications, and complementary medicine modalities such as acupuncture.

En Route Care

En route care involves the medical management of a patient during movement from one echelon of care to the next. Depending on the type of transport and level of care required for the evacuating patient, en route care providers can range from medics to nurses and intensive care physicians. Each stage of patient transport can continue the modalities initiated at the originating echelon of care. For example, the evacuation asset that collects a casualty from the Role 1 can continue to manage the interventions and analgesic modalities initiated by the Role 1 providers, and the transportation asset from a Role 3 includes critical care nurses and providers who can continue the interventions initiated at the Role 3 facility for the evacuation of patients out of theater.[47]

Patients are transported through the JTS using a variety of vehicles. These assets fall into two main categories: casualty evacuation (CASEVAC) and medical evacuation (MEDEVAC). CASEVAC assets are vehicles of opportunity for the transportation of casualties; these can be ground transport or aircraft assets and do not have medical attendants organic to the platform. CASEVAC is most commonly used for moving patients from the point of injury to Role 1 sites but can be used to transport casualties directly to a Role 2 or 3 location. MEDEVAC assets are vehicles dedicated to the transport of patients. They include tactical ambulances, helicopters, and fixed-wing aircraft, equipped and staffed such that they can continue care initiated at the point of pickup. These assets can collect casualties from the point of injury and move patients between echelons of care. Depending on the vehicle, roles of care may be skipped (e.g., Role 1 direct to Role 3) within theater depending on conditions and acuity of the casualties. The U.S. Marine Corps and U.S. Navy lack dedicated air MEDEVAC capability and doctrinally treat all transport aircraft in theater as potential CASEVAC assets, whereas the U.S. Army and U.S. Air Force maintain dedicated MEDEVAC aircraft. Helicopters are used to move casualties within the theater of operations, whereas fixed-wing aircraft configured as flying ICUs evacuate casualties from Role 3 to treatment facilities outside the theater of operations. These fixed-wing assets have equipment cleared for flight used to continue PCA infusions and RA infusions during transport to a Role 4 5 facility (Figure 17.3).

Challenges for Pain Management in the Joint Trauma System

Despite the robust scope of the JTS, barriers exist that can limit its full implementation and potential. Available therapeutics are dependent on the proper personnel and resources in theater. The nature of the operation and logistical constraints can reduce interventions available to treat casualties. For example, a Special Forces operation may only consist of a dozen or less personnel in total, to include medical assets, and the supplies may be limited to that which can be carried in a backpack. The ability to control airspace or shoreline may also impact on medical capabilities: It may not be possible to establish a Role 2 or 3 facility until control of one or both are secured. Complexities and constraints of the logistical chain may limit when and what can be supplied, restricting providers in how they manage casualties.

The training and comfort level of providers may also impact on battlefield pain management. A 2015 study examining pain management at point of injury and Role 1 between 2013 and 2014, following the revised TCCC guidelines, found that 53% of

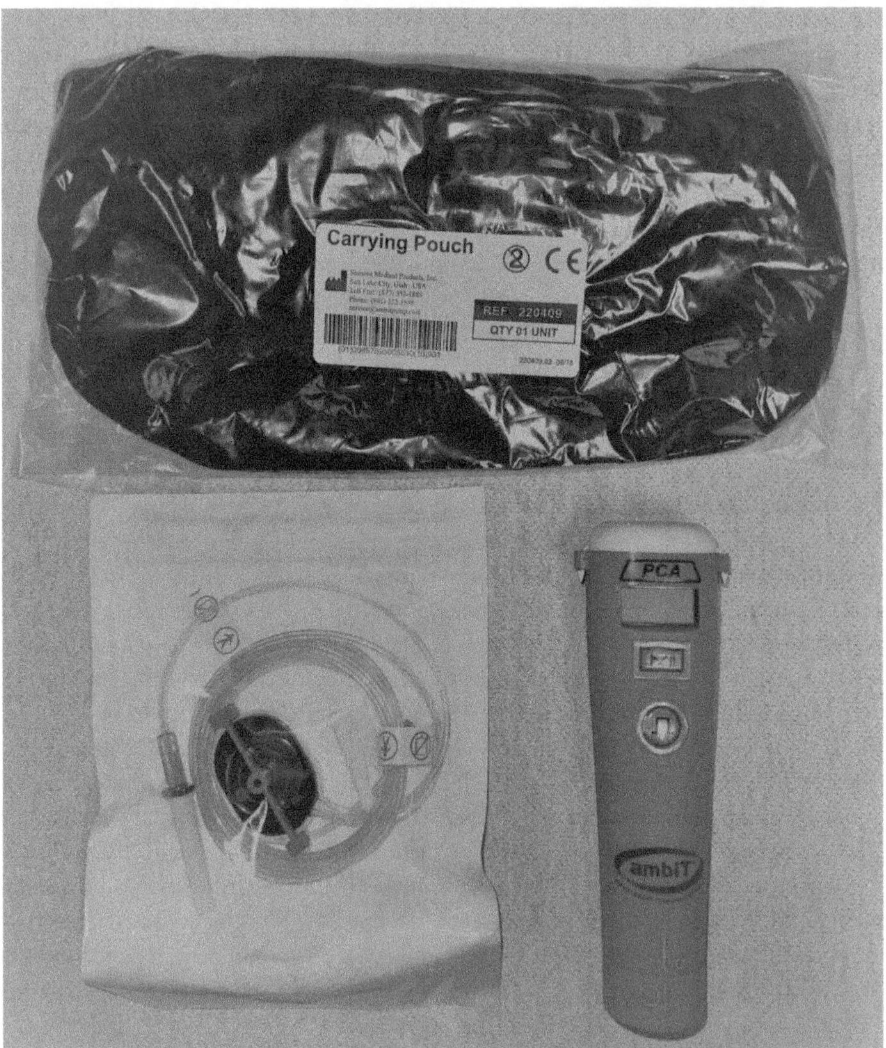

Figure 17.3 Patient controlled infusion pump system (ambIT, Summit Medical Products, Inc. USA)

casualties received no pain medication, 29% received analgesia per the guidelines, and 18% received a medication not listed in the guidelines.[47] A study examining an earlier data set found that 61% of patients received no pain medication at the point of injury, with 92% receiving analgesics during MEDEVAC from the point of injury.[41] A study of battlefield pain management in the Israeli Defense Forces between 1997 and 2014 found that only 12.3% of casualties received prehospital analgesia, and of those who did, 90.5% were administered by paramedics or physicians.[48] All these studies conclude that it is the variability in the training and resources given to first responders that limited the extent to which analgesia was provided and that better training of these lowest level caregivers would improve adherence to guidelines and treatment of casualties.

Future Directions for the Joint Trauma System

The JTS Clinical Practice Guidelines are reviewed annually and revised as warfare evolves and new evidence that impacts the management of war wounded advances. This ensures that the most up-to-date evidence-based practices are disseminated through the military health care system and the equipment and training are updated to reflect any changes. The following are some therapeutic avenues under development:

Intravenous meloxicam: This formulation would be included in the TCCC guidelines as an alternative for use in patients unable to tolerate oral medications.[49]

Sublingual sufentanil: This medication would replace oral transmucosal fentanyl citrate (OTFC) due to its more favorable safety profile.[50] The single-dose applicator device allows the medication to be self-administered,[51] it has a rapid onset of less than 15 min with a duration of 2 or 3 h,[51] there has been no observed respiratory depression or cognitive impairment associated with the 30-μg oral dose, and it has a reduced euphoric state compared to OTFC.[50]

Ketamine autoinjector: Ketamine has been the principal analgesic of the TCCC guidelines since 2013; however, there are no formulations available in concentrations suitable for analgesic administration, resulting in the need to dilute the medication before administration. The U.S. Department of Defense is funding the development of a U.S. Food and Drug Administration–approved formulation and autoinjector system for analgesic use.

Percutaneous peripheral nerve stimulators: A promising area of investigation is the neuromodulation of peripheral nerve plexi using percutaneous leads implanted under ultrasound guidance.[52] This technique stimulates peripheral large-fiber non-noxious afferent nerves, overwhelming peripherally generated nociceptive inputs. The advantage of this modality is that it is does not impact motor function and is nonpharmacologic, reducing risk. Preliminary studies have shown clinically significant reductions in opioid use and pain scores with this modality.[53] It remains to be determined if this technique can be utilized in the battlefield environment.

Complementary medicine modalities: In addition to BFA, which has been widely adopted within the JTS,[33] additional modalities are being studied for possible incorporation into battlefield pain management.[45] Such interventions include immersion virtual reality systems, acupuncture, and massage therapy.

Telemedicine: Advances in battlefield communication and the realities of conflicts have highlighted the need for telemedicine capabilities to address potential gaps and provide advanced care as far forward as possible.[54] Trials have been performed using the Warfighter Information Network–Tactical Increment 2 Tactical Communications Node, liking aid stations to the Joint Readiness Training Center that allowed video calls to be made.[54] Most telehealth systems address routine or non-urgent care issues such as disease and non-battle injury; however, regional programs have been implemented to bring telehealth services to more acutely ill.[55]

Acute and Chronic Pain in Military Personnel

The mental and physical challenges of military duty, ongoing readiness training, and injuries associated with prior engagements all place soldiers at a unique risk for acute and chronic pain. [56] This population is especially susceptible to the development of chronic pain due to their unique injury patterns, concomitant psychological stressors, and systems that may delay their initial care. From the moment of injury, soldiers are immediately at risk for the development of chronic pain. Whether it is delay in evacuation, a need to avoid analgesic medications due to hemodynamic instability, or complex injuries requiring multiple trips to the operating room, battle-wounded patients have multiple risk factors for poorly controlled pain.

The treatment of battlefield patients relies heavily on their respective militaries' ability to evacuate patients safely and rapidly. Movement of these patients may be significantly delayed due to tactical limitations, and this postponement of care or access to more specialized pain management is a unique vulnerability of war-wounded patients. In a retrospective case series, patients reported significantly worse pain at earlier levels of care and during transport compared to care at Roles 4 and 5, and they endorsed that this contributed to psychological stress and anxiety. [25] Access to analgesic options is limited at lower roles by supplies, availability, and staffing. Numerous studies have identified an association between the early use of continuous peripheral nerve catheters and a decrease in chronic post-traumatic amputation pain. [57–59] A prospective cohort study of battle-injured U.S. patients from Operation Enduring Freedom (OEF)/Operation Iraqi Freedom (OIF) during 2007–2013 evaluated chronic pain outcomes in patients who received early RA for extremity injuries. The patients who received RA within 7 days of their combat-related extremity injury had improved pain and quality of life scores at 6 months. At 24 months, patients reported greater pain relief, decreased neuropathic pain intensity, and higher satisfaction with pain outcomes.[60] Like civilian trauma, RA and other multimodal methods of pain control are clearly useful in reducing pain scores while limiting the side effects of opioid monotherapy. [61] Unfortunately, continuous peripheral nerve blocks are often only available in later roles of care when central sensitization may have already occurred and the development of chronic pain has begun. Opioid medications are often the only ones available for moderate to severe pain at the point of injury, with the risk of hypotension, altered mental status, and airway compromise a significant concern. Battlefield casualties are not only susceptible to undercontrolled pain but also particularly vulnerable given the complex injury patterns observed in war.

The improvement in battlefield medicine has led to increased survivability but has also created a generation of patients with increasingly complex injuries. These patients can often expect to undergo multiple surgeries due to their elaborate and often contaminated injuries. One survey of patients with soft tissue injuries in Iraq noted that the mean time from injury to wound closure was 4.24 days.[31] From 2009 to 2012, the overall infection rate in U.S. combat casualties from time of injury through initial U.S. hospitalization was 34%. Infection can worsen pain severity directly and indirectly due to frequent washout or debridement surgeries.[62] The sheer number of surgeries may also predispose this population to the development of chronic pain, and perioperative analgesia can be difficult to manage. In addition to the prevalence of polytrauma, these compound injuries often include crush or ischemic mechanisms for which analgesia can be difficult to achieve.

The correlation between war and psychological trauma has been described in history's conflicts as "shell shock," "combat fatigue," and PTSD. The earliest accounts of PTSD were recorded from battlefields in what is modern-day Iraq in 1300 BCE by the Mesopotamians, with symptoms including flashbacks, sleep disturbance, and depressed mood. [63] During the 21st-century conflicts in that region, service members have experienced increased rates of depression and PTSD, independent of known pain issues.[4] Soldiers returning from Iraq and Afghanistan reporting both pain and psychological changes endorsed higher average pain scores than those reporting pain alone.[2] There is also evidence that patients who suffer polytrauma have an association with increased pain scores and PTSD. [61] One study found that soldiers who experienced combat trauma during OEF/OIF were more likely to be diagnosed with PTSD than the general OEF/OIF veteran population. Chronic and worsening PTSD trajectories were associated with greater pain intensity following combat injury, even when accounting for early RA for pain management.[64] Unfortunately, psychologic harm can be further compounded by a reluctance to seek help. Of military members reporting psychiatric symptoms, less than one-third seek treatment for these symptoms.[65] There is a long-standing stigma that perceived toughness and the ability to endure suffering are hallmarks of a good solider. For many, seeking help with psychiatric concerns runs counter to the warrior mindset, and those who remain on active duty are concerned about the effect treatment may have on career progression.[4]

It is also possible that increased pain intensity near the point of injury may be associated with psychologic harm. A large retrospective cohort of TBI patients suggested that early use of morphine following battlefield injuries led to lower incidences of PTSD. [66] Because most battlefield injuries involve the extremities, many wounded also suffer from functional loss and the inability to continue their occupation, serving as another significant psychologic stressor. In addition to the individual toll on soldiers, there are also repercussions for their continued care as veterans in U.S. health care systems. Almost 80% of active-duty soldiers who developed chronic pain after a deployment during 2008–2014 utilized care from the Veterans Health Administration (VHA). Of those VHA enrollees, 62% of military members who separated from the military between 2011 and 2015 were diagnosed with PTSD, TBI, or other psychological health conditions (e.g., adjustment disorder and alcohol use disorder) in the 2 years before separation.[67]

Socioeconomic Impacts in Veteran Populations

In the United States, military personnel receive care through distinctive health care systems as veterans in both civilian and federal treatment facilities. In general, eligibility for health care covered by the U.S. Department of Veterans Affairs (VA) requires that a veteran has served in the military for at least 24 months and met criteria with respect to service-connected disability rating, income, and other factors. Because both the active-duty soldier and the veteran may utilize these federally funded systems, understanding of the socioeconomic trends and impact on greater society remains imperative.

In a cross-sectional evaluation of VA patients, investigators discovered that out of the roughly 17 million total veterans receiving medical care, only 35–40% utilize the VHA. However, those who did use the VA system accumulated annual medical expenses approximately 65% higher per veteran than their non-VA counterparts. VA users were also more likely to be non-Hispanic, Black, elderly, have lower income, be in poorer health, and live in nonmetropolitan areas.[68]

VA patients are unfortunately also more likely to have unique pain and treatment complications. In the VA health care population, diagnosed opioid use disorder (OUD) is almost sevenfold higher than in non-veteran counterparts. The most vulnerable population appears to be patients with chronic noncancerous pain who are prescribed opioids. [69] Demographic studies illustrate that VA patients diagnosed with OUD are likely to be male (>90%), with higher representation among White, Black, or Native American veterans. The most common comorbidities associated with OUD in this population are psychiatric problems, other substance abuse, arthritis, and low back pain. Analyses reveal that adjusted annual health care costs for patients diagnosed with OUD are significantly higher than those for patients without OUD, and the treatment for opioid-specific health care is on the order of thousands of dollars annually per patient.[69]

Although veterans face a higher burden of chronic pain compared to the civilian population, this can be addressed with the addition of intensive treatment programs, potentially involving nonpharmacologic complementary care. In 2015, researchers compared OIF/OEF war veterans with chronic and disabling musculoskeletal pain who received standard care to those who received an intensive 24-week staged treatment process. Those who underwent the 24-week program reported significantly decreased pain intensity and pain interference with their lives.[70] In another investigation, VA patients with chronic musculoskeletal pain who utilized complementary and integrative health services (acupuncture, massage, and chiropractic) had decreased health care costs and pain on average. However, the subset of patients who utilized more than eight integrative health visits annually accumulated significantly increased health care costs.[71]

The treatment of chronic pain is complex and costly to health care systems. Beyond the VA system, these findings are paralleled in European studies of the health care burden of chronic pain in civilian populations. The severity and frequency of pain were found to be the most significant determinants of quality-of-life measures and the utilization of health care resources.[72,73] Further investigation is warranted to understand the significant differences in outcomes among various veteran demographics. Moreover, because the veteran population stands apart in their injury patterns, treatment options, and costs, there are existing opportunities to improve their care and treatment.

Conclusion

Management of pain during humanitarian response operations and on the battlefield represents a unique challenge in the context of austere medical operations and complex injury patterns. The experience with 21st-century conflict has identified pain management as one of the fundamental pillars to the successful treatment and rehabilitation of casualties. Failure to adequately address pain during the early phases of treatment risks increasing morbidity and mortality, the development of chronic pain syndromes, and a reduction in quality of life and recovery. Freedom from intrusive pain can be the single most important long-term determinant of overall outcome in the combat and disaster wounded.

References

1. United Nations Office for Disaster Risk Reduction. Disaster. 2022. https://www.undrr.org/terminology/disaster
2. Clark ME, Walker RL, Gironda RJ, Scholten JD. Comparison of pain and emotional symptoms in soldiers with polytrauma: Unique aspects of blast exposure. *Pain Med.* 2009;10(3):447–455.
3. Werner MU, Mjöbo HN, Nielsen PR, Rudin Å. Prediction of postoperative pain: A systematic review of predictive experimental pain studies. *Anesthesiology.* 2010;112(6):1494–1502.
4. Watrous JR, McCabe CT, Jones G, et al. The relationships between self-reported pain intensity, pain interference, and quality of life among injured U.S. service members with and without low back pain. *J Clin Psychol Med Settings.* 2021;28(4):746–756.
5. Levine AC, Teicher C, Aluisio AR, et al. Regional Anesthesia for Painful Injuries after Disasters (RAPID): Study protocol for a randomized controlled trial. *Trials.* 2016;17(1):542.
6. Institute for Economics & Peace. Ecological Threat Register 2020: Understanding ecological threats, resilience, and peace. 2020. https://reliefweb.int/report/world/ecological-threat-register-2020-understanding-ecological-threats-resilience-and-peace
7. Lam D. How the world survived the population bomb: Lessons from 50 years of extraordinary demographic history. *Demography.* 2011;48(4):1231–1262.
8. World population. Worldometer. May 6, 2022. https://www.worldometers.info
9. Bournay E. Trends in natural disasters. *Environment and Poverty Times.* 2006;3.
10. Intergovernmental Panel on Climate Change. Climate change widespread, rapid, and intensifying [Press release]. August 9, 2021. https://www.ipcc.ch/2021/08/09/ar6-wg1-20210809-pr
11. World Health Organization. Health emergency and disaster risk management fact sheets. 2017. https://cdn.who.int/media/docs/default-source/disaster-mngmt/risk-management-safe-hospitals-december2017bc5b1106-594d-46a8-9d86-248e69342150.pdf?sfvrsn=3a422e1d_1&download=true
12. Aluisio AR, Teicher C, Wiskel T, Guy A, Levine A. Focused training for humanitarian responders in regional anesthesia techniques for a planned randomized controlled trial in a disaster setting [published correction appears in PLoS Curr. 2017 Feb 6;9]. *PLoS Curr.* 2016;8:ecurrents.dis.e75f9f9d977ac8adededb381e3948a04.
13. Pan ST, Cheng YY, Wu CL, et al. Association of injury pattern and entrapment location inside damaged buildings in the 2016 Taiwan earthquake. *J Formos Med Assoc.* 2019;118(1 Pt 2):300–323.
14. Missair A, Pretto EA, Visan A, et al. A matter of life or limb? A review of traumatic injury patterns and anesthesia techniques for disaster relief after major earthquakes. *Anesth Analg.* 2013;114(4):934–941.
15. Bieler D, Franke A, Kollig E, et al. Terrorist attacks: Common injuries and initial surgical management. *Eur J Trauma Emerg Surg.* 2020;46(4):683–694.
16. Yang Y, Zeng W, Lu B, Wen J. The contributing factors of delayed-onset post-traumatic stress disorder symptoms: A nested case–control study conducted after the 2008 Wenchuan earthquake. *Front Public Health.* 2021;9:682714.
17. Yuan G, Shi W, Lowe S, Chang K, Jackson T, Hall BJ. Associations between posttraumatic stress symptoms, perceived social support and psychological distress among disaster-exposed Chinese young adults: A three-wave longitudinal mediation model. *J Psychiatr Res.* 2021;137:491–497.

18. Cubano M. *Emergency War Surgery, 5th US Revision*. Department of the Army, The Borden Institute; 2018.
19. Khorram-Manesh A, Goniewicz K, Burkle F, Robinson Y. Review of military casualties in modern conflicts: The re-emergence of casualties from armored warfare. *Military Medicine*. 2022:187(3–4):e313–e321.
20. Stefanopoulos PK, Pinialidis DE, Hadjigeorgiou GF, Filippakis KN. Wound ballistics 101: The mechanisms of soft tissue wounding by bullets. *Eur J Trauma Emerg Surg*. 2017;43(5):579–586.
21. U.S. Department of Defense Blast Injury Research Coordinating Office. What is blast injury? 2019. https://blastinjuryresearch.health.mil/index.cfm/blast_injury_101/what_is_blast_injury
22. Loddo M, Hart M. *Landmine Monitor 2021*. International Campaign to Ban Landmines; 2021. http://www.the-monitor.org/media/3318354/Landmine-Monitor-2021-Web.pdf
23. Hogg IV. Artillery. Britannica; 2020. https://www.britannica.com/technology/artillery
24. The National Academies and the Department of Homeland Security. IED attack: Improvised explosive devices. News and Terrorism: Communicating in a Crisis. 2022. https://www.dhs.gov/xlibrary/assets/prep_ied_fact_sheet.pdf
25. Buckenmaier CC III, Rupprecht C, McKnight G. Pain following battlefield injury and evacuation: A survey of 110 casualties from the wars in Iraq and Afghanistan. *Pain Med*. 2009;10(8):1487–1496.
26. Eastridge B, Mabry R, Seguin P, et al. Death on the battlefield (2001–2011): Implications for the future of combat casualty care. *J Trauma Acute Care Surg*. 2012;73:S431–S437.
27. Savage E, Forestier C, Withers N, Tien H, Pannell D. Tactical combat casualty care in the Canadian Forces: Lessons learned from the Afghan war. *Can J Surg*. 2011;54(6):S118–S123.
28. Ramasamy A, Hill A, Clasper J. Improvised explosive devices: Pathophysiology, injury profiles and current medical management. *J R Army Med Corps*. 2009;155:265–272.
29. Mitchell SL, Hayda R, Chen AT, et al. The Military Extremity Trauma Amputation/Limb Salvage (METALS) study: Outcomes of amputation compared with limb salvage following major upper-extremity trauma. *J Bone Joint Surg Am*. 2019;101(16):1470–1478.
30. Kragh JF Jr, Wade CE, Baer DG, et al. Fasciotomy rates in Operations Enduring Freedom and Iraqi Freedom: Association with injury severity and tourniquet use. *J Orthop Trauma*. 2011;25(3):134–139.
31. Leininger BE, Rasmussen TE, Smith DL, Jenkins DH, Coppola C. Experience with wound VAC and delayed primary closure of contaminated soft tissue injuries in Iraq. *J Trauma*. 2006;61(5):1207–1211.
32. Gelfand HJ, Kent ML, Buckenmaier CC III. Management of acute pain of the war wounded during short and long-distance transport and "casevac." *Techniques Orthop*. 2017;32(4):263–269.
33. Committee on Tactical Casualty Combat Care. Tactical casualty combat care (TCCC) guidelines for medical personnel. 2021. https://learning-media.allogy.com/api/v1/pdf/1045f287-baa4-4990-8951-de517a262ee2/contents
34. Gurney J, Onifer D, Pamplin J, et al. Pain, anxiety and delirium (CPG ID: 29). 2021. https://jts.health.mil/assets/docs/cpgs/Pain_Anxiety_Delirium_26_Apr_2021_ID29.pdf
35. Buckenmaier C III, Mahoney P, Anton T, Kwon N, Polomano R. Impact of an acute pain service on pain outcomes with combat-injured soldiers at Camp Bastion, Afghanistan. *Pain Med*. 2012;13(7):919–926.
36. U.S. Air Force Acupuncture and Integrative Medical Center. Battlefield acupuncture handbook. 2021. https://jts.health.mil/assets/docs/education/Battlefield_Acupuncture_Handbook.pdf
37. Taylor SL, Giannitrapani KF, Ackland PE. The implementation and effectiveness of battlefield auricular acupuncture for pain. *Pain Med*. 2021;22(8):1721–1726.
38. Jan AL, Aldridge ES, Rogers IR. Does ear acupuncture have a role for pain relief in the emergency setting? A systematic review and meta-analysis. *Med Acupunct*. 2017;29(5):276–289.

39. Yang J, Ganesh R, Wu Q. Battlefield acupuncture for adult pain: A systematic review and meta-analysis of randomized controlled trials. *Am J Chinese Med.* 2020;49(1):25–40.
40. Giannitrapani KF, Ackland PE, Holliday J, et al. Provider perspectives of battlefield acupuncture: Advantages, disadvantages and its potential role in reducing opioid use for pain. *Med Care.* 2020;58(9):S88–S93.
41. Shackelford SA, Fowler M, Schultz K, et al. Prehospital pain medication use by U.S. forces in Afghanistan. *Mil Med.* 2015;180(3):304–309.
42. de Rocquigny G, Dubecq C, Martinez T, et al. Use of ketamine for prehospital pain control on the battlefield: A systematic review. *Trauma Acute Care Surg.* 2020;88(1):180–185.
43. Remley M, Loos P, Riesberg J. Prolonged casualty care guidelines. *J Spec Oper Med.* 2022;22(1):18–47.
44. Pamplin J, Fisher A, Penny A., et al. Analgesia and sedation management during prolonged field care. *J Spec Oper Med.* 2017;17(1):106–120.
45. Cliford JL, Fowler M, Hansen JJ. State of the science review: Advances in pain management in wounded service members over a decade at war. *J Trauma Acute Care Surg.* 2014;77(3):S228–S236.
46. Buckenmaier CC. Regional anesthesia in austere environment medicine. In: Hadzic A, ed. *Hadzic's Textbook of Regional Anesthesia and Acute Pain Management.* 2nd ed. McGraw-Hill; 2017; 1004–111.
47. Schauer SG, Robinson JB, Mabry RL, Howard JT. Battlefield analgesia: TCCC guidelines are not being followed. *J Spec Oper Med.* 2015;15(1):85–89.
48. Benov A, Salas MM, Nakar H. Battlefield pain management: A view of 17 years in Israel Defense Forces. *J Trauma Acute Care Surg.* 2017;83(1):S150–S155.
49. Berkowitz RD, Mack RJ, McCallum SW. Meloxicam for intravenous use: Review of its clinical efficacy and safety for management of postoperative pain. *Pain Manag.* 2021;11(3):249–258.
50. Kim SY, Buckenmaier CC III, Howe EG, Choi KH. The newest battlefield opioid, sublingual sufentanil: A proposal to refine opioid usage in the U.S. military. *Mil Med.* 2022;187(3–4):77–83.
51. Reardon CE, Kane-Gill SL, Smithburger PL. Sufentanil sublingual tablet: A new option for acute pain management. *Ann Pharmacother.* 2021;53(12):1220–1226.
52. Ilfeld B, Gelfand H, Dhanjal S, et al. Ultrasound-guided percutaneous peripheral nerve stimulation: A pragmatic effectiveness trial of a nonpharmacologic alternative for the treatment of postoperative pain. *Pain Med.* 2020;21(Suppl):S53–S61.
53. Ilfeld B, Plunkett A, Vijjeswarapu A, et al.; PAINfRE Investigators. Percutaneous peripheral nerve stimulation (neuromodulation) for postoperative pain: A randomized, sham-controlled pilot study. *Anesthesiology.* 2021;135(1):95–110.
54. April MD, Stednick PJ, Landry C, Brady DP, Davidson M. Telemedicine at the Joint Readiness Training Center: Expanding forward medical capability. *Med J (Ft Sam Houst Tex).* 2021;(PB 8-21-04/05/06):9–13.
55. Nettesheim N, Powell D, Vasios W, et al. Telemedical support for military medicine. *Mil Med.* 2018;183(11–12):e462–e470.
56. Reif S, Adams RS, Ritter GA, Williams TV, Larson MJ. Prevalence of pain diagnoses and burden of pain among active duty soldiers, FY2012. *Mil Med.* 2018;183(9–10):e330–e337.
57. Kent M, Hsia H, Van de Ven T, Buchheit T. Perioperative pain management strategies for amputation: A topical review. *Pain Med.* 2017;18(3):504–519.
58. Laloo R, Ambler G, Locker D, Twine C, Bosanquet D. Systematic review and meta-analysis of the effect of perineural catheters in major lower limb amputations. *Eur J Vasc Endovasc Surg.* 2021;62(2):295–303.
59. Borghi B, D'Addabbo M, White P, et al. The use of prolonged peripheral neural blockade after lower extremity amputation: The effect on symptoms associated with phantom limb syndrome. *Anesth Analg.* 2010;111(5):1308–1315.
60. Gallagher RM, Polomano RC, Giordano NA, et al. Prospective cohort study examining the use of regional anesthesia for early pain management after combat-related extremity injury [Published online ahead of print]. *Reg Anesth Pain Med.* 2019;100773.

61. Carness JM, Wilson MA, Lenart MJ, Smith DE, Dukes SF. Experiences with regional anesthesia for analgesia during prolonged aeromedical evacuation. *Aerosp Med Hum Perform.* 2017;88(8):768–772.
62. Weintrob AC, Murray CK, Xu J, et al. Early infections complicating the care of combat casualties from Iraq and Afghanistan. *Surg Infect (Larchmt).* 2018;19(3):286–297.
63. Abdul-Hamid WK, Hughes JH. Nothing new under the sun: Post-traumatic stress disorders in the ancient world. *Early Sci Med.* 2014;19(6):549–557.
64. Giordano NA, Richmond TS, Farrar JT, Buckenmaier CC III, Gallagher RM, Polomano RC. Differential pain presentations observed across post-traumatic stress disorder symptom trajectories after combat injury. *Pain Med.* 2021;22(11):2638–2647.
65. Campbell M, Auchterlonie J, Andris Z, Cooper DC, Hoyt T. Mental health stigma in Department of Defense policies: Analysis, recommendations, and outcomes. *Mil Med.* 2023;188(5–6):e1171–e1177.
66. Holbrook T, Galarneau M, Dye J, Quinn K, Dougherty A. Morphine use after combat injury in Iraq and post-traumatic stress disorder. *N Engl J Med.* 2010;362(2):110–117.
67. Adams R, Meerwijk E, Larson M, Harris A. Predictors of Veterans Health Administration utilization and pain persistence among soldiers treated for postdeployment chronic pain in the Military Health System. *BMC Health Serv Res.* 2021;21(1):494.
68. Machlin SR, Muhuri P. Characteristics and health care expenditures of VA health system users versus other veterans, 2014–2015 (combined). Statistical brief No. 508. Agency for Healthcare Research and Quality. 2018. https://www.ncbi.nlm.nih.gov/books/NBK476413
69. Baser O, Xie L, Mardekian J, Schaaf D, Wang L, Joshi AV. Prevalence of diagnosed opioid abuse and its economic burden in the Veterans Health Administration. *Pain Pract.* 2014;14(5):437–445.
70. Bair MJ, Ang D, Wu J, et al. Evaluation of Stepped Care for Chronic Pain (ESCAPE) in veterans of the Iraq and Afghanistan conflicts: A randomized clinical trial. *JAMA Intern Med.* 2015;175(5):682–689.
71. Herman PM, Yuan AH, Cefalu MS, et al. The use of complementary and integrative health approaches for chronic musculoskeletal pain in younger US veterans: An economic evaluation. *PLoS One.* 2019;14(6):e0217831.
72. Langley P, Muller-Schwefe G, Nicolaou A, Liedgens H, Pergolizzi J, Varrassi G. The societal impact of pain in the European Union: Health-related quality of life and healthcare resource utilization. *J Med Econ.* 2010;13(3):571–581.
73. Langley PC. The societal burden of pain in Germany: Health-related quality-of-life, health status and direct medical costs. *J Med Econ.* 2012;15(6):1201–1215.

18
Pain in Low-Income Nations

Rediet Shimeles Workneh, Gaston Nyirigira, Fola Faponle, Olivia Sutton, Steven Amaefuna, Oluwakemi Tomobi, Allen Finley, and John Sampson

Introduction

> Pain and suffering, illness and the lack of health care, is still as present as it was in the past. While others watch and wait, Africa's children are suffering.[1]

Pain is an enormous problem globally. Estimates suggest that 20% of adults suffer from pain globally, and 10% are newly diagnosed with chronic pain each year.[1] The International Association for the Study of Pain estimates that 1 in 5 patients experiences pain and that 1 in 10 patients is diagnosed with chronic pain every year.[2] Musculoskeletal conditions, including osteoarthritis, rheumatoid arthritis, and osteoporosis, and traumatic injury are among the leading causes of pain.[2] In Africa, there are higher incidences of postoperative pain, with poor postoperative pain management.[3] Data from across the continent demonstrate a widespread incidence of poorly controlled postoperative pain, with an incidence as low as 49.7% and as high as 88.2% in countries such as Nigeria, Kenya, and Ethiopia.[4–7]

Chronic pain currently affects one in five adults, is more prevalent among women and the elderly, and is associated with physically demanding work and lower education.[8]

In a 2016 review by Jackson et al.,[9] an attempt was made to assess the burden of chronic pain in general, elderly, and working populations of low- and middle-income countries (LMICs). The systematic review included 119 publications in 28 LMICs. The meta-analysis confirms the prevalence of unspecified persistent pain (headache, low back pain, dental pain, migraine, and unspecified pain) to be 34% in the general population in LMICs and even higher in the elderly and working population.[9] However, Jackson et al. concluded that steps should be taken to reduce heterogeneity in the assessment of global chronic pain because heterogeneity has led to difficulties in characterizing the disease burden and management. Possible actions may include standardization of the definition of chronic pain; widespread adoption of validated questionnaires across cultures; attention to inequitably burdened populations; and inclusion of queries regarding known associations of chronic pain with social and psychological factors that, in combination, increase the global burden of noncommunicable disease and disability.[10]

There is also a growing prevalence of chronic pain from known causes such as cancer, injuries, and HIV infection and AIDS.[11] An estimated 25% of the burden of chronic pain results from surgery and trauma, 60–70% of patients with advanced cancer and late-stage AIDS experience moderate to severe pain, and 70% of the pain experienced by elderly patients is chronic in nature.[14]

Gathering epidemiologic data regarding the prevalence of chronic pain has been a consistent challenge in LMICs. In a systematic review on the prevalence of chronic pain in countries with a Human Development Index of less than 0.9, it was noted that prevalence of chronic pain in the general population was "high." However, there was insufficient reliable data to estimate with any certainty the quantitative prevalence of chronic pain in such countries. Subtle differences in review and survey methodology appeared to impact estimates markedly.[11,12] It is interesting to note that there is no correlation between the Human Development Index and the prevalence of pain. It will be necessary to standardize pain-related definitions so that more valid and reliable epidemiologic data can be gathered and analyzed to define the extent of the problem.

This chapter on chronic pain in LMICs includes the experiences and lessons learned from leading global health chronic pain experts, including top experts from Ethiopia, Rwanda, Nigeria, and Canada.

Socioeconomic Burden

Chronic pain is often accompanied by depression, anxiety, anorexia, sleep disturbance, decreased mobility, and a host of social challenges related to family, work, costs, and finances.[13,14] It has been estimated that 1 million working days are lost in Denmark yearly due to chronic pain.[15] In the United Kingdom, health care costs for back pain are estimated to be 1 billion pounds per year.[16] It is difficult to estimate the economic costs of chronic pain in LMICs including sub-Saharan Africa, but they are likely to be considerable.[3] It is especially difficult to estimate these costs due to the involvement of multidisciplinary health care practitioners in chronic pain management and particularly the importance placed on alternative medicine in many of these countries. Due to the poorly developed health care systems in many developing countries, most expenses are borne by patients and their families.

Sociocultural Factors

In many areas of the world, the cultural expression of pain is associated with weakness or lack of courage. Pain is viewed as a natural part of a disease, birth, or injury, with resultant suffering and pain syndrome development. For example, perception of labor pain by pregnant women in Nigeria was the focus of a study in 2004. The women who were interviewed within 2 h of delivery perceived labor pain as being very painful. Although more than 70% of them viewed labor pain as being moderately to severely painful, 32% did not want any treatment.[8]

A systematic review on the impact of sociocultural factors on pain management approaches in sub-Saharan Africa showed that pain assessment and management are underrecognized because of sociocultural influences. It also suggested that gender differences in pain expression were linked to societal perceptions of courage and endurance.[9] This may impair clinicians' ability to interpret the nonverbal and verbal language of pain.[10] It is important to note that because the majority of studies on LMICs have examined the cultural expression of pain in environments with limited access to pain control, the environment itself may be a factor in maintaining these differences.

Access to Care

There are many barriers to effective pain management in Africa. The barriers may vary from country to country depending on the strength of the health care system, but most of the countries in sub-Saharan Africa fall on the lower end of the spectrum compared to developed countries. Medical tourism to other locations therefore prospers in many countries in sub-Saharan Africa.

As one of the world's poorest countries, The Gambia has an estimated per capita income of less than $1,000 per person per year, according to the World Bank. In The Gambia, barriers to effective pain management include shortage of health care personnel, shortage of strong opioids and other pain medications, and the role of sociocultural influences. In certain cultures in The Gambia, patients expect to bear their own pain, and at times, health care workers also expect their patients to live through some degree of pain. Various medications, including painkillers, are often in short supply at public clinics in the country. The most common medications for treating postoperative pain are acetaminophen, aspirin, and ibuprofen. No analgesia is administered for childbirth because health care practitioners in the labor rooms do not have the expectation of administering analgesia and are often hindered by the non-availability of medications.

In Nigeria, the situation is different. There is more awareness about pain management due mostly to the efforts of pain societies and some nongovernmental agencies to provide training and advocacy for pain management in the hospitals. The government of Nigeria has taken bold steps to ensure that pain management is adequately addressed, and this is demonstrated by the publication of a widely available national guideline for pain management. It was produced after several years of consultation and deliberations with governmental and nongovernmental agencies. Strong opioids and non-opioid analgesics are available in the country, although the supply of the strong opioids can sometimes be erratic, and stakeholders have to continually advocate for governmental agencies to ensure the provision. The supply is usually centrally controlled, and often, provision of the medications can be difficult due to paucity of funds.[17]

Many African countries have very low opioid consumption. As a continent, Africa has the lowest opioid consumption per capita of any continent in the world. For example, Zambia's morphine consumption was 0.0704 mg/capita, and that of Uganda was 0.4001 mg/capita. Compared to South Africa (2004), which had a morphine consumption of 3.7694 mg/capita, Tanzania's morphine consumption was 0.3250 mg/capita.[6]

The World Health Organization (WHO) (2006) has listed reasons for low opioid use in Africa, which include concerns regarding opioid addiction, strict national laws, misuse of drugs, and lack of knowledge.[7] Many countries in Africa have also severely restricted opioid formularies. A report from the Global Opioid Policy Initiative, which collected data from 25 of the 52 African countries, demonstrated that only 15 of the 25 had morphine available in their formularies.[8] Widespread overregulation of opioids has made access to pain management extremely difficult.

In Ethiopia, there is a significant shortage of opioids for treatment of acute as well as chronic pain. As is common in most countries, narcotic diversion and drug abuse exist. In Ethiopia, even a weak opioid such as tramadol was found to be abused by high school students, having been sold without proper prescription. However, in 2022, the Ethiopian Food and Drug Authority responded by limiting access and has put in place a strict monitoring control system to prevent negative health, social, economic, and political effects caused by misuse of tramadol.

Education of Providers

It has been demonstrated that there is an enormous knowledge gap in pain management in Africa and, thus, inadequate and ineffective care of patients in pain. This is brought about by limited access to short- or long-term pain education, undergraduate and postgraduate curricular deficiencies in pain management, lack of exemplary pain management centers that can potentially maximize exposure of medical professionals and students, and lack of literature regarding pain from LMICs.

The knowledge and practices among clinicians regarding assessment and management of pain in Africa are inadequate. A multicenter cross-sectional study in Cameroon showed that 77.6% of emergency department physicians rated "poor" in level of knowledge of pain management.[18] In an Ethiopian study at Jimma University, "unacceptable" levels of knowledge deficit, poor pain management judgment, and poor attitudes toward pain management were demonstrated.[17] A Ghanaian study showed similar results, with a demonstration of poor baseline pain knowledge and poor attitude toward postoperative management among surgical ward nurses.[19]

The knowledge gaps in pain management can be traced back to undergraduate as well as postgraduate program curriculum deficiencies in pain management. A study in South Africa on pain knowledge, especially with regard to the pharmacology of pain, noted important deficiencies in final-year medical students. The study demonstrated that the undergraduate curriculum and teaching would benefit from a review of the pain curriculum.[20] Supporting pain management curricula with clinical exposure is of vital importance. A prospective, multicenter study conducted across five medical colleges in Nigeria on e-learning platforms for pain management aimed to increase user uptake and engagement to incorporate pain education into medical school curriculum.[21]

Historical Role of Herbal Medicine

The continent of Africa—especially sub-Saharan Africa—is abundant with rich vegetation. Among the plants that naturally grow on the continent, there are many that are used to treat a variety of diseases. Herbal medicines are one of the oldest methods used for healing in Africa, even before the European invasion. Globally, the use of traditional medicine (TM), particularly herbal medicines, has surged during the past two decades. For example, in Europe, the use of TM ranges from 42% in Belgium to 90% in the United Kingdom; TM use by adults in the United States and Canada is 42% and 70%, respectively. In Africa, TM usage ranges from 60% in Uganda and the United

Republic of Tanzania to 70% in Ghana and Rwanda, 80% in Benin, and 90% in Burundi and Ethiopia.[22] According to the WHO, 70–80% of the population uses some form of TM, with herbal medicines standing out in particular. Within Africa, the knowledge regarding which plants are safe to be used for healing has been orally transmitted from the elders. Currently, most regions combine herbal and modern medicines according to the patient's presentation and the plants available.[23]

According to the WHO 1996 guidelines, herbal medicine comprises active end products that contain underground or aerial parts of either plants or plant materials or a combination of both. Most herbal medicines affect eicosanoid metabolism by inhibiting one or both of the lipoxygenase and cyclooxygenase pathways.[24] Their use is generally based on traditional methods, and the ideal extract dose and treatment duration for most herbal medicines have yet to be determined.

Herbal medicine plays an important role in pain treatment in Africa. Most of the information about the medications is passed down by oral rituals, although there is some increasing understanding that this type of treatment should also be based on scientific evidence. Very few studies have been conducted to determine the efficacy of traditional medications, and it is necessary that conditions of use be better defined and that patients be informed of potential adverse effects of the plants.

Research on herbal medicine for pain has significantly advanced in the past 30 years and is currently broadly distributed across multiple research disciplines. However, in a bibliometric analysis by Wang and Meng in 2021,[25] focusing on the global research trends of herbal medicine for pain in three decades (1990–2019), no African country featured in the top 10 countries worldwide in publications on herbal medications for pain management. China, the United States, and South Korea were the leading countries in terms of publications on herbal medicine. Although many plants are used in Africa as herbal treatments, knowledge of their use is passed by oral tradition and clinical research on such plants is not as well-established compared to that in Western countries.[25]

Research and use of TMs are gaining increased attention, particularly in Africa. The 2014–2023 traditional medicine strategic document, published by WHO,[26] laid out two major objectives: (1) to support countries seeking to understand the contribution of traditional medicine to health and well-being and (2) to promote the safe and effective use of traditional medicine through regulation.

The *West African Herbal Pharmacopoeia*, first published by the West African Health Organisation in 2013 and revised in 2020, contains the details of various herbal preparations for treatment of various common infections.[27] The publication, although quite detailed on the uses of various plants, herbs, and roots, did not include any traditional medication for treating pain. With continuous engagement of clinicians and scientists on this important topic, it is hoped that the benefits of available TMs to treat pain will be investigated beyond the oral knowledge and documented to share their usefulness.

Pediatric Chronic Pain in Africa

Multiple studies have shown a prevalence of chronic or complex persistent pain in children and adolescents of up to 20%, with severe, disabling pain of at least 5% or 6%.[28–30]

These studies have been primarily undertaken in high-income countries, and there is no evidence that the prevalence is any lower in LMICs. It is well recognized that patients, especially children, will show less behavioral pain response over time, especially if the pain continues without treatment or relief, despite ongoing positive reports of pain intensity.[31] This is especially true for the majority of patients seen in high-income country pain clinics, who generally do not have tissue-damaging disease but, rather, nociplastic or neuropathic conditions such as chronic widespread pain (e.g., fibromyalgia), headache, recurrent abdominal pain, or peripheral nerve injuries. Of note, one has to assume that the population in LMICs will have not only pain without tissue damage but also an additional number of other painful chronic conditions, including HIV/AIDS, sickle cell disease, untreated cancer, parasitic diseases, etc., depending on the region and living conditions.

The standard of care for multimodal, multidisciplinary care of chronic pain in children includes psychological and physical therapy, especially focusing on education and skill development, rather than active treatment.[32] It requires specific training and skills to provide tailored physiotherapy or psychological care for chronic pain in children—these are not usually in the curriculum for general clinicians in these fields. The medications required are usually nonsteroidal anti-inflammatories, tricyclic antidepressants, or serotonin–noradrenaline reuptake inhibitors, and/or anticonvulsants, especially gabapentinoids. Opioids are rarely appropriate or helpful, unless the patient has tissue injury from cancer, sickle cell disease, severe rheumatoid arthritis, etc. Unfortunately, both non-opioid medications and nonpharmacological approaches can be in very short supply or prohibitively expensive in LMICs.

The combination of these factors results in a large, but hidden, cohort of children with ongoing suffering, who may lose out on education, physical activity, and socialization. It is recognized that youth with chronic pain have a high risk of becoming adults with chronic pain, with the consequent and well-known impacts on their own lives and social and economic costs to society.[33] There is no quick and easy fix for this. Solutions will require broad-based government support to develop pain management resources, including, but not limited to, multidisciplinary clinics focused on pediatric pain care.

Lessons Learned

Pioneers leading pain management efforts in Africa realize that the journey to change does not come without resistance. A lack of local support from institutions and governments can seem just as burdensome and isolating to the pioneer as a shortage of health care workers in the subspecialty, which ultimately affects disparities in access to much-needed care. Here are some lessons learned from pioneers in the field:

- Persistence is key; pain management skills and leadership skills become necessary when implementing change. Despite the challenges faced in LMICs, pioneers in the field are empowered to manage pain.
- Forming alliances and collaborations with other experts throughout the world, especially those with shared challenges in lower resource settings, creates a strong

global community for addressing pain as a global public health issue and allows for a more meaningful experience.

- Realize that patients may wait and delay care before seeing a specialist, and when they do see a specialist, the underlying disease process may be advanced or the pain level will be quite complicated. Nevertheless, it is important to encourage patients to freely express their pain feelings in order to improve assessment and management. Also, once patients are educated about their pain, it becomes easier to assess and treat.
- Nonpharmacological approaches should be encouraged, especially in LMICs, where access to appropriate pain medications is problematic and knowledge about the use of opioids is limited.
- Protocols and guidelines help improve every aspect of medical practice.
- Having pain focal points in every unit of the hospital plays a major role in compliance to local protocols and guidelines.
- Training of more faculty anesthesiologists is essential to achieve the best possible pain practice.
- Quality improvement initiatives also aid in addressing pain management.
- Alliances with other specialties help advance the pain medicine field. Anesthesiology and pain management are not practiced in silos; forming alliances with obstetrics and surgery specialists is key to addressing global health inequities. In addition, a multidisciplinary approach with other care providers, such as nurses and pharmacists, is necessary to deliver quality effective pain management.

References

1. Goldberg DS, McGee SJ. Pain as a global public health priority. *BMC Public Health.* 2011;11:770.
2. Breivik H., Collett B., Ventafridda V., et al. Survey of chronic pain in Europe: Prevalence, impact on daily life, and treatment. *Eur J Pain.* 2006;10:287–333.
3. Faponle A, Soyannwo O, Ajayi I. Post-operative pain therapy: A survey of prescribing patterns and adequacy of analgesia in Ibadan, Nigeria. *Cent Afr J Med.* 2001;47:70–74.
4. Mwaka G, Thikra S, Mung'ayi V. The prevalence of postoperative pain in the first 48 hours following day surgery at a tertiary hospital in Nairobi. *Afr Health Sci.* 2013;13:768–776.
5. Eshete MT, Baeumler PI, Siebeck M, et al. Quality of postoperative pain management in Ethiopia: A prospective longitudinal study. *PLoS One.* 2019;14:e0215563.
6. Argaw F, Berhe T, Assefa S, et al. Acute postoperative pain management at a tertiary hospital in Addis Ababa, Ethiopia: A prospective cross-sectional study. *East Cent Afr J Surg.* 2019; 24:82–88.
7. Admassu W, Hailekiros A, Abdissa Z. Severity and risk factors of post-operative pain in University of Gondar Hospital, northeast Ethiopia. *J Anesth Clin Res.* 2016; 7:675.
8. Faponle AF, Kuti O. Perception of labour pain by pregnant women in south-western Nigeria. *Trop J Obstetrics Gynaecol.* 2004;21(2):153–155.
9. Jackson T, Thomas S, Stabile V, Shotwell M, Han X, McQueen KA. A systematic review and meta-analysis of the global burden of chronic pain without clear etiology in low- and middle-income countries: Trends in heterogeneous data and a proposal for new assessment methods. *Anesth Analg.* 2016;123:739–748.
10. Woolf AD, Pfleger B. Burden of major musculoskeletal conditions. *Bull World Health Organ.* 2003;81:646–656.

11. Tsang A, Von Korff M, Lee S, et al. Common chronic pain conditions in developed and developing countries: Gender and age differences and comorbidity with depression–anxiety disorders. *J Pain.* 2008;9:883–891.
12. Elzahaf RA, Tashani OA, Unsworth BA, et al. The prevalence of chronic pain with an analysis of countries with a Human Development Index less than 0.9: A systematic review without meta-analysis. *Curr Med Res Opin.* 2012;28(12):211–229.
13. Brennan F, Carr DB, Cousins M. Pain management: A fundamental human right. *Anesth Analg.* 2007;105:205–221.
14. King NB, Fraser V. Untreated pain, narcotics regulation, and global health ideologies. *PLoS Med.* 2013;10:e1001411.
15. Phillips CJ. The cost and burden of chronic pain. *Rev Pain.* 2009;3:2–5.
16. Maniadakis N, Gray A. The economic burden of back pain in the UK. *Pain.* 2000;84:95–103.
17. Eyob T, Mulatu A, Abrha H. Knowledge and attitude towards pain management among medical and paramedical students of an Ethiopian university. *J Pain Relief.* 2013;3:Article 127.
18. Etoundi PO, Mbengono JAM, Ntock FN, et al. Knowledge, attitudes, and practices of Cameroonian physicians with regards to acute pain management in the emergency department: A multicenter cross-sectional study. *BMC Emerg Med.* 2019;19:Article 45.
19. Adams SM, Varaei S, Jalalinia F. Nurses' knowledge and attitude towards postoperative pain management in Ghana. *Pain Res Manag.* 2020;7:4893707.
20. Mashanda-Tafaune B, Van Nugteren J, Parker R. Pain knowledge and attitudes of final-year medical students at the University of Cape Town: A cross-sectional survey. *Afr J Prim Health Care Fam Med.* 2020;30;12(1):e1–e6.
21. Onyeka TC, Iloanusi N, Namisango E, et al. Project OPUS: Development and evaluation of an electronic platform for pain management education of medical undergraduates in resource-limited settings. *PLoS One.* 2020;15(12):e0243573.
22. Pain & Policy Studies Group. (2006). Availability of morphine and pethidine in the world and Africa, with a special focus on: Botswana, Ethiopia, Kenya, Malawi, Nigeria, Rwanda, Tanzania, Zambia.
23. Jahromi B, Pirvulescu I, Candido KD, Knezevic NN. Herbal medicine for pain management: Efficacy and drug interactions. *Pharmaceutics.* 2021;13(2):Article 251.
24. Weiner DK, Ernst E. Complementary and alternative approaches to the treatment of persistent musculoskeletal pain. *Clin J Pain.* 2004;20:244–255.
25. Wang C, Meng Q. Global research trends of herbal medicine for pain in three decades (1990–2019): A bibliometric analysis. *J Pain Res.* 2021;4(14):1611–1626.
26. World Health Organization. *WHO Traditional Medicine Strategy: 2014–2023.* 2013. https://iris.who.int/bitstream/handle/10665/92455/9789241506090_eng.pdf?Sequence=1
27. West African Health Organisation. *West African Herbal Pharmacopoeia.* 2020. https://www.wahooas.org/web-ooas/sites/default/files/publications/2318/west-african-herbal-pharmacopoeia.PDF
28. Perquin CW, Hazebroek-Kampschreur AAJM, Hunfield JAM, et al. Pain in children and adolescents: A common experience. *Pain.* 2000;87:51–58.
29. Stanford EA, Chambers CT, Biesanz JC, Chen E. The frequency, trajectories and predictors of adolescent recurrent pain: A population-based approach. *Pain.* 2008;138(1):11–21.
30. Huguet A, Miró J. The severity of chronic pediatric pain: An epidemiological study. *J Pain.* 2008;9(3):226–236.
31. Beyer JE, McGrath PJ, Berde CB. Discordance between self-report and behavioral pain measures in children aged 3–7 years after surgery. *J Pain Symptom Manage.* 1990;5(6):360–366.
32. Miró J, McGrath PJ, Finley GA, Walco GA. Pediatric chronic pain programs: Current and ideal practice. *Pain Rep.* 2017;2(5):e613.
33. Walker LS, Sherman AL, Bruehl S, et al. Functional abdominal pain patient subtypes in childhood predict functional gastrointestinal disorders with chronic pain and psychiatric comorbidities in adolescence and adulthood. *Pain.* 2012;153(9):1798–1806.

19
Pain in Patients with Substance Use Disorders

Martin D. Cheatle

Introduction

There has been substantial scholarly, political, and health policy focus on the opioid crisis due to the burgeoning rate of opioid-related deaths during the past decade. This has fostered devising new practice standards and polices such as the Centers for Disease Control and Prevention's (CDC) opioid guideline published in 2016,[1] which has been recently revised in response to numerous criticisms. The 2016 guideline recommendations were instituted by many states, insurance companies, and retail pharmacies as more law than guidance, such as having a mandated upper limit on opioid dosing, a mandated duration of use even for acute pain, and mandating that only certain medical specialties could prescribe opioids long term (pain physicians, physiatrists, and addiction psychiatrists). This led to many patients suffering unnecessarily. Many patients who were on stable doses of opioids and functioning well were rapidly tapered and in some cases discharged from care. The *CDC Clinical Practice Guideline for Prescribing Opioids for Pain—United States, 2022*[2] strongly emphasized that the guideline provides "voluntary clinical practice recommendations for clinicians that should not be used as inflexible standards of care" and that care should be individualized. Other practice standards and policies included the development of state prescription drug monitoring programs, educational programs on safe opioid prescribing (e.g., the Risk Evaluation and Mitigation Strategies program), and institutional stewardship programs for opioid prescribers such as "academic detailing" or one-to-one education on proper opioid prescribing[3] to curb unnecessary opioid prescribing. These efforts have resulted in a significant reduction in prescription of opioids to patients in the acute phase but also patients with chronic non-cancer pain (CNCP).[4] There is consensus agreement that opioids are typically not first-line therapy for patients with CNCP and that many pain conditions can be managed with non-opioid therapies, such as antiepileptic drugs (pregabalin and gabapentin) for neuropathically mediated pain disorders, nonsteroidal anti-inflammatory drugs and acetaminophen for certain musculoskeletal conditions, and antidepressants for fibromyalgia pain. There is also consensus that the most clinically efficacious, evidenced-based approach to chronic pain is multidisciplinary care to include coordinated medical, rehabilitative, and psychological services.[5] In real-world practice, access to multidisciplinary pain care is limited,[6,7] and although there has been an emerging effort to develop online multidisciplinary pain interventions to bridge this gap in need and access,[8] the vast majority of patients with chronic pain have limited pain treatment options.

There has been an ongoing debate on the efficacy and safety of opioids for patients with CNCP,[1,2,9–12] with evidence that in well-selected patients, who have not responded or only partially responded to first-line therapies, short-term opioid therapy can be efficacious in relieving pain and promoting increased function and quality of life.[10–13] Poorly managed pain and tapering of opioids can lead to deleterious outcomes. Using a retrospective cohort study design, Agnoli et al.[13] evaluated associations between opioid dose tapering and rates of overdose and mental health crisis among patients prescribed stable, long-term, higher dose opioids. Opioid tapering was defined as at least a 15% relative reduction in mean daily dose during any of six overlapping 60-day windows within a 7-month follow-up period. Primary outcomes were emergency department or hospital encounters for drug overdose or withdrawal and mental health crisis (depression, anxiety, and suicide attempt) during up to 12 months of follow-up. Results revealed that post-tapering patient periods were associated with an adjusted incidence rate of 9.3 overdose events per 100 person-years compared with 5.5 events per 100 person-years in nontapered periods and an adjusted incidence rate of 7.6 mental health crisis events per 100 person-years compared with 3.3 events per 100 person-years among nontapered periods. The authors concluded that these results suggest that tapering events in patients on stable, high-dose opioids were significantly associated with increased risk of overdose and mental health crisis. Another recent retrospective study examined the effect of rapid opioid dose reduction after high-dose, long-term opioid therapy on suicide, overdose, or other opioid-related adverse events extracted from a large insurance claims database.[14] It was discovered that both abrupt and dose reduction were significantly associated with increased risk of suicide compared to that for patients on stable or increasing doses, and patients abruptly discontinued had a higher risk of overdose on heroin (not prescription opioids) compared to other groups. In a comparative effectiveness study, the association of opioid tapering or abrupt discontinuation with opioid overdose and suicide in patients receiving stable long-term opioid therapy without evidence of opioid misuse was evaluated. Results revealed a small increase in risk of harms associated with opioid tapering compared with a stable opioid dosage.[15] In contrast, a systematic review of the literature on the risks and benefits of opioid tapering in patients on long-term opioid therapy revealed mixed results and suggested that clinics should closely monitor patients during an opioid reduction.[16]

This national focus on the risks and benefits of opioid therapy for patients with pain and need for tapering of opioids has obscured the vulnerability of patients with pain who are susceptible to discrimination based on opioid use or having a co-occurring opioid use disorder (OUD) and to developing other forms of non-opioid use disorders. This chapter discusses the myths and facts of opioids in the pain population, the prevalence of pain and both nicotine use disorder and alcohol use disorder, and assessment and mitigation strategies.

Definitions of Misuse, Abuse, and Substance Use Disorder

The terms misuse, abuse, and substance use disorder (addiction) are often used interchangeably. *Misuse* can be defined as taking a substance for a therapeutic intent (opioids for pain relief) but not as prescribed (prescribed one tablet of oxycodone twice daily for pain but using three or four tablets for pain relief). *Abuse* can be operationalized as taking a substance for nontherapeutic purposes of obtaining psychotropic effects, such as managing anxiety, causing sedation, inducing sleep, or for euphoria.[17] *Substance use disorder* can be characterized by the four C's: out of *c*ontrol use, *c*ompulsive use, *c*raving for non-pain use, and use causing negative *c*onsequences.[18]

Pain and Opioid Use Disorder

Etiology of the Opioid Crisis

The root cause of the opioid crisis is a confluence of a number of factors. Starting in the 1980s, several influential articles were published touting the potential efficacy and safety of opioids in managing pain in patients with low probability of developing an OUD (addiction). Several articles were based on results from a small sample size,[19] case reports, and surveys. Many were opinion/commentary pieces, such as Melzack's 1990 article in *Scientific American* titled "The Tragedy of Needless Pain,"[20] which supported the notion that taking opioids solely for pain is not addictive and that undertreating pain was causing unnecessary suffering. These publications fostered a change in standard practice, extrapolating end-of-life pain care to patients with CNCP. This position was supported by numerous professional societies and experienced pain clinicians.[21–27] These were well-meaning professionals who were rendering opinions based on the available data with the purpose of improving the quality of life of countless numbers of patients with agonizing CNCP. A second factor contributing to the opioid crisis was the pharmaceutical industry, which propagated through often paid or incentivized educational programs that opioids were safe and effective, opioid addiction was rare in patients with CNCP, clinicians were allowing patients to suffer due to "opioidphobia," and that patients could easily be tapered off opioids. A 2018 retrospective cohort study by Zezza and Bachhuber[28] linked the Open Payments database and Medicare Part D drug utilization data and discovered an association between physician payments from opioid pharmaceutical companies and higher volume and more expensive opioid analgesic prescribing. Other causative factors of the opioid crisis are the general lack of core competencies on pain management in medical school curricula[29] and health care insurance companies not covering or limiting more expensive non-opioid therapies.[30]

Myths and Facts of Pain and Opioid Use Disorder

There has been ongoing debate regarding the role of prescription opioids in the increase in OUD and opioid-related deaths. One myth is that patients with chronic pain receiving long-term opioid therapy are at high risk for developing OUD, and another myth is that the prescribing of opioids to patients with pain directly contributed to the opioid crisis. In fact, there were more than 100,000 drug-related deaths in 2021, which represented a 28% increase in deaths since 2020.[31] There have been three waves of the opioid crisis. In the 1990s, there was a significant increase in prescription opioid overdose deaths. In 2010, there was a rise in heroin-related deaths, and currently most opioid-related deaths are attributable to synthetic opioids, particularly illicit fentanyl,[32] and the vast majority of these deaths are not in patients with pain. Since the 2016 release of the CDC guideline,[1] there has been a 66% reduction in opioid prescribing and a 253% increase in opioid-related overdoses.[32] In the 1990s, prescribing opioids for CNCP was considered the standard of care. This resulted in a large quantity of opioids being available in the community reservoir for diversion to individuals susceptible to OUDs. The prevalence of actual OUD in patients with chronic pain prescribed opioids is 8.8–10.7%,[33–35] which is similar to the prevalence of other substance use disorders (SUDs) in the United States (14% overall, 10.2% alcohol use disorder [AUD], and 6.6% drug use disorders). The conflation of the prevalence of OUD in the pain population is related to error in diagnosing OUD, which may represent tolerance, misuse, or abuse but not meeting criteria for true OUD.

Key Points

- The opioid crisis is the result of a confluence of factors, including the overprescribing of opioids to patients with chronic pain.
- There are patients with pain who would benefit from opioid therapy, which requires patient selection based on risk–benefit analysis and close monitoring.
- The rate of OUD in patients with chronic pain is similar to that of other drugs of abuse at 8–10%, but this is not inconsequential.

Pain and Alcohol Use Disorder

The national attention on the opioid crisis has obscured other substances of abuse that can also cause significant harm to vulnerable patients with chronic pain, such as alcohol.

Alcohol Use Disorder

The 2020 National Survey on Drug Use and Health revealed that 50.0% of people aged 12 years or older (or 138.5 million people) used alcohol in the past month. Of the 138.5 million people who used alcohol, 61.6 million people (or 44.4%) were classified as binge drinkers, 17.7 million people (28.8% of current binge drinkers and 12.8% of current alcohol users) were classified as heavy drinkers, and approximately 14.5 million people aged 12 years or older developed an AUD.[36] The CDC reports that 29 people in the United States die every day in motor vehicle accidents that involve an alcohol-impaired driver.[37] Statistics on past month general substance use among people aged 12 years or older in 2020 revealed that alcohol was most used (138.5 million people), followed by tobacco products (51.7 million), marijuana (32.8 million), and prescription pain reliever misuse (2.5 million).[36]

Pain and Alcohol

There is a noteworthy relationship between pain, alcohol use, and AUD. McDermott et al.[38] employed data from the National Epidemiologic Survey on Alcohol and Related Conditions and conducted logistic regression analyses examining the association between pain interference and concurrent and prospective AUD and nicotine use disorder. Moderate pain interference predicted the development of AUD (moderate: odds ratio [OR] = 1.56; 95% confidence interval [CI], 1.39–1.75; $p < .001$) and nicotine use disorder (OR = 1.37; 95% CI, 1.14–1.65; $p < .001$). Imtiaz et al.[39] evaluated longitudinal alcohol consumption patterns and health-related quality of life and found that decreases in alcohol consumption were associated with reductions in ratings of acute pain severity 3 years later, and another study revealed that acute pain frequency (i.e., days with pain) was associated with the diagnosis of AUD.[38] Patients with chronic pain have a tendency to report higher levels of alcohol use and AUD than the general population,[39] and individuals with chronic pain report using alcohol to medicate acute pain symptoms.[40–42] Last, one-third to more than one-half of individuals seeking treatment for AUD report chronic, recurrent pain.[43,44]

Key Points

- Pain reduction during alcohol treatment is associated with lower alcohol relapse risk. Heavier drinking is associated with greater pain severity, pain interference, and less pain coping among chronic pain patients receiving long-term opioid therapy.
- Treatment should focus on the interconnection of pain and alcohol use, as well as aberrant opioid use among patients prescribed opioid therapy in order to improve long-term treatment outcomes in patients dealing with pain and AUD.
- Comorbidity of pain and AUD is extremely concerning and important to target given that alcohol is commonly taken along with opioids and other substances among individuals experiencing chronic pain.
- The combined use of alcohol, opioids, and sedatives increases the risk for overdose.

Pain and Nicotine and Tobacco

There is a robust and evolving literature on the interrelationship of pain, nicotine, and tobacco smoking. In a seminal review article by LaRowe and Ditre,[45] a number of salient facts on pain and nicotine/tobacco smoking were highlighted. Although the current prevalence of cigarette smoking has declined to approximately 14% in the general population,[46] the smoking rates remain substantially higher among individuals with co-occurring pain (24–68%).[46–48] It has been estimated that 60% of patients who meet criteria for tobacco use disorder have concomitant chronic pain.[49]

Pain and smoking are reciprocal. Smoking can lead to the development of chronic pain, and pain can encourage nicotine/tobacco use and impede cessation. It has been postulated that the pain/nicotine mechanisms related to tobacco smoking may lead to dysregulated pain processing and poorer outcomes through both nicotine/tobacco-specific (e.g., tissue degeneration/healing impairment) and general neurobiological effects (e.g., allostatic load on overlapping pain, stress, and reward neurocircuitry). Furthermore, pain is often associated with anxiety; smokers report increased smoking in response to anxiety, thus leading to a pain–anxiety–increased smoking cycle.[50] Avoidance of pain or relief of pain or both may be powerful reinforcers in the maintenance of nicotine abuse. It has also been identified that patients with pain endorse smoking/tobacco use as a means to cope with pain.[51] In addition, poor pain coping is a major factor in nicotine/tobacco relapse, and smokers with pain versus no pain are more likely to cite pain as a barrier to quitting.[52] There is also evidence that current smoking status and nicotine dependence are both independently associated with an increased risk for chronic low back pain and/or chronic radicular neuropathic leg pain.[53] Last, tobacco use has been identified as a risk factor for the development of OUD in patients with chronic pain.[54]

Key Points

- Nicotine use and abuse are common in patients with chronic pain.
- Smoking and pain are reciprocal: Pain can cause increased smoking, and smoking can be a risk factor for developing chronic pain.
- Patients with chronic pain who smoke tend to have poorer outcomes with regard to function, mood, and pain intensity.

Assessment

Assessing the potential of patients with chronic pain to misuse or abuse substances and the risk of developing a SUD is important in managing these typically complex patients. A comprehensive evaluation should include mental health screening (depression and anxiety) and screening for nicotine abuse, alcohol abuse, risk of OUD or aberrant drug-related behavior (ADRB), and other substances of abuse.

Mental Health Screening

There are a variety of validated and reliable mental health screening tools. The Beck Depression Inventory (BDI)[55] and the Profile of Mood States (POMS)[56] are two measures that have been recommended by an expert consensus group on measuring emotional functioning in chronic pain.[57] The BDI is a 21-question self-report measure of depression severity over the past week. The POMS has a full-length version (65 items) and a shorter version (35 questions), both comprising seven scales, three of which are particularly relevant to the pain population: anger/hostility, depression/dejection, and tension/anxiety.

Opioid Use Disorder and Aberrant Drug-Related Behavior

A number of assessment tools have been developed and validated to assess the risk of a patient engaging in ADRB either prior to initiating long-term opioid therapy (LTOT), such as the Opioid Risk Tool[58] or the Screener and Opioid Assessment for Patients with Pain,[59] or when patients are on LTOT, such as the Current Opioid Misuse Measure[60] or the Prescription Drug Use Questionnaire.[61] Although screening for ADRBs can be useful, ADRBs are not necessarily surrogates for OUD. Common ADRBs include a patient requesting an early refill of an opioid, being seen in urgent care with increased pain requesting opioids, or frequent phone calls to the clinic regarding their pain. The Opioid Risk Tool–OUD is based on data comparing patients with chronic pain with and without co-occurring OUD, thus allowing to risk stratify for OUD.[62]

Alcohol Abuse/Alcohol Use Disorder

Two commonly employed screeners for alcohol abuse are the Alcohol Use Disordered Identification Test (AUDIT), which has 10 weighted yes/no questions,[63] and the CAGE (Cut Down, Annoyed, Guilty, Eye Opener) and the CAGE-AID, which was adapted to assess for both alcohol and drugs.[64] The AUDIT has greater sensitivity for detecting alcohol abuse than the CAGE.

Nicotine Dependence

The Fagerström Test for Nicotine Dependence (FTND) is a standard instrument for assessing the intensity of physical dependence to nicotine.[65] It contains six items that evaluate the quantity of cigarette consumption, the compulsion to use, and dependence. The FTND has six questions that yield a total score of 0–10. The higher the total Fagerström score, the more intense is the patient's physical dependence on nicotine.

Universal Screening for Alcohol, Drugs, Nicotine, and Other Substances of Abuse

The Tobacco, Alcohol, Prescription Medication, and Other Substance Use (TAPS) tool has two components. The first component (TAPS-1) is a four-item screen for tobacco, alcohol, illicit drugs, and nonmedical use of prescription drugs. If a patient screens positive on TAPS-1, it triggers the second component (TAPS-2), which consists of brief substance-specific assessment questions to arrive at a risk level for each substance.[66]

Treatment Strategies

Managing SUDs in patients with chronic pain includes both pharmacologic and nonpharmacologic interventions, which are briefly discussed.

Pharmacologic Interventions

Opioid Use Disorder and Pain

There are three medications for OUD: methadone, buprenorphine, and naltrexone. Methadone is a full μ-opioid agonist and blocks *N*-methyl-D-aspartate receptor and monoamine reuptake, which is efficacious for neuropathically mediated pain disorders. The pharmacokinetic and pharmacodynamic effects of methadone give it an advantage over other opioids in that methadone is long-acting and development of tolerance is low, thus potentially leading to lower dosing long term. Patients on methadone maintenance for OUD who do experience CNCP require higher dosing of opioids for pain relief. Methadone for OUD can only be dispensed from a federally licensed facility.

Buprenorphine is a partial opioid agonist, thus producing a ceiling effect to opioid effects (euphoria and respiratory depression), and it is safer with patients on concurrent benzodiazepine therapy. Buprenorphine is dosed daily to weekly; take-home doses are allowed without time-in-treatment requirement. Patients can switch from methadone to buprenorphine. Buprenorphine is as effective as moderate doses of methadone, but for patients with high levels of physical dependency, methadone may be a better choice. There are three buprenorphine formulations for OUD (sublingual, implant, and injection) and two buprenorphine formulations for pain (transdermal patch and buccal).

Naltrexone, which is an antagonist at the opioid receptor, is approved for treating both OUD and AUD. Naltrexone comes in a pill form or as an injectable. The pill form of naltrexone can be taken at 50 mg once per day. The injectable extended-release form of the drug is administered typically at 380 mg intramuscularly once a month. Extended-release naltrexone in alcohol-dependent adults has been shown to increase initial and 6-month abstinence. In OUD, following detoxification, extended-release naltrexone shows efficacy for maintaining abstinence, improving retention, decreasing craving, and preventing relapse.

Nicotine and Pain

The current pharmacotherapy interventions approved by the U.S. Food and Drug Administration for the treatment of tobacco smoking dependence and abuse in adults include nicotine replacement therapy (NRT; (e.g., nicotine transdermal patches, lozenges, gum, inhalers, or nasal spray), bupropion hydrochloride sustained-release (SR), and varenicline. All three types of pharmacotherapy increase tobacco smoking cessation rates. Using a combination of NRT products (in particular, combining short-acting and long-acting forms of NRT) has been found to be more effective than using a single form of NRT. Based on a smaller number of studies, varenicline appears to be more effective than NRT or bupropion SR in maintaining abstinence.[66]

Alcohol Use Disorder and Pain

There are three medications for AUD: acamprosate, disulfiram, and naltrexone. Acamprosate is appropriate for people in recovery, who are no longer drinking alcohol and want to avoid relapse. Acamprosate comes as a delayed-release tablet taken orally. Acamprosate acts to normalize dysregulation in neurochemical systems that have been implicated in the biological mechanisms of alcohol dependence and abuse. It prevents people from drinking alcohol, but it does not prevent withdrawal symptoms after people drink alcohol. It has not been shown to work in people who continue drinking alcohol, consume illicit drugs, and/or engage in prescription drug misuse and abuse.

Disulfiram is a type of aversive therapy intended to treat chronic alcoholism and is most effective in people who have already gone through detoxification or are in the initial stage of abstinence. Disulfiram blocks the conversion of acetaldehyde to acetic acid, resulting in an upsurge of acetaldehyde. This upsurge is toxic and causes the individual to become ill when consuming alcohol. Offered in a tablet form and taken once a day, disulfiram should never be taken while intoxicated, and it should not be taken for at least 12 h after drinking alcohol because it will cause severe illness, nausea, flushing, and tachycardia. Disulfiram is most effective in maintaining abstinence when coupled with psychosocial interventions.

Naltrexone blocks the euphoric effects and feelings of intoxication, and it allows people with AUDs to reduce alcohol use and remain motivated to continue to take the medication, stay in treatment, and avoid relapses. Once the patient has sustained abstinence, naltrexone can be discontinued, but there are no long-term adverse effects of continued naltrexone.

Nonpharmacologic Treatments

A number of nonpharmacologic interventions can be efficacious in managing pain and comorbid SUD, including fostering social support such as attending Alcoholics Anonymous or Narcotics Anonymous, complementary and alternative medicine such as acupuncture for pain, smoking cessation and cognitive–behavioral therapy (CBT), and acceptance and commitment therapy (ACT).

CBT is a well-established therapy for a number of mental health conditions and chronic pain. CBT targets maladaptive thinking (catastrophizing) and maladaptive behavior (kinesiophobia). A program of CBT includes having individuals reconceptualize their role in the healing process; promoting a proactive mental state rather than a reactive state; and acquiring skills such as relaxation therapy, pacing, CBT for insomnia, cognitive restructuring, effective communication, behavioral activation, and stress management followed by skill consolidation and rehearsal and relapse training.

ACT is a form of CBT that is a directive and experiential type of therapy based on rational frame theory. The goal of ACT is to experience life mindfully and reinforce psychological flexibility, fostering increased activity and function—finding ways around life's barriers, including pain. There are six core processes in ACT: contact with the present moment, self-as-context, defusion, acceptance, values, and committed action.

There is an evolving literature on the efficacy of CBT/ACT in treating pain and concomitant SUD. For example, Wachholtz et al.[67] evaluated the efficacy and feasibility of an integrated cognitive–behavioral, 90-min, 12-week outpatient group therapy called STOP (Self-Regulation Therapy for Opioid Addiction and Pain). Results revealed STOP had high attendance rates (80%) and active patient engagement; urine toxicology showed no illicit drug use after Week 8, and pre-intervention to a 3-month follow-up showed significant functional improvement ($F(1, 12) = 45.82$; $p < .01$) and decreased pain severity levels ($F(1, 12) = 37.62$; $p < .01$). The Pain and Smoking Study (PASS) was a comparative effectiveness trial of a telephone-delivered, cognitive–behavioral intervention among veterans with chronic pain who smoked cigarettes. PASS participants were randomized to a standard telephone counseling intervention that includes five sessions focusing on motivational interviewing, craving and relapse management, rewards, and nicotine replacement therapy versus the same components with the addition of a cognitive–behavioral intervention for pain management.[68]

Given the barriers of obtaining behavioral health care, there has been an effort to develop more remote delivery approaches. For example, Tetreault et al.[69] performed a randomized clinical trial evaluating feasibility, satisfaction, and substance use outcomes for 58 individuals with SUD who were randomized to standard care or standard care plus access to a Web-based SUD intervention (computer-based training in CBT or CBT4CBT). Self-reported substance use and urine toxicology screens were assessed at 8 weeks after randomization. Of those assigned to this condition, 77% accessed the program at least once; of those, 77% completed all seven modules. Satisfaction with the program was very high. Participants reported greater than 90% days of abstinence for all classes of drugs, with no significant differences between conditions.

Managing the Patient with Pain and Substance Use Disorder

Managing patients with pain and comorbid SUDs can be highly challenging. Clinicians who prescribe opioids should have a well-vetted process for patient selection (risks–benefits of opioids), use of an opioid agreement, and initial and ongoing monitoring of ADRB (routine urine drug testing, risk assessment tools, and querying the state Prescription Drug Monitoring Program). Because alcohol and nicotine use are more prevalent in the pain population than opioids, it is prudent to extend risk assessment and monitoring to all possible substances of abuse (e.g., using TAPS, which assesses for tobacco, alcohol, and other substances of abuse) and have a plan of action if a patient is actively abusing opioids, alcohol, or other substances of abuse. This includes having an established referral network for local substance abuse treatment centers and a list of local Alcoholics Anonymous and Narcotic Anonymous meetings. Basic resources for treating patients with SUDs can be found through organizations such as the American Society of Addiction Medicine (https://www.asam.orghttps://) and the American Academy of Addiction Psychiatry (http://www.aaap.org). Last, the Substance Abuse and Mental Health Services Administration has a treatment locator website that can help clinicians quickly locate an appropriate treatment facility (https://findtreatment.samhsa.gov).

Summary

- The opioid crisis has obscured the equally important issue of pain and other SUDs.
- Opioid-related overdoses are primarily related to illicit heroin and fentanyl use; they rarely occur in legitimate patients suffering from chronic pain.
- Alcohol and nicotine use and abuse are common in patients with chronic pain, and both alcohol and nicotine have an analgesic effect on pain that complicates recovery.

- Clinicians caring for patients with chronic pain should be cognizant of other SUDs beyond opioids.
- It is critical to develop a multimodal approach to treatment that includes both pharmacologic and nonpharmacologic interventions which can be easily accessed.

References

1. Dowell D, Haegerich TM, Chou R. CDC guideline for prescribing opioids for chronic pain—United States, 2016. *JAMA*. 2016;315(15):1624–1645. doi:10.1001/jama.2016.1464
2. Dowell D, Ragan KR, Jones CM, Baldwin GT, Chou R. CDC clinical practice guideline for prescribing opioids for pain—United States, 2022. *MMWR Recomm Rep*. 2022;71(3):1–95.
3. Trotter Davis M, Bateman B, Avorn J. Educational outreach to opioid prescribers: The case for academic detailing. *Pain Physician*. 2017;20(2S):S147–S151.
4. Townsend T, Cerdá M, Bohnert A, Lagisetty P, Haffajee RL. CDC guideline for opioid prescribing associated with reduced dispensing to certain patients with chronic pain. *Health Aff*. 2021;40(11):1766–1775. doi:10.1377/hlthaff.2021.00135
5. Kamper SJ, Apeldoorn AT, Chiarotto A, et al. Multidisciplinary biopsychosocial rehabilitation for chronic low back pain: Cochrane systematic review and meta-analysis. *BMJ*. 2015;350:h444. doi:10.1136/bmj.h444
6. Choinière M, Peng P, Gilron I, et al. Accessing care in multidisciplinary pain treatment facilities continues to be a challenge in Canada. *Reg Anesth Pain Med*. 2020;45(12):943–948. doi:10.1136/rapm-2020-101935
7. Leonard C, Ayele R, Ladebue A, et al. Barriers to and facilitators of multimodal chronic pain care for veterans: A national qualitative study. *Pain Med*. 2021;22(5):1167–1173. doi:10.1093/pm/pnaa312
8. Smith J, Faux SG, Gardner T, et al. Reboot online: A randomized controlled trial comparing an online multidisciplinary pain management program with usual care for chronic pain. *Pain Med*. 2019;20(12):2385–2396. doi:10.1093/pm/pnz208
9. Ballantyne JC, Shin NS. Efficacy of opioids for chronic pain: A review of the evidence. *Clin J Pain*. 2008;24(6):469–478. doi:10.1097/AJP.0b013e31816b2f26
10. Chou R, Clark E, Helfand M. Comparative efficacy and safety of long-acting oral opioids for chronic non-cancer pain: A systematic review. *J Pain Symptom Manage*. 2003;26(5):1026–1048. doi:10.1016/j.jpainsymman.2003.03.003
11. Petzke F, Klose P, Welsch P, Sommer C, Häuser W. Opioids for chronic low back pain: An updated syswtematic review and meta-analysis of efficacy, tolerability and safety in randomized placebo-controlled studies of at least 4 weeks of double-blind duration. *Eur J Pain*. 2020;24(3):497–517. doi:10.1002/ejp.1519
12. Sommer C, Klose P, Welsch P, Petzke F, Häuser W. Opioids for chronic non-cancer neuropathic pain: An updated systematic review and meta-analysis of efficacy, tolerability and safety in randomized placebo-controlled studies of at least 4 weeks duration. *Eur J Pain*. 2020;24(1):3–18. doi:10.1002/ejp.1494
13. Agnoli A, Xing G, Tancredi DJ, Magnan E, Jerant A, Fenton JJ. Association of dose tapering with overdose or mental health crisis among patients prescribed long-term opioids [Erratum in JAMA. 2022 Feb 15;327(7):688]. *JAMA*. 2021;326(5):411–419. doi:10.1001/jama.2021.11013.
14. Hallvik SE, El Ibrahimi S, Johnston K, et al. Patient outcomes after opioid dose reduction among patients with chronic opioid therapy [Erratum in: Pain. 2022 Apr 1;163(4):e613]. *Pain*. 2022;163(1):83–90. doi:10.1097/j.pain.0000000000002298
15. Larochelle MR, Lodi S, Yan S, Clothier BA, Goldsmith ES, Bohnert ASB. Comparative effectiveness of opioid tapering or abrupt discontinuation vs no dosage change for opioid

overdose or suicide for patients receiving stable long-term opioid therapy. *JAMA Netw Open.* 2022;5(8):e2226523. doi:10.1001/jamanetworkopen.2022.26523
16. Mackey K, Anderson J, Bourne D, Chen E, Peterson K. Benefits and harms of long-term opioid dose reduction or discontinuation in patients with chronic pain: A rapid review. *J Gen Intern Med.* 2020;35(Suppl 3):935–944. doi:10.1007/s11606-020-06253-8
17. Smith SM, Dart RC, Katz NP, et al. Classification and definition of misuse, abuse, and related events in clinical trials: ACTTION systematic review and recommendations. *Pain.* 2013;154(11):2287–2296.
18. Cheatle MD, O'Brien CP. Opioid therapy in patients with chronic noncancer pain: Diagnostic and clinical challenges. *Adv Psychosom Med.* 2011;30:61–91.
19. Portenoy RK, Foley KM. Chronic use of opioid analgesics in non-malignant pain: Report of 38 cases. *Pain.* 1986;25(2):171–186. doi:10.1016/0304-3959(86)90091-6
20. Melzack R. The tragedy of needless pain. *Sci Am.* 1990;262(2):27–33. doi:10.1038/scientificamerican0290-27
21. Portenoy RK. Opioid therapy for chronic nonmalignant pain: A review of the critical issues. *J Pain Symptom Manage.* 1996;11(4):203–217. doi:10.1016/0885-3924(95)00187-5
22. The use of opioids for the treatment of chronic pain: A consensus statement from the American Academy of Pain Medicine and the American Pain Society. *Clin J Pain.* 1997;13(1):6–8.
23. Savage SR. Opioid use in the management of chronic pain. *Med Clin North Am.* 1999;83(3):761–786. doi:10.1016/s0025-7125(05)70133-4
24. The Federation of State Medical Boards of the United States, Inc. Model guidelines for the use of controlled substances for the treatment of pain. 1998. https://www.cpmission.com/main/model.html
25. McQuay H. Opioids in pain management. *Lancet.* 1999;353:2229–2232.
26. Ballantyne JC, Mao J. Opioid therapy for chronic pain. *N Engl J Med.* 2003;349(20):1943–1953. doi:10.1056/NEJMra025411
27. Fishbain DA, Cole B, Lewis J, Rosomoff HL, Rosomoff RS. What percentage of chronic nonmalignant pain patients exposed to chronic opioid analgesic therapy develop abuse/addiction and/or aberrant drug-related behaviors? A structured evidence-based review. *Pain Med.* 2008;9(4):444–459. doi:10.1111/j.1526-4637.2007.00370.x
28. Zezza MA, Bachhuber MA. Payments from drug companies to physicians are associated with higher volume and more expensive opioid analgesic prescribing. *PLoS One.* 2018;13(12):e0209383. doi:10.1371/journal.pone.0209383
29. Fishman SM, Carr DB, Hogans B, et al. Scope and nature of pain- and analgesia-related content of the United States Medical Licensing Examination (USMLE). *Pain Med.* 2018;19(3):449–459. doi:10.1093/pm/pnx336
30. Cheatle MD. Facing the challenge of pain management and opioid misuse, abuse and opioid-related fatalities. *Expert Rev Clin Pharmacol.* 2016;9(6):751–754. doi:10.1586/17512433.2016.1160776
31. Centers for Disease Control and Prevention. Drug overdose deaths in the U.S. top 100,000 annually. 2021. Accessed September 11, 2022. https://www.cdc.gov/nchs/pressroom/nchs_press_releases/2021/20211117.htm
32. Centers for Disease Control and Prevention. Data overview. 2022. Accessed September, 11, 2022. https://www.cdc.gov/opioids/data/index.html#:~:text=Overdose%20deaths%20involving%20opioids%2C%20including,than%20eight%20times%20since%201999.&text=Overdoses%20involving%20opioids%20killed%20nearly,those%20deaths%20involved%20synthetic%20opioids
33. Vowles KE, McEntee ML, Julnes PS, Frohe T, Ney JP, van der Goes DN. Rates of opioid misuse, abuse, and addiction in chronic pain: A systematic review and data synthesis. *Pain.* 2015;156(4):569–576. doi:10.1097/01.j.pain.0000460357.01998.f1
34. Volkow ND, McLellan AT. Opioid abuse in chronic pain—Misconceptions and mitigation strategies. *N Engl J Med.* 2016;374(13):1253–1263. doi:10.1056/NEJMra1507771

35. Cheatle MD, Gallagher RM, O'Brien CP. Low risk of producing an opioid use disorder in primary care by prescribing opioids to prescreened patients with chronic noncancer pain. *Pain Med.* 2018;19(4):764–773. doi:10.1093/pm/pnx032
36. Substance Abuse and Mental Health Services Administration. Alcohol, tobacco, and other drugs. n.d. Accessed November 5, 2022. https://www.samhsa.gov/find-help/atod#:~:text=SAMHSA%E2%80%99s%202020%20National%20Survey%20on%20Drug%20Use%20and,past%20month%20%28i.e.%2C%20current%20alcohol%20users%29%20%282020%20NSDUH%29
37. Centers for Disease Control and Prevention. Alcohol-induced death rates in the United States, 2019–2020. 2022. Accessed December 20, 2022. https://www.cdc.gov/nchs/products/databriefs/db448.htm
38. McDermott KA, Joyner KJ, Hakes JK, Okey SA, Cougle JR. Pain interference and alcohol, nicotine, and cannabis use disorder in a national sample of substance users. *Drug Alcohol Depend.* 2018;186:53–59.
39. Imtiaz S, Loheswaran G, Le Foll B, Rehm J. Longitudinal alcohol consumption patterns and health-related quality of life: Results from the National Epidemiologic Survey on Alcohol and Related Conditions. *Drug Alcohol Rev.* 2018;37(1):48–55.
40. Edlund MJ, Sullivan MD, Han X, Booth BM. Days with pain and substance use disorders: is there an association? Clin J Pain. 2013 Aug;29(8):689–695.
41. Vowles KE, Witkiewitz K, Pielech M, et al. Alcohol and opioid use in chronic pain: A cross-sectional examination of differences in functioning based on misuse status. *J Pain.* 2018;19(10):1181–1188.
42. Alford DP, German JS, Samet JH, Cheng DM, Lloyd-Travaglini CA, Saitz R. Primary care patients with drug use report chronic pain and self-medicate with alcohol and other drugs. *J Gen Intern Med.* 2016;31(5):486–491.
43. Brennan PL, Schutte KK, SooHoo S, Moos RH. Painful medical conditions and alcohol use: A prospective study among older adults. *Pain Med.* 2011;12(7):1049–1059.
44. Riley JL 3rd, King C. Self-report of alcohol use for pain in a multi-ethnic community sample. *J Pain.* 2009;10(9):944–952.
45. LaRowe LR, Ditre JW. Pain, nicotine, and tobacco smoking: Current state of the science. *Pain.* 2020;161(8):1688–1693.
46. Boissoneault J, Lewis B, Nixon SJ. Characterizing chronic pain and alcohol use trajectory among treatment-seeking alcoholics. *Alcohol.* 2019;75:47–54.
47. Jakubczyk A, Ilgen MA, Bohnert AS, et al. Physical pain in alcohol-dependent patients entering treatment in Poland—Prevalence and correlates. *J Stud Alcohol Drugs.* 2015;76(4):607–614.
48. Michna E, Ross EL, Hynes WL, et al. Predicting aberrant drug behavior in patients treated for chronic pain: Importance of abuse history. *J Pain Symptom Manage.* 2004;28:250–258.
49. Orhurhu VJ, Pittelkow TP, Hooten WM. Prevalence of smoking in adults with chronic pain. *Tob Induc Dis.* 2015;13: Article 17.
50. Elman I, Borsook D. Common brain mechanisms of chronic pain and addiction. *Neuron.* 2016;89(1):11–36.
51. John W, Wu LT. Chronic non-cancer pain among adults with substance use disorders: Prevalence, characteristics, and association with opioid overdose and healthcare utilization. *Drug Alcohol Depend.* 2020;209:107902.
52. Patterson AL, Gritzner S, Resnick MP, Dobscha SK, Turk DC, Morasco BJ. Smoking cigarettes as a coping strategy for chronic pain is associated with greater pain intensity and poorer pain-related function. *J Pain.* 2012;13:285–292.
53. Schembri E, Massalha V, Camilleri L, Lungaro-Mifsud S. Is chronic low back pain and radicular neuropathic pain associated with smoking and a higher nicotine dependence? A cross-sectional study using the DN4 and the Fagerström Test for Nicotine Dependence. *Agri.* 2021;33(3):155–167.

54. Cheatle MD, Falcone M, Dhingra L, Lerman C. Independent association of tobacco use with opioid use disorder in patients of European ancestry with chronic non-cancer pain. *Drug Alcohol Depend*. 2020;209:107901.
55. Beck A, Ward C, Mendelson M, Mock J, Erbaugh J. An inventory for measuring depression. *Arch Gen Psychiatry*. 1961;4:561–571.
56. McNair D, Lorr M, Droppleman L. *Profile of Mood States*. Educational and Industrial Testing Service; 1971.
57. Dworkin R, Turk DC, Farrar JT, et al.; IMMPACT. Core outcome measures for chronic pain trials: IMMPACT recommendations. *Pain*. 2005;113(1–2):9–19.
58. Webster LR, Webster RM. Predicting aberrant behaviors in opioid-treated patients: Preliminary validation of the Opioid Risk Tool. *Pain Med*. 2005;6:432–442.
59. Butler S, Budman S, Fernandez K, Jamison R. Validation of a screener and opioid assessment measure for patients with chronic pain. *Pain*. 2004;112(1–2): 65–75.
60. Butler S, Budman SH, Fernandez KC, et al. Development and validation of the Current Opioid Misuse Measure. *Pain*. 2007;130(1–2):144–156.
61. Compton P, Darakjian J, Miotto K. Screening for addiction in patients with chronic pain and "problematic" substance use: Evaluation of a pilot assessment tool. *J Pain Symptom Manage*. 1998;16(6):355–363.
62. Cheatle MD, Compton PA, Dhingra L, Wasser TE, O'Brien CP. Development of the revised Opioid Risk Tool to predict opioid use disorder in patients with chronic nonmalignant pain. *J Pain*. 2019;20(7):842–851.
63. Reinert DF, Allen JP. The Alcohol Use Disorders Identification Test: An update of research findings. *Alcohol Clin Exp Res*. 2007;31:185–199.
64. Ewing JA. Detecting alcoholism. The CAGE questionnaire. *JAMA*. 1984;252(14):1905–1907.
65. Heatherton TF, Kozlowski LT, Frecker RC, Fagerström KO. The Fagerström Test for Nicotine Dependence: A revision of the Fagerström Tolerance Questionnaire. *Br J Addict*. 1991;86(9):1119–1127.
66. McNeely J, Wu L, Subramaniam G, et al. Performance of the Tobacco, Alcohol, Prescription Medication, and Other Substance Use (TAPS) tool for substance use screening in primary care patients. *Ann Intern Med*. 2016;165:690–699.
67. .U.S. Preventive Services Task Force. Tobacco smoking cessation in adults, including pregnant persons: Interventions. 2021. Accessed December 29, 2222. https://www.uspreventiveservicestaskforce.org/uspstf/document/RecommendationStatementFinal/tobacco-use-in-adults-and-pregnant-women-counseling-and-interventions#citation46
68. Wachholtz A, Robinson D, Epstein E. Developing a novel treatment for patients with chronic pain and opioid user disorder. *Subst Abuse Treat Prev Policy*. 2022;17(1): Article 35.
69. Tetreault JM, Holt SR, Cavallo DA, et al. Computerized cognitive behavioral therapy for substance use disorders in a specialized primary care practice: A randomized feasibility trial to address the RT component of SBIRT. *J Addict Med*. 2020;14(6):e303–e309.

20

Pain and Mental Health

Focus on Depression and Anxiety

Snehal Bhatt, Maya Armstrong, and Vanessa Jacobsohn

Case Example: J.M.

J.M. is a 28-year-old woman being evaluated by Dr. Sam for treatment of her chronic pain. As a teen, J.M. experienced gradually worsening symptoms of severe neck pain and "excruciating" headaches. She was diagnosed with Chiari malformation and tethered cord. She was treated by her primary care provider with gradually increasing doses of opioids. Eventually, she was diagnosed with cervical instability and underwent an occiput through C5 posterior instrumented fusion at age 18 years.

Following this surgery, her pain initially improved, and pain medications were discontinued. However, over the next several years, her pain again began to worsen. She reports that over the past year, in addition to neck pain and headaches, she has also developed right fourth and fifth finger numbness and tingling and pain radiating down the right fifth finger. Very rarely, she has taken "pills off the street" to help relieve her pain. She is worried that unless her pain gets better, she will wind up using these pills regularly.

J.M. reports a long history of depression and anxiety beginning in childhood, and she notes both have worsened as a result of her pain. She carries diagnoses of major depressive disorder (MDD) and generalized anxiety disorder (GAD). She had one prior suicide attempt at age 16 years for which she was hospitalized but denies any history of manic or psychotic episodes. At present, she reports "depressed mood," with anhedonia, loss of interest, as well as insomnia. Her chronic anxiety contributes to her insomnia as well as muscle tightness. She states that due to pain and depression, "I don't do anything . . . don't go anywhere," and this has led to weight gain. She denies current thoughts of harm to self or others.

J.M. reports that her mother also had "severe untreated depression." Her father left the family when she was 6 years old. The family frequently moved around and struggled financially. She graduated high school and started college but did not complete it. At present, she lives with her dog and is on disability.

She denies other medical problems; her only medications are fluoxetine 60 mg daily and clonazepam 1 mg BID, as prescribed by her provider. She does not endorse any particular benefit from these medications.

Physical exam is significant for limited range of motion of the cervical spine and tender palpable spasms along the paraspinals, upper trapezius, sternocleidomastoids, and scalenes. There is reduced strength in right biceps, triceps, and wrist extensor and flexor muscles. Lower extremity strength is intact. She has a body mass index of 29. No recent imaging is available.

J.M. reports that in her view, "everything is related to my pain." She describes feeling very stigmatized, especially about her opioid use and "people thinking I am making all this up." She reports this has led to her avoiding seeking care or leaving treatment prematurely. She expresses fear that her pain will never get better and "I will wind up alone and unable to make anything of myself."

Introduction

The case example highlights several important topics encountered by clinicians caring for patients with chronic pain. The remainder of this chapter explores the following questions in depth: How common is the co-occurrence of chronic pain, depression, and anxiety? How do these illnesses impact each other and the overall outcomes for the patient? What are some mechanisms that may explain the interactions among these conditions? What are best practices for evaluation and treatment of patients with co-occurring chronic pain, anxiety, and depression?

Prevalence

According to estimates from the Centers for Disease Control and Prevention (CDC), 20.4% of U.S. adults (50 million) have chronic pain, and 8.0% of U.S. adults (19.6 million) have high-impact chronic pain associated with limitations in major life domains.[1] These prevalence rates are similar to those reported globally.[1,2] Chronic pain is increasingly recognized as a major health problem, impacting daily activities and interpersonal relationships; resulting in poor perceived health, poor emotional health, and reduced quality of life; and causing a significant financial burden on patients, caregivers, health care systems, and national economies.[2]

Similarly, depression and anxiety are two leading causes of disability as well as societal, economic, and health burden.[2,3] According to the World Health Organization, the number of people experiencing depression and anxiety increased by 50% worldwide between 1990 and 2013.[2] Alarmingly, the COVID-19 pandemic seems to have further contributed to rising rates of these conditions and associated disability globally.[3]

Chronic Pain and Depression

Up to 61% of patients with chronic pain have co-occurring depression.[4,5] Compared to people without pain, the odds ratio for depression is 1.8 with single-site pain and 3.7 with multisite pain.[6] Risk for depression seems to increase with longer duration of pain, more frequent pain episodes, greater pain severity, greater pain-related dysfunction, and lack of improvement in pain.[5] The interaction between chronic pain and depression appears to be bidirectional, with recent studies showing that individuals with depression are 1.9 times more likely to develop a chronic pain diagnosis.[7]

Chronic Pain and Anxiety

Chronic pain and anxiety also often co-occur, with up to 50% of patients with chronic pain having co-occurring anxiety disorder.[8] The interaction between chronic pain and anxiety also appears to be bidirectional, with anxiety disorders contributing to the risk for chronic pain development.[9] It appears that the development of anxiety disorders is mediated by the severity of pain. Importantly, it is the severity of the anxiety and the total number of anxiety disorders, as opposed to a specific anxiety disorder, that appear to mediate the negative impact on chronic pain and health-related quality of life.[8]

Table 20.1, based on data presented by Velly and Mohit,[9] lists the odds ratios for depression and anxiety for various chronic pain syndromes.

Additive Impact

Studies have supported the idea that chronic pain, depression, and anxiety have additive impact on adverse outcomes. The presence of pain might reduce the proper recognition and treatment of co-occurring depression. Co-occurrence of chronic pain and depression is associated with more severe depression, poorer quality of life, higher costs of health care utilization, poorer self-rated health, higher unemployment rate, higher number of doctor visits and hospitalization days, greater functional limitations, more pain complaints, greater pain intensity, longer duration of pain, more persistent pain, more future pain episodes, social impairments, less satisfaction with treatment, and higher rates of disability.[5] Although literature evaluating the additive impact of chronic pain and anxiety is less robust, it does show that co-occurrence is associated with worse health-related quality of life, worse psychological functioning, greater pain-related functional impairment, greater pain severity, poorer treatment response, worse

Table 20.1 Odds Ratios for Depression and Anxiety for Various Types of Chronic Pain

Type of Pain	OR for Depression	OR for Anxiety
Chronic back/neck pain	1.4–2.3	1.5–2.3
Arthritis	1.4–2.0	1.5–2.2
Headache	1.7–4.0	2.0–10.4
Chronic orofacial pain	1.6–4.6	1.5–5.1
Chronic widespread pain	3.3	2.9
Fibromyalgia	2.7–8.4	4.7–6.7
Irritable bowel syndrome	3.9	3.5

OR, odds ratio.

long-term pain outcomes, and greater rates of disability.[8] Concurrence of all three conditions seems to be associated with additional burden, with greater pain severity and disability days compared to individuals with one or two of the three conditions.[10]

Considering the devastating impact of the ongoing opioid epidemic in the United States, it is especially relevant that having co-occurring depression or anxiety increases the likelihood of opioid analgesic use by a patient with chronic pain.[2,5] It has been reported that the 16% of U.S. adults with depression and anxiety disorders receive 51.4% of all opioid prescriptions, making them twice as likely as those without a mental health disorder to receive an opioid prescription.[11] Multidisciplinary treatment of chronic pain that addresses underlying mental illnesses and psychological factors has the potential to reduce opioid use.

Finally, the risk for suicidality in patients with co-occurring chronic pain, anxiety, and depression must be considered. Depression, anxiety, and chronic pain each are risk factors for suicide. In combination, the associated excess risk appears to be more than additive.[12] It has been hypothesized that mechanisms such as catastrophic thinking, along with poor coping mechanisms, hopelessness, increased social isolation, and reduced self-efficacy to manage symptoms, serve as psychological mechanisms that increase the risk for suicidal thoughts and behaviors in people suffering with these chronic conditions.[12]

Biopsychosocial Model

The interactions among pain, depression, and anxiety are complex, and they are mediated in part by psychological and social factors. The International Association for the Study of Pain (IASP) defines pain as "an unpleasant sensory and emotional experience associated with, or resembling that associated with, actual or potential tissue damage."[13p1977] IASP notes that pain is a personal experience shaped by biopsychosocial factors; the pain experience is far more than nociception alone such that pain cannot be "inferred solely from activity in sensory neurons" and that individuals learn the concept of pain through life experiences.[13p1977] IASP further states that pain in turn can impact an individual's functioning as well as social and psychological health.[13] This understanding of pain is remarkably consistent with the concept of "total pain," which was initially proposed by Dame Cicely Saunders, the founder of the modern hospice movement, in 1993. This concept emphasizes that an individual's experience of pain is shaped not only by physical pain but also by emotional pain (including the impact of illness on self-concept and self-worth), social pain (changing social roles and social isolation), as well as existential pain (the meaning of illness, fear of dying, and spiritual concerns).[14]

In the case example, the pain experienced by the patient is shaped not only by her tethered cord and bilateral radiculopathy but also by her fear of isolation and of chronic disability; by ongoing depressive symptoms contributing to hopelessness about the future; by fear of activities that may cause pain, leading to further deconditioning and weight gain; as well as by multiple losses related to her illnesses. Casey et al.[15] showed that depression was the strongest independent predictor of pain chronicity in patients with acute back pain. Depression as well as pain constancy and beliefs about pain permanence also were associated with disability. Other factors that are associated with worsened pain outcomes include kinesiophobia (fear of movement, closely associated with catastrophizing and avoidance) and prior experiences with pain.[4]

The pain matrix model helps shed light on the influence of emotional and cognitive factors on the pain experience.[16] In this model, first-order processing of pain occurs with the nociceptive activation of the spinothalamic tract, which carries the pain stimulus from the dorsal horn of the spinal cord to the posterior thalamus. However, pain then undergoes second-order processing in the anterior cingulate cortex (ACC), insula, prefrontal cortex (PFC), and posterior parietal cortex, during which the pain stimulus is subjected to attentional and cognitive modulation. Next, third-order processing occurs in the orbitofrontal cortex, perigenual ACC, and anterolateral PFC; the emotional context of the pain generator as well as the patient's own unique psychological factors and memories add further meaning to the pain experience. From a psychological perspective, the fear avoidance model of chronic pain suggests that in patients with high levels of pain catastrophizing, the fear of pain leads to avoidant behaviors, such as lack of activity, which in turn may contribute to physical deconditioning and disability.

In the following section, we explore the tiers of the pain matrix, expanding the discussion beyond the nervous system to include the neuroendocrine and immune systems as well as certain aspects of personality and development. Interestingly, when describing the development and maintenance of depression and anxiety, parallel categories often are invoked.

The concept of allostatic load is central to subsequent discussion of matrix elements. Allostatic load refers to the cumulative burden of chronic stress and life events. Allostasis is the ability of an organism to achieve stability despite a constantly changing environment. In simple organisms, this requires adjustments that are primarily physiologic and behavioral. In humans, this also requires cognitive, emotional, and social strategies. As reviewed by Guidi et al.,[17] "when environmental challenges exceed the individual ability to cope, then allostatic overload ensues" (p. 11). Allostatic overload results not only from external stressors but also from the sequelae of maladaptive responses. In the context of this chapter, chronic pain, anxiety, and depression all can be understood as resulting from allostatic overload in the absence of sufficient moderating factors. It also is important to acknowledge the effects of chronicity with respect to any form of stress. Whereas acute stress can lead to behaviors that mitigate dangers and contribute to survival, chronic stress generally is seen as maladaptive.

Physiological Influences

Autonomic Dysfunction

Chronic stress and its associated physiologic responses shift the homeostatic balance, resulting in sustained sympathetic stimulation (i.e., increased "sympathetic tone") and diminished vagal or parasympathetic tone. Researchers have found evidence of autonomic dysregulation in individuals with anxiety,[18] depression,[19] and a variety of chronic pain states,[20] contributing to symptoms such as muscular tension, headache, abdominal discomfort, nervousness, and fatigue.

Hypothalamic–Pituitary–Adrenal Axis

The hypothalamic–pituitary–adrenal axis plays a critical role in the maintenance of stress-related homeostasis. The relationships between cortisol levels and chronic pain, depression, and anxiety appear to be aberrant among those with more severe psychopathology.[21]

Inflammation

Inflammation can be seen not only in people with inflammatory pain conditions, such as the inflammatory arthritides or inflammatory bowel disease, but also in conditions such as chronic low back pain,[22] fibromyalgia,[23] and migraine headaches.[24] It also is well established that a significant proportion of patients with mood and anxiety-related disorders have elevated inflammatory markers.[25] In fact, inflammation appears to be a causal agent of depression in at least some patients, leading to the characterization of "inflammatory depression," in which innate immune activation and inflammatory cytokines preferentially affect brain regions relevant to reward and threat sensitivity.[26]

Central Sensitization

Central sensitization has been defined as "an amplification of neural signaling within the CNS [central nervous system] that elicits pain hypersensitivity,"[27pS5] leading to the perception of a normally benign afferent input as a noxious stimulus. Although defined with respect to pain, this phenomenon likely contributes to anxiety states as well, resulting in hypervigilance and heightened emotional response to relatively benign stimuli.

Perception/Attention

Interoception

Interoception refers to an awareness of a wide array of physical and physiological states of one's body; it is critical to the maintenance of bodily homeostasis[28] and to one's "sense of self."[29] The flow of this type of information often is categorized as "bottom-up." That is, sensory data from the cells, tissues, and organ systems provide information to the brain about one's internal state. However, it appears that individuals with chronic pain conditions, mood disorders, and anxiety disorders rely on sources other than bottom-up homeostatic data and instead give more weight to top-down, self-referential, cognitive–emotional schemes of interpretation.[29] This may lead to overinterpretation of bodily sensations, which is integral to the cognitive-perceptual[30] and fear-avoidance[31] models of anxiety and chronic pain. On the other hand, blunted interoception may be characteristic of depression, especially in individuals experiencing dysthymia, alexithymia, or dissociative states.

Salience and Default Mode Networks

Two large-scale brain networks that appear to be relevant in chronic pain, affective disorders, and anxiety disorders are the default mode network (DMN) and salience network (SN). The DMN is associated with self-referential processing, rumination, and thinking about the thoughts and emotions of others.[32] The SN has been implicated in response to homeostatically relevant stimuli[33] as well as in modulating the switch between the internally directed cognition of the DMN and the externally directed cognition of the central executive network. A relatively extreme example of the aforementioned switch is the change in attentional states when a nearby loud noise interrupts (via the SN) the almost dreamlike imaginative state that occurs while reading a good book (DMN-dominant). However, far more subtle switches affect not only the dominance of these core networks but also their functional connectivity with other brain regions.

Although much remains to be elucidated about these networks, their functions, and their relationship with pathologic conditions, existing data point toward differing connectivity patterns when comparing controls to individuals with fibromyalgia,[34] chronic low back pain,[35] migraines,[36] GAD,[37] post-traumatic stress disorder,[38] and depression[39]—conditions associated with homeostatic stress, hypervigilance, self-focused attention, rumination, and catastrophizing. For example, resting functional magnetic resonance imaging in patients with fibromyalgia with active pain shows greater connectivity (compared to that seen in patients with active pain but without fibromyalgia) of the DMN to the bilateral anterior insula,[40] a region of the cortex known to be involved with emotional awareness and interoception. Importantly, interventions such as mindfulness practices and exposure therapy, as well as emerging therapies incorporating psychedelic medicine, have been shown to affect these brain networks and their functional connectivity.[41]

Sleep

Subjective complaints of poor sleep are practically ubiquitous among our populations of interest, suggesting another shared vulnerability that is poorly understood. Research suggests that patients with chronic pain experience frequent nighttime awakenings, fragmented sleep, and poor sleep quality,[42] contributing to heightened sensitivity to pain, more intense pain, and greater disability.[43] Pertinently, this may be mediated by co-occurring depression, anxiety, and other psychological factors such as catastrophizing.[44]

Cognitive/Emotional Appraisal

Personality Traits and Worldview

Locus of control, which is represented by a continuum of internal to external, is another potentially modifiable factor related to our topic. External locus of control has been associated with depression, anxiety, and pain-related distress[45,46]; external health locus of control after low back injury has been shown to predict lower rates of return to work 6 months later.[47] Related to locus of control is belief permanence. Strong permanence of beliefs (sometimes referred to as "fixed" mindset) predicts distress in a variety of chronic conditions.[48] For example, in children with chronic migraines, those with "fixed" health mindsets were more likely to appraise setbacks as threatening and to endorse decreased quality of life. Children with higher "growth" mindsets reported lower functional disability and higher life satisfaction.[49]

Role of Developmental Trauma and Epigenetics

Since the original study by Felitti et al.[50] was published in the late 1990s, there has been much interest in the role of adverse childhood experiences in a wide variety of health conditions and outcomes. Epigenetic changes may be induced by high stress states, especially during critical periods of development, including prenatal periods and early childhood.[51,52] These changes, although potentially reversible, may provide the foundation of many of the aforementioned mechanisms of vulnerability common to chronic pain, anxiety, and affective states.

Implications

If one attempts to represent these multidirectional influences and interrelated outcomes, the result is a complex, multidimensional matrix that is not elegantly reproduced on a two-dimensional page. Indeed, the concept of "mutual maintenance" is central to the approach and management of these comorbid, often debilitating conditions and highlights the futility of single-target approaches. Although potentially overwhelming, the complexity of these conditions and their etiologic matrices is encouraging in that there are many entry points for influencing these processes and, ultimately, improving anxiety, depression, and the experience of pain.

Assessment

All patients with chronic pain should be screened for depression and anxiety with validated questionnaires, such as the Patient Health Questionnaires (PHQs) for depression, and the General Anxiety Disorder–7 (GAD-7) for anxiety.[53,54] For depression, an evidence-based clinical approach is to begin by administering the two-question PHQ-2. If this is positive (a score of ≥2), the nine-question PHQ-9 should be administered. If the screening tests are positive, more thorough assessments should be conducted to clarify the diagnoses and, importantly, to elicit and appreciate how these symptoms may interact with the patient's chronic pain to impact their life.

The clinician should proceed with an appreciation for the concept of total pain. In addition to the traditional assessment that includes the seven dimensions of pain, psychiatric history, and physical/mental status examinations, the clinician should also assess the various psychosocial factors that can impact the pain experience. *Suicidality should be assessed at initial and all follow-up visits.* The entire assessment should proceed with a compassionate approach. Because patients may have experienced stigma related to their chronic pain and/or mental health conditions, it is of utmost importance to acknowledge and validate the pain experience. An empathic interview, using open-ended questions and being attentive to the patient's goals and personal motivation, is most conducive to accurately assessing the impact of chronic pain and engaging the patient in needed treatments for co-occurring depression and/or anxiety.

The following questions can be useful to increase the patient's trust and engagement in treatment:

Acknowledge and express curiosity/interest in the patient's pain experience:
- How does the pain affect your life?
- What are your goals for pain management and for everyday function?
- How do you feel I [the provider] can most be of help?
- What has your experience been with prior treatments?

Assess the psychosocial elements of the pain:
- Does the pain lead to feelings of depression and/or anxiety?
- Does the pain impact the quality of sleep?
- Has the pain experience led you to feel that life is not worth living?
- How has the pain affected your home life? Your work? Your hobbies? Your relationships?
- In order to control the pain, have you used prescription medications that were not prescribed to you, or substances obtained illicitly?
- Have you experienced any adverse childhood experiences or other traumas?
- Can you identify chronic stressors that contribute to your pain, depression, and/or anxiety? (This may include racism, intimate partner violence, homophobia, and other social contexts.)

Establish the patient's functional objectives and goals:
- If your pain were better controlled, how would your life be different?
- What are some of your short-term and long-term goals? How can we work toward them?

Throughout the patient assessment, the provider should use the principles of motivational interviewing (MI), a reflective approach that embraces the stages of change and recognizes the patient as guide. This approach affirms the patient's autonomy and is most likely to allow for beneficial outcomes of treatment.[55]

Treatments

Once the initial assessment of the patient has been completed, the provider's primary role is to recognize the patient's autonomy and help guide the patient toward their established goals, incorporating the spirit of MI. The clinician should share knowledge of pain pathophysiology appropriate to the patient's understanding and level of interest. Importantly, the clinician should emphasize the need for a multimodal approach to treatment to empower the patient to understand pain within their own life context.[56] Pain self-management programs, which encourage active participation by individuals with chronic pain toward achieving their optimal health and wellness, have been shown to decrease both pain interference and depression severity.[57] Active involvement in the decision-making process has been found to improve outcomes of treatment in ethnically diverse populations.[58] This point of view is consistent with the CDC guidelines for prescribing opioids to treat chronic pain,[59] which emphasize interdisciplinary care focusing on functional goals and improvement that allows patients to engage actively in their own pain management.

Psychological Treatments

A variety of psychotherapeutic methods have shown promising evidence for addressing pain, especially in the context of depression and/or anxiety. Cognitive–behavioral therapy (CBT) has the largest body of evidence as a psychological therapy for chronic pain and is a mainstay of treatment for depression and anxiety. CBT for pain utilizes the fear-avoidance model described previously. Consistent with this approach, CBT targets catastrophizing and avoidant beliefs/behaviors, confronts perceived threats related to pain, and builds skills to cope with the pain and related symptoms. CBT may be delivered in individual or group settings, typically over a course of 2–4 months. It has been associated with small but consistent long-term improvements in pain intensity, pain-related distress, disability, quality of life, pain-related coping, depression, and health care–seeking behaviors.[4,60]

Mindfulness-based approaches, including acceptance and commitment therapy and mindfulness-based stress reduction, are useful in the treatment of individuals with chronic pain. These approaches focus on mindful awareness and nonjudgmental acceptance of the pain experience, while identifying core values and building commitment to pursue goals consistent with these values. These interventions are typically delivered over a 6- to 8-week period. Data on efficacy have been more mixed compared to CBT but in general have shown small to moderate effects for improvements in pain, depression, anxiety, physical well-being, and quality of life.[4]

Also rooted in evidence are multidisciplinary pain rehabilitation programs, which utilize a biopsychosocial approach to treating individuals with chronic pain. They typically combine group-based CBT with group-based physical therapy/occupational therapy and demonstrate improvements in pain intensity, functional disability, and sustained employment, in addition to reduced medical costs. They may be particularly useful in helping patients taper off opioid pain medications.[4]

Multiple nonpharmacologic interventions are endorsed by the American College of Physicians specifically for the treatment of low back pain, including exercise, acupuncture, relaxation, biofeedback, tai chi, yoga, spinal manipulation, and laser therapy. Often, such practices are underutilized in the medical community due to cost, limited access, or lack of provider knowledge.

Pharmacologic Treatments

In this section, we consider the overlap in pharmacologic treatments for chronic pain and depression/anxiety; in an effort to minimize the risks of polypharmacy, we strive to identify treatments that have evidence of effectiveness in both conditions. The SCAMP trial showed that in patients with co-occurring chronic pain and depression, optimizing antidepressant therapy along with following a pain self-management program can lead to significant reductions in depression and pain severity.[6]

Tricyclic antidepressants (TCAs) act mainly through inhibition of the reuptake of serotonin and norepinephrine. They have a long history in the management of depression, and more recently they have been associated with benefit in neuropathic pain syndromes.[61] Amitriptyline and its active metabolite, nortriptyline, are the most frequently prescribed TCAs. Meta-analyses have focused on the effectiveness of amitriptyline, showing a number needed to treat of 5.1 for painful diabetic neuropathy, post-herpetic neuralgia, and mixed neuropathic pain.[62] Due to its higher potential for toxicity and side effects particularly in older adults, amitriptyline should be used cautiously. Nortriptyline, which has less potential for sedation, is considered the preferred TCA in the setting of chronic pain. It is essential to counsel patients on potential side effects and to be aware of the risk for fatal overdose. Due to their anticholinergic effects, small therapeutic index, and their potential to cause negative cardiac effects, including QTc prolongation, TCAs are no longer considered as first-line treatments for depression. The following is a table of the dosing of these medications for depression versus pain[61]:

Medication	Antidepressant Dose (mg/day)	Pain Dose (mg/day)
Amitriptyline	100–300	25–150
Nortriptyline	75–150	25–150

Serotonin and norepinephrine reuptake inhibitors (SNRIs) are considered first-line treatment for neuropathic pain and are mainstays in the treatment of depression and anxiety.[61] Duloxetine 60 mg/day has the most evidence for treatment of painful diabetic neuropathy and fibromyalgia and some evidence of effectiveness for treatment of knee pain associated with chronic osteoarthritis. Venlafaxine, at doses of 50–225 mg/day, has a smaller body of evidence supporting its use for treatment of neuropathic pain and fibromyalgia, and it may work better as an analgesic at doses greater than 150 mg/day. In the case of a patient with depression/anxiety and chronic pain who is taking an antidepressant of a different class (as in the case example), transitioning to an SNRI may be considered if the patient is willing to do so and has not derived optimal benefit from the other antidepressant. If the patient is not currently on any antidepressants, an SNRI may be considered the first-line antidepressant.[6]

With both SNRIs and TCAs, caution is advised to ensure that interactions with other medications do not contribute to serotonin syndrome. The following is a list of commonly encountered serotonin interactions:

Psychiatric medications that increase risk for serotonin syndrome
- Selective serotonin reuptake inhibitors, SNRIs, monoamine oxidase inhibitors
- St. John's wort, trazodone, valproate, carbamazapine

Non-psychiatric medications that increase risk for serotonin syndrome
- Triptans, ondansetron, cyclobenzaprine
- Tramadol, hydromorphone
- Isonicotinic acid hydrazide, linezolid

Other substances that also may increase risk
- Methamphetamine, cocaine, MDMA, LSD

Gabapentinoids (gabapentin and pregabalin) also are considered first-line treatment for chronic neuropathic pain and may be used in combination with TCAs or duloxetine.[61] In addition, they have shown benefit in the treatment of GAD. A Cochrane review found that gabapentin dosed 400 mg three times daily showed benefit in the treatment of neuropathic pain syndromes, specifically postherpetic neuralgia and painful diabetic neuropathy. For pregabalin, a dose of 600 mg daily was found to be more effective than 300 mg daily. In addition to reviewing potential side effects such as sedation, prescriptive caution should be used because both pregabalin and gabapentin may have increased potential for misuse, especially if patients screen positive for co-occurring substance use disorders.

Opioids

Although it would be unethical to completely withhold opioids in this patient population, additional consideration is warranted. For example, psychiatric illnesses and use of psychotropic medications are risk factors for opioid misuse in patients with chronic pain on long-term opioid therapy.[63] Similarly, opioid use may worsen some of the neurovegetative symptoms of depression. Once again, this points toward the appropriateness of a multidisciplinary approach to treatment of co-occurring chronic pain and depression/anxiety because this approach may allow the use of opioid pain medications to be minimized. If opioids are used, appropriate patient education and a thorough analysis of potential risks/benefits are required, with ongoing monitoring for aberrant behaviors and co-prescription of naloxone.

Benzodiazepines

As discussed previously, anxiety is a common experience of individuals living with chronic pain. Although treatment with benzodiazepines can be a seductive treatment option, it is important to recognize that this treatment strategy carries significant risk to the patient and little evidence of long-term benefit. As per the U.S. Department of Health and Human Services Pain Management Best Practice Inter-Agency Task Force,[64] benzodiazepines increase an individual's risk of developing a substance use disorder; increase risk of fatal overdose if taken with opioids; and, especially when used chronically, may worsen one's cognitive abilities, which in turn can decrease coping mechanisms for pain management. Therefore, these medications are never considered first-line treatments for pain or anxiety and should be used with utmost caution if deemed necessary for treatment.[64]

Importance of a Team-Based Approach

In order to recognize and address as many contributing factors as possible, a patient-centered team generally should consist of a primary care provider knowledgeable of the complexity and multidisciplinary management of chronic pain, a psychologist or therapist, and a physical therapist with experience working with individuals with chronic pain syndromes. Other valuable team members may include a pain specialist, sleep medicine specialist, addiction specialist (if relevant), dietician, and case manager when available. Peer support also may be useful. Ideally, these practitioners would be recruited to the team as early as possible after the diagnosis of a chronic pain syndrome to prevent the entrenchment of maladaptive patterns and to optimize the cumulative benefits of interdisciplinary interventions. Unfortunately, the typical current approach is limited not only by provider awareness but also by insurance limitations and patient resources. Fortunately, patient education and empowerment are at the center of this approach, and several groups have developed helpful materials that may guide patients and practitioners through many of these topics.[65]

Case Example: J.M.'s Management Plan

After thanking J.M. for coming in and sharing the story of her pain experience, Dr. Sam emphasizes that J.M.'s pain is real and acknowledges that it has affected her life in profound ways. He also acknowledges that to treat her pain most effectively, they will need to address her depression and anxiety as well, as this generally improves outcomes. Finally, Dr. Sam takes time to explain that opioids typically are not the best initial choice for treatment and to discuss other potentially helpful options that have not yet been explored.

Over the next several visits, Dr. Sam continues to establish a trusting therapeutic relationship with J.M, who begins a journal to record observations about her pain experience and how it may be affected by mood, sleep, physical activity, and stress. She is encouraged to explore these factors as well as maladaptive cognitions in her CBT sessions, and she works to improve her sleep hygiene. She begins graded physical therapy with a therapist specializing in chronic pain syndromes. Through this work, her kinesiophobia decreases, and she increases the amount and variety of daily physical activity. She expresses interest in trigger point injections to address her neck pain and continues gentle stretches at home. Her fluoxetine is tapered and switched to duloxetine, which is titrated to 60 mg daily. Her clonazepam is lowered to 0.5 mg TID with a plan to taper and discontinue, while gabapentin is initiated and titrated to a dose of 300 mg in the morning and 600 mg at bedtime. Finally, should opioids continue to be part of J.M.'s treatment plan, she agrees to switch to buprenorphine, which has a better safety profile.

Conclusion

As this chapter highlights, chronic pain, anxiety, and depression often co-occur, likely due to shared vulnerabilities with complex interactions. Given this overlap of prevalence and mechanisms, a multidisciplinary approach that aims to actively engage, educate, and empower the patient, create an accepting and nonstigmatizing environment, and treat these conditions in a holistic manner using evidence-based nonpharmacologic and pharmacologic interventions is most appropriate. Finally, although beyond the scope of this discussion, exciting new frontiers continue to be explored, including the roles of neuroinflammation, gut microbiota, and nutrition in co-occurring chronic pain and depression,[66] as well as the potential utility of cannabinoids and ketamine.[67]

References

1. Dahlhamer J, Lucas J, Zelaya, C, et al. Prevalence of chronic pain and high-impact chronic pain among adults—United States, 2016. *MMWR Morb Mortal Wkly Rep.* 2018;67:1001–1006.
2. Khan WU, Michelini G, Battaglia M. Twin studies of the covariation of pain with depression and anxiety: A systematic review and re-evaluation of critical needs. *Neurosci Biobehav Rev.* 2020;111:135–148.
3. Santomauro DF, Herrera AM, Shadid J, et al. Global prevalence and burden of depressive and anxiety disorders in 204 countries and territories in 2020 due to the COVID-19 pandemic. *Lancet.* 2021;398(10312):1700–1712.
4. Hooten WM. Chronic pain and mental health disorders: Shared neural mechanisms, epidemiology, and treatment. *Mayo Clin Proc.* 2016;91(7):955–970.
5. Bair MJ, Robinson RL, Katon W, et al. Depression and pain comorbidity: A literature review. *Arch Intern Med.* 2003;163(20):2433–2445.
6. Kroenke K, Bair MJ, Damush TM, et al. Optimized antidepressant therapy and pain self-management in primary care patients with depression and musculoskeletal pain: A randomized controlled trial. *JAMA.* 2009;301(20):2099–2110.
7. Onwumere J, Stubbs B, Stirling M, et al. Pain management in people with severe mental illness: An agenda for progress. *Pain.* 2022;163(9):1653–1660.
8. Kroenke K, Outcalt S, Krebs E, et al. Association between anxiety, health-related quality of life and functional impairment in primary care patients with chronic pain. *Gen Hosp Psychiatry.* 2013;35(4):359–365.
9. Velly AM, Mohit S. Epidemiology of pain and relation to psychiatric disorders. *Prog Neuropsychopharmacol Biol Psychiatry.* 2018;87:159–167.
10. Bair MJ, Wu J, Damush TM, et al. Association of depression and anxiety alone and in combination with chronic musculoskeletal pain in primary care patients. *Psychosom Med.* 2008;70(8):890–897.
11. Davis MA, Lin LA, Liu H, et al. Prescription opioid use among adults with mental health disorders in the United States. *J Am Board Fam Med.* 2017;30(4):407–417.
12. Racine M. Chronic pain and suicide risk: A comprehensive review. *Prog Neuropsychopharmacol Biol Psychiatry.* 2018;87:269–280.
13. Raja SN, Carr DB, Cohen M, et al. The revised IASP definition of pain: Concepts, challenges, and compromises. *Pain.* 2020;161(9):1976–1982.
14. Mehta A, Chan LS. Understanding of the concept of "total pain": A prerequisite for pain control. *J Hosp Palliat Nurs.* 2008;10(1):26–32.
15. Casey CY, Greenberg MA, Nicassio PM, et al. Transition from acute to chronic pain and disability: A model including cognitive, affective, and trauma factors. *Pain.* 2008;134(1–2):69–79.
16. Garcia-Larrea L, Peyron R. Pain matrices and neuropathic pain matrices: A review. *Pain.* 2013;154:S29–S43.
17. Guidi J, Lucente M, Sonino N, et al. Allostatic load and its impact on health: A systematic review. *Psychother Psychosom.* 2021;90(1):11–27.
18. Chalmers JA, Quintana DS, Abbott MJ, et al. Anxiety disorders are associated with reduced heart rate variability: A meta-analysis. *Front Psychiatry.* 2014;5, 80.
19. Paniccia M, Paniccia D, Thomas S, et al. Clinical and non-clinical depression and anxiety in young people: A scoping review on heart rate variability. *Auton Neurosci.* 2017;208:1–14.
20. Evans S, Seidman LC, Tsao JC, et al. Heart rate variability as a biomarker for autonomic nervous system response differences between children with chronic pain and healthy control children. *J Pain Res.* 2013;6:449–457.
21. Turner AI, Smyth N, Hall SJ, et al. Psychological stress reactivity and future health and disease outcomes: A systematic review of prospective evidence. *Psychoneuroendocrinology.* 2020;114:104599.
22. Teodorczyk-Injeyan JA, Triano JJ, Injeyan HS. Nonspecific low back pain: Inflammatory profiles of patients with acute and chronic pain. *Clin J Pain.* 2019;35(10):818–825.

23. Theoharides TC, Tsilioni I, Bawazeer M. Mast cells, neuroinflammation and pain in fibromyalgia syndrome. *Front Cell Neurosci.* 2019;13: Article 353.
24. Conti P, D'Ovidio C, Conti C, et al. Progression in migraine: Role of mast cells and pro-inflammatory and anti-inflammatory cytokines. *Eur J Pharmacol.* 2019;844:87–94.
25. Felger JC. Imaging the role of inflammation in mood and anxiety-related disorders. *Curr Neuropharmacol.* 2018;16(5):533–558.
26. Suneson K, Lindahl J, Chamli Hårsmar S, et al. Inflammatory depression—Mechanisms and non-pharmacological interventions. *Int J Mol Sci.* 2021;22(4):1640.
27. Woolf CJ. Central sensitization: Implications for the diagnosis and treatment of pain. *Pain.* 2011;152(3):S2–S15.
28. Di Lernia D, Serino S, Riva G. Pain in the body: Altered interoception in chronic pain conditions: A systematic review. *Neurosci Biobehav Rev.* 2016;71:328–341.
29. Paulus MP, Stein MB. Interoception in anxiety and depression. *Brain Struct Funct.* 2010;214(5):451–463.
30. Clark DM, Salkovskis PM, Öst LG, et al. Misinterpretation of body sensations in panic disorder. *J Consult Clin Psychol.* 1997;65(2):203–213.
31. Vlaeyen JW, Crombez G, Linton SJ. The fear-avoidance model of pain. *Pain.* 2016;157(8):1588–1589.
32. Shen HH. Resting-state connectivity. *Proc Natl Acad Sci USA.* 2015;112(46):14115–14116.
33. Seeley WW. The salience network: A neural system for perceiving and responding to homeostatic demands. *J Neurosci.* 2019;39(50):9878–9882.
34. van Ettinger-Veenstra H, Lundberg P, Alföldi P, et al. Chronic widespread pain patients show disrupted cortical connectivity in default mode and salience networks, modulated by pain sensitivity. *J Pain Res.* 2019;12:1743–1755.
35. Tu Y, Jung M, Gollub RL, et al. Abnormal medial prefrontal cortex functional connectivity and its association with clinical symptoms in chronic low back pain. *Pain.* 2019;160(6):1308–1318.
36. Veréb D, Szabó N, Tuka B, et al. Temporal instability of salience network activity in migraine with aura. *Pain.* 2020;161(4):856–864.
37. Xiong H, Guo RJ, Shi HW. Altered default mode network and salience network functional connectivity in patients with generalized anxiety disorders: An ICA-based resting-state fMRI study. *Evid Based Complement Alternat Med.* 2020;2020:4048916.
38. Viard A, Mutlu J, Chanraud S, et al. Altered default mode network connectivity in adolescents with post-traumatic stress disorder. *Neuroimage Clin.* 2019;22:101731.
39. Hamilton JP, Farmer M, Fogelman P, et al. Depressive rumination, the default-mode network, and the dark matter of clinical neuroscience. *Biol Psychiatry.* 2015;78(4):224–230.
40. Čeko M, Frangos E, Gracely J, et al. Default mode network changes in fibromyalgia patients are largely dependent on current clinical pain. *NeuroImage.* 2020;216:116877.
41. Smigielski L, Scheidegger M, Kometer M, et al. Psilocybin-assisted mindfulness training modulates self-consciousness and brain default mode network connectivity with lasting effects. *NeuroImage.* 2019;196:207–215.
42. Finan PH, Goodin BR, Smith MT. The association of sleep and pain: An update and a path forward. *J Pain.* 2013;14(12):1539–1552.
43. Evans S, Djilas V, Seidman LC, et al. Sleep quality, affect, pain, and disability in children with chronic pain: Is affect a mediator or moderator? *J Pain.* 2017;18(9):1087–1095.
44. Campbell CM, Buenaver LF, Finan P, et al. Sleep, pain catastrophizing, and central sensitization in knee osteoarthritis patients with and without insomnia. *Arthritis Care Res.* 2015;67(10):1387–1396.
45. Hovenkamp-Hermelink JH, Jeronimus BF, Spinhoven P, et al. Differential associations of locus of control with anxiety, depression and life-events: A five-wave, nine-year study to test stability and change. *J Affect Disord.* 2019;253:26–34.
46. Wong HJ, Anitescu M. The role of health locus of control in evaluating depression and other comorbidities in patients with chronic pain conditions, a cross-sectional study. *Pain Pract.* 2017;17(1):52–61.

47. Gallagher RM, Rauh V, Haugh LD, et al. Determinants of return-to-work among low back pain patients. *Pain*. 1989;39(1):55–67.
48. Mullarkey MC, Schleider JL. Contributions of fixed mindsets and hopelessness to anxiety and depressive symptoms: A commonality analysis approach. *J Affect Disord*. 2020;261:245–252.
49. Caruso A, Grolnick W, Mueller C, et al. Health mindsets in pediatric chronic headache. *J Pediatr Psychol*. 2022;47(4):391–402.
50. Felitti VJ, Anda RF, Nordenberg D, et al. Relationship of childhood abuse and household dysfunction to many of the leading causes of death in adults: The Adverse Childhood Experiences (ACE) study. *Am J Prev Med*. 1998;14(4):245–258.
51. Soltani S, Kopala-Sibley DC, Noel M. The co-occurrence of pediatric chronic pain and depression. *Clin J Pain*. 2019;35(7):633–643.
52. Van den Bergh BR, van den Heuvel MI, Lahti M, et al. Prenatal developmental origins of behavior and mental health: The influence of maternal stress in pregnancy. *Neurosci Biobehav Rev*. 2020;117:26–64.
53. Levis B, Sun Y, He C, et al. Accuracy of the PHQ-2 alone and in combination with the PHQ-9 for screening to detect major depression: Systematic review and meta-analysis. *JAMA*. 2020;323(22):2290–2300.
54. Plummer F, Manea L, Trepel D, et al. Screening for anxiety disorders with the GAD-7 and GAD-2: A systematic review and diagnostic metaanalysis. *Gen Hosp Psychiatry*. 2016;39:24–31.
55. Alperstein D, Sharpe L. The efficacy of motivational interviewing in adults with chronic pain: A meta-analysis and systematic review. *J Pain*. 2016;17(4):393–403.
56. Moseley GL, Butler DS. Fifteen years of explaining pain: The past, present, and future. *J Pain*. 2015;16(9):807–813.
57. Damush TM, Kroenke K, Bair MJ, et al. Pain self-management training increases self-efficacy, self-management behaviours and pain and depression outcomes. *Eur J Pain*. 2016;20(7):1070–1078.
58. Patel SR, Bakken S. Preferences for participation in decision making among ethnically diverse patients with anxiety and depression. *Community Ment Health J*. 2010;46(5):466–473.
59. Dowell D, Ragan KR, Jones CM, Baldwin GT, Chou R. CDC clinical practice guideline for prescribing opioids for pain—United States, 2022. *MMWR Recommend Rep*. 2022;71(3):1.
60. de C Williams AC, Fisher E, Hearn L, et al. Psychological therapies for the management of chronic pain (excluding headache) in adults. *Cochrane Database Syst Rev*. 2020;2020(8):CD007407.
61. Sutherland AM, Nicholls J, Bao J, et al. Overlaps in pharmacology for the treatment of chronic pain and mental health disorders. *Prog Neuropsychopharmacol Biol Psychiatry*. 2018;87:290–297.
62. Moore RA, Kalso EA, Wiffen PJ, et al. Antidepressant drugs for neuropathic pain: An overview of Cochrane reviews. *Cochrane Database Syst Rev*. 2017;2017(1):CD011606.
63. Boscarino JA, Rukstalis M, Hoffman SN, et al. Risk factors for drug dependence among outpatients on opioid therapy in a large US health-care system. *Addiction*. 2010;105(10):1776–1782.
64. U.S. Department of Health and Human Services Pain Management Best Practices Inter-Agency Task Force. Pain Management Best Practices Inter-Agency Task Force Report: Updates, Gaps, Inconsistencies, and Recommendations. Final Report. 2019. Accessed August 28, 2022. https://www.hhs.gov/opioids/prevention/pain-management-options/index.html
65. Zoffness R. *The Pain Management Workbook: Powerful CBT and Mindfulness Skills to Take Control of Pain and Reclaim Your Life*. New Harbinger; 2020.
66. Li S, Hua D, Wang Q, et al. The role of bacteria and its derived metabolites in chronic pain and depression: Recent findings and research progress. *Int J Neuropsychopharmacol*. 2020;23(1):26–41.
67. IsHak WW, Wen RY, Naghdechi L, et al. Pain and depression: A systematic review. *Harv Rev Psychiatry*. 2018;26(6):352–363.

21

Pain and Suicide

The Silent Epidemic

Martin D. Cheatle

Introduction

Suicide has become a global epidemic. The Word Health Organization's publication, "Suicide Worldwide 2019,"[1] reports some very alarming facts: More than 700,000 people die due to suicide every year; every 40 s, someone in the world dies by suicide, and for every suicide there are many more people who attempt suicide; and 77% of global suicides occur in low- and middle-income countries, where the most vulnerable populations live. Experiencing conflict, disaster, violence, abuse, or loss and a sense of isolation are strongly associated with suicidal behavior. Suicide rates are also high among vulnerable groups who experience discrimination.

In 2020, suicide was the 12th leading cause of death in the United States.[2] Suicide is the second leading cause of death in people aged 10–34 years and the fifth leading cause in people aged 35–54 years.[2] Certain populations are at high risk for suicide, including individuals who suffer from chronic pain, as many patients with chronic pain experience isolation, personal and vocational losses, and at times do not feel validated by family or their health care providers.

Chronic Pain and Suicide

There is a robust literature on the prevalence of suicidal ideation in patients with pain, which has revealed that the risk of suicide in this patient population is not inconsequential.[3–18] For example, Hitchcock et al.[4] found that 50% of patients with chronic pain endorsed experiencing suicidal ideation directly related to pain intensity. Tang and Crane[15] completed a systematic review of the literature on pain and risk of suicide and discovered that the risk of successful suicide was doubled in patients with chronic pain compared to non-pain controls. Campbell et al.[17] examined the prevalence and correlates of suicidal ideation and suicidal behavior in a sample of 1,514 community-based subjects with chronic non-cancer pain (CNCP) receiving opioid therapy. Past 12-month suicidal ideation was endorsed by 36.5% of the sample, and 16.4% reported a lifetime suicide attempt subsequent to the onset of their pain. Cheatle et al.[13] assessed risk of suicide and possible predictors of suicidal ideation in a sample of 466 patients with CNCP entering a behaviorally based pain program. Rate of suicidal ideation was high (26%), and logistic regression revealed that history of sexual abuse (β = 0.825;

$p < .020$; odds ratio [OR] = 2.657; 95% confidence interval [CI]: 1.447–4877), family history of suicidal ideation ($\beta = 0.471$; $p < .006$; OR = 1.85; 95% CI: 1.234–3.070), and being socially withdrawn ($\beta = 0.482$; $p < .001$; OR = 2.226; 95% CI: 1.413–3.505) were predictive of suicidal ideation.

Pain and Suicide: Risk Factors and Mediators

General risk factors for suicide include gender (female); age (>45 years old); having co-occurring mental disorders (especially depression, suicidal ideation, and substance use disorder); acute losses and stressors (relationships, job, and finances); enduring chronic medical illnesses; experiencing conflict, disaster, and discrimination; past psychiatric hospitalizations; frequency of suicidal ideation; severity of psychiatric disorder; poor social support; and a previous suicide attempt, which is the strongest predictor of suicide.[1,18] Although patients with pain share a number of the risk factors of the general population (personal and vocational losses, isolation, mood, and anxiety disorders), there are risk factors that are more specific to patients with pain.

Chronic Pain and Suicide: Risk Factors

Chronic pain–specific risk factors for suicide include pain type, sleep disturbance, pain intensity, pain duration, and opioid dosing and cessation.

Pain Type

Research on the effect of pain on current and lifetime suicidal ideation and suicidal behavior found that any type of physical pain (headache, spine, chest, musculoskeletal, pelvic, fibromyalgia, abdominal, or pain of an occult etiology) is an independent risk factor for suicidality.[19,20] Patients experiencing persistent fibromyalgia, migraine, and complex regional pain syndromes are especially vulnerable to suicidal ideation and suicidal behavior. Jimenez-Rodriguez et al.[21] assessed the risk of suicidal ideation and suicidal behavior in patients with fibromyalgia syndrome (FMS) compared to non-pain controls and patients with chronic low back pain (LBP). Suicidal ideation in the control group was 4%, that for LBP patients was 18.8% (OR = 4.583; 95% CI: 0.826–25.432; $p = 0.082$), and that for patients with FMS was 41% (OR = 26.889; 95% CI: 5.72–126.42; $p < .0001$). In a systematic review and meta-analysis by Adawi et al.[22] on the prevalence of suicidal ideation in patients with FMS, 13 studies met inclusion criteria that included 394,087 patients with FMS. Results revealed that the overall prevalence of suicide ideation was 29.57% (95% CI: 1.84–72.07), with an OR of 9.12 (95% CI: 1.42–58.77), ranging from 2.34 (95% CI: 1.49–3.66) to 26.89 (95% CI: 5.72–126.42). Pooled prevalence of suicide behavior was 5.69% (95% CI: 1.26–31.34), with an OR of 3.12 (95% CI: 1.37–7.12). Suicide risk was higher with respect to the general population, with an OR of 36.77 (95% CI, 15.55–96.94), as well as suicide behavior, with a hazard ratio (HR) of 1.38 (95% CI: 1.17–1.71). Nović et al.[23] conducted a systematic review of the literature on the relationship between migraine and suicidal ideation. Seventeen papers met inclusion criteria. Results indicated that there was a strong association between migraine and suicidal ideation and suicidal behavior, especially in the subtype of migraine with aura. In a more recent systematic review and meta-analysis of the prevalence of suicidal ideation and behavior, 15 studies involving 2,247,648 participants with migraine met inclusion criteria. Pooled prevalence estimates of suicidal ideation were 15.5% (95% CI: 10.4–21.3%) and 3.9% (95% CI: 0.9–8.8%) for suicidal behavior.[24]

Patients with migraine and comorbid FMS have a particularly high risk of suicide. A sample of 1,318 patients with migraine, with 10.1% of this cohort having concomitant FM, were assessed for suicidal ideation and suicidal behavior. Patients experiencing both migraine and FMS had a higher rate of headache frequency and headache-related disability, poorer sleep, and were more depressed and anxious compared to patients who experienced only migraine. Patients with both headache and FMS had a statistically higher rate of suicidal ideation (58.3% vs. 24%) and suicidal behavior (17.6% vs. 5.7%).[25] In a study by Do-Hyeong Lee et al.,[26] patients with complex regional pain syndrome (CRPS) type 1 and type 2 were evaluated for suicidality. They found that 74.9% of patients with CRPS were at high risk compared to 25.6% who were at low risk for suicidal ideation. Risk factors associated with suicidal ideation in this sample included depression, pain severity, and low functionality.

Sleep Disturbance

Sleep disturbance is highly prevalent in patients with chronic pain, ranging from 50% to 80%,[27,28] and sleep disturbance has been identified as a risk factor for suicidal ideation in this patient population. Smith et al.[29] assessed 51 outpatients with chronic pain and found that 24% endorsed current suicidal ideation. A discriminant analysis revealed that sleep-onset insomnia and pain intensity accounted for greater than 84% of the cases of patients with suicidal ideation, which was independent of depression severity. Racine et al.[12] evaluated 88 patients with chronic pain. The patients completed a self-administered questionnaire at intake to three large pain clinics in Canada. Similar to the findings of Smith et al.,[29] 24% of this cohort acknowledged experiencing suicidal ideation. Poor sleep quality was the only significant variable predicting suicidal ideation. A more recent systematic review of pain and sleep disturbance corroborated findings from earlier studies that patients with both pain and sleep disorders are more likely to have concurrent depression, catastrophizing, anxiety, and suicidal ideation.[30] Although sleep disturbance is common in patients with pain, it is often not evaluated or effectively treated.[27]

Pain Intensity

In a study by Ilgen et al.,[16] a large cohort of Veterans Affairs' medical records and the National Death Index ($N = 260{,}254$) were analyzed evaluating the association between self-assessed pain severity and suicidal behavior in veterans. The authors found that after controlling for demographic and psychiatric factors, veterans with severe pain were more likely to die by suicide than veterans with mild or moderate pain (HR: 1.33; 95% CI: 1.15–1.54).

Opioid Dosing and Opioid Cessation

Ilgen et al.[31] evaluated the risk of suicide stratified by different opioid doses in a retrospective analysis of veterans with CNCP. After controlling for demographic and other psychiatric comorbidities, they discovered that higher opioid doses were associated with increased risk of suicide mortality. Compared with individuals who received 20 mg morphine equivalent daily dose (MEDD) or less, those prescribed 20–50 MEDD had an HR of 1.48 (95% CI: 1.25–1.75), those prescribed 50–100 MEDD had an HR of 1.69 (95% CI: 1.33–2.14), and those prescribed 100 MEDD or more had an HR of 2.15 (95% CI: 1.64–2.81). Although opioid dosing may be related to risk of suicide, opioid cessation is also of concern. Oliva et al.[32] employed a cohort from the Veterans Health Administration examining the association between discontinuing opioid therapy, duration of treatment, and death from overdose or suicide. Results revealed that patients were at greater risk of death from overdose or suicide after ceasing opioid therapy, with an even greater risk the longer patients had been treated before opioids were discontinued. Clinicians should be cognizant of the risk of overdose or suicide when considering an opioid taper.

Chronic Pain and Suicide: Mediators

Identified mediators of pain and suicide include pain catastrophizing, burdensomeness, mental defeat, and social isolation.

Pain Catastrophizing

Patients with CNCP tend to engage in maladaptive thinking—pain catastrophizing—which can be theorized as magnified, exaggerated negative focus on pain that can contribute to depression and disability.[33] For example. Brown et al.[34] evaluated the longitudinal association between two styles of pain coping, catastrophizing and hoping/praying, as predictors of subsequent suicidal ideation in patients with CNCP on long-term opioid therapy. Catastrophizing was a statistically significant predictor of increased subsequent suicidal ideation, whereas hoping/praying did not protect against future suicidal ideation or behavior. The relationship between catastrophizing and future suicidal ideation was mediated by depression but not by social support or pain interference.[34] Reducing pain catastrophizing is a primary objective of cognitive–behavioral therapy (CTB; discussed later).

Burdensomeness and Social Isolation

One theory of suicidal ideation and behavior is based on the interpersonal theory of suicide,[35,36] which postulates that there are two primary factors which greatly contribute to the context that leads to suicidal ideation and possible suicidal behavior: thwarted belongingness, which is the unfulfilled need for social interaction and connectedness, and perceived burdensomeness, which is perceiving oneself as a burden or a liability to others, particularly family members. In a study by Wilson et al.,[37] 260 patients with CNCP enrolled in an interdisciplinary chronic pain treatment program were administered two validated scales assessing burdensomeness (the Self-Perceived Burden Scale and the Interpersonal Needs Questionnaire Perceived Burdensomeness Scale), the Beck Scale for Suicide Ideation, and the thoughts of self-harm item of the Patient Health Questionnaire-9 (PHQ-9). The patients who perceived that they had become "a burden to others" were at increased risk for suicidal ideation. Cheatle et al.[13]

also discovered that social withdrawal and isolation were predictive of suicidal ideation in a cohort of 466 patients enrolled in a behavioral pain clinic. It is important to assist patients who express being a burden and/or feeling isolated to pursue a sense of purpose and being with others (e.g., volunteering).

Mental Defeat

A novel construct for increased risk of suicidal ideation in patients with CNCP is mental defeat, defined as a state of mind marked by a loss of autonomy, agency, and human integrity.[38] Phenomenological studies have revealed that patients suffering from CNCP often report a sense of "defeat of the mind" and that "the pain is taking over," resulting in them "unable to cope with what [they are] supposed to do" and "feeling less like a human being."[39] These thoughts are associated with greater symptom interference, distress, physical and psychosocial disability, breakdowns in self-management of pain, and increased treatment seeking and precipitating suicidal ideation and behavior.[40,41]

Assessment of Risk for Suicide

Assessment of risk for suicide in patients with CNCP should include general mental health screening and specific suicide assessment tools, but also pain coping (pain catastrophizing) and sleep disturbance because both of these are known risk factors for suicide in this patient population. Assessing these factors for suicide also provides the clinician targets for intervention for risk mitigations. A number of validated and reliable measures of depression and anxiety are available. Often employed depression tools include the Beck Depression Inventory[42] and the PHQ-9,[43] both of which include a question on suicidal intent. Clinicians should not only consider the total score but also, in a potentially high-risk patient (see "Risk Stratification"), examine the response to the suicide question. There are a number of sleep assessment scales that asses different aspects of sleep disturbance. The Pittsburgh Sleep Quality Scale[44] and the Patient-Reported Outcome Measures for Sleep Disturbance and Sleep-Related Impairments Scale[45] are common assessment tools. Sullivan et al.[46] developed the Pain Catastrophizing Scale, which provides a global score and subscale scores. There are also a number of suicide risk scales. The Columbia-Suicide Severity Rating Scale (C-SSRS) has been frequently used for clinical trials on new medications and in clinical practice. The C-SSRS assesses a number of domains, including ideation, intensity, behaviors, severity of self-injury, and potential lethality of suicide attempts.[47] All these tools are relatively rapid screeners of pertinent risk factors that should be administered every office visit (they can be completed online prior to the scheduled visit) because risk factors are dynamic as patients face new stressors and challenges.

Risk Stratification

There are risk factors for suicide that are applicable to the general population and others more specific to patients suffering from pain. General risk factors include gender (female); age (>45 years old); having co-occurring mental disorders; acute losses and

Table 21.1 Rapid Risk Stratification

	Low	High
Plans	Vague	Specific
Means	No	Yes (lethal supply of prescription opioids, antidepressants, access to firearms/guns)
History of suicide attempts	No	Yes
Level of support	High	Low
Coping abilities	Good	Poor
Relationship with health care provider	Good	Poor
Willingness to contract	Yes	No

stressors (relationships, job, and finances); coping with chronic medical illnesses; experiencing conflict, disaster, and discrimination; past psychiatric hospitalizations; frequency of suicidal ideation; severity of psychiatric disorder; poor social support; and a previous suicide attempt, which is the strongest predictor of suicide.[1,18] Individuals with pain commonly have a number of these general risk factors (loss of vocational and home roles, isolation, and depression) related to their pain[48] but also pain-specific risk factors noted above (pain type, pain duration, pain intensity, sleep disturbance, pain coping, and opioid dosing). General clinical factors to consider in stratification of risk for suicide are outlined in Table 21.1. Note that one key factor in mitigating risk is the therapeutic relationship a health care provider has with their patient, which can be challenging to establish in busy clinics and with overworked clinicians.

Pharmacologic and Nonpharmacologic Interventions

Mitigating the risk of suicidal ideation and suicidal behavior requires both pharmacologic and nonpharmacologic strategies that address mood, sleep, pain, and pain coping.

Pharmacologic Interventions

The pharmacologic approach to reducing the risk of suicide in patients with CNCP includes targeting depression and anxiety, improving sleep disturbance, and reducing pain. If opioid or benzodiazepine use is medically necessary in a patient at risk for suicide, these potentially lethal medications should be prescribed judiciously, in small amounts, and should be held and administered by a family member.

Antiepileptic drugs such as gabapentin and pregabalin have been found to be effective in managing fibromyalgia and neuropathic pain conditions (diabetic neuralgia and complex regional pain syndrome), and they may also provide mood stabilization and improve sleep. Several antidepressant medications are clinically indicated for treating co-occurring depression and pain, including serotonin–norepinephrine reuptake inhibitor (SNRI) antidepressants venlafaxine, duloxetine, and milnacipran (not approved by the U.S. Food and Drug Administration for the treatment of depression), in addition to desvenlafaxine and tricyclic antidepressants, some of which also have sedating qualities to improve sleep (e.g., amitriptyline, nortriptyline, and doxepin). There is evidence of the analgesic properties of tricyclics and certain SNRIs, which, like opioids, are used to modulate descending inhibitory pain pathways. There is equivocal literature regarding the association between suicide and antidepressant and antiepileptic medication.[49] When initiating antidepressant or antiepileptic drug therapy, the clinician should closely monitor a patient for increased risk of suicide.

Buprenorphine is a partial agonist at the μ-opioid receptors and an antagonist at the κ receptors, with formulations indicated for both opioid use disorder and pain. There is emerging evidence of buprenorphine reducing suicidal ideation.[50] For example, Yovell et al.[51] conducted a randomized, double-blind, placebo-controlled trial of ultra-low-dose sublingual buprenorphine in severely suicidal patients without substance abuse. Patients who received ultra-low-dose buprenorphine had a greater reduction in Beck Suicide Ideation Scale scores than patients who received placebo, both after 2 weeks and after 4 weeks. Last, there is encouraging evidence supporting the use of ketamine for pain reduction (especially neuropathically mediated pain), mood improvement, and in reducing suicidal ideation.[52,53]

Nonpharmacologic Interventions

Patients with CNCP often experience concomitant depression, anxiety, and sleep disturbance, which can increase the risk of suicidal ideation and suicidal behavior. The most effective approach in managing pain and comorbid conditions is combining rational pharmacotherapy and nonpharmacologic evidenced-based interventions such as cognitive–behavioral therapy (CBT) and acceptance commitment therapy (ACT).

Cognitive–Behavioral Therapy

There is a robust literature supporting the efficacy of CBT in improving mood and anxiety disorders, pain, and sleep disturbance.

CBT-Pain

Patients experiencing CNCP often engage in maladaptive thinking patterns, most commonly catastrophizing (a significant risk factor for suicidal ideation in patients with chronic pain) and maladaptive behaviors (e.g., kinesiophobia/fear of movement), which can result in deconditioning, increased pain, social isolation, worsening depression, and an increased risk of suicide. CBT consists of specific evidenced-based techniques to support the patient in identifying maladaptive behaviors and dysfunctional thought patterns that may lessen the patient's ability to cope with their chronic pain, contributing to concomitant depression and anxiety. The objective of CBT is to promote the patient being more proactive than reactive in managing their pain, reinforcing a sense of competence and self-efficacy. CBT techniques can include mindfulness-based stress reduction, progressive muscle relaxation training, pacing, behavioral activation, effective communication, and cognitive restructuring, followed by skill consolidation, rehearsal, and relapse training.[54]

There is persuasive literature supporting the clinical efficacy and cost-effectiveness of CBT in improving function and mood in a number of chronic pain disorders, including chronic low back pain, arthritis, lupus, fibromyalgia, and sickle cell disease.[55–61]

CBT-Sleep Disturbance

Cognitive–behavioral therapy for insomnia (CBT-I) has been demonstrated to be effective in improving sleep disturbance, sleep efficiency, and sleep quality, and its effectiveness is equal or superior to that of sleep medications.[62] Sleep disturbance is highly prevalent in patients with CNCP and, as noted previously, is a known risk factor for suicide in patients with CNCP.[12,29,30]

A program of CBT-I typically includes psychoeducation about sleep and insomnia; stimulus control; sleep restriction; sleep hygiene; relaxation training; and cognitive restructuring. CBT-I can be delivered in an individual, group, and computer-assisted format with generally equal effectiveness. There has been some effort to combine CBT-Pain and CBT-I into a hybrid program to target both pain and insomnia, with promising results in improving sleep, mood, and function.[63]

Acceptance and Commitment Therapy

Acceptance and commitment therapy is a mindfulness-based therapy that is directive and experiential. The core processes of ACT include contact with the present moment, self as context, cognitive defusion, acceptance, values, and committed action. The goal of ACT is for the patient to strive for psychological flexibility to cope with pain more effectively, thus supporting improvement in mood and function. Numerous randomized clinical trials have demonstrated treatment efficacy and long-term durability of ACT in patients with CNCP. For example, Vowles et al.[64] demonstrated improvement in physical and emotional well-being in a cohort of patients with chronic musculoskeletal pain who completed a course of ACT for pain, and these improvements were maintained 3 years after treatment by 64.8% of these patients. ACT for pain has also been adapted to be delivered in a primary care setting, allowing for greater dissemination and accessibility.[65]

Key Points for Clinicians

- Clinicians caring for patients with chronic pain should be cognizant of the risk factors for suicide.
- Suicidal ideation in this patient population should be routinely monitored, which can be assessed discretely by checking the suicide question on the clinic's routine depression screening tool.
- Monitoring should be dynamic, not static, because conditions may change in a patient's life placing them at higher risk for suicide, such as losing a job, going through a divorce, developing other medical disorders, or any added life stressor.
- Clinicians and their staff should complete training on suicide assessment and prevention and have an established action plan if a patient endorses suicidal ideation.

One resource is Zero Suicide Institute (https://zerosuicide.edc.org), which is a nonprofit organization that provides Web-based training in suicide assessment and mitigation strategies.

Conclusion

Patients who suffer from chronic pain are vulnerable to a myriad of medical and psychological comorbidities, including depression; anxiety; the development of secondary medical conditions; sleep disorders; and suicidal ideation, which is highly prevalent in this patient population. There is a robust and evolving literature on the risk factors and mediators of suicidal ideation and suicidal behavior in patients with chronic pain. Many of these factors are amenable to both pharmacologic and nonpharmacologic interventions. Clinicians managing patients with CNCP should be vigilant in assessing for risk of suicide and be mobilized with a plan of action if a patient is identified as high risk for suicide. Future directions in this field include developing and testing novel delivery systems for CBT/ACT and other nonpharmacologic interventions to expand access, investigating phenotypic and genotypic characteristics of suicidal ideation and behavior in patients with pain, and further exploring the potential efficacy of buprenorphine formulations and ketamine to co-treat pain and suicidal ideation.

References

1. World Health Organization. Suicide worldwide 2019. https://www.who.int/publications/i/item/9789240026643
2. Centers for Disease Control and Prevention. About multiple cause of death, 1999–2020. 2021. https://wonder.cdc.gov/wonder/help/mcd.html. Accessed 12/23/2022.
3. Centers for Disease Control and Prevention. WONDER online database. 2021. https://wonder.cdc.gov. Accessed 12/23/2022.
4. Hitchcock L, Ferrell B, McCaffery M. The experience of chronic nonmalignant pain. *J Pain Symptom Manage*. 1994;9:312–318.
5. Stenager EN, Stenager E, Jensen K. Attempted suicide, depression and physical diseases: A 1-year follow-up study. *Psychother Psychosom*. 1994;61:65–73.
6. Fishbain DA. The association of chronic pain and suicide. *Semin Clin Neuropsychiatry*. 1999;4:221–227.
7. Smith MT, Edwards RR, Robinson RC, Dworkin RH. Suicidal ideation, plans and attempts in chronic pain patients: Factors associated with increased risk. *Pain*. 2004;111:201–208.
8. Braden JB, Sullivan MD. Suicidal thoughts and behavior among adults with self-reported pain conditions in the National Comorbidity Survey Replication. *J Pain*. 2008;9:1106–1115.
9. Ilgen MA, Zivin K, McCammon RJ, Valenstein M. Pain and suicidal thoughts, plans and attempts in the United States. *Gen Hosp Psychiatry*. 2008;30:521–527.
10. Ratcliffe GE, Enns MW, Belik SL, Sareen J. Chronic pain conditions and suicidal ideation and suicide attempts: An epidemiologic perspective. *Clin J Pain*. 2008;24:204–210.
11. Substance Abuse & Mental Health Services, Administration Office of Applied Studies. Drug Abuse Warning Network, 2022: Estimates of drug-related emergency department visits. https://store.samhsa.gov/sites/default/files/pep23-07-03-001.pdf. Accessed 12-27-2023.
12. Racine M, Choinière M, Nielson WR. Predictors of suicidal ideation in chronic pain patients: An exploratory study. *Clin J Pain*. 2014;30(5):371–378.

13. Cheatle M, Wasser T, Foster C, Olugbodi A, Bryan J. Prevalence of suicidal ideation in patients with chronic noncancer pain referred to a behaviorally based pain program. *Pain Phys.* 2014;17(3):E359–E367.
14. Edwards RR, Smith MT, Kudel I, Haythornthwaite J. Pain-related catastrophizing as a risk factor for suicidal ideation in chronic pain. *Pain.* 2006;126: 272–279.
15. Tang NK, Crane C. Suicidality in chronic pain: A review of the prevalence, risk factors and psychological links. *Psychol Med.* 2006;36:575–586.
16. Ilgen MA, Zivin K, Austin KL, et al. Severe pain predicts greater likelihood of subsequent suicide. *Suicide Life Threat Behav.* 2010;40(6):597–608.
17. Campbell G, Bruno R, Darke S, et al. Prevalence and correlates of suicidal thoughts and suicide attempts in people prescribed pharmaceutical opioids for chronic pain. *Clin J Pain.* 2016;32(4):292–301.
18. Centers for Disease Control and Prevention. National Center for Injury Prevention and Control 2022. Accessed December 27, 2023. https://www.cdc.gov/suicide/suicide-data-statistics.html
19. Calati R, Laglaoui Bakhiyi C, Artero S, Ilgen M, Courtet P. The impact of physical pain on suicidal thoughts and behaviors: Meta-analyses. *J Psychiatr Res.* 2015;71:16–32.
20. Racine M. Chronic pain and suicide risk: A comprehensive review. *Prog Neuropsychopharmacol Biol Psychiatry.* 2018;87(Pt B):269–280.
21. Jimenez-Rodríguez I, Garcia-Leiva JM, Jimenez-Rodriguez BM, Condés-Moreno E, Rico-Villademoros F, Calandre EP. Suicidal ideation and the risk of suicide in patients with fibromyalgia: A comparison with non-pain controls and patients suffering from low-back pain. *Neuropsychiatr Dis Treat.* 2014;10:625–230.
22. Adawi M, Chen W, Bragazzi NL, et al. Suicidal behavior in fibromyalgia patients: Rates and determinants of suicide ideation, risk, suicide, and suicidal attempts—A systematic review of the literature and meta-analysis of over 390,000 fibromyalgia patients. *Front Psychiatry.* 2021;12:629417.
23. Nović A, Kõlves K, O'Dwyer S, De Leo D. Migraine and suicidal behaviors: A systematic literature review. *Clin J Pain.* 2016;32(4):351–364.
24. Pei JH, Wang XL, Yu Y, et al. Prevalence of suicidal ideation and suicide attempt in patients with migraine: A systematic review and meta-analysis. *J Affect Disord.* 2020;277:253–259.
25. Liu HY, Fuh JL, Lin YY, Chen WT, Wang SJ. Suicide risk in patients with migraine and comorbid fibromyalgia. *Neurology.* 2015;85(12):1017–1023.
26. Lee DH, Noh EC, Kim YC, et al. Risk factors for suicidal ideation among patients with complex regional pain syndrome. *Psychiatry Investig.* 2014;11(1):32–38.
27. Cheatle MD, Foster S, Pinkett A, Lesneski M, Qu D, Dhingra L. Assessing and managing sleep disturbance in patients with chronic pain. *Anesthesiol Clin.* 2016;34(2):379–393.
28. Husak AJ, Bair MJ. Chronic pain and sleep disturbances: A pragmatic review of their relationships, comorbidities, and treatments. *Pain Med.* 2020;21(6):1142–1152.
29. Smith MT, Perlis ML, Haythornthwaite JA. Suicidal ideation in outpatients with chronic musculoskeletal pain: An exploratory study of the role of sleep onset insomnia and pain intensity. *Clin J Pain.* 2004;20(2):111–118.
30. Racine M, Sánchez-Rodríguez E, Gálan S, et al. Factors associated with suicidal ideation in patients with chronic non-cancer pain. *Pain Med.* 2017;18(2):283–293.
31. Ilgen MA, Bohnert AS, Ganoczy D, Bair MJ, McCarthy JF, Blow FC. Opioid dose and risk of suicide. *Pain.* 2016;157(5):1079–1084.
32. Oliva EM, Bowe T, Manhapra A, et al. Associations between stopping prescriptions for opioids, length of opioid treatment, and overdose or suicide deaths in US veterans: observational evaluation. BMJ. 2020;368:m283.
33. Turner JA, Aaron LA. Pain-related catastrophizing: What is it? *Clin J Pain.* 2001;17(1):65–71.
34. Brown LA, Lynch KG, Cheatle M. Pain catastrophizing as a predictor of suicidal ideation in chronic pain patients with an opiate prescription. *Psychiatry Res.* 2020;286:112893.
35. Joiner T. *Why People Die by Suicide.* Harvard University Press; 2005.

36. Van Orden KA, Witte TK, Cukrowicz KC, Braithwaite SR, Selby EA, Joiner TE. The interpersonal theory of suicide. *Psychol Rev.* 2010;117:575–600.
37. Wilson KG, Kowal J, Caird SM, Castillo D, McWilliams LA, Heenan A. Self-perceived burden, perceived burdensomeness, and suicidal ideation in patients with chronic pain. *Can J Pain.* 2017;1(1):127–136.
38. Tang NK, Salkovskis PM, Hanna M. Mental defeat in chronic pain: Initial exploration of the concept. *Clin J Pain.* 2007;23(3):222–232.
39. Tang NK, Salkovskis PM, Hodges A, Soong E, Hanna MH, Hester J. Chronic pain syndrome associated with health anxiety: A qualitative thematic comparison between pain patients with high and low health anxiety. *Br J Clin Psychol.* 2009;48(Pt 1):1–20.
40. Tang NKY, Goodchild CE, Hester J, Salkovskis PM. Mental defeat is linked to interference, distress and disability in chronic pain. *Pain.* 2010;149(3):547–554.
41. Tang NK, Beckwith P, Ashworth P. Mental defeat is associated with suicide intent in patients with chronic pain. *Clin J Pain.* 2016;32(5):411–419.
42. Beck A, Ward C, Mendelson M, Mock J, Erbaugh J. An inventory for measuring depression. *Arch Gen Psychiatry.* 1961;4:561–571.
43. Kroenke K, Spitzer RL, Williams JB. The PHQ-9: Validity of a brief depression severity measure. *J Gen Intern Med.* 2001;16(9):606–613.
44. Buysse DJ, Reynolds CF 3rd, Monk TH, Berman SR, Kupfer DJ. The Pittsburgh Sleep Quality Index: A new instrument for psychiatric practice and research. *Psychiatry Res.* 1989;28(2):193–213.
45. Buysse DJ, Yu L, Moul DE, et al. Development and validation of patient-reported outcome measures for sleep disturbance and sleep-related impairments. *Sleep.* 2010;33(6):781–92.
46. Sullivan MJL, Bishop SR, Pivik J. The Pain Catastrophizing Scale: Development and validation. *Psychol Assess.* 1995;7(4):524–532.
47. Posner K, Brown GK, Stanley B, et al. The Columbia-Suicide Severity Rating Scale: Initial validity and internal consistency findings from three multisite studies with adolescents and adults. *Am J Psychiatry.* 2011;168(12):1266–1277.
48. Cheatle MD. Depression, chronic pain, and suicide by overdose: On the edge. *Pain Med.* 2011;12(Suppl 2):S43–S48.
49. Bailly F, Belaid H. Suicidal ideation and suicide attempt associated with antidepressant and antiepileptic drugs: Implications for treatment of chronic pain. *Joint Bone Spine.* 2021;88(1):105005.
50. Cameron CM, Nieto S, Bosler L, et al. Mechanisms underlying the anti-suicidal treatment potential of buprenorphine. *Adv Drug Alcohol Res.* 2021;1:10009. doi:10.3389/adar.2021.10009
51. Yovell Y, Bar G, Mashiah M, et al. Ultra-low-dose buprenorphine as a time-limited treatment for severe suicidal ideation: A randomized controlled trial. *Am J Psychiatry.* 2016;173(5):491–498.
52. Wilkinson ST, Ballard ED, Bloch MH, et al. The effect of a single dose of intravenous ketamine on suicidal ideation: A systematic review and individual participant data meta-analysis. *Am J Psychiatry.* 2018;175(2):150–158.
53. Tran K, McCormack S. Ketamine for Chronic Non-Cancer Pain: A Review of Clinical Effectiveness, Cost-Effectiveness, and Guidelines [Internet]. Ottawa (ON): Canadian Agency for Drugs and Technologies in Health; 2020 May 28. PMID: 33231962.
54. Turk DC, Flor H. Etiological theories and treatments for chronic back pain: II. Psychological models and interventions. *Pain.* 1984;19(3):209–233.
55. Lamb SE, Hansen Z, Lall R, Castelnuovo E, Withers EJ, Nichols V. Group cognitive behavioral treatment for low-back pain in primary care: A randomized controlled trial and cost-effectiveness analysis. *Lancet.* 2010;375:916–923.
56. Linton SJ. A 5-year follow-up evaluation of the health and economic consequences of an early cognitive behavioral intervention for back pain: A randomized, controlled trial. *Spine.* 2006;31(8):853–858.
57. Keefe FJ, Caldwell DS. Cognitive behavioral control of arthritis pain. *Med Clin North Am.* 1997;81:277–290.

58. Greco CM, Rudy TE, Manzi S. Effects of a stress-reduction program on psychological function, pain, and physical function of systemic lupus erythematosus patients: A randomized controlled trial. *Arthritis Rheum.* 2004;51(4):625–634.
59. Thieme K, Flor H, Turk D. Psychological pain treatment in fibromyalgia syndrome: Efficacy of operant behavioral and cognitive behavioral treatments. *Arthritis Res Ther.* 2006;8(4):R121.
60. Chen E, Cole SW, Kato PM. A review of empirically supported psychosocial interventions for pain and adherence outcomes in sickle cell disease. *J Pediatr Psychol.* 2004;29:1997–2009.
61. Bernardy K, Klose P, Busch AJ, Choy EH, Häuser W. Cognitive behavioral therapies for fibromyalgia. *Cochrane Database Syst Rev.* 2013;2013(9):CD009796.
62. Svertsen B, Omvik S, Pallesen S, et al. Cognitive behavioral therapy vs zopiclone for treatment of chronic primary insomnia in older adults: A randomized controlled trial. *JAMA.* 2006;295(24):2851–2858.
63. Tang NK, Goodchild CE, Salkovskis PM. Hybrid cognitive–behavior therapy for individuals with insomnia and chronic pain: A pilot randomized controlled trial. *Behav Res Ther.* 2012;50(12):814–821.
64. Vowles KE, McCracken LM, O'Brien JZ. Acceptance and values-based action in chronic pain: A three-year follow-up analysis of treatment effectiveness and process. *Behav Res Ther.* 2011;49(11):748–755.
65. Kanzler KE, Robinson PJ, McGeary DD, et al. Addressing chronic pain with focused acceptance and commitment therapy in integrated primary care: Findings from a mixed methods pilot randomized controlled trial. *BMC Prim Care.* 2022;23(1):Article 77.

22
Pain in Seriously Mental Ill Populations

Ashli A. Owen-Smith and Jeffrey F. Scherrer

Definition of Serious Mental Illness

The National Institute of Mental Health[1] defines serious mental illness (SMI), also called severe mental illness, as a mental, behavioral, or emotional disorder resulting in serious functional impairment that interferes with life activities. Per this definition, 5.6% of adults in the United States had an SMI in 2020.[1] SMI is also defined by diagnoses of psychotic disorders (schizophrenia), bipolar disorder and major depression with psychotic features, or treatment-resistant depression (TRD).[2]

Schizophrenia: Background, Definition, and Epidemiology

Compared to the substantial literature on the association between pain and depression,[3–6] relatively little has been reported on the prevalence of pain, risk for pain, and the impact of pain among persons with schizophrenia or bipolar disorder. This may be partly explained by the relative rarity of these conditions compared to depression. Less than 1% of persons in the United States have schizophrenia. From a variety of data sources, it is estimated that 0.25–0.64% of the U.S. population has schizophrenia or similar psychotic disorders,[1] similar to the 0.33–0.75% estimated prevalence worldwide.

Schizophrenia onsets in late adolescence to early adulthood and is a thought and information processing disorder that includes psychotic symptoms such as hallucinations and delusions.[1] Hallucinations involve hearing, tasting, seeing, or feeling things that are not present. Delusions are beliefs that are not true, such as believing messages meant for the individual are being sent through the radio or that a person or group is watching them. Problems organizing thoughts occur and can make speech difficult to follow. Other symptoms include blunted emotional expression, low motivation, and motor and cognitive impairment, and often patients experience challenges in social relationships.[1] Antipsychotics are often effective front-line treatments, and psychotherapies can help patients understand their disease and adopt behaviors that enable problem-solving and symptom management. Patients often have comorbid psychiatric disorders, poor quality of life, and a shortened life span that is partly explained by the high rate of physical comorbidities (diabetes and heart disease) observed in this population.[1]

Pain in Schizophrenia

The association between both experimental and clinical pain and schizophrenia is unique compared to pain comorbid with other psychiatric disorders. Specifically, there is substantial evidence that persons with schizophrenia have muted pain expression, which could explain the lower pain prevalence observed in this population compared to those with other psychiatric disorders.[7,8] This is consistent with evidence that clinically recognized pain conditions are less common among patients with schizophrenia compared to patients with depression and bipolar disorder.[7] A cross-sectional study of U.S. veterans revealed any pain occurred in 65.6% of patients with depression, 61.3% of those with bipolar disorder, and 46.9% of those with schizophrenia.[7] Similarly, approximately 3.3% of depressed and bipolar patients had chronic pain, but only 1.8% of schizophrenics reported chronic pain. The prevalence of chronic pain does not significantly differ between schizophrenics and the general population in the United States[8] and other countries.[9]

Experimental Pain and Schizophrenia

Experimental pain involves exposing study participants to objective pain stimuli in a controlled laboratory setting. For example, the cold pressure test measures pain tolerance by having subjects place their forearm in an ice bath to measure how long they can tolerate the painful stimuli. This type of research has led to some mixed evidence regarding differences between patients with schizophrenia and healthy controls in nociception.[10,11] Similarly, mixed findings have been reported on heat pain tolerance in treated and untreated patients with schizophrenia.[10–13]

Two experimental pain studies observed no difference in nociception between patients with and without schizophrenia.[10,11] In addition, heat pain tolerance did not differ within subjects tested prior to initiating treatment and 3 days after starting antipsychotics.[10,11] In contrast, two pilot studies investigating the neurophysiology of experimental pain tolerance in patients with schizophrenia reported greater heat pain tolerance among unmedicated patients with schizophrenia compared to healthy controls.[12,13] This was correlated with less activation in pain affective–cognitive processing areas of the brain and hyperactivity in sensory discriminative pain processing regions.[13] Higher heat pain tolerance was observed in unmedicated patients compared to healthy controls, and this did not differ between treated, stable patients with schizophrenia and healthy controls despite non-normal neural pain processing, similar to that observed in unmedicated patients.[12]

Although there have been inconsistent findings regarding experimental pain sensitivity in schizophrenia, the best evidence comes from a large 2015 meta-analyses of 17 studies involving 387 subjects.[14] This work revealed that patients with schizophrenia, compared to healthy controls, had greater pain tolerance, reduced physiological response to adverse stimuli, and lower pain intensity ratings.[14] These findings were similar in treated and untreated patients.[14]

Because antipsychotics, such as haloperidol, bind to opioid receptors, several studies have compared pain response in patients with versus without antipsychotic treatment.[8]

A systematic review of laboratory studies concluded that there is a moderate effect size for diminished pain response, and this is independent of whether patients are receiving antipsychotics.[15] Based on laboratory studies, antipsychotics do not generate sufficient analgesia to change pain perception.

Overall, most evidence supports the conclusion that patients with schizophrenia experience greater pain tolerance and report less severe pain when exposed to experimental pain stimuli. Antipsychotic treatment does not significantly change pain perception. Both conclusions are consistent with results from the few studies of clinical pain in schizophrenia.

Clinical Pain and Schizophrenia

Clinical pain in schizophrenia raises additional questions. The most common pain locations in schizophrenia are the head, face, abdomen, and lower spinal column.[8] It is alarming that schizophrenic patients with severe burns, fractures, and myocardial infarction report only minor pain.[8,16,17] Patients with schizophrenia experiencing a heart attack are more likely than persons without schizophrenia to present without pain.[8,17]

Bipolar Disorder: Background, Definition, and Epidemiology

Bipolar disorder involves changes in mood and energy or activity. Bipolar I disorder is characterized by cycling between depressive and manic episodes. Manic episodes can be extremely severe and involve delusions and hallucinations, hypersexuality, and anger. Bipolar II involves cycles of depressive episodes and hypomanic episodes that are of shorter duration and less severe than manic episodes. Bipolar disorder is much more common than schizophrenia but still relatively rare: Among adults, the 12-month prevalence of bipolar disorder in the United States is 2.8%, and the lifetime prevalence is 4.4%. The 12-month prevalence of bipolar disorder in young adults is nearly 5%. As with schizophrenia, onset of bipolar disorder occurs in adolescence and young adulthood. With appropriate treatment, patients with bipolar disorder can experience long periods of remission.[1]

Pain in Bipolar Disorder

Meta-analysis of prevalence studies found that "clinically relevant" pain (*any* documented pain condition) occurs in nearly 30% and chronic pain is present in 23.7% of patients with bipolar disorder.[18] In a cross-sectional study of the associations between pain and schizophrenia, and depression and bipolar disorder among Veterans Health Affairs patients, Birgenheir et al.[7] observed pain conditions were most common among those with depression, followed by bipolar disorder, and least common in schizophrenia. In contrast, analyses of more than 149,000 patients in the UK Biobank revealed chronic pain was most prevalent (54.8%) among those with bipolar I and II, followed by depression (50.4%) and controls (38.2%).[19] This study also observed increasing prevalence of bipolar disorder as the number of pain sites increased.[19] Owen-Smith and colleagues'[20] analysis of multiple large private sector health care systems in the United States revealed that compared to patients without a mental health diagnosis, there was a 90% greater risk for a pain diagnoses among those with depression, 86% greater risk in schizophrenia, and a 71% greater risk in bipolar disorder. Others have observed nearly a fivefold increased risk for chronic pain in bipolar compared to controls and nearly a fourfold increase among those with schizophrenia.[21] Although there is variation in whether pain is more common in major depression, bipolar, or schizophrenia, most evidence indicates those with bipolar disorder have a markedly higher risk for pain compared to persons without mental illness.

Moderate to severe pain interference—that is, the degree to which pain impairs activities of daily living—worsens mental health and functioning in bipolar disorder and is more common in this patient population compared to depression and pain.[22] Risch et al.[22] note the long-term adverse consequences of this association given the stable high prevalence of pain in bipolar disorder. Interestingly, a qualitative study revealed that for some patients with bipolar disorder, pain appears to be less severe during manic or euphoric states while worsening during periods of irritability or anger.[23] Patients also reported feeling disconnected from pain,[23] which is consistent with evidence of abnormal pain processing in patients with bipolar disorder.[24]

Bipolar Disorder and Migraine

There is evidence that migraine is a unique burden for patients with bipolar disorder. Migraine headache is twice as common among those with bipolar disorder compared to the general population, and it is associated with worse outcomes.[25] Results from the Canadian Community Health Survey of more than 36,000 participants revealed that men with bipolar and comorbid migraine compared to bipolar disorder alone were more likely to have low income, require social assistance and welfare, have earlier age of onset of bipolar, have high lifetime comorbid anxiety, and use more mental and physical health care.[25] Women with comorbid bipolar disorder and migraine compared to bipolar alone required personal and instrumental support in activities of daily living.[25] Oedegaard and Fasmer[26] suggest migraine headaches are a bipolar trait because the clinical characteristics of comorbid migraine and depression resemble some bipolar symptoms, such as high rates of irritability and affective temperaments. Additional research is needed to determine the type of pain and pain locations that might distinguish comorbid pain in bipolar disorder from pain comorbid in depression and schizophrenia.

Treatment-Resistant Depression: Background, Definition, and Epidemiology

Treatment-resistant depression is typically characterized by a poor response (e.g., failure to achieve remission) to an adequate course of treatment for individuals with major depressive disorder.[27] Prevalence rates of TRD are dictated, in part, by the patient's stage of treatment (e.g., Stage 1 involves failure of one class of a major antidepressant; Stage 2 involves failure of two different classes of antidepressants; Stage 3 involves failure of an additional tricyclic antidepressant; Stage 4 involves failure of an additional trial of a monoamine oxidase inhibitor; and Stage 5 involves failure of an additional course of electroconvulsive therapy) and depend on the specific treatment setting. However, some estimates suggest that Stage 1 TRD has been reported to have a prevalence of approximately 50%.[27]

Pain in Treatment-Resistant Depression

Pain conditions are common in individuals with TRD, with some studies documenting a prevalence of up to 73% in TRD populations[28] and consistent evidence that individuals with TRD are significantly more likely to suffer from pain compared to those without TRD.[29] One explanation for these findings is that patients with chronic pain may not respond as well to antidepressants (compared to those without chronic pain), which can subsequently increase the risk of TRD. For example, in one controlled trial in which clinically depressed patients were randomized to one of four selective serotonin reuptake inhibitor (SSRI) treatments, the odds of a poor depression treatment response were twice as high in patients with moderate pain at baseline and three or four times as high in those with severe pain at baseline, even after controlling for demographics (age, gender, and race) and other covariates (SSRI type, clinic site, treating physician, non-pain somatic symptoms, and baseline depression score).[30]

Barriers to Pain Identification and Management in Populations with SMI

Pain is associated with increased disability and poor quality of life among persons both with and without SMI.[25,31] However, there may be individual, interpersonal, and system-level factors that uniquely contribute to this association for persons with SMI.

Although some evidence suggests a lower prevalence of pain among individuals with schizophrenia (described previously), this may be due to the fact that patients are less able to report pain in clinical settings. Impaired executive functioning, attention, and vigilance in individuals with schizophrenia, for example, may contribute to a blunted pain expression.[10] Thus, these patients may experience pain at the same level as healthy controls, as indicated in experimental pain studies, or even at increased levels compared to healthy controls, but they may be unable to communicate it effectively to their health care providers.[8] Given that pain is most commonly assessed through self-report—and requires that the patient (1) understand a physician or other health care provider's request for a pain rating, (2) accurately recall pain events in the given time frame, and (3) accurately interpret the experience of noxious stimuli as a painful event[32]—individuals with SMI are often unable to adequately describe physical symptoms due to social communication impairments.[33] They may also have lower motivation to report pain to health care providers, perhaps due to concerns about how they will be treated by them. For example, Kuritzky and colleagues reported that a large percentage of people (~40%) with schizophrenia who had pain-related complaints indicated that they never reported these complaints in order to avoid being perceived a burden to providers and/or to avoid hospitalization.[8,34] This leads to the possibility that clinical pain is underestimated in schizophrenics because these patients do not seek care for pain.[16] Patients who have experienced inadequate pain management may be reluctant to seek medical care for other health problems as well.[35]

Clinicians also may not proactively assess and diagnose pain in patients with SMI as often as with individuals without SMI, and thus pain is likely underrecognized and underdiagnosed in this population. Mental health clinicians may be less likely to assign pain-related diagnoses for individuals with schizophrenia because many have limited training in physical symptom management[36] and are more focused on treating psychiatric than medical concerns[37–39]; primary care clinicians may be less likely to assign pain-related diagnoses because their short consultation times make it difficult to both assess mental symptoms and conduct physical assessments. In addition, less experienced physicians or other health care providers may be uncomfortable with SMI and may avoid intensifying their interaction with a patient by asking probing questions about physical symptoms and performing a physical exam.[36]

Furthermore, individuals with SMI often experience fragmented health care, which likely further contributes to underestimating pain in this population.[16] Uncoordinated care between primary and mental health services can lead to uncertainty regarding which provider carries the responsibility for the physical health issues of those with SMI.[40] Mental health providers may lack the skills to diagnose and manage physical health-related comorbidities, and primary and specialty care providers may be unfamiliar with the management of mental illness.[41] Even with access to health services, the quality of care delivered to persons with SMI often is subpar relative to that seen in the general population.[42] Additional research is needed to develop, implement, and evaluate collaborative care interventions that better integrate primary care, specialty/pain management, and behavioral health care for individuals with SMI.

Finally, there also continues to be profound perceived stigma associated with both mental illness and chronic pain. One recent study reported that individuals with comorbid depression and chronic pain reported higher levels of chronic pain stigma compared to those with chronic pain alone.[43] This combined stigma may further increase the burden of each condition[44] and dissuade patients from seeking care.[45–47] Stigma has a disproportionate impact on help-seeking for mental health specifically among Black, Indigenous, and people of color[47]; thus, given that people who identify as non-Hispanic Black are diagnosed with schizophrenia at higher rates[48] and with certain health conditions in which pain is a primary feature (e.g., sickle cell disease),[49] stigma is likely to play an important role in identifying and managing pain in this population.

Consequences of Undiagnosed and Untreated/Undertreated Pain in SMI Populations

Undiagnosed and untreated/undertreated pain has myriad negative interpersonal, financial, and health-related consequences for both the individual with pain and their loved ones.

Living in pain can affect relationships with others in profound ways. Pain can make it difficult for individuals to initiate or maintain social relationships and engage in social activities,[50] Misplaced anger, one of the most salient emotional correlates of pain,[51] and codependence[52] can introduce conflict into close relationships for individuals living with pain. These problems are likely further exacerbated for individuals with SMI because core features of SMI include social withdrawal and avoidance of social contacts, resulting in social isolation. Evidence also suggests that individuals with SMI have difficulties in developing and maintaining social relationships,[53] have smaller social networks,[54,55] and have more disrupted marital interactions/greater marital dissatisfaction compared to individuals without mental health conditions.[56,57] Caregivers for those in pain[50] and those with SMI[58] may experience significant psychological and physiological stress, thus adding to the potential for interpersonal difficulties.

Financially, living in pain affects one's ability to maintain employment and is associated with a host of negative employment-related outcomes, including increased sick leave,[59] absenteeism and reduced productivity,[60–62] and unemployment and lost work days.[63–65] One study that specifically examined the independent and interactive effects of mental illness and chronic pain conditions on employment and work outcomes found that each was independently associated with a doubling of the likelihood of reported work limitations.[66] Furthermore, for female participants in particular, there was a significant synergistic effect of the presence of a mental disorder combined with the presence of a chronic pain condition on the outcome of no work in the past 12 months and of number of days of work missed in the past month, suggesting mental disorders have a greater effect on how much a person is able to work when a chronic pain condition is also present.[66]

Physically, untreated pain can interfere with a person's ability to eat and sleep, leading to reduced mobility and subsequent loss of strength and resulting in immune system impairment and increased susceptibility to disease.[52] Among individuals with mental illness, specifically, chronic pain is also associated with greater functional incapacitation.[25,67] Reduced patient and clinician identification of pain in individuals with SMI may contribute to the delayed diagnosis and timely treatment of conditions that present with pain (e.g., appendicitis and cardiovascular disease),[68] thus partly explaining the well-documented significant morbidity and mortality-related disparities in this population.[16,69–71] With respect to mental health–related sequelae, chronic pain among individuals with mental illness is associated with worsening of psychiatric symptoms, impaired recovery/poor therapeutic response, and increased risk of suicidal ideation and suicide attempt.[7,72,73]

Opportunities to Improve Pain Identification and Management in SMI Populations

The overreliance on self-report assessments of pain disadvantages those with communication-related impairments and likely results in individuals with SMI being underdiagnosed and undertreated for their pain. Thus, there have been recent calls for implementing more holistic pain assessment procedures based on several core principles.[32,68] First, an assessment of pain should always include a standardized behavioral observation rating scale that requires the clinician to observe the patient and note the presence or absence of key indicators of pain, including facial expressions (e.g., grimacing and rapid blinking), vocalizations (e.g., sighing and moaning), body movements (e.g., rigid, guarding, fidgeting, pacing, and mobility changes), changes in interpersonal interactions (e.g., resisting care, disruptive, and withdrawn), changes in activity patterns (e.g., appetite or sleep changes), and mental status changes (e.g., crying, irritability, and distress). Second, in addition to self-report, whenever possible, obtaining reports from others—particularly a significant other or family member—can be informative. Third, document any relevant issues related to the patient's current medical condition; pain can be assumed to be present when patients have undergone a procedure that is typically painful or if they have a condition for which pain-related comorbidities are common (e.g., cancer). Fourth, assess for other physiological indicators of pain, such as increased heart rate or blood pressure, diaphoresis, or pupil dilation, although these features may not be present with more chronic forms of pain.[32] These strategies have been utilized more frequently in other populations with communication deficiencies (e.g., those with dementia), and thus additional work is needed to determine the validity of these tools for individuals with comorbid SMI and pain. Additional research is also needed to further understand differences in pain-related communication between individuals with versus without SMI; any differences identified need to be more systematically included in health care provider education and training.

There is a growing body of evidence documenting the efficacy of several behavioral and pharmacological interventions for individuals with comorbid SMI and pain. Cognitive–behavioral therapy (CBT), which focuses on helping patients use both cognitive and behavioral strategies to manage distorted or distressing thoughts, enhance problem-solving and coping skills, and set realistic goals, can be independently effective for treating symptoms of SMI[74–77] and pain.[78–80] However, given that complex conditions such a chronic pain often co-occur with other physical and mental comorbidities, there have been repeated calls to provide a more hybrid approach when delivering CBT such that the clinician is deliberately treating the myriad issues linked to and exacerbated by pain as opposed to solely focusing on pain management.[81] This approach focuses on treating the patient more holistically, avoids prioritizing the treatment of one condition over the other and reinforcing artificial boundaries between physical and mental health, and addresses problems associated with fractured health care systems (described previously) by simplifying and better integrating health care access and delivery.[81] CBT may also be an important therapeutic approach for caregivers of those with comorbid SMI and pain because pain and mental health issues, including depression and insomnia, are common in this population. Thus, delivering CBT jointly to SMI patients and their caregivers may help both develop more adaptive responses to pain and facilitate a healthier caregiving relationship.[68] Additional research is needed to explore the efficacy of interventions aimed at the unit of the family as opposed to focusing solely on the individual.

There is significant overlap in the pharmacological management of pain and mental health disorders, presenting both opportunities and risks of managing these frequently co-occurring conditions. In patients with comorbid mood disorders and pain, evidence suggests that serotonin and norepinephrine reuptake inhibitors (SNRIs), gabapentinoids, or opioids with SNRI effects (e.g., tramadol and tapentadol) may improve both conditions.[82] Interestingly, there is some evidence that having a major depressive disorder or bipolar disorder diagnosis is associated with increased odds of receiving opioid medications compared to having no mental health-related diagnoses, perhaps due to the fact that these individuals may present with greater pain severity, thereby increasing the likelihood that clinicians will prescribe an opioid and at a higher dose.[20] However, there are compelling data that mental illness is a risk factor for opioid misuse and addiction[83,84]; thus, caution is warranted when considering including any opioids in a treatment plan for this population. Second-generation antipsychotics and anticonvulsants, commonly prescribed for individuals with SMI, can also have analgesic effects on certain pain disorders, including cancer, musculoskeletal pain, migraine, and fibromyalgia.[85,86] Studies examining the impact of ketamine, historically used for treatment-resistant depression and pain management,[87] have consistently demonstrated robust antidepressant and anti-suicidal effects,[88–90] but a recent meta-analysis reported worsened positive and negative symptoms in patients with schizophrenia.[91] Similarly, although cannabinoid, cannabis, and cannabidiol are promising tools in the field of pain management,[92,93] beneficial effects may be significantly offset by serious harms particularly among individuals at risk of SMI (including reduced age of onset of psychosis and increased risk of any psychotic outcome, schizophrenia/other psychotic disorder diagnosis, and psychotic symptoms) or among individuals with SMI (including nonadherence to antipsychotic medication and increased risk of relapse of psychosis and rehospitalization).[94]

One of the most significant barriers to improving pain management in SMI populations is the widespread exclusion of these individuals from behavioral and pharmacological intervention research studies. In their systematic review examining rates of exclusion for psychiatric conditions on clinicaltrials.gov, Harris et al.[95] found that 16% of chronic pain studies explicitly excluded people with SMI, 55% had broader exclusion criteria that could be used to exclude people with SMI, and that people with SMI were more likely to be excluded than people managing depression alone. Harris and colleagues rightly note that "overuse of exclusion based on psychiatric conditions is likely leading to a) less than representative samples and b) studies that don't inform clinical care for people who are managing psychiatric conditions."[95p140] Thus, although there are promising treatments for individuals with chronic pain *or* individuals with SMI—including, but not limited to, the use of companion animals,[96] acceptance and commitment therapy,[97,98] virtual reality,[99] transcranial direct current stimulation,[100–102] monoclonal antibodies,[103] peripheral nerve field stimulation,[104] and mindfulness meditation[105,106]—more research is needed to examine their effectiveness specifically among people managing *co-occurring pain and SMI.*

Conclusion

Persons with SMI represent a unique and vulnerable pain population. Physiological responses to pain can be impaired in this patient population and may result in underdetection and undertreatment. Collaborative care models may improve pain assessment and treatment while also reducing stigma. Patients are much more likely to seek mental health care in a primary care setting in which co-located behavioral health and psychiatry can collaborate with pain management. It is also clear that patients with SMI benefit from caregivers' involvement in treatment. To advance appropriate and safe pain therapies, physicians and other health care providers should consider including caregivers in treatment planning. It is critical to implement improved models of care and assessment tools to detect and treat pain in patients with SMI because poor pain outcomes can contribute to worse mental health and vice versa.

References

1. National Institute of Mental Health. Mental illness. n.d. Accessed June 14, 2022. https://www.nimh.nih.gov/health/statistics/mental-illness
2. Evans TS, Berkman N, Brown C, Gaynes B, Weber RP. Disparities within serious mental illness. Technical Briefs, No. 25. Agency for Healthcare Research and Quality; 2016.
3. Kroenke K, Wu J, Bair MJ, Krebs EE, Damush TM, Tu W. Reciprocal relationship between pain and depression: A 12-month longitudinal analysis in primary care. *J Pain*. 2011;12:964–973.
4. Fishbain D, Cutler R, Rosomoff H, Rosomoff RS. Chronic pain-associated depression: Antecedent or consequence of chronic pain? A review. *Clin J Pain*. 1997;13:116–137.
5. Bair MJ, Robinson RL, Katon W, Kroenke K. Depression and pain comorbidity: A literature review. *Arch Intern Med*. 2003;163(20):2433–2445.
6. Pinheiro MB, Ferreira ML, Refshauge K, et al. Symptoms of depression and risk of new episodes of low back pain: A systematic review and meta-analysis. *Arthritis Care Res*. 2015;67(11):1591–1603.
7. Birgenheir DG, Ilgen MA, Bohnert AS, et al. Pain conditions among veterans with schizophrenia or bipolar disorder. *Gen Hosp Psychiatry*. 2013;35(5):480–484.
8. Engels G, Francke AL, van Meijel B, et al. Clinical pain in schizophrenia: A systematic review. *J Pain*. 2014;15(5):457–467.
9. Kishi T, Matsuda Y, Mukai T, et al. A cross-sectional survey to investigate the prevalence of pain in Japanese patients with major depressive disorder and schizophrenia. *Compr Psychiatry*. 2015;59:91–97.
10. Jochum T, Letzsch A, Greiner W, Wagner G, Sauer H, Bar KJ. Influence of antipsychotic medication on pain perception in schizophrenia. *Psychiatry Res*. 2006;142(2–3):151–156.
11. Guieu R, Samuelian JC, Coulouvrat H. Objective evaluation of pain perception in patients with schizophrenia. *Br J Psychiatry*. 1994;164(2):253–255.
12. de la Fuente-Sandoval C, Favila R, Gomez-Martin D, Leon-Ortiz P, Graff-Guerrero A. Neural response to experimental heat pain in stable patients with schizophrenia. *J Psychiatr Res*. 2012;46(1):128–134.
13. de la Fuente-Sandoval C, Favila R, Gomez-Martin D, Pellicer F, Graff-Guerrero A. Functional magnetic resonance imaging response to experimental pain in drug-free patients with schizophrenia. *Psychiatry Res*. 2010;183(2):99–104.
14. Stubbs B, Thompson T, Acaster S, Vancampfort D, Gaughran F, Correll CU. Decreased pain sensitivity among people with schizophrenia: A meta-analysis of experimental pain induction studies. *Pain*. 2015;156(11):2121–2131.
15. Potvin S, Marchand S. Hypoalgesia in schizophrenia is independent of antipsychotic drugs: A systematic quantitative review of experimental studies. *Pain*. 2008;138(1):70–78.
16. Stubbs B, Mitchell AJ, De Hert M, et al. The prevalence and moderators of clinical pain in people with schizophrenia: A systematic review and large scale meta-analysis. *Schizophr Res*. 2014;160(1–3):1–8.
17. Kim DJ, Mirmina J, Narine S, et al. Altered physical pain processing in different psychiatric conditions. *Neurosci Biobehav Rev*. 2022;133:104510.
18. Stubbs B, Eggermont L, Mitchell AJ, et al. The prevalence of pain in bipolar disorder: A systematic review and large-scale meta-analysis. *Acta Psychiatr Scand*. 2015;131(2):75–88.

19. Nicholl BI, Mackay D, Cullen B, et al. Chronic multisite pain in major depression and bipolar disorder: Cross-sectional study of 149,611 participants in UK Biobank. *BMC Psychiatry.* 2014;14: Article 350.
20. Owen-Smith A, Stewart C, Sesay MM, et al. Chronic pain diagnoses and opioid dispensings among insured individuals with serious mental illness. *BMC Psychiatry.* 2020;20(1):Article 40.
21. Bahorik AL, Satre DD, Kline-Simon AH, Weisner CM, Campbell CI. Serious mental illness and medical comorbidities: Findings from an integrated health care system. *J Psychosom Res.* 2017;100:35–45.
22. Risch N, Dubois J, M'Bailara K, et al. Self-reported pain and emotional reactivity in bipolar disorder: A prospective FACE-BD study. *J Clin Med.* 2022;11(3): Article 893.
23. Travaglini LE, Kuykendall L, Bennett ME, Abel EA, Lucksted A. Relationships between chronic pain and mood symptoms among veterans with bipolar disorder. *J Affect Disord.* 2020;277:765–771.
24. Minichino A, Delle Chiaie R, Cruccu G, et al. Pain-processing abnormalities in bipolar I disorder, bipolar II disorder, and schizophrenia: A novel trait marker for psychosis proneness and functional outcome? *Bipolar Disord.* 2016;18(7):591–601.
25. McIntyre RS, Konarski JZ, Wilkins K, Bouffard B, Soczynska JK, Kennedy SH. The prevalence and impact of migraine headache in bipolar disorder: Results from the Canadian Community Health Survey. *Headache.* 2006;46(6):973–982.
26. Oedegaard KJ, Fasmer OB. Is migraine in unipolar depressed patients a bipolar spectrum trait? *J Affect Disord.* 2005;84(2–3):233–242.
27. Nemeroff CB. Prevalence and management of treatment-resistant depression. *J Clin Psychiatry.* 2007;68(Suppl 8):17–25.
28. Mrazek DA, Hornberger JC, Altar CA, Degtiar I. A review of the clinical, economic, and societal burden of treatment-resistant depression: 1996–2013. *Psychiatr Serv.* 2014;65(8):977–987.
29. Cepeda MS, Reps J, Ryan P. Finding factors that predict treatment-resistant depression: Results of a cohort study. *DepressAnxiety.* 2018;35(7):668–673.
30. Bair MJ, Robinson RL, Eckert GJ, Stang PE, Croghan TW, Kroenke K. Impact of pain on depression treatment response in primary care. *Psychosom Med.* 2004;66(1):17–22.
31. Stubbs B, Gardner-Sood P, Smith S, et al. Pain is independently associated with reduced health related quality of life in people with psychosis. *Psychiatry Res.* 2015;230(2):585–591.
32. Snow AL, Shuster JL Jr. Assessment and treatment of persistent pain in persons with cognitive and communicative impairment. *J Clin Psychol.* 2006;62(11):1379–1387.
33. Bonnot O, Anderson GM, Cohen D, Willer JC, Tordjman S. Are patients with schizophrenia insensitive to pain? A reconsideration of the question. *Clin J Pain.* 2009;25(3):244–252.
34. Kuritzky A, Mazeh D, Levi A. Headache in schizophrenic patients: A controlled study. *Cephalalgia.* 1999;19(8):725–727.
35. Wells N, Pasero C, McCaffery M. Improving the quality of care through pain assessment and management. In: Hughes RG, ed. *Patient Safety and Quality: An Evidence-Based Handbook for Nurses.* Agency for Healthcare Research and Quality; 2008:1–48.
36. Phelan M, Stradins L, Morrison S. Physical health of people with severe mental illness. *BMJ.* 2001;322(7284):443–444.
37. Dickerson FB, Brown CH, Daumit GL, et al. Health status of individuals with serious mental illness. *Schizophr Bull.* 2006;32(3):584–589.
38. Fleischhacker WW, Cetkovich-Bakmas M, De Hert M, et al. Comorbid somatic illnesses in patients with severe mental disorders: Clinical, policy, and research challenges. *J Clin Psychiatry.* 2008;69(4):514–519.
39. Heald A. Physical health in schizophrenia: A challenge for antipsychotic therapy. *Eur Psychiatry.* 2010;25(Suppl 2):S6–S11.
40. Melamed OC, Fernando I, Soklaridis S, Hahn MK, LeMessurier KW, Taylor VH. Understanding engagement with a physical health service: A qualitative study of patients with severe mental illness. *Can J Psychiatry.* 2019;64(12):872–880.

41. Lawrence D, Kisely S. Inequalities in healthcare provision for people with severe mental illness. *J Psychopharmacol.* 2010;24(4 Suppl):61–68.
42. Mitchell AJ, Malone D, Doebbeling CC. Quality of medical care for people with and without comorbid mental illness and substance misuse: Systematic review of comparative studies. *Br J Psychiatry.* 2009;194(6):491–499.
43. Naushad N, Dunn LB, Munoz RF, Leykin Y. Depression increases subjective stigma of chronic pain. *J Affect Disord.* 2018;229:456–462.
44. Leventhal H, Ethan H, Horowitz C, Leventhal E, Ozakinci G. Living with chronic illness: A contextualized, self-regulation approach. In: Sutton S, Baum A, Johnston M, eds. *The SAGE Handbook of Health Psychology.* SAGE; 2004:197–240.
45. Earnshaw VA, Quinn DM. The impact of stigma in healthcare on people living with chronic illnesses. *J Health Psychol.* 2012;17(2):157–168.
46. Barney LJ, Griffiths KM, Jorm AF, Christensen H. Stigma about depression and its impact on help-seeking intentions. *Aust N Z J Psychiatry.* 2006;40(1):51–54.
47. Clement S, Schauman O, Graham T, et al. What is the impact of mental health-related stigma on help-seeking? A systematic review of quantitative and qualitative studies. *Psychol Med.* 2015;45(1):11–27.
48. Coleman KJ, Stewart C, Waitzfelder BE, et al. Racial–ethnic differences in psychiatric diagnoses and treatment across 11 health care systems in the mental health research network. *Psychiatr Serv.* 2016;67(7):749–757.
49. Piel FB, Steinberg MH, Rees DC. Sickle cell disease. *N Engl J Med.* 2017;376(16):1561–1573.
50. Solberg Nes L, Roach AR, Segerstrom SC. Executive functions, self-regulation, and chronic pain: A review. *Ann Behav Med.* 2009;37(2):173–183.
51. Fernandez E, Turk DC. The scope and significance of anger in the experience of chronic pain. *Pain.* 1995;61(2):165–175.
52. Brennan F, Carr DB, Cousins M. Pain management: A fundamental human right. *Anesth Analg.* 2007;105(1):205–221.
53. Mueser K, Tarrier N. *Handbook of Social Functioning in Schizophrenia.* Allyn & Bacon; 1998.
54. Albert M, Becker T, McCrone P, Thornicroft G. Social networks and mental health service utilisation: A literature review. *Int J Soc Psychiatry.* 1998;44(4):248–266.
55. Klug G. Change in social networks due to psychoses. *Fortschr Neurol Psyc.* 2005;73:S66–S73.
56. Nelson GM, Beach SR. Sequential interaction in depression: Effects of depressive behaviour on spouse aggression. *Behav Ther.* 1990;21:167–182.
57. Whisman MA. Marital dissatisfaction and psychiatric disorders: Results from the National Comorbidity Survey. *J Abnorm Psychol.* 1999;108(4):701–706.
58. Saunders JC. Families living with severe mental illness: A literature review. *Issues Ment Health Nurs.* 2003;24(2):175–198.
59. Fiane I, Haugland ME, Stovner LJ, Zwart JA, Bovim G, Hagen K. Sick leave is related to frequencies of migraine and non-migrainous headache: The HUNT Study. *Cephalalgia.* 2006;26(8):960–967.
60. Clarke CE, MacMillan L, Sondhi S, Wells NE. Economic and social impact of migraine. *QJM.* 1996;89(1):77–84.
61. Hu XH, Markson LE, Lipton RB, Stewart WF, Berger ML. Burden of migraine in the United States: Disability and economic costs. *Arch Intern Med.* 1999;159(8):813–818.
62. Patel AS, Farquharson R, Carroll D, et al. The impact and burden of chronic pain in the workplace: A qualitative systematic review. *Pain Pract.* 2012;12(7):578–589.
63. Duquesnoy B, Allaert FA, Verdoncq B. Psychosocial and occupational impact of chronic low back pain. *Rev Rhum Engl Ed.* 1998;65(1):33–40.
64. Latham J, Davis BD. The socioeconomic impact of chronic pain. *Disabil Rehabil.* 1994;16(1):39–44.
65. Maetzel A, Li L. The economic burden of low back pain: A review of studies published between 1996 and 2001. *Best Pract Res Clin Rheumatol.* 2002;16(1):23–30.
66. Braden JB, Zhang L, Zimmerman FJ, Sullivan MD. Employment outcomes of persons with a mental disorder and comorbid chronic pain. *Psychiatr Serv.* 2008;59(8):878–885.

67. Hirschfeld RM, Calabrese JR, Weissman MM, et al. Screening for bipolar disorder in the community. *J Clin Psychiatry.* 2003;64(1):53–59.
68. Onwumere J, Stubbs B, Stirling M, et al. Pain management in people with severe mental illness: An agenda for progress. *Pain.* 2022;163(9):1653–1660.
69. Cooke BK, Magas LT, Virgo KS, Feinberg B, Adityanjee A, Johnson FE. Appendectomy for appendicitis in patients with schizophrenia. *Am J Surg.* 2007;193(1):41–48.
70. Firth J, Siddiqi N, Koyanagi A, et al. The Lancet Psychiatry Commission: A blueprint for protecting physical health in people with mental illness. *Lancet Psychiatry.* 2019;6(8):675–712.
71. Solmi M, Fiedorowicz J, Poddighe L, et al. Disparities in screening and treatment of cardiovascular diseases in patients with mental disorders across the world: Systematic review and meta-analysis of 47 observational studies. *Am J Psychiatry.* 2021;178(9):793–803.
72. Ratcliffe GE, Enns MW, Belik SL, Sareen J. Chronic pain conditions and suicidal ideation and suicide attempts: An epidemiologic perspective. *Clin J Pain.* 2008;24(3):204–210.
73. Kroenke K, Shen J, Oxman TE, Williams JW Jr, Dietrich AJ. Impact of pain on the outcomes of depression treatment: Results from the RESPECT trial. *Pain.* 2008;134(1–2):209–215.
74. Rathod S, Kingdon D, Weiden P, Turkington D. Cognitive–behavioral therapy for medication-resistant schizophrenia: A review. *J Psychiatr Pract.* 2008;14(1):22–33.
75. Rector NA, Beck AT. Cognitive behavioral therapy for schizophrenia: An empirical review. *J Nerv Ment Dis.* 2001;189(5):278–287.
76. Turkington D, Dudley R, Warman DM, Beck AT. Cognitive–behavioral therapy for schizophrenia: A review. *J Psychiatr Pract.* 2004;10(1):5–16.
77. Chiang KJ, Tsai JC, Liu D, Lin CH, Chiu HL, Chou KR. Efficacy of cognitive–behavioral therapy in patients with bipolar disorder: A meta-analysis of randomized controlled trials. *PLoS One.* 2017;12(5):e0176849.
78. Eccleston C, Hearn L, Williams AC. Psychological therapies for the management of chronic neuropathic pain in adults. *Cochrane Database Syst Rev.* 2015;2015(10):CD011259.
79. Eccleston C, Palermo TM, Williams AC, et al. Psychological therapies for the management of chronic and recurrent pain in children and adolescents. *Cochrane Database Syst Rev.* 2012;12:CD003968.
80. Eccleston C, Williams AC, Morley S. Psychological therapies for the management of chronic pain (excluding headache) in adults. *Cochrane Database Syst Rev.* 2009;(2):CD007407.
81. Tang NKY. Cognitive behavioural therapy in pain and psychological disorders: Towards a hybrid future. *Prog Neuropsychopharmacol Biol Psychiatry.* 2018;87(Pt B):281–289.
82. Sutherland AM, Nicholls J, Bao J, Clarke H. Overlaps in pharmacology for the treatment of chronic pain and mental health disorders. *Prog Neuropsychopharmacol Biol Psychiatry.* 2018;87(Pt B):290–297.
83. Liebschutz JM, Saitz R, Weiss RD, et al. Clinical factors associated with prescription drug use disorder in urban primary care patients with chronic pain. *J Pain.* 2010;11(11):1047–1055.
84. Wasan AD, Butler SF, Budman SH, Benoit C, Fernandez K, Jamison RN. Psychiatric history and psychologic adjustment as risk factors for aberrant drug-related behavior among patients with chronic pain. *Clin J Pain.* 2007;23(4):307–315.
85. Coronado B, Dunn J, Veronin MA, Reinert JP. Efficacy and safety considerations with second-generation antipsychotics as adjunctive analgesics: A review of literature. *J Pharm Technol.* 2021;37(4):202–208.
86. Fishbain DA, Cutler RB, Lewis J, Cole B, Rosomoff RS, Rosomoff HL. Do the second-generation "atypical neuroleptics" have analgesic properties? A structured evidence-based review. *Pain Med.* 2004;5(4):359–365.
87. Morgan CJA, Curran HV. Ketamine use: A review. *Addiction.* 2012;107(1):27–38.
88. Bahji A, Vazquez GH, Zarate CA Jr. Comparative efficacy of racemic ketamine and esketamine for depression: A systematic review and meta-analysis. *J Affect Disord.* 2021;278:542–555.
89. McIntyre RS, Rosenblat JD, Nemeroff CB, et al. Synthesizing the evidence for ketamine and esketamine in treatment-resistant depression: An international expert opinion on the available evidence and implementation. *Am J Psychiatry.* 2021;178(5):383–399.

90. Xiong J, Lipsitz O, Chen-Li D, et al. The acute antisuicidal effects of single-dose intravenous ketamine and intranasal esketamine in individuals with major depression and bipolar disorders: A systematic review and meta-analysis. *J Psychiatr Res.* 2021;134:57–68.
91. Beck K, Hindley G, Borgan F, et al. Association of ketamine with psychiatric symptoms and implications for its therapeutic use and for understanding schizophrenia: A systematic review and meta-analysis. *JAMA Netw Open.* 2020;3(5):e204693.
92. Boyaji S, Merkow J, Elman RNM, Kaye AD, Yong RJ, Urman RD. The role of cannabidiol (CBD) in chronic pain management: An assessment of current evidence. *Curr Pain Headache Rep.* 2020;24(2): Article 4.
93. Urits I, Gress K, Charipova K, et al. Use of cannabidiol (CBD) for the treatment of chronic pain. *Best Prac Res Clin Anaesthesiol.* 2020;34(3):463–477.
94. Mohiuddin M, Blyth FM, Degenhardt L, et al. General risks of harm with cannabinoids, cannabis, and cannabis-based medicine possibly relevant to patients receiving these for pain management: An overview of systematic reviews. *Pain.* 2021;162(Suppl 1):S80–S96.
95. Harris JI, Hanson D, Leskela J, et al. Reconsidering research exclusion for serious mental illness: Ethical principles, current status, and recommendations. *J Psychiatr Res.* 2021;143:138–143.
96. Bradley L, Bennett PC. Companion-animals' effectiveness in managing chronic pain in adult community members. *Anthrozoos.* 2015;28(4):635–647.
97. Baranoff J, Hanrahan S, Burke A, Connor J. Changes in acceptance in a low-intensity, group-based acceptance and commitment therapy (ACT) chronic pain intervention. *Int J Behav Med.* 2016;23(1):30–38.
98. Montgomery KL, Kim JS, Franklin C. Acceptance and commitment therapy for psychological and physiological illnesses: A systematic review for social workers. *Health Social Work.* 2011;36(3):169–181.
99. Cieślik B, Mazurek J, Rutkowski S, Kiper P, Turolla A, Szczepańska-Gieracha J. Virtual reality in psychiatric disorders: A systematic review of reviews. *Complement Ther Med.* 2020;52:102480.
100. Fregni F, El-Hagrassy MM, Pacheco-Barrios K, et al. Evidence-based guidelines and secondary meta-analysis for the use of transcranial direct current stimulation in neurological and psychiatric disorders. *Int J Neuropsychopharmacol.* 2021;24(4):256–313.
101. Janice Jimenez-Torres G, Weinstein BL, Walker CR, et al. A study protocol for a single-blind, randomized controlled trial of adjunctive transcranial direct current stimulation (tDCS) for chronic pain among patients receiving specialized, inpatient multimodal pain management. *Contemp Clin Trials.* 2017;54:36–47.
102. Pridmore S, Oberoi G, Marcolin M, George M. Transcranial magnetic stimulation and chronic pain: Current status. *Australas Psychiatry.* 2005;13(3):258–265.
103. Giamberardino MA, Affaitati G, Curto M, Negro A, Costantini R, Martelletti P. Anti-CGRP monoclonal antibodies in migraine: Current perspectives. *Intern Emerg Med.* 2016;11(8):1045–1057.
104. Gorp EJ, Eldabe S, Slavin KV, et al. Peripheral nerve field stimulation for chronic back pain: Therapy outcome predictive factors. *Pain Practice.* 2020;20(5):522–533.
105. Hilton L, Hempel S, Ewing B, et al. Mindfulness meditation for chronic pain: Systematic review and meta-analysis. *Ann Behav Med.* 2017;51(2):199–213.
106. Parra-Delgado M, Latorre-Postigo J. Effectiveness of mindfullness-based cognitive therapy in the treatment of fibromyalgia: A randomised trial. *Cognit Ther Res.* 2013;37(5):1015–1026.

23
Cancer Pain

Shuran Ma and Sandy Christiansen

Introduction

Pain is a common symptom of cancer, with a prevalence of 52–86%.[1] In fact, 62% of patients reporting to the emergency room for cancer-related symptoms reported pain as their primary concern.[2] All stages of cancer may be associated with pain, but pain is most prevalent in patients with metastatic disease. Up to one-third of surveyed oncology patients report moderate to severe pain with impairment of daily function.[1]

Certain types of cancer are associated with pain more than other types (Figure 23.1). For example, studies report head and neck cancers as well as bone cancers to be painful in up to 51–88% of patients.[1] On the contrary, leukemia is less commonly associated with pain and is reported in 5–66% of patients.[3,4]

The pathophysiology of cancer-related pain is complex because it may be associated with tumor invasion, compression and expansion of structures, as well as the oncological treatment.[5] Second, there is evidence that cancer creates an inflammatory state by release of various cytokines that promote both peripheral and central sensitization to pain.[6] Third, the patient may also have chronic pain prior to the diagnosis of cancer-related pain, which may further complicate treatment. For example, patients who have been on chronic opioid therapy for non-cancer pain may have developed tolerance or opioid-induced hyperalgesia, thus complicating opioid treatment for cancer pain.

Despite these challenges, it is critically important to control cancer-related pain because even moderate pain scores (visual analog scale [VAS] = 5–7) disrupt quality of life.[7] At severe levels (VAS >7), pain becomes the primary focus of the patient's life. Furthermore, the presence of cancer-related pain causes significant psychological distress not only to the patient but also to the supporting family members. Last, as advancements in oncological therapies have prolonged survival, more patients are likely to have chronic cancer-related pain, such as chemotherapy and radiation-induced neuropathic pain.

Disparity of Care in Cancer Pain

Despite the advancements in cancer-related pain treatment, specific populations remain vulnerable to inadequate pain management and thus reduced quality of life. Patients often have multiple reasons for vulnerability. For instance, extremes of age may limit access to care by nature of dependency on caretakers.[6] Researchers have found that racial minorities are more likely than Caucasians to be of a lower socioeconomic status, and

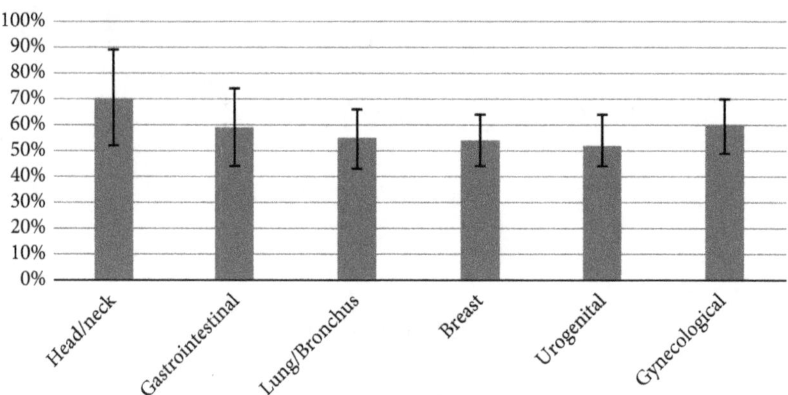

Figure 23.1 Prevalence of cancer pain by cancer type. Error bars depict 95% confidence intervals. The total sample included 3,300 patients, with exclusion of patients cured of cancer.

Adapted with permission from van den Beuken-van Everdingen et al.[1]

both race and low-income vulnerabilities are independently associated with increased cancer-related morbidity. This chapter examines several of these vulnerabilities in detail and proposes remediation strategies as they relate to the treatment of cancer-related pain.

Age

Pediatric Patients

Young age is a health care vulnerability and thus an important consideration when providing cancer-related pain care. Young children may be (1) unable to describe their level of pain, (2) unlikely to understand and make independent decisions related to their care process, and (3) dependent on their caretakers to manage their medications and treatments.

The treatment for pediatric cancer has improved dramatically in the past decade, and as such, 80% of pediatric cancer patients have a prognosis of 5 years or longer.[8] Pain associated with pediatric cancers can last from the time of diagnosis through survivorship. The most commonly reported cancer pain source is secondary to active oncological treatments, such as chemotherapy, radiation, or surgery (79.7%). The second most common source of pain occurs from procedures, such as blood draws. At the end of life, the most commonly reported cancer-related symptom in children is pain.[9] Even when cured, up to 60% of survivors report ongoing chronic pain.

Children with active cancer report heightened pain and distress caused by recurrent diagnostic and therapeutic procedures, such as bone marrow aspiration, lumbar puncture, and intravenous line placement. In fact, compared to adults, children are more likely to become increasingly anxious with repeat procedures.[10] If a physician or health care provider fails to treat a child's procedural pain, it could lead to significant psychological stress to both the child and caregivers. However, although there is limited evidence that pharmacological interventions can reduce the psychological aftereffects of recurrent procedures, cognitive–behavioral therapy is efficacious.[11]

In terms of assessing pain levels in this vulnerable population, physicians and other health care providers may observe behavior and physiologic measures, such as heart rate and blood pressure. However, even when clinicians diagnose pain, it is challenging and sometimes impossible to differentiate between neuropathic and nociceptive pain, which have different treatment strategies. Whereas opioid medications may be helpful for nociceptive pain, neuropathic pain may respond better to neuromodulators such as gabapentin. Neuropathic pain is present in 30–40% of pediatric cancer patients, and thus providers should consider neuropathic pain treatments, particularly in patients who are not responding to opioids.[8]

In addition, although opioids remain standard of care for moderate to severe cancer pain in children, it is important to note that children may have altered metabolism for this class of medications. Codeine, for example, is converted to morphine by the CYP2D6 enzyme. Children who have slow CYP2D6 metabolism may achieve limited pain relief, whereas those with rapid CYP2D6 metabolism are at risk of overdose.[12] Similarly, neonates have an overall immature hepatic metabolism, which increases the half-life of all hepatically cleared medications.[12]

Another medication challenge for pediatric oncology patients relates to transitioning from pain medication hospital regimens to home regimens. Pain at home may be more difficult to control because it is less likely to be procedure related and thus more difficult to anticipate the optimal timing of medication administration. Furthermore, many caregivers report not feeling confident with their ability to administer medications and express fear of potential side effects and addiction. Parents who report feeling less confident in their abilities to treat pain often report a higher pain score for their child,[8] which may be secondary to restricting medication administration.[12]

Finally, pediatric survivors of cancer often experience chronic pain as a complication of surgical and oncological treatments. In one study that compared adult survivors of pediatric cancers to their cancer-free siblings, the survivors were more likely to report pain and frequent headaches.[13] Furthermore, 17.9% of survivors reported using prescription analgesics compared to 12.6% of siblings.[13]

Geriatric Patients

In many ways, the geriatric population may face similar challenges as the pediatric population. Similar to young patients, elderly patients may be unable to (1) articulate their pain, (2) make informed decisions related to their care, and (3) independently manage their medications and treatments. However, unlike pediatric patients, cancer disproportionally affects geriatric patients because the median age of cancer diagnosis is 66 years, and the average age at death from cancer is 72 years. Elderly patients are also more sensitive to the side effects of medications and polypharmacy, and they are more likely to have multiple comorbidities and cognitive impairment complicating their pain care.

A study by Bernabei[14] found that 26% of elderly patients who reported having daily cancer-related pain received no analgesics. Furthermore, patients aged 85 years or older were less frequency prescribed opioids by 33% compared to patients aged 65–74 years. Despite these findings, no study to date has indicated that elderly patients have physiologic changes leading to decreased pain perception. On the contrary, older adults may experience more pain than younger people.[15]

Rather than decreased pain perception, underreporting of pain is more likely to explain suboptimal pain care in the elderly population. The presence of multiple medical problems, cognitive impairment, and depression may all contribute to underreporting of pain.[16] Furthermore, elderly patients may be less likely to report pain because they perceive pain as concomitant with aging and thus a normal life experience. The relationship between cognitive impairment and pain reporting is controversial because some studies suggest a connection, whereas others refute such a link.[16,17] With regard to depression, some evidence suggests that depression is related to a hypersensitivity to pain, whereas other studies connect depression with underreporting.[17]

When cancer pain is not treated, it can lead to depression and physical deconditioning, which in turn puts these patients at an increased risk of falls and subsequent morbidity.[15] The sleep disturbances caused by pain may also exacerbate cognitive decline. As such, it is important that clinicians recognize the specific vulnerabilities of the older adult population and develop multimodal treatment plans to address their cancer-related pain. The combination of medications, interventions, and complementary therapies may enable elderly patients to have improved pain control, thus limiting their sole reliance on medications, which may lead to polypharmacy and subsequent cognitive, sedative, gastrointestinal, and other side effects.

Race

Having a cultural understanding of perceptions and attitudes related to cancer and cancer pain is important in designing an appropriate treatment plan. Non-Caucasian cultures may be more or less likely to (1) report their pain, (2) fear medication side effects or addiction, and (3) prefer complementary therapies to manage pain. Failing to address individual culture beliefs may result in undertreatment of pain due to lack of recognition of strategies that are culturally acceptable for individual patients.

In a study by Crombez et al.,[18] racial minorities were more likely to "accept" their pain because they described pain as something they cannot control. However, even after adjustment for stage of cancer and comorbidities, Hispanic (49%) and Black (50%) people were more likely than Caucasians (33%) to report severe pain at the time of diagnosis. Similarly, although Chinese Americans report more frequent and intense pain, they are more likely to be satisfied with the pain care provided compared to Caucasians.[19] Interestingly, Chinese Americans who were more fluent in English were more likely to complain of poorly managed pain. Dhingra et al.[19] postulated that this result may be due to Chinese Americans' acclimatization to Western culture. Conversely, some Asian cultures associate "bad karma" with cancer and will often minimalize their pain because they fear worsening pain would reflect poorly on their moral character.[20]

According to a study by Vallerand et al.,[21] the African American community reports higher pain and distress levels, and lower functional status, compared to Caucasian patients. For instance, 42% of African American patients reported barriers to obtaining opiate pain medication, with 25% reporting a reluctance to prescribe by physicians.[22] In terms of taking pain medications, 25% of African Americans reported they never filled a prescribed opiate analgesic, and 42% filled the pain medication but never took it. The reasons given for not taking their medications were reported fear of opioid medications, not finding the medication useful, and spontaneous improvement of pain.[21]

Poverty, fear of addiction, and cultural stoicism are all common barriers to cancer pain care identified in qualitative studies of the Hispanic population.[23] In one study, 76% of Hispanic cancer patients agreed that they should "be strong and not lean on pain medication," and 71% were concerned about addiction.[23] Furthermore, more than 40% of Hispanic patients did not take their medications as prescribed, with the majority failing to take their analgesics around the clock, resulting in breakthrough pain. Similarly, patients from some developing countries, such as the Philippines, are also more likely to have a cultural stigma against opioids.

For those patients who are amenable to taking opiate pain medications, 29% of Hispanics reported the most common barriers to receiving pain medications as cost (6%) and limited availability of drugs (12%).[24] Racial minorities, in particular, may have difficulty obtaining prescribed opioids from their pharmacies because pharmacies located in minority neighborhoods reported a lower stock of opioid medications due to fear of break-ins and robberies.[25]

Patients across all cultural backgrounds are likely to use complementary/alternative medicine to control their cancer pain, especially if they are concerned about the side effects of more traditional medications, such as opioids. However, data are currently lacking on whether these alternative therapies are effective in controlling cancer pain. The studies that have been performed suggest that there might be some benefit to music therapy, acupuncture, reflexology, Chinese medicine, and cupping; however, the overall quality of evidence is low. One study found that sham or real acupuncture plus medication therapy was better than medication therapy alone.[26] However, there was no difference between sham acupuncture and real acupuncture. Nevertheless, the use of complimentary/alternative medicine for cancer pain is growing, and some modalities could be favored by various cultures.

Income

Low-income patients face similar hardships as racial minorities in terms of lack of access to health care and lower health care literacy.[27] Compared to patients of higher socioeconomic status, economically disadvantaged patients have a higher risk for (1) a diagnosis of cancer, (2) late cancer stage at time of diagnosis, and (3) more difficulty managing pain.[27] Furthermore, patients of lower socioeconomic status are more hesitant to engage with palliative care because they fear participation is equivalent to life-saving treatment. Lower health literacy is associated with higher levels of unmet informational needs and dissatisfaction with the information provided.

Many multimodal approaches for cancer pain are also unavailable to those of lower income, including interventions and complementary alternative medicine (CAM) therapies.[22] Those of lower socioeconomic status, however, utilize more no-cost therapies, such as prayer, deep breathing, and relaxation techniques. Many patients listed cost as a direct barrier to receiving CAM therapies, such as massage and chiropractic care.[22]

Likewise, insurance coverage is a major determinant of cancer care and pain control. For instance, women with high-deductible health insurance plans were more likely to experience delays in breast cancer diagnosis and treatment.[28] Although both low-income and high-income women with high-deductible health insurance waited longer than the control group, there were greater delays in the low-income group. Cancer patients with Medicaid were more likely to receive long-acting opioids, such as extended-release oxycodone and fentanyl patches, compared to patients who self-paid, and they were more likely to be prescribed lower doses of long-acting opioids or only short-acting opioids.[29] Prescribing short-acting opioids alone may lead to worse pain control in the self-pay population due to more peak-trough fluctuations in opioid plasma concentrations that lead to greater periods of inadequate pain control.

Low socioeconomic status also influences cancer treatment in the pediatric population. Pediatric cancer patients from lower socioeconomic groups are more likely to have disease recurrence and less likely to be compliant in their cancer care; they are also more likely to have a higher incidence of pain.[9] In addition, these patients are also more likely to report lower quality of life because of their symptoms and higher levels of stress. Similar to their adult counterparts, pediatric patients from low-income families are less likely to have access to opiates and be compliant with prescriptions for pain medications.

Access to Health Care

Populations in inner cities, rural areas, and developing countries may have (1) difficulties with access to comprehensive cancer pain care, (2) decreased access to educational resources for clinicians, and (3) barriers to obtaining recommended treatments.

Regarding access to health care, rural communities and developing countries may have limited public or affordable transportation options. For Americans living in rural areas of the country, transportation costs were reported as one of the highest barriers to receiving palliative care.[25] Globally, health care systems in many regions, such as South America, Africa, and Russia, simply do not offer palliative care.[30] Patients without access to these services have shorter survival times, more pain, and worse quality of life.

Even in areas of the world with regional cancer pain options, locally patients may experience a lack of hospitals with specialized pain physicians or other providers.[31] Rural pain specialists are also less likely to have access to educational resources because most in-person continued education programs occur in urban areas. However, since the start of the COVID-19 pandemic, there has been a substantial increase in availability of online, continued medical education content, which has improved accessibility for all physicians and providers.

There are knowledge gaps between the physicians and health care providers in high-income countries and those in low-income countries. In one study comparing physicians training in oncology, physiatry, and anesthesiology at academic institutions in Ghana to those training in the United States, 45.7% of the doctors in the United States felt competent in using opiate analgesics for pain compared to 29.5% in Ghana.[32] Yet, both groups of physicians considered treatment of cancer-related pain important or very important. Among the surveyed physicians, 50% of those in Ghana stated their training was inadequate for cancer-related pain compared to 44% of those in the United States. Both groups of doctors felt inadequate in their training in interventional pain procedures, palliative care, and managing procedural and postoperative pain. Interestingly, these specialists from the United States felt more uncomfortable managing palliative care needs. Physicians in Ghana, however, reported feeling more comfortable addressing palliative care needs; they likely developed more experience in palliative care from treating more patients with late-stage cancer diagnoses that led to palliative rather than curative measures.[32]

In terms of access to treatment, although cancer is more prevalent in developing nations, opioid prescriptions for pain are less common. In fact, only 15% of the world's population consumes 95% of the world's prescription opioids.[31] Furthermore, many countries have laws and regulations in place that create barriers to prescribing opioids. For example, in the Philippines, doctors have to pay for special prescription forms for opioids, and in China only tertiary hospitals dispense opioids.

In many underdeveloped countries, greater than 90% of patients will die with untreated pain. One hypothesis for untreated pain relates to the high cost of opiates. In a cost analysis of oral morphine in three countries—Uganda, Romania, and Chile—the cost ranged from $216 to $420 per year to achieve adequate pain control.[30]

Consequences of Disparities

The prevalence of chronic pain in cancer patients is almost double that of the general population in the United States.[33] Vulnerable populations are not only more likely to have cancer but also more likely to have untreated cancer-related pain.

Overall, children who have higher pain scores are more likely to have worse physical, emotional, and social health. In terms of pediatric oncology patients in particular, those with untreated cancer pain are more likely to be emotionally distressed, do worse in school, and have delayed social development, which can have long-term economic, social, and mental health implications.[34] They are also more likely to report disturbances in sleep; general fatigue; and cognitive fatigue that is associated with difficulty paying attention, remembering, and thinking.

Procedural pain can also be traumatic for both patients and caregivers, with long-lasting social and mental ramifications. In one study, 97% of children undergoing a bone marrow aspiration displayed signs of anxiety such as crying, rigidity, screaming, verbal expressions, and refusal of the procedure.[35] Furthermore, children do not appear to become less anxious with repeated procedures. Some of these children go on to develop depression and anxiety with skin rashes and insomnia. After the procedure, children can become withdrawn and embarrassed by their behavior. These children may develop fear of hospitals and medical staff and post-traumatic stress disorder.[13] Furthermore, adolescents and female children with cancer pain displayed larger disturbances in emotion and mood.[12] The non-cancer chronic pain literature has shown that mood and sleep disturbances can cyclically lead to worsening pain.[35] Adult survivors of pediatric cancers are more likely to experience pain compared to their siblings. Unfortunately, even as survival of cancer has increased globally, there has been a lack of proportional improvement in pain treatments for survivors.

When cancer pain is not adequately treated, it leads to negative effects on all aspects of a patient's quality of life, even in adult patients. This occurs regardless of the patient's cultural beliefs and coping strategies given that patients throughout the world have reported worsened sleep, appetite, mood, familial support, financial status, and enjoyment of life with increased pain.[4]

Due to limited access to health care, inexperienced caretakers may ultimately care for cancer patients. A Turkish study found that up to 62.6% of caregivers experienced health problems, 17.7% experienced hopelessness, and 16.8% experienced financial burden.[36] Caregivers were also more likely to experience pain compared to the general population.

Uncontrolled cancer pain also creates an economic burden, not only for the patients and their families but also for their health care systems. Cancer pain can incur three categories of costs: direct costs from medical care and rehabilitation, indirect costs from productivity loss, and psychological costs from reduced quality of life and suffering.[31] At MD Anderson Cancer Center, up to 14% of unscheduled admissions were for poorly controlled pain. Each stay averaged 10.5 days, with a cost of approximately $1,200 per day.[2] These challenges are especially difficult for vulnerable patients because they are more likely to have out-of-pocket expenses and have limited health insurance.

Solutions

World Health Organization

In 1986, the World Health Organization (WHO) created the WHO analgesic ladder to guide physicians on how to provide adequate pain relief for cancer patients (Figure 23.2). The ladder was part of a program that included educational campaigns, shared

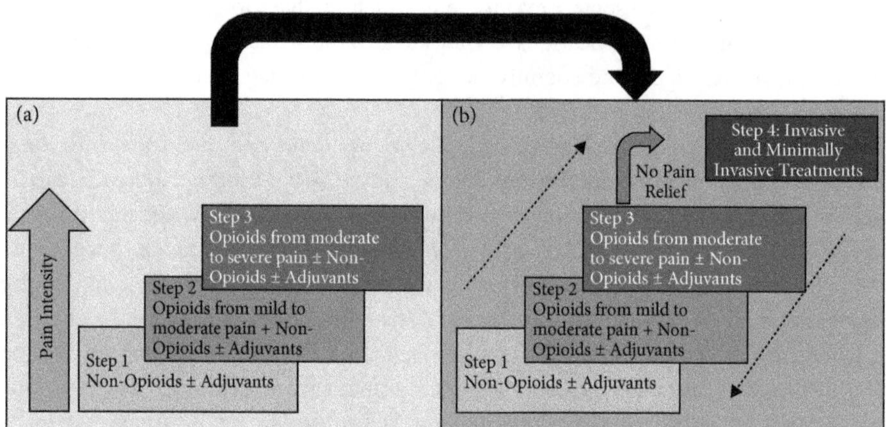

Figure 23.2 Revised WHO analgesic ladder. Transition from the original WHO three-step analgesic ladder (A) to the revised WHO four-step form (B). The additional Step 4 is an "interventional" step and includes invasive and minimally invasive techniques. This updated WHO ladder provides a bidirectional approach.

Reproduced from Anekar and Cascella.[38]

strategies, and a global network of support. Although the purpose of this strategy was to reduce untreated cancer-related pain, the utility of this initiative has been questioned because the WHO analgesic ladder does not differentiate between different types of pain (nociceptive vs. neuropathic) and does not elaborate on nonpharmacologic modalities to treat pain.[37] The benefit of the ladder, however, is that it provides a basic systematic approach to cancer-related pain that can be useful when physicians or other providers are unsure of the appropriate next steps.

Patient Education and Psychosocial Support

Patient education is effective in reducing cancer pain intensity.[11] Common barriers that patient education addresses are concerns about medication side effects, addiction potential, proper use of medication, nonmedical interventions, and attitudes about pain control. Research shows that patient education increases adherence to medication; however, it is not able to decrease reported side effects.[39] Although education does decrease pain, there does not appear to be a subsequent decrease in pain interference. These surprising findings may be because patients who benefit from education feel encouraged to report more medication side effects and pain interference. Interestingly, this review[39] demonstrated that education was able to decrease pain scores by 1 point on the 0–10 pain scale after 1 week of therapy, whereas acetaminophen and gabapentin prescriptions of 1 week were only able to decrease pain scores by 0.8 and 0.5 points, respectively.

Vulnerable populations more likely have low health care literacy, lower levels of education, and lower socioeconomic status.[25] Overall, minorities are less likely to have pain resolution with increased education.[40] These populations may benefit from intensive techniques, such as one-on-one coaching and longer session times. For example, one study of adults with cancer pain showed that the most effective educational interventions included face-to-face and lasted 30–60 min. The least successful interventions included 20-min video sessions and online support groups.[39]

Likewise, terminal cancer pain patients who have comorbid substance use disorders may also require tailored education. The recommended goal in palliative patients is to reduce substance use rather than complete cessation because complete cessation may be associated with heighten stress and subsequent relapse.[41]

Despite the benefit of education and psychosocial support, these interventions are not able to eliminate all barriers to care, such as the expense of medications and access to care.

Pain Inventory Scales

In many cultures, such as Asian and Hispanic cultures, there is a stigma associated with cancer pain that leads to decreased reporting of pain and decreased health-seeking behaviors.[19,23] Furthermore, non-White people express pain differently. For example, African American patients report more trouble with the numeric rating scores compared to the facial pain scales.[6] Comprehensive pain inventory scales, such as the

Brief Pain Inventory, may identify more cultural variants of expression of pain and are validated for cultures outside of the United States. As such, clinicians should consider more frequent use of inventory scales rather than rating scores.

Complementary Medicine

Those of diverse cultures may also be more reluctant to use traditional pain medications, such as opioids, because of cultural stigma attached to the medications. They instead may opt for complementary medicine strategies, such as traditional Chinese medicine or acupuncture. Although the literature is limited, Bao et al.[26] found that some therapies, such as acupuncture, in combination with Western medicine are superior to Western medicine alone. Although this benefit may be due to the placebo effect, physicians should consider recommending complementary alternative therapies, if available, and help patients identify these therapies in their community.

Automated Pain Interventions/Telehealth

Telehealth represents another solution for vulnerable cancer pain populations. For example, one study used an automated response system to assess the pain of low-income Black and Hispanic breast cancer patients for 8 weeks, and it found that patients were able to achieve better levels of pain control.[40] These patients would receive biweekly automated calls to assess their pain control and discuss any perceived barriers to pain care. If their pain was above a 5/10 or if they expressed any barriers, the researchers would send a message to their oncologist to address pain control, or a member of the research staff would contact the patient with information on how to overcome the barrier. Thus, employing these automated assessments of pain control may be a cost-effective strategy to help alert health care professionals of increased pain or perceived barriers.

Telehealth is an expanding area of health care, particularly since the start of the COVID-19 pandemic. Because many people in rural areas have limited access to palliative care, telehealth is one solution to expand care to these populations. One difficulty of assessing the value of telehealth relates to its many definitions, which encompass anything from phone calls or after-hour services to full video clinic visits.[42] However, despite the variations, the access to direct physician or provider care in otherwise remote locations is invaluable.

Telehealth also improves caregiver burden for patients receiving palliative care services. For example, one review found that telehealth with a caregiver was especially effective in decreasing caregiver anxiety; however, caregiver quality of life was not significantly influenced.[43] Caregivers who received telehealth visits endorsed less negative mood and perceived stress. Overall, the caregivers were satisfied with telehealth treatment. Given the novelty of telehealth, the future applications and impact require further research.

Telehealth presents possible limitations in that it may not be appropriate for all vulnerable populations. For example, patients who are in extreme age groups or those who do not speak the native language may be unable to navigate the technology to access the telehealth visit. Similarly, patients of low income may not have access to computers, telephones, or the internet, thus preventing them from participating in the telehealth visit.

Conclusion

It is critical that physicians and other health care providers appreciate barriers to appropriate cancer pain management in vulnerable populations. These vulnerabilities relate to extremes of age, race, income level, and access to health care. The awareness of barriers coupled with the recognition of solutions will help both physicians and patients overcome these obstacles.

Pediatric oncology patients are more likely to have undertreated pain because of their dependency on adult caregivers. Because they are less mature, they are also more likely to experience heightened anxiety from their cancer-related treatments. The consequence is a population at risk of long-term deleterious effects, including social withdrawal and poor school and job performance, which may persist into survivorship.

Older adults are more commonly diagnosed with cancer compared to the pediatric population and still face barriers to adequate pain management. These patients are more likely to have complex treatment plans due to multiple comorbidities and less likely to report their pain. Consequently, older adults with cancer are more likely to die with undertreated pain.

Different races may express varying beliefs and wishes regarding their cancer pain management. Across all races and cultures, it is important that clinicians appreciate poverty, fear of addiction, and cultural stoicism as factors that may influence an individual's pain treatment plan. Certain races may also be more open to complementary medicine strategies.

Last, both low income and lack of access to appropriate health care are independently associated with lack of cancer pain control. Patients with low income may be unable to afford certain cancer pain treatments. Similarly, patients who lack access to health care may be unable to establish care with experienced providers to manage their pain.

Failure to treat cancer-related pain is no longer acceptable and should be considered a first-line indicator of poor quality of medical care. Worsened sleep, appetite, mood, familial support, financial status, and enjoyment of life are all outcomes of poorly managed cancer pain that can further negatively influence cancer treatment.[15] By using pain inventory scales, tailored education and psychosocial support, telehealth tools, and complementary therapies, physicians and other health care providers can bridge the gaps in managing pain among these vulnerable populations of patients.

References

1. van den Beuken-van Everdingen MHJ, de Rijke JM, Kessels AG, Schouten HC, van Kleef M, Patijn J. Prevalence of pain in patients with cancer: A systematic review of the past 40 years. *Ann Oncol*. 2007;18(9):1437–1449. doi:10.1093/annonc/mdm056

2. Caterino JM, Adler D, Durham DD, et al. Analysis of diagnoses, symptoms, medications, and admissions among patients with cancer presenting to emergency departments. *JAMA Netw Open*. 2019;2(3):e190979. doi:10.1001/jamanetworkopen.2019.0979
3. Foley KM. Pain syndromes in patients with cancer. In: Swerdlow M, Ventafridda V, eds. Cancer Pain. Springer; 1987:45–54. doi:10.1007/978-94-010-9139-8_5
4. Breivik H, Cherny N, Collett B, et al. Cancer-related pain: A pan-European survey of prevalence, treatment, and patient attitudes. *Ann Oncol.* 2009;20(8):1420–1433. doi:10.1093/annonc/mdp001
5. Yoon SY, Oh J. Neuropathic cancer pain: Prevalence, pathophysiology, and management. *Korean J Intern Med.* 2018;33(6):1058–1069. doi:10.3904/kjim.2018.162
6. McNeill JA, Reynolds J, Ney ML. Unequal quality of cancer pain management: Disparity in perceived control and proposed solutions. *Oncol Nurs Forum.* 2007;34(6):1121–1128. doi:10.1188/07.ONF.1121-1128
7. Serlin RC, Mendoza TR, Nakamura Y, Edwards KR, Cleeland CS. When is cancer pain mild, moderate or severe? Grading pain severity by its interference with function. *Pain.* 1995;61(2):277–284. doi:10.1016/0304-3959(94)00178-H
8. Fortier MA, Wahi A, Bruce C, Maurer EL, Stevenson R. Pain management at home in children with cancer: A daily diary study. *Pediatr Blood Cancer.* 2014;61(6):1029–1033. doi:10.1002/pbc.24907
9. Ilowite MF, Al-Sayegh H, Ma C, et al. The relationship between household income and patient-reported symptom distress and quality of life in children with advanced cancer: A report from the PediQUEST study. *Cancer.* 2018;124(19):3934–3941. doi:10.1002/cncr.31668
10. Kuppenheimer WG, Brown RT. Painful procedures in pediatric cancer. *Clin Psychol Rev.* 2002;22(5):753–786. doi:10.1016/S0272-7358(02)00105-8
11. Lovell MR, Luckett T, Boyle FM, Phillips J, Agar M, Davidson PM. Patient education, coaching, and self-management for cancer pain. *J Clin Oncol.* 2014;32(16):1712–1720. doi:10.1200/JCO.2013.52.4850
12. Duffy EA, Dias N, Hendricks-Ferguson V, et al. Perspectives on cancer pain assessment and management in children. *Semin Oncol Nurs.* 2019;35(3):261–273. doi:10.1016/j.soncn.2019.04.007
13. Lu Q, Krull KR, Leisenring W, et al. Pain in long-term adult survivors of childhood cancers and their siblings: A report from the Childhood Cancer Survivor Study. *Pain.* 2011;152(11):2616–2624. doi:10.1016/j.pain.2011.08.006
14. Bernabei R. Management of pain in elderly patients with cancer. *JAMA.* 1998;279(23):1877. doi:10.1001/jama.279.23.1877
15. Sengstaken EA, King SA. The problems of pain and its detection among geriatric nursing home residents. *J Am Geriatr Soc.* 1993;41(5):541–544. doi:10.1111/j.1532-5415.1993.tb01892.x
16. Herr KA, Garand L. Assessment and measurement of pain in older adults. *Clin Geriatr Med.* 2001;17(3):457–478. doi:10.1016/S0749-0690(05)70080-X
17. Cohen-Mansfield J, Creedon M. Nursing staff members' perceptions of pain indicators in persons with severe dementia. *Clin J Pain.* 2002;18(1):64–73. doi:10.1097/00002508-200201000-00010
18. Crombez P, Bron D, Michiels S. Multicultural approaches of cancer pain. *Curr Opin Oncol.* 2019;31(4):268–274. doi:10.1097/CCO.0000000000000547
19. Dhingra L, Lam K, Homel P, et al. Pain in underserved community-dwelling Chinese American cancer patients: Demographic and medical correlates. *Oncologist.* 2011;16(4):523–533. doi:10.1634/theoncologist.2010-0330
20. Im EO, Liu Y, Kim YH, Chee W. Asian American cancer patients' pain experience. *Cancer Nurs.* 2008;31(3):E17–E23. doi:10.1097/01.NCC.0000305730.95839.83
21. Vallerand AH, Hasenau S, Templin T, Collins-Bohler D. Disparities between Black and White patients with cancer pain: The effect of perception of control over pain. *Pain Med.* 2005;6(3):242–250. doi:10.1111/j.1526-4637.2005.05038.x

22. Ludwick A, Corey K, Meghani S. Racial and socioeconomic factors associated with the use of complementary and alternative modalities for pain in cancer outpatients: An integrative review. *Pain Manag Nurs*. 2020;21(2):142–150. doi:10.1016/j.pmn.2019.08.005
23. Im EO, Guevara E, Chee W. The pain experience of Hispanic patients with cancer in the United States. *Oncol Nurs Forum*. 2007;34(4):861–868. doi:10.1188/07.ONF.861-868
24. Juarez G, Ferrell B, Borneman T. Influence of culture on cancer pain management in Hispanic patients. *Cancer Pract*. 1998;6(5):262–269. doi:10.1046/j.1523-5394.1998.00020.x
25. Anderson KO, Richman SP, Hurley J, et al. Cancer pain management among underserved minority outpatients. *Cancer*. 2002;94(8):2295–2304. doi:10.1002/cncr.10414
26. Bao Y, Kong X, Yang L, et al. Complementary and alternative medicine for cancer pain: An overview of systematic reviews. *Evid Based Complement Alternat Med*. 2014;2014:1–9. doi:10.1155/2014/170396
27. Lewis JM, DiGiacomo M, Currow DC, Davidson PM. Dying in the margins: Understanding palliative care and socioeconomic deprivation in the developed world. *J Pain Symptom Manage*. 2011;42(1):105–118. doi:10.1016/j.jpainsymman.2010.10.265
28. Wharam JF, Zhang F, Wallace J, et al. Vulnerable and less vulnerable women in high-deductible health plans experienced delayed breast cancer care. *Health Aff*. 2019;38(3):408–415. doi:10.1377/hlthaff.2018.05026
29. Bryan M, de La Rosa N, Hill AM, Amadio WJ, Wieder R. Influence of prescription benefits on reported pain in cancer patients. *Pain Med*. 2008;9(8):1148–1157. doi:10.1111/j.1526-4637.2008.00427.x
30. Are M, McIntyre A, Reddy S. Global disparities in cancer pain management and palliative care. *J Surg Oncol*. 2017;115(5):637–641. doi:10.1002/jso.24585
31. Li Z, Aninditha T, Griene B, et al. Burden of cancer pain in developing countries: A narrative literature review. *Clinicoecon Outcomes Res*. 2018;10:675–691. doi:10.2147/CEOR.S181192
32. Odonkor CA, Osei-Bonsu E, Tetteh O, Haig A, Mayer RS, Smith TJ. Minding the gaps in cancer pain management education: A multicenter study of clinical residents and fellows in a low- versus high-resource setting. *J Glob Oncol*. 2016;2(6):387–396. doi:10.1200/JGO.2015.003004
33. Jiang C, Wang H, Wang Q, Luo Y, Sidlow R, Han X. Prevalence of chronic pain and high-impact chronic pain in cancer survivors in the United States. *JAMA Oncol*. 2019;5(8):1224. doi:10.1001/jamaoncol.2019.1439
34. Schulte FSM, Patton M, Alberts NM, et al. Pain in long-term survivors of childhood cancer: A systematic review of the current state of knowledge and a call to action from the Children's Oncology Group. *Cancer*. 2021;127(1):35–44. doi:10.1002/cncr.33289
35. Katz ER, Kellerman J, Siegel SE. Behavioral distress in children with cancer undergoing medical procedures: Developmental considerations. *J Consult Clin Psychol*. 1980;48(3):356–365. doi:10.1037/0022-006X.48.3.356
36. Ovayolu N, Ovayolu Ö, Serçe S, Tuna D, Pirbudak Çöçelli L, Sevinç A. Pain and quality of life in Turkish cancer patients. *Nurs Health Sci*. 2013;15(4):437–443. doi:10.1111/nhs.12047
37. Yang J, Bauer BA, Wahner-Roedler DL, Chon TY, Xiao L. The modified WHO analgesic ladder: Is it appropriate for chronic non-cancer pain? *J Pain Res*. 2020;13:411–417. doi:10.2147/JPR.S244173
38. Anekar A, Cascella M. The revised WHO analgesic ladder. In: StatPearls. StatPearls Publishing; 2022.
39. Bennett MI, Bagnall AM, Closs JS. How effective are patient-based educational interventions in the management of cancer pain? Systematic review and meta-analysis. *Pain*. 2009;143(3):192–199. doi:10.1016/j.pain.2009.01.016
40. Anderson KO, Palos GR, Mendoza TR, et al. Automated pain intervention for underserved minority women with breast cancer. *Cancer*. 2015;121(11):1882–1890. doi:10.1002/cncr.29204
41. Passik SD, Theobald DE. Managing addiction in advanced cancer patients. *J Pain Symptom Manage*. 2000;19(3):229–234. doi:10.1016/S0885-3924(00)00109-3

42. Kidd L, Cayless S, Johnston B, Wengstrom Y. Telehealth in palliative care in the UK: A review of the evidence. *J Telemed Telecare*. 2010;16(7):394–402. doi:10.1258/jtt.2010.091108
43. Finucane AM, O'Donnell H, Lugton J, Gibson-Watt T, Swenson C, Pagliari C. Digital health interventions in palliative care: A systematic meta-review. *NPJ Digit Med*. 2021;4(1): Article 64. doi:10.1038/s41746-021-00430-7

24
Pain in Sickle Cell Disease

Siddika S. Mulchan, Megan Coco, and Donna Boruchov

Pathophysiology of Sickle Cell Pain

Sickle cell disease (SCD) is a group of genetic hemoglobin disorders that affect approximately 100,000 Americans, mostly of Black or African descent.[1] A mutation in the hemoglobin gene causes the red blood cell (RBC) to polymerize, or become a sickle shape, when deoxygenated. The effect of the polymerization causes the RBC to become more fragile and hemolyze, or break apart, triggering an inflammatory cascade and anemia. It also causes adherence of the RBC to other cells and vaso-occlusion. The vaso-occlusion and inflammation cause the hallmark pain associated with SCD.[2] Pain in SCD can begin in infancy and is unpredictable and severe.[3] Often, the pain requires emergency department (ED) utilization or hospitalization, and high rates of readmission exist in this patient population.[4] In addition, patients have frequent episodes of moderate pain managed at home. Pain in young children can greatly impair quality of life, including mood, sleep, school performance, and social development, and place them at risk for chronic pain conditions later in life.[4] Pain in SCD also leads to difficulties in adult life with advanced education and maintaining employment.

Complications in Sickle Cell Disease

Medical Complications

In addition to pain, patients with SCD are also at risk for many other physical problems because of the chronic hemolysis in their blood vessels.[5] Nearly every organ in the body can be affected. Patients are at greater risk of avascular necrosis of the large joints and skin ulcers. Nocturnal enuresis, kidney disease, and priapism are complications of the illness. People with SCD are at increased risk of life-threatening infections due to immunodeficiency. Acute chest syndrome is a leading cause of morbidity and mortality in both children and adults with SCD. Chronic lung disease as well as pulmonary hypertension and cardiac dysfunction can develop. The development of cholelithiasis, pancreatitis, and hepatopathy can complicate SCD.

Growth and sexual development are often delayed. Short stature and delayed puberty can be especially stressful for adolescent boys and can contribute to bullying and social stigmatization.[6] SCD affects the central nervous system with an increased risk of stroke and retinopathy.

Fatigue is also a significant symptom of SCD. Chronic anemia, hypoxemia inflammation, and sleep disruption all contribute to SCD fatigue.[7] The relationship between sleep, SCD pain, and fatigue is especially important. Valrie et al.[8] showed that greater daytime pain was related to poor sleep that night, which in turn was related to greater pain the following day. Ameringer and Smith[7] found a significant association between fatigue and anxiety and depression; the associations among 60 adolescents and young adults were moderate to strong.

Psychological Complications

Children with SCD are at risk for psychological dysfunction due to both their pain and medical complications.[6] Vasculopathy in the vessels of the brain can lead to stroke. By age 18 years, nearly 30% of children with SCD have had a silent or overt stroke, which can cause physical and cognitive challenges.[9] Executive function and memory are especially affected; this cognitive impairment, especially without overt physical signs, can pose a challenge in adolescence during the transition to adult care and have a major impact on adherence to medical care and function.[6]

Similar to other chronic pain conditions, SCD mutually exists with surrounding psychosocial factors.[10] Many studies have found higher rates of depression and anxiety in children and adolescents with greater frequency and intensity of SCD pain.[11] In their study of 75 children and adolescents, Graves et al.[12] found that overall there was a greater incidence of anxiety than in the general population and that quality of life scores were negatively associated with depression, anxiety, and school avoidance.

What Is the Evidence for Vulnerability?

Previous research has documented several vulnerability factors affecting health outcomes for individuals with SCD.[13] Vulnerability in health care has been defined as "being more likely to have one's interests unjustly considered."[14] Factors associated with vulnerability risk include financial resources, housing and location, health status, age, personal characteristics, functional or developmental considerations, effective communication ability, and the presence of a chronic illness or disability.[15] Vulnerable populations are likely to experience health disparities, where significant differences in disease incidence, prevalence, morbidity, mortality, and survival exist among specific groups compared to the general population.[16] As described above, patients with SCD are affected by both physiological and psychosocial vulnerabilities that can impact pain management and treatment.[10] Given the multiple vulnerability factors affecting patients with SCD, we propose a biopsychosocial (BPS) model for conceptualizing vulnerability of SCD pain.

A BPS model is the overarching framework to conceptualize pain in SCD. The BPS model was adapted from the widely used BPS approach to pain developed by Turk and Gatchel with additional input from Taylor and colleagues in the BPS-spiritual model for chronic SCD pain.[17,18] This model approaches pain from a holistic perspective, including the social, biological, psychological, and spiritual factors that contribute to the pain experience.

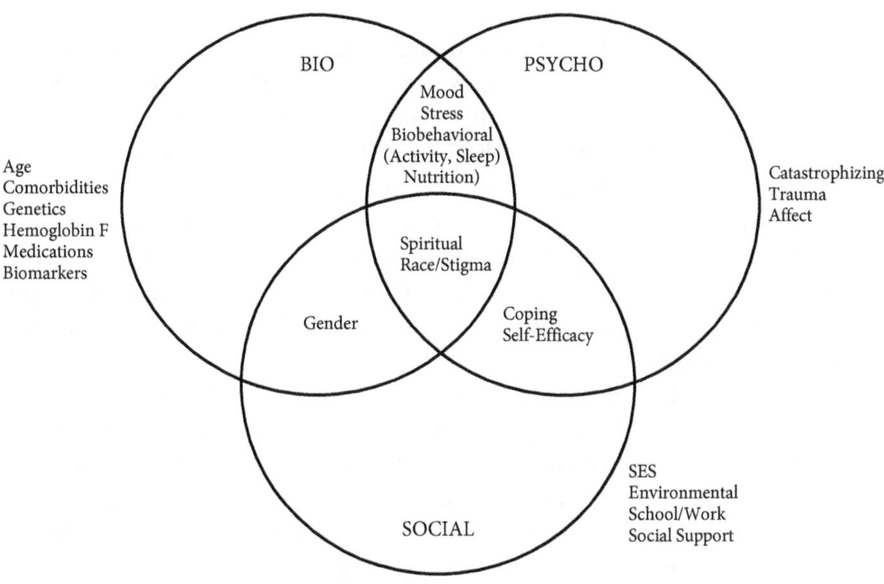

Biological

Biological factors include genetic predispositions, age, gender, and the central and peripheral processes in the nervous system as well as several physical comorbidities that are common in SCD. Genetic differences in SCD modify disease severity, leading to phenotypic diversity. Co-inheritance of α-thalassemia and persistence of hereditary fetal hemoglobin have both been described to ameliorate complications of SCD.

Psychological

The contribution of psychosocial factors to pain among patients with SCD has been well-documented.[19] These include sociodemographic variables, psychological functioning, and social determinants of health (SDoH).[10] Individuals with SCD are also at risk for psychological dysfunction due to neurocognitive impairment secondary to disease-related complications.[6] In addition to neurocognitive impairment, patients with SCD are also at risk of lower educational attainment due to missed school secondary to pain and other disease-related complications.[20] These psychological considerations increase this population's vulnerability when coupled with the stress of seeking pain treatment.[21]

Race and Perceived Injustice

Many social and political forces complicate pain care for patients with SCD. Patients with SCD are often people of color affected by health care disparities; this can create an imbalance between their health care providers who are typically White, middle class, and highly educated.[22] Race and ethnicity have been implicated in SCD pain and may affect pain treatment and clinical decision-making.[23,24] SCD predominantly affects Black, Latinx, Middle Eastern, and Mediterranean populations, and concerns for perceived discrimination, health-related stigma, and racial bias from health care providers and others in their community (school personnel, law enforcement officials, etc.) have been reported by patients with SCD and their families.[25–28] These experiences contribute to feelings of mistrust and may lead to poor adherence and negative health outcomes for individuals with SCD.[29,30] Inadequate communication between provider and patient is more likely if the patient's gender, race, or ethnicity is different from that of the provider.[22] It has been shown that health care providers often have an unconscious bias and negative attitude about SCD, pain, and use of opioids for the treatment of chronic nonmalignant pain.

Pack-Mabien et al.[31] studied the practices, knowledge, and attitudes of nurses in both the ED and medical surgical floor. The study found that nurses taking care of patients with SCD were frustrated, had difficulty understanding sickle cell pain, and overestimated addiction, even though the data do not support a high incidence of addiction among this population. Other researchers found that nurses have difficulty understanding the chronicity of sickle cell pain and sympathizing with patients when they do not fit the stereotypical sick role.[32] Jenerette et al.[33] measured ED, intensive care unit, and medical surgical nurses' attitudes and stigma toward patients with SCD, and they found that nurses had a less negative attitude when they judged that the patient had been using their pain medication appropriately. Providers (physicians, physician assistants, and nurse practitioners) can also have negative attitudes and beliefs toward patients with SCD and chronic pain.[34] Studies have documented that physician, physician assistant, and nurse practitioner attitudes were less negative than those of nurses, possibly due to the greater exposure nurses had to these patients.[34] These negative attitudes of nurses in the acute care setting can impact multiple aspects of a clinical encounter, including the assessment and delivery of pain medications, the patient–clinician relationship, and the health care experience of the patient.[33]

The attitudes and unconscious bias that providers have toward patients with SCD have many implications. For example, they have the potential to impact the delivery of pain medications to patients in the acute care setting. Patients may experience a delay in receiving needed pain medications or not receive the appropriate treatments at all due to attitudes and unconscious bias. These are also a considerable factor in the development of a trusting health care relationship. The resulting dysfunctional relationship that develops between the patient with SCD and the health care provider can further exacerbate an already complicated disease. If patients perceive that they have been stigmatized, whether based on race, ethnicity, social status, or disease, they may begin to delay seeking care for their pain.[33] Decreased access to health care and adherence to appropriate screening may lead to poorer outcomes and increased morbidity and mortality.

Many studies have examined the perceived injustice felt by patients with SCD. Haywood et al.[35] studied the experience of perceived race and disease-based injustice from health care providers. They found that patients had a greater burden of race-based discrimination than what had been reported in earlier studies. Surprisingly, they also found that disease-based discrimination was more prevalent, and for SCD patients reporting perceived disease-based injustice, there was an increase in the report of chronic pain, days of severe pain, and a decrease in "good" pain days. Ezenwa et al.[36] also showed that perceived injustice can lead to stress and pain in adults with SCD.

Opioid Crisis

In the United States, the opioid crisis has manifested with a marked increase in opioid addiction and overdose. There has been increased scrutiny and regulation of opioid prescribing practices, which inadvertently have had a negative effect on access to pain medications for SCD. The use of opioids in the management of SCD pain requires a comprehensive balance of the risks and benefits of opioid use in individual patients.[37] Care by a team familiar with the complexities of SCD is crucial.

Mood

Depression and anxiety in sickle cell patients are estimated to be very prevalent; rates of depression can range from 4% to 46%, with higher rates associated with increased disease severity.[38] In addition, Connolly et al.[39] found that patients with persistent pain reported lower health-related quality of life and decreased scores on neurocognitive tests. Youth with chronic pain also have higher levels of pain burden and disability, as well as more pain catastrophizing.[40]

Pain Catastrophizing

Catastrophizing is an exaggerated negative mental state seen in response to real or anticipated pain.[40] In response to pain, there is a heightened focus on pain, greater emotional response, and component of fear that in turn all amplify the pain experience. It is seen frequently in chronic pain states such as fibromyalgia and functional abdominal pain.[40] There is conflicting evidence regarding whether the phenomenon of catastrophizing contributes to SCD. Some studies have shown a modest correlation between pain but no correlation between adjustment disorder and mood and catastrophizing.[41] Interestingly, there has been an association between parental catastrophizing and children's pain and functional disability; for instance, Sil and colleagues[40] studied 100 youth with SCD and their parents and found that when youth had low scores on a pain catastrophizing scale, functional disability was decreased more if the parental catastrophizing score was high. Conversely, youth with high levels of catastrophizing had greater disability even if their parents had low levels on the same scale. Both findings show that there is an interaction occurring between parent and child that uniquely affects the ability of the youth to cope with pain that is independent of their own perceptions. Sil et al.'s findings also reinforce the need for a thorough family assessment of pain, functioning, and coping. Families can also affect coping based on their response to the child's distress, their ability to model coping behaviors, and the degree to which they can coach their child through stress.[42]

Coping and Adjustment in Sickle Cell Disease

Many patients with SCD live full and productive lives, although some have severe disease and incur high health care utilization. Both physical and psychological health can impact quality of life and functional ability of the patient with SCD. Often, the difference is how well the patient can process and cope with the many challenges of SCD.

According to Sarafino and Smith,[43] "coping is the process by which people try to manage the perceived discrepancy between the demands and resources they appraise in a stressful situation" (p. 113). Furthermore, the coping process is not a single event but, rather, a constant cognitive and behavioral negotiation with the environment.[43]

Coping can be grouped into emotion-focused and problem-focused along with behavioral and cognitive approaches. Emotion-focused coping controls the emotional response to the stressor. Behavioral approaches include seeking support; engaging in activities; and using stress management techniques such as relaxation, deep breathing, or yoga. Cognitive approaches include appraisals of the stressor and defense mechanisms such as denial or avoidance.[43] Finding the resources to cope with the stressor represents problem-focused coping, and it includes such approaches as seeking treatment and learning new skills.[43]

Self-Efficacy

To adapt and cope with SCD and prevent complications, patients need to promote positive health behaviors. Motivation and self-efficacy are important considerations in improving health behavior. Self-efficacy is the belief that one can achieve a certain health outcome.[44] Furthermore, it emphasizes the individuals' belief that they can exert control over their behaviors and internal and external environment.[44] Studies have shown that higher self-efficacy in patients with SCD is associated with improved coping, lower incidence of symptoms, and decreased pain intensity.[44]

Social Factors

Social factors increasing vulnerability among individuals with SCD include the high burden of SDoH in this population.[45] SDoH are defined as the conditions in which people work, live, and age and the wider systems shaping these conditions of daily life.[46] SDoH have been identified as "mostly responsible" for health inequities, which are systematic differences in the health status of different population groups.[46] Food insecurity, inadequate housing, and limited access to medication have been associated with worse health outcomes and a lower quality of life.[47,48] In fact, overall health outcomes may be more influenced by SDoH than medical care received.[49] SDoH, including structural racism and injustice, have been found to disproportionately affect people of color, including the SCD population.[45] As such, individuals with SCD experience vulnerabilities related to the intersection of their health status and racial identity. High rates of poverty and public health insurance have been associated with higher health care utilization, lower quality of life, and an increased risk of medical complications among youth with SCD.[50–52]

Vocational outcomes are another important social consideration for patients with SCD. A striking 25–60% of adults with SCD are unemployed.[53] Studies have documented several factors affecting these outcomes, including cognitive deficits, demographic variables (i.e., gender), perceived impact of SCD, and assertiveness. Specifically, lower IQ scores and educational attainment increased the odds of being unemployed, whereas female gender and a positive perception of SCD decreased the odds of being unemployed.[54] Employment is often critical for adults to access affordable health insurance in the United States; therefore, considering vocational rehabilitation services for patients with SCD should be a part of multidisciplinary care.

All of the above complications and characteristics associated with SCD have led to difficulty in access to medical and psychological care in both children and adults. In addition, funding of research for SCD and the development of novel therapies has been lacking in large part due to the economic disadvantage of persons with SCD.[55]

Remediation and Treatment

Remediation and treatment of pain in SCD utilize the overarching framework of the BPS model in improving the lives of people with SCD and their family and friends. It is crucial that physicians, medical providers, and caregivers care for the entire person—body, mind, and soul. Pain medications, including opioids, remain the mainstay of treatment for vaso-occlusive crises in conjunction with hydration and supportive care measures, including warmth, massage, distraction, and relaxation. Comprehensive sickle cell programs address the biological, psychological, and social factors that contribute to the pain experience. There is great hope for improvement in all of these factors in the upcoming years.

The most effective treatments for pain in SCD are those that prevent the painful complications of the disease. Clinical research for a cure for SCD is promising and now involves hematopoietic stem cell transplantation and gene therapy. In addition, medical treatments for SCD have advanced rapidly in the past decade with more therapeutics available as well as improvements in supportive care for complications. Hydroxyurea is routinely prescribed for all people with severe SCD beginning in infancy. It has been used for many years and decreases pain episodes. Voxelotor is a medication that inhibits hemoglobin S polymerization and reduces hemolysis to improve anemia. Crizanlizumab is an intravenous medication that is indicated to reduce the frequency of vaso-occlusive crises in patients aged 16 years or older. Both voxelotor and crizanlizumab were approved by the U.S. Food and Drug Administration in 2019. Clinicians continue to optimize their use in SCD.

Psychological care and support have also improved with an increase in mental health awareness and acceptance. Strategies promoting wellness are needed to begin at a young age and continue throughout the life span.

Socially, the stigma surrounding the pain of SCD must be eliminated, and many institutions are refocusing their efforts to address the specific needs of this population.

Currently, pain remains the hallmark of SCD. With advancements in the treatments of biological, psychological, and social factors, pain will diminish and the quality of life of people living with SCD will improve.

References

1. Centers for Disease Control and Prevention. Data & statistics on sickle cell disease. 2016. http://www.cdc.gov/ncbddd/sicklecell/data.html. Accessed March 8, 2023.
2. National Heart, Lung, and Blood Institute. Health topics. n.d. Accessed February 13, 2023. http://www.nhlbi.nih.gov/health/health-topics
3. Kavanagh PL, Fasipe TA, Wun T. Sickle cell disease. JAMA. 2022;328(1):57–68.
4. Dobson CE, Byrne MW. Original research: Using guided imagery to manage pain in young children with sickle cell disease. *Am J Nurs.* 2014;114(4):26–36.
5. Piel FB, Steinberg MH, Rees DC. Sickle cell disease. *N Engl J Med.* 2017;376(16):1561–1573.
6. Anie KA. Psychological complications in sickle cell disease. *Br J Haematol.* 2005;129(6):723–729.
7. Ameringer S, Smith WR. Emerging biobehavioral factors of fatigue in sickle cell disease. *J Nurs Scholarsh.* 2011;43(1):22–29.
8. Valrie CR, Gil KM, Redding-Lallinger R, Daeschner C. The influence of pain and stress on sleep in children with sickle cell disease. *Children's Health Care.* 2007;36(4):335–353.
9. Verduzco LA, Nathan DG. Sickle cell disease and stroke. *Blood.* 2009;114(25):5117–5125.
10. Edwards AL, Abbott RD. Relationships among the Edwards Personality Inventory Scales, the Edwards Personality Preference Schedule, and the Personality Research Form Scales. *J Consult Clin Psychol.* 1973;40(1):27–32.
11. Benton TD, Boyd R, Ifeagwu J, Feldtmose E, Smith-Whitley K. Psychiatric diagnosis in adolescents with sickle cell disease: A preliminary report. *Curr Psychiatry Rep.* 2011;13(2):111–115.
12. Graves JK, Hodge, C, Jacob, E. Depression, anxiety, and quality of life in children and adolescents with sickle cell disease. *Pediatr Nurs.* 2016;42(3):113–119.
13. Jenerette CM, Murdaugh C. Testing the theory of self-care management for sickle cell disease. *Res Nurs Health.* 2008;31(4):355–369.
14. Sossauer L, Schindler M, Hurst S. Vulnerability identified in clinical practice: A qualitative analysis. *BMC Med Ethics.* 2019;20(1): Article 87.
15. Dorsey CJ, Murdaugh, CL. The theory of self-care management for vulnerable populations. *J Theory Construct Test.* 2003;7(2):43–49.
16. Institute of Medicine (US) Committee on the Review and Assessment of the NIH's Strategic Research Plan and Budget to Reduce and Ultimately Eliminate Health Disparities; Thomson GE, Mitchell F, Williams MB, Eds. *Examining the Health Disparities Research Plan of the National Institutes of Health: Unfinished Business.* National Academies Press; 2006.
17. Taylor LEV, Stotts NA, Humphreys J, Treadwell MJ, Miaskowski C. A biopsychosocial-spiritual model of chronic pain in adults with sickle cell disease. *Pain Manag Nurs.* 2013;14(4):287–301.
18. Gatchel RJ, Peng YB, Peters ML, Fuchs PN, Turk DC. The biopsychosocial approach to chronic pain: Scientific advances and future directions. *Psychol Bull.* 2007;133(4):581–624.
19. Schlenz AM, Schatz J, Roberts CW. Examining biopsychosocial factors in relation to multiple pain features in pediatric sickle cell disease. *J Pediatr Psychol.* 2016;41(8):930–940.
20. Crosby LE, Joffe NE, Irwin MK, et al. School performance and disease interference in adolescents with sickle cell disease. *Phys Disabil.* 2015;34(1):14–30.
21. Mulchan SS, Hinderer KA, Walsh J, McCool A, Becker J. Feasibility and use of a transition process planning and communication tool among multiple subspecialties within a pediatric health system. *J Spec Pediatr Nurs.* 2022;27(1):e12355.

22. Todd KH, Green C, Bonham VL, Haywood C, Ivy E. Sickle cell disease related pain: Crisis and conflict. *J Pain*. 2006;7(7):453–458.
23. Mathur VA, Kiley KB, Carroll CP, et al. Disease-related, nondisease-related, and situational catastrophizing in sickle cell disease and its relationship with pain. *J Pain*. 2016;17(11):1227–1236.
24. Nelson SC, Hackman HW. Race matters: Perceptions of race and racism in a sickle cell center. *Pediatr Blood Cancer*. 2012;60(3):451–454.
25. Abdallah K, Buscetta A, Cooper K, et al. Emergency department utilization for patients living with sickle cell disease: Psychosocial predictors of health care behaviors. *Ann Emerg Med*. 2020;76(3, Suppl):S56–S63.
26. Blake A, Asnani V, Leger RR, et al. Stigma and illness uncertainty: Adding to the burden of sickle cell disease. *Hematology*. 2017;23(2):122–130.
27. Hood AM, Crosby LE, Hanson E, et al. The influence of perceived racial bias and health-related stigma on quality of life among children with sickle cell disease. *EthnHealth*. 2022;27(4):833–846.
28. Wakefield EO, Pantaleao A, Popp JM, et al. Describing perceived racial bias among youth with sickle cell disease. *J Pediatr Psychol*. 2018;43(7):779–788.
29. Aisiku IP, Smith WR, McClish DK, et al. Comparisons of high versus low emergency department utilizers in sickle cell disease. *Ann Emerg Med*. 2009;53(5):587–593.
30. Booker MJ, Blethyn KL, Wright CJ, Greenfield SM. Pain management in sickle cell disease. *Chronic Illness*. 2006;2(1):39–50.
31. Pack-Mabien A, Labbe E, Herbert D, Haynes J. Nurses' attitudes and practices in sickle cell pain management. *Appl Nurs Res*. 2001;14(4):187–192.
32. Alleyne J, Thomas VJ. The management of sickle cell crisis pain as experienced by patients and their carers. *J Adv Nurs*. 1994;19(4):725–732.
33. Jenerette CM, Pierre-Louis BJ, Matthie N, Girardeau Y. Nurses' attitudes toward patients with sickle cell disease: A worksite comparison. *Pain Manag Nurs*. 2015;16(3):173–181.
34. Glassberg JA, Tanabe P, Chow A, et al. Emergency provider analgesic practices and attitudes toward patients with sickle cell disease. *Ann Emerg Med*. 2013;62(4):293–302.
35. Haywood C Jr, Bediako S, Lanzkron S, et al. An unequal burden: Poor patient–provider communication and sickle cell disease. *Patient Educ Couns*. 2014;96(2):159–164.
36. Ezenwa MO, Molokie RE, Wilkie DJ, Suarez ML, Yao Y. Perceived injustice predicts stress and pain in adults with sickle cell disease. *Pain Manag Nurs*. 2015;16(3):294–306.
37. Schatz J, Schlenz AM, McClellan CB, et al. Changes in coping, pain, and activity after cognitive–behavioral training. *Clin J Pain*. 2015;31(6):536–547.
38. Moody KL, Mercer K, Glass M. An integrative review of the prevalence of depression among pediatric patients with sickle cell disease. *Soc Work Public Health*. 2019;34(4):343–352.
39. Connolly ME, Bills SE, Hardy SJ. Neurocognitive and psychological effects of persistent pain in pediatric sickle cell disease. *Pediatr Blood Cancer*. 2019;66(9):e27823.
40. Sil S, Cohen LL, Dampier C. Psychosocial and functional outcomes in youth with chronic sickle cell pain. *Clin J Pain*. 2016;32(6):527–533.
41. Citero VA, Levenson JL, McClish DK, et al. The role of catastrophizing in sickle cell disease: The PiSCES project. *Pain*. 2007;133(1):39–46.
42. Hildenbrand AK, Barakat LP, Alderfer MA, Marsac ML. Coping and coping assistance among children with sickle cell disease and their parents. *J Pediatr Hematol Oncol*. 2015;37(1):25–34.
43. Sarafino EP, Smith TW. *Health Psychology: Biopsychosocial Interactions*. 8th ed. Wiley; 2014.
44. Ahmadi M, Shariati A, Jahani S, Tabesh H, Keikhaei B. The effectiveness of self-management programs on self-efficacy in patients with sickle cell disease. *Jundishapur J Chronic Dis Care*. 2014;3(3):1–7.
45. Power-Hays A, Patterson A, Sobota A. Household material hardships impact emergency department reliance in pediatric patients with sickle cell disease. *Pediatr Blood Cancer*. 2020;67(10):e28587.
46. World Health Organization. Social determinants of health. 2022. Accessed August 1, 2022. https://www.who.int/health-topics/social-determinants-of-health

47. Gundersen C, Kreider B. Bounding the effects of food insecurity on children's health outcomes. *J Health Econ.* 2009;28(5):971–983.
48. Mojtabai R, Olfson M. Medication costs, adherence, and health outcomes among Medicare beneficiaries. *Health Aff.* 2003;22(4):220–229.
49. Daniel H, Bornstein SS, Kane GC. Addressing social determinants to improve patient care and promote health equity: An American College of Physicians position paper. *Ann Intern Med.* 2018;168(8):577–578.
50. Panepinto JA, Walters MC, Carreras J, et al. Matched-related donor transplantation for sickle cell disease: Report from the Center for International Blood and Transplant Research. *Br J Haematol.* 2007;137(5):479–485.
51. Raphael JL, Dietrich CL, Whitmire D, Mahoney DH, Mueller BU, Giardino AP. Healthcare utilization and expenditures for low income children with sickle cell disease. *Pediatr Blood Cancer.* 2009;52(2):263–267.
52. Robinson MR, Daniel LC, O'Hara EA, Szabo MM, Barakat LP. Insurance status as a sociodemographic risk factor for functional outcomes and health-related quality of life among youth with sickle cell disease. *J Pediatr Hematol Oncol.* 2014;36(1):51–56.
53. Sanger M, Jordan L, Pruthi S, et al. Cognitive deficits are associated with unemployment in adults with sickle cell anemia. *J Clin Exp Neuropsychol.* 2016;38(6):661–671.
54. Bediako SM. Predictors of employment status among African Americans with sickle cell disease. *J Health Care Poor Underserved.* 2010;21(4):1124–1137.
55. Farooq F, Mogayzel PJ, Lanzkron S, Haywood C, Strouse JJ. Comparison of US federal and foundation funding of research for sickle cell disease and cystic fibrosis and factors associated with research productivity. *JAMA Netw Open.* 2020;3(3):e201737.

25

Pain in Chronic Gastrointestinal Disease

Irritable Bowel Syndrome and Inflammatory Bowel Disease

David A. Edwards and Jeffrey M. Lackner

Introduction

Irritable bowel syndrome (IBS) and inflammatory bowel disease (IBD) affect millions of people worldwide.[1,2] These bowel disorders are some of the most prevalent medical conditions for which people present for medical care, and pain is a common initial and persistent complaint.[3,4] IBS is diagnosed by the presence of recurrent abdominal pain in the absence of gastrointestinal (GI) disease, whereas IBD is confirmed by the presence of noninfectious inflammatory lesions in the GI tract after presenting with a variety of symptoms often including pain. Treatment of GI disease has improved greatly in the past several decades with advances in medical and surgical interventions directed at disease pathophysiology; however, tools for treatment or prevention of pain have not advanced in parallel. Sixty percent of patients with IBD report abdominal pain, half continue to have pain for at least 5 years, and 30–50% continue to have pain even after treatment and disease remission.[3,5] In IBS, pain is the most disruptive symptom, and there are few effective treatments.[6]

One reason pain in GI disease has been a challenge to treat is that the disease itself is complex and the mechanisms underlying visceral pain in GI disease are poorly understood. As a result, medical pain treatments are nonspecific, limited by side effects, and simply not very effective.[6] Overall, pain is underassessed and undertreated in GI disease, and although there are several validated clinical assessment tools for IBD, there are no fully tested assessment tools for pain in IBD.[5] In one recent study, 24% of patients with IBD were not treated specifically for pain.[3]

Nevertheless, advances in understanding GI disease have resulted in better treatments and fewer disease symptoms, including pain.[7,8] This underscores the importance of a mechanistic approach to understanding and treating visceral pain, whereby treatment of inflammatory disease with immunomodulators results in prevention and alleviation of pain symptoms.[9] But treatment of the disease alone is insufficient to control pain, especially when disease-related complications occur or surgery is needed. In IBS, there is no GI pathology to which treatment can be targeted. Similarly, IBD patients in remission show no gut inflammation and yet 30–50% report significant pain.[5] This chapter reviews the presentation and pathophysiology of IBS and IBD and discusses the pain experience and psychosocial factors involved, with a focus on points of vulnerability to pain in GI disease.

Irritable Bowel Syndrome

Irritable bowel syndrome has been called a functional gastrointestinal disorder (FGID) because it has historically been defined by symptomatology in the absence of GI tract pathology. More recently, the FGIDs have been renamed disorders of gut–brain interaction (DGBI), recognizing the important bidirectional interaction between the brain and the gut. In DGBIs, there is dysregulation of the interaction of cognitive and emotional centers of the central nervous system (CNS) with the gut, presenting with irritable bowel symptoms.[10]

Frequent recurrent abdominal pain and changes in stool frequency and form are the most prominent presenting symptoms of IBS and the ones by which IBS is diagnosed. By Rome IV criteria, IBS is diagnosed by the presence of recurrent abdominal pain, on average, at least 1 day per week in the past 3 months, with defecation or associated with a change in the frequency or form of stool, and symptoms must have started at least 6 months prior.[2,11] Pain is typically located in the lower abdomen and described as aching, cramping, stabbing, or sharp with associated feelings of bloating, abdominal distention, or urgency.

IBS is classified by stool form according to the Bristol Stool Form Scale.[12] There exist four subtype classifications: IBS with predominant diarrhea (IBS-D) if loose stools occur more than 25% of the time, IBS with predominant constipation (IBS-C) if hard stools occur more than 25% of the time, IBS with mixed diarrhea and constipation (IBS-M) when diarrhea and hard stool occur more than 25% of the time, and IBS unclassified when bowel habits do not fit these categories.

IBS is estimated to affect 5–10% of the global general population.[2,11,13] Studies demonstrate wide variability in prevalence estimates between time periods and countries depending on the methodology, diagnostic criteria used, and the availability of data. Variability may also reflect true differences in populations with differential risk factors. A Rome Foundation global survey is underway to improve prevalence estimates of DGBIs across 34 countries using Rome IV diagnostic criteria, taking into account cultural and language differences. In one recent population-based survey, the prevalence of IBS in Canada, the United States, and the United Kingdom was 4.4–4.8% by Rome IV criteria, approximately half as prevalent as when assessed by Rome III criteria.[14] In Western countries, there is a consistently slightly higher prevalence of IBS in women compared to men, but this difference does not exist when measured in South Asia, South America, or Africa.[2]

Inflammatory Bowel Disease

Inflammatory bowel diseases were described as early as 1761.[15] In 1932, Burrill Bernard Crohn submitted the name "regional enteritis" to the American Medical Association for consideration as a unique disease entity in which noninfectious inflammation of the bowel could be seen.[16] Over time, two unique presentations were better distinguished, ultimately being called Crohn's disease (CD) and ulcerative colitis (UC). A third category exists called indeterminate colitis, when the diagnosis is unclear. IBD presents with abdominal pain, cramps, diarrhea, feelings of urgency, rectal bleeding, and weight loss in a relapsing and remitting pattern.

CD is diagnosed by endoscopic visual exam and biopsy-identified inflammatory patches, called skip lesions, in any portion of the GI tract. The Montreal classification divides CD into the most common regions affected: the terminal ilium (L1), the colon (L2), ileocolonic (L3), and the upper GI tract (L4).[17] Of these, the most common regions are the distal ileum and the proximal colon. This classification by region is important because there appears to be a difference in risk of disease progression or of complications depending on where the disease is located. Notably, however, there is a low likelihood CD will spread outside of the region where it was initially identified.[18] All layers of the bowel wall can be involved in CD, and occasionally the disease penetrates the bowel and fistulas form. UC, on the other hand, is limited to the colon. Inflammation commonly starts in the rectum and spreads in a continuous fashion, extending up the colon, and the ulcers and inflammation are generally limited to the superficial mucosa.

Worldwide, there are approximately 7 million people affected by IBD, most prevalent in Western countries such as the United States, Canada, and the United Kingdom, and less so in Asia or Africa. However, incidence is rising in non-Western countries possibly due to environmental risk factors, standardization of diagnostic criteria, and improved data collection.[19] There was an increased global crude prevalence of IBD from 68.6/100,000 in 1990 to 89.6/100,000 in 2017 (31% increase).[1]

What Makes People with Gastrointestinal Disease More Vulnerable to Pain?

A person with greater risk for experiencing and suffering from pain is considered vulnerable. Pain vulnerability can be the result of intrapersonal factors determined by one's own biologic or psychologic predispositions. Biological risk factors may include one's genetics, epigenetics, comorbid diseases, and environmental exposures. Psychological risk factors may include the presence of mood disorders or adaptive or maladaptive traits. Social factors for pain vulnerability include inadequate social systems or resources for health care and treatment. Considering disease through this lens is known as the biopsychosocial model and is useful as a framework for discussing pain vulnerability in GI disease as well.[20–22]

Biology of Visceral Pain

Mechanistically speaking, there are three supercategories of pain.[9] The first is nociceptive pain, where sensory neurons (nociceptors) sense pain-evoking (noxious) stimuli, such as excessive stretch, distention, or impingement. Nociceptive pain is somatic if the nociceptors are found in musculoskeletal tissue or visceral if found within visceral organs. A second type of pain is inflammatory pain, in which the presence of an inflammatory milieu of cytokines, prostaglandins, and growth factors directly activates transducer molecules on nociceptor terminals and also increases the excitability of neurons.

A third type of pain, neuropathic pain, is a type of pathologic pain due to direct damage or malfunction of the nerve itself, in the peripheral or central nervous system. Central pain is pathologic pain, where synaptic remodeling in the spinal cord or brain results in increased pain sensitivity that may be present even without macroscopic structural abnormality or inflammation. Notably, central pain may be perceived to originate from a peripheral organ or body part in the absence of identifiable disease there.

The bowel is innervated by the vagus nerve and by bilateral sensory spinal nerves. The cell bodies of the primary visceral afferents from the vagus nerve are located in the nodose and rostral jugular ganglia. The central terminals of the vagus extend to the nucleus of the solitary tract in the dorsal medulla or to the upper cervical spinal cord.[23] Vagal input likely contributes to the unpleasant and aversive feelings associated with visceral pain, such as nausea and bloating.[24]

Primary afferent spinal sensory axons project from the viscera, traverse the prevertebral ganglia (celiac, superior mesenteric, inferior mesenteric, or pelvic ganglia) and the paravertebral ganglia, and then enter the spinal cord. The cell bodies of the spinal visceral afferents are in the dorsal root ganglia, and they project centrally to the dorsal column laminae I, II, X; the interomediolateral cell column; and the sacral parasympathetic plexus. Visceral pain afferents, like somatic pain afferents, transit pain via thinly myelinated Aδ fibers and unmyelinated C fibers. They have complex nerve endings, can have several receptive fields per neuron, and have branching networks within the visceral wall.[24] In the CNS, second-order neurons receive input from both visceral and somatic primary afferents (viscerosomatic convergence) and from multiple visceral regions (viscero-visceral convergence).[25] This peripheral and central complexity contributes to the poor localization of visceral pain and the sense of referred pain.

Pain is processed in the CNS, where it is perceived and experienced. Converging evidence from functional magnetic resonance imaging and positron emission tomography studies demonstrates that visceral pain processing starts in the thalamus, which acts as an integrative relay station to the anterior cingulate cortex, the insular cortex, the somatosensory cortex (for discriminatory sense), the frontal and parietal lobes (presumably for cognitive appraisal), and the amygdala and locus coeruleus (for emotional arousal).[26,27]

Inflammatory Bowel Disease and Biological Pain Vulnerability

The exact cause of IBD is not known, but leading evidence implicates an interaction between an individual's genetics, the immune system, the microbiome, and environmental triggers. Possibly in response to an environmental trigger, an initial localized inflammatory reaction occurs in the GI tract. Part of the immune response is directed at commensal homeostatic microbiota within the gut. When dysbiosis, or a nonhomeostatic makeup of the microbiome, exists in genetically susceptible individuals, a maladaptive and exaggerated immune response occurs.[28] Hundreds of gene loci have been associated with IBD, and many are related to the immune response, but these explain less than one-third of the variance for the development of IBD.[29,30] Exaggerated inflammatory responses and histologic and cellular changes lead to mucosal erosion and ulceration.[31]

In CD, a nonpenetrating, nonstricturing inflammatory phenotype occurs first, and this may or may not be symptomatic. This can progress to a penetrating phenotype, with shallow and deep ulcers that erode through the bowel wall, creating fistulas. In severe disease, with significant histologic changes, a stricturing phenotype can develop.[18] Perianal lesions occur in 20–30% of patients, with a cumulative risk of developing perianal fistulas of 45%–50% at 20 years. Seventy percent develop strictures or penetrating complications, and many require surgical drainage.[32–34]

In UC, superficial inflammatory lesions occur in the rectum and colon. One-third present with colitis of the rectum, one-third with colorectal disease distal to the splenic flexure, and one-third with disease proximal to the splenic flexure.[35] At 20 years, 25% of patients have pancolitis.[36] UC flare-ups occur that range from mild in severity to treatment-refractory colitis requiring surgical resection. Flare-ups are interrupted by periods of remission usually associated with healing of the mucosa. Remission occurs in 50% one year after the onset of UC, and one-third have no recurrence at 10 years.[37]

The complexity of visceral innervation and the multiple mechanisms by which pain can be triggered in IBD explain the complexity of IBD presentation. IBD is a waxing and waning disease, with flare-ups coinciding with periods of acute pain.[38] Persistent inflammation will evoke inflammatory pain and peripheral nerve sensitization.[39,40] Visceral nociceptive pain is triggered with bowel distention. Although it is generally presumed that flare-ups represent increased disease and inflammation, this is not always the case: 20% of patients in complete remission still have periods of pain.[41,42] Changes in the CNS result in a persistently sensitized state in which pain is chronically amplified.[9,43]

Irritable Bowel Syndrome and Biological Pain Vulnerability

Abdominal pain in IBS may be a symptom of early disease or a sign of disordered brain–gut communication. In 10% of patients, IBS onset occurs after a period of acute gastroenteritis from bacterial, viral, or fungal infection. Acute inflammatory GI pain may persist in patients in whom chronic low-grade inflammation exists.[44,45] Bowel distention or irregular or overactive peristalsis can trigger visceral nociceptive pain.[46] In laboratory studies, some patients with IBS exhibit sensitization to pain with bowel distention (visceral hyperalgesia), evidence that peripheral and central thresholds for pain detection are lowered.[47] Descending pain modulatory pathways in IBS are also dysfunctional, resulting in visceral hypersensitivity.[48]

Psychology and Pain Vulnerability in Inflammatory Bowel Disease

Symptom severity or level of disability from IBD does not directly correlate with the risk factors a patient presents with or the endoscopic status of their disease.[49] Similar discordance between symptom burden and biomarkers of disease is common in diseases in which chronic pain is present, and it underscores the importance of considering psychological contributions that amplify pain. The experience of pain is subjective and increased with stress, anxiety, and depression, the most frequent mood disorders in

IBD. Thirty-two percent of patients with IBD have anxiety and 25% have depression.[50,51] Stress amplifies pain nearly 40% in IBD patients.[52] Mood disorders worsen pain in IBD, and vice versa, pain worsens symptoms of anxiety and depression in IBD.[53–56]

Effective management of GI symptoms and treatment side effects depends on not only adjustments to medical care but also strengthening self-management skills. Cognitive–behavioral therapy (CBT) is a more effective and durable treatment overall than medical treatment or changes in diet for improving symptoms in GI disease.[57] This not only validates the influence of central factors on maintaining GI symptoms but also highlights that formalized cultivation of specific behavioral skills through CBT is a key component of treatment. Patient self-efficacy—confidence in their own ability to head off symptoms if they recognize them early enough—is a potential CBT-specific factor by which improvement is mediated.[57] Pain catastrophizing (the tendency to magnify the threat of pain and feeling helpless managing pain) functions as a marker of the pain experience predicting worse outcomes in IBD (and other pain conditions); it is not a mechanism by which behavioral treatments achieve symptom relief in IBD.[57,58]

Psychology and Pain Vulnerability in Irritable Bowel Syndrome

Brain–gut communication in IBS is bidirectionally altered. Psychological disorders are risk factors for IBS and for pain. IBS is more common in patients with other functional somatic syndromes such as chronic fatigue, chronic pelvic pain, and fibromyalgia (chronic overlapping pain disorders) and DGBIs such as pelvic floor dyssynergia, functional dyspepsia, and gastroesophageal reflux disease.[11,59] Psychiatric comorbidities are common in those with IBS, with anxiety disorders and depression being the most common.[60] Early life adversity, trauma, and sexual and emotional abuse are strong environmental factors associated with IBS that suggest a relationship between trauma and overwhelmed coping mechanisms in the expression of persistent irritable bowel symptoms.[61–65]

Epidemiology and Pain Vulnerability in Irritable Bowel Syndrome

In best estimates, IBS affects 1 in 10 people globally, but this is surely an undercount because many countries do not provide data.[66] Moreover, prevalence is increasing in newly industrialized countries and stabilized at high rates in Western industrialized nations.[67] This suggests that there exist ongoing stable vulnerability to pain associated with IBS in industrialized nations and increasing vulnerability to pain throughout the world as potential environmental factors lead to disease. In addition, ethnic psychosocial makeup and genetic factors play an important role in pain susceptibility. Recognizing these specific risk factors is a crucial first requirement before being able to allocate resources to prevent or treat pain in IBS. Availability and access to treatment are the best chance for symptom control, and unfortunately, on average, it takes 4 years before people with IBS are diagnosed in the best circumstances—long enough for pain to become chronic, centralized, and difficult to treat.[2]

Environmental risk factors for development of GI disease have overlap with those for development of chronic pain. Stress as a result of the individual burdens of disease or external social factors are well-described risks for development of chronic pain.[68] Stressful social upheaval in ethnic minority populations has been implicated in higher prevalence of IBS in these groups.[69,70] Trauma-related stress, depression, anxiety, and psychological traits such as catastrophizing behavior and poor coping skills all contribute to pain severity and disability from GI diseases.[56,68,71–75]

Environmental risk factors may provide some insight into triggers for IBS. Potential risk factors for IBS include diet, gut dysbiosis, GI infection, psychological factors, and genetics. Two-thirds of IBS patients associate symptoms with food.[76] Western diets high in fat and sugar are associated with IBS.[77,78] The most common dietary intervention used to reduce symptoms of IBS is to restrict intake of poorly absorbed carbohydrates—fermentable oligo-, di-, and monosaccharides and polyols (FODMAPs).[76,79] It is hypothesized that FODMAPs result in an osmotic load and, after fermentation by intestinal bacteria, production of short-chain fatty acids and gases that trigger bowel symptoms.[76] The low FODMAPs diet involves an initial highly restrictive elimination phase after which foods are reintroduced to identify those that may be contributing to symptoms.[79] When evaluated in meta-analyses, low-FODMAPs, gluten-free, and lactose-restrictive diets have not demonstrated consistent outcomes, and the quality of studies is low.[16,76,79–81]

Epidemiology and Pain Vulnerability in Inflammatory Bowel Disease

It has been hypothesized that IBD is an overactive immune response to environmental triggers in susceptible individuals and that region-specific increases in IBD prevalence are the result of rising exposure to environmental risk factors such as a hygienic, low-fiber, and high-protein diet common in Western countries.[1,82] This may be why offspring of immigrants to Western countries have similar increased incidence of IBD.[1] Other potential risk factors for IBD include smoking in CD, use of antibiotics and nonsteroidal anti-inflammatory drugs (NSAIDs), stress, and poor hygiene.

The IBD burden among countries and the shifting epidemiological patterns were most thoroughly described in the Global Burden of Disease Study 2017 (Table 25.1).[1] Like IBS, IBDs are most prevalent in Western industrialized nations, where a high burden of disease exists. The prevalence of IBD in the United States is approximately 465.5 per 100,000 (95% uncertainty interval: 438.6–490.9) and in the United Kingdom is 449 per 100,000.[1] From 1990 to 2017, there has been an 85% increase in global estimates of IBD from 3.7 million in 1990 to 6.8 million in 2017; this is mostly the result of increasing prevalence of IBD in previously low-prevalence countries in South America, Asia, Africa, and eastern Europe, possibly due to changes in diet and other exposures in recent decades. There were slightly more females (3.9 million, 57%) than males (3.0 million, 43%) living with IBD worldwide in 2017.[1] Onset of IBD most commonly occurs at ages 20–30 years for CD and ages 30–40 years for UC, with peak prevalence at ages 60–64 years for women and ages 70–74 years for men.[1,34] With the onset during the most productive years of adulthood, incomplete understanding of the

Table 25.1 Epidemiology of Inflammatory Bowel Disease

Peak prevalence age (years)	20–40
Global prevalence	6.8 million
Age-standardized global prevalence	84.3 (79.2–89.9)/100,000
Female global prevalence	3.9 million (57%)
Age-standardized global female prevalence	93.8 (87.8–100)/100,000
Female age-specific peak (years)	60–64
Male age-specific peak (years)	70–74
High-income North America age-standardized prevalence	422.0 (398.7–466.1)/100,000

Source: Data from GBD 2017 Inflammatory Bowel Disease Collaborators.[1]

disease etiology, and no cure, the significant growing global burden that IBD represents cannot be understated.

Treatment and Pain Vulnerability in Inflammatory Bowel Disease

The goal of IBD treatment is disease remission, resulting in mucosal healing and decrease in symptoms, improving quality of life.[83] The tools for treatment of IBD are medical, surgical, and psychological, and best outcomes are obtained when these are integrated into a cohesive treatment plan (Box 25.1).[75] Treatment of acute pain with active disease and chronic pain after disease remission was identified by providers and patients as an important priority.[84] The International Organization for the Study of IBD recently updated guidelines and therapeutic goals for treatment of IBD, encapsulated in the STRIDE-II initiative, Selecting Therapeutic Targets in Inflammatory Bowel Disease.[83] Pain control was recognized as a relevant treatment target defining clinical response in CD.[83] Currently, pain and psychosocial health care are considered undertreated in IBD, procedures and surgery for IBD treatment may result in increased pain and stress, and medical pain treatments for IBD are not very effective.[3,75,84,85]

Medical treatment of IBD involves medications and surgery. Treatment aims to suppress inflammation using anti-inflammatories (sulfasalazine, mesalamine, and diazo-bonded 5-ASA) and immunosuppressants (corticosteroids) and to achieve remission and mucosal healing.[86] Early aggressive medical treatment may stop progression of the disease before irreversible bowel damage occurs.[87] Induction and maintenance with anti-tumor necrosis factor-α treatment (infliximab and adalimumab) is strongly recommended for adult outpatients with severe CD.[88] For progressive disease severity and worsening symptoms, systemic corticosteroids, biologic therapies, and immunomodulators should be used to induce remission.[86] In ambulatory patients with moderate to severe UC, biologics (infliximab, adalimumab, golimumab, vedolizumab, and ustekinumab) are strongly recommended for induction and maintenance, whereas consideration is given to intravenous methylprednisolone, infliximab, or cyclosporine in hospitalized patients.[89]

Box 25.1 Integrative Pain Management Options for Gastrointestinal Disease

Psychological Treatment
- Cognitive–behavioral therapy
- Gut-directed hypnotherapy
- Mindfulness
- Psychodynamic–interpersonal therapy

Medical Treatment
- Neuromodulators
- Tricyclic antidepressants
- Serotonin–norepinephrine reuptake inhibitors
- Antispasmodics
- Non-antimuscarinics
- Hyoscine
- Otilonium
- Alverine
- Drotaverine
- Mebeverine
- Pinaverium
- Pargeverine
- Antimuscarinics
- Cimetropium
- Pirenzipine
- Rociverine
- Trimebutine
- Calcium channel blockers
- Gabapentin
- Pregabalin
- Opioids
- loperamide
- Asimadoline
- Eluxadoline

In severe disease, abscesses, fistulae, strictures, and bacterial overgrowth can all be painful and may require surgical intervention. Partial bowel resection may result in disease and symptom remission in CD, and total colectomy can be curative for UC. Repeated interventions and surgery can be traumatic in patients with IBD who are already sensitized to pain, and even hospitalized patients may continue to suffer without measurable improvement of pain.[73] Patients with IBD are vulnerable to the development of postoperative chronic pain by virtue of high baseline preoperative pain level, surgical trauma, and ongoing psychological stress.[5,90]

STRIDE-II recommends a prompt treat-to-target approach once IBD is diagnosed so that the disease is quickly put into remission and the patient is spared chronic complications, including pain and psychological distress. In many cases, medical treatment of IBD will improve the subjective measure of pain; however, disease treatment is not itself analgesic, so concurrent pain control is crucial.[7,8] Uncontrolled acute pain, if left untreated, can progress to chronic pain that can persist even after IBD is in remission.[42] Likewise, unaddressed psychological distress worsens dysfunction in active IBD, and disability can persist long after IBD remission.

Pain treatment in IBD benefits from an integrative approach that considers multiple available options over time. Pain management clinicians and psychologists with knowledge and skill in treating GI acute and chronic pain with pharmacologic and nonpharmacologic therapies can be helpful partners in supportive care for IBD primary services.[75] Pharmacologic treatment of pain in IBD is challenging because many common analgesics have gut-related side effects. Although it makes mechanistic sense to use anti-inflammatory medications to treat an inflammatory disease, regular NSAID use can exacerbate IBD.[91] There are no controlled trials investigating the use of the calcium channels blockers, pregabalin and gabapentin, or the tricyclic antidepressants (TCAs) or serotonin–norepinephrine reuptake inhibitors (SNRIs) for treatment of pain in IBD.[5] The limited number of studies investigating cannabinoids for IBD demonstrate improvement in subjective, but not objective, outcomes of disease.[92] Opioid use in IBD is associated with poorer clinical outcomes, does not improve pain in the long term, and can have significant bowel-related side effects.[93]

Treatment and Pain Vulnerability in Irritable Bowel Syndrome

The biopsychosocial model of disease has been useful in guiding an integrative approach to IBS treatment (see Box 25.1). Medical treatment is directed at underlying biological variables of the disease and at stabilizing comorbid physical and psychological conditions that exacerbate IBS symptoms. For instance, stool softeners are used to treat constipation, and anti-diarrheal medications are used to stop diarrhea. Pain is treated by considering the predominant mechanism. Antispasmodics (e.g., hyoscine and alverine) treat cramps and spasticity-related pain. A recent meta-analysis showed that antispasmodics relieve IBS symptoms better than placebo (61% vs. 44%, $p < .001$).[94] In addition to their benefit for depression, some antidepressants (e.g., amitriptyline and duloxetine) treat central and neuropathic pain. Calcium channel blockers (e.g., pregabalin and gabapentin) are useful for treatment of neuropathic pain and anxiety. A systematic review of several antidepressants and calcium channel blockers (collectively called anti-neuropathic agents) used for treatment of pain in IBS identified 13 studies that used the TCA amitriptyline, the SNRI desipramine, and the calcium channel antagonists gabapentin and pregabalin.[95] There was significant heterogeneity in the studies, so meta-analysis was limited to only 3 studies. The pooled relative risk for not improving pain with anti-neuropathic agents versus controls was 0.5 (95% confidence interval: 0.38–0.66). There was no consistent benefit of pregabalin or gabapentin on pain outcomes. TCAs appeared beneficial and SSRIs no better than placebo for IBS pain in three recent systematic reviews.[95–97] All pain medications are used off-label for IBS.

Psychological intervention is a key component of IBS treatment with strong empirical support.[57,98] CBT and gut-directed hypnotherapy are the most supported among behavioral treatments (see Box 25.1).[99,100] CBT addresses maladaptive thoughts and responses to disease, including pain, and helps patients feel they can more effectively manage symptoms before they become uncontrollable.[57,98,100] CBT has been helpful in adults and children in decreasing the impact of pain in IBS on function.[101]

Conclusion

The GI disorders, IBS and IBD, are some of the most prevalent diseases globally, and the number of people who meet criteria is growing. GI disease can profoundly alter a patient's life, setting them on a course of chronic disease and symptom management. With treatment, including behavioral support, and access to psychological therapies as well as medical and surgical care, a patient can achieve the best outcomes, which are disease remission and symptom control.

However, even with available treatments, up to 50% of patients in remission live with chronic pain.[3,4] Individual pain experiences vary widely, being subject to modification by one's own biological, psychological, and social history. Effective assessment and treatment of pain depend on both the source of the pain and to what degree pain interferes in normal behaviors. In chronic illness, such as with GI disease, the context of biological, psychological, and social risk contributes to the severity of the impact of the disease for each patient. These risk factors create vulnerability, which is susceptibility to the disease and its progression, and susceptibility to the impact of pain on function. No one risk factor predicts with great odds the likely development of IBS or IBD or in whom severe or prolonged pain will be involved. This unpredictability makes preventative efforts challenging, and targeted treatment approaches based on the putative mechanism of disease still inadequate. While advances are being made in medical and surgical treatment of GI disease, no targeted and effective pain medicine or procedural intervention outside of bowel resection is labeled for GI pain in IBS or IBD. Cognitive–behavioral intervention, however, is effective at reducing symptom burden, including pain, with one-third of IBS patients showing a rapid response to CBT with durable symptom improvement.[57] An integrative treatment approach involving medical and psychological therapy is the most effective buttress against the detrimental effects of chronic pain in GI disease. Further research is necessary to identify prognostic factors that can inform clinical decisions, conserve clinical resources, and optimize patient and provider satisfaction around shared goals. Box 25.2 identifies clinically useful strategies that can support clinicians' ability to direct patients who may—or may not—be strong candidates for CBT and other behavioral treatments.

Box 25.2 When to Consider CBT

Is CBT right for your patient?

- If they are interested in learning to control problems on their own
- If they are willing and interested in practicing change strategies ("homework") between sessions
- If they are not interested in focusing exclusively on past issues or "talk therapy"

When to consider CBT

- Persistent IBS without significant relief from first-line medications or dietary changes
- Preference for non-drug option
- Moderate to severe symptoms (>2 days a week, life interference)
- Diminished quality of life
- Illness behaviors (e.g., reassurance seeking, request for diagnostic testing, etc.)
- Symptom onset corresponds with major stressors (e.g., life transitions)
- Poor social support
- Accompanying distress (anxiety, depression) or chronic anxiety
- **DON'T WAIT FOR DISTRESS TO ESCALATE!**

References

1. GBD 2017 Inflammatory Bowel Disease Collaborators. The global, regional, and national burden of inflammatory bowel disease in 195 countries and territories, 1990–2017: A systematic analysis for the Global Burden of Disease Study 2017. *Lancet Gastroenterol Hepatol.* s2020;5(1):17–30. doi:10.1016/S2468-1253(19)30333-4
2. Black CJ, Ford AC. Global burden of irritable bowel syndrome: Trends, predictions and risk factors. *Nat Rev Gastroenterol Hepat.* 2020;17(8):473–486. doi:10.1038/s41575-020-0286-8
3. Zeitz J, Ak M, Muller-Mottet S, et al. Pain in IBD patients: Very frequent and frequently insufficiently taken into account. *PLoS One.* 2016;11(6):e0156666. doi:10.1371/journal.pone.0156666
4. Coates MD, Johri A, Gorrepati VS, et al. Abdominal pain in quiescent inflammatory bowel disease. *Int J Colorectal Dis.* 2021;36(1):93–102. doi:10.1007/s00384-020-03727-3
5. Bakshi N, Hart AL, Lee MC, et al. Chronic pain in patients with inflammatory bowel disease. *Pain.* 2021;162(10):2466–2471. doi:10.1097/j.pain.0000000000002304
6. BouSaba J, Sannaa W, Camilleri M. Pain in irritable bowel syndrome: Does anything really help? *Neurogastroenterol Motil.* 2022;34(1):e14305. doi:10.1111/nmo.14305
7. Torres J, Mehandru S, Colombel JF, Peyrin-Biroulet L. Crohn's disease. *Lancet.* 2017;389(10080):1741–1755. doi:10.1016/S0140-6736(16)31711-1
8. Panes J, Vermeire S, Lindsay JO, et al. Tofacitinib in patients with ulcerative colitis: Health-Related quality of life in Phase 3 randomised controlled induction and maintenance studies. *J Crohns Colitis.* 2019;13(1):139–140. doi:10.1093/ecco-jcc/jjy135
9. Vardeh D, Mannion RJ, Woolf CJ. Toward a mechanism-based approach to pain diagnosis. *J Pain.* 2016;17(9 Suppl):T50–T69. doi:10.1016/j.jpain.2016.03.001
10. Lackner JM. The role of psychosocial factors in functional gastrointestinal disorders. *Front Gastroint Res.* 2014;33:104–116. doi:10.1159/000356785

11. Ford AC, Sperber AD, Corsetti M, Camilleri M. Functional gastrointestinal disorders 2: Irritable bowel syndrome. *Lancet.* 2020;396(10263):1675–1688. doi:10.1016/S0140-6736(20)31548-8
12. Heaton KW, Odonnell LJD. An office guide to whole-gut transit-time: Patients' recollection of their stool form. *J Clin Gastroenterol.* 1994;19(1):28–30. doi:10.1097/00004836-199407000-00008
13. Schmulson MJ, Drossman DA. What is new in Rome IV. *J Neurogastroenterol.* 2017;23(2):151–163. doi:10.5056/jnm16214
14. Palsson OS, Whitehead W, Tornblom H, Sperber AD, Simren M. Prevalence of Rome IV functional bowel disorders among adults in the United States, Canada, and the United Kingdom. *Gastroenterology.* 2020;158(5):1262–1273. doi:10.1053/j.gastro.2019.12.021
15. Mulder DJ, Noble AJ, Justinich CJ, Duffin JM. A tale of two diseases: The history of inflammatory bowel disease. *J Crohns Colitis.* 2014;8(5):341–348. doi:10.1016/j.crohns.2013.09.009
16. Catassi C, Alaedini A, Bojarski C, et al. The overlapping area of non-celiac gluten sensitivity (NCGS) and wheat-sensitive irritable bowel syndrome (IBS): An update. *Nutrients.* 2017;9(11):1268. doi:10.3390/nu9111268
17. Silverberg MS, Satsangi J, Ahmad T, et al. Toward an integrated clinical, molecular and serological classification of inflammatory bowel disease: Report of a Working Party of the 2005 Montreal World Congress of Gastroenterology. *Can J Gastroenterol.* 2005;19(Suppl A):5A–36A. doi:10.1155/2005/269076
18. Louis E, Collard A, Oger AF, Degroote E, Aboul Nasr El Yafi FA, Belaiche J. Behaviour of Crohn's disease according to the Vienna classification: Changing pattern over the course of the disease. *Gut.* 2001;49(6):777–782. doi:10.1136/gut.49.6.777
19. Kaplan GG. The global burden of IBD: From 2015 to 2025. *Nat Rev Gastroenterol Hepatol.* 2015;12(12):720–727. doi:10.1038/nrgastro.2015.150
20. Sullivan MD, Sturgeon JA, Lumley MA, Ballantyne JC. Reconsidering Fordyce's classic article, "Pain and Suffering: What Is the Unit?" to help make our model of chronic pain truly biopsychosocial. *Pain.* 2023;164(2):271–279. doi:10.1097/j.pain.0000000000002748
21. Dibley L, Khoshaba B, Artom M, et al. Patient strategies for managing the vicious cycle of fatigue, pain and urgency in inflammatory bowel disease: Impact, planning and support. *Dig Dis Sci.* 2021;66(10):3330–3342. doi:10.1007/s10620-020-06698-1
22. Klossika I, Flor H, Kamping S, et al. Emotional modulation of pain: A clinical perspective. *Pain.* 2006;124(3):264–268. doi:10.1016/j.pain.2006.08.007
23. Foreman RD, Garrett KM, Blair RW. Mechanisms of cardiac pain. *Compr Physiol.* 2015;5(2):929–960. doi:10.1002/cphy.c140032
24. Gebhart GF, Bielefeldt K. Physiology of visceral pain. *Compr Physiol.* 2016;6(4):1609–1633. doi:10.1002/cphy.c150049
25. Giamberardino MA, Costantini R, Affaitati G, et al. Viscero-visceral hyperalgesia: Characterization in different clinical models. *Pain.* 2010;151(2):307–322. doi:10.1016/j.pain.2010.06.023
26. Silverman DH, Munakata JA, Ennes H, Mandelkern MA, Hoh CK, Mayer EA. Regional cerebral activity in normal and pathological perception of visceral pain. *Gastroenterology.* 1997;112(1):64–72. doi:10.1016/s0016-5085(97)70220-8
27. Labus JS, Naliboff BN, Fallon J, et al. Sex differences in brain activity during aversive visceral stimulation and its expectation in patients with chronic abdominal pain: A network analysis. *NeuroImage.* 2008;41(3):1032–1043. doi:10.1016/j.neuroimage.2008.03.009
28. Walker AW, Sanderson JD, Churcher C, et al. High-throughput clone library analysis of the mucosa-associated microbiota reveals dysbiosis and differences between inflamed and non-inflamed regions of the intestine in inflammatory bowel disease. *BMC Microbiol.* 2011;11: Article 7. doi:10.1186/1471-2180-11-7
29. Jostins L, Ripke S, Weersma RK, et al. Host–microbe interactions have shaped the genetic architecture of inflammatory bowel disease. *Nature.* 2012;491(7422):119–124. doi:10.1038/nature11582

30. Glocker EO, Kotlarz D, Boztug K, et al. Inflammatory bowel disease and mutations affecting the interleukin-10 receptor. *N Engl J Med.* 2009;361(21):2033–2045. doi:10.1056/NEJMoa0907206
31. Kaur A, Goggolidou P. Ulcerative colitis: Understanding its cellular pathology could provide insights into novel therapies. *J Inflamm.* 2020;17: Article 15. doi:10.1186/s12950-020-00246-4
32. Schwartz DA, Loftus EV Jr, Tremaine WJ, et al. The natural history of fistulizing Crohn's disease in Olmsted County, Minnesota. *Gastroenterology.* 2002;122(4):875–880. doi:10.1053/gast.2002.32362
33. Vermeire S, Van Assche G, Rutgeerts P. Perianal Crohn's disease: Classification and clinical evaluation. *Dig Liver Dis.* 2007;39(10):959–962. doi:10.1016/j.dld.2007.07.153
34. Cosnes J, Gower-Rousseau C, Seksik P, Cortot A. Epidemiology and natural history of inflammatory bowel diseases. *Gastroenterology.* 2011;140(6):1785–1794. doi:10.1053/j.gastro.2011.01.055
35. Moum B, Ekbom A, Vatn MH, Elgjo K. Change in the extent of colonoscopic and histological involvement in ulcerative colitis over time. *Am J Gastroenterol.* 1999;94(6):1564–1569. doi:10.1111/j.1572-0241.1999.01145.x
36. Langholz E, Munkholm P, Davidsen M, Nielsen OH, Binder V. Changes in extent of ulcerative colitis: A study on the course and prognostic factors. *Scand J Gastroenterol.* 1996;31(3):260-266. doi:10.3109/00365529609004876
37. Froslie KF, Jahnsen J, Moum BA, Vatn MH, Group I. Mucosal healing in inflammatory bowel disease: Results from a Norwegian population-based cohort. *Gastroenterology.* 2007;133(2):412–422. doi:10.1053/j.gastro.2007.05.051
38. Best WR, Becktel JM, Singleton JW, Kern F Jr. Development of a Crohn's disease activity index: National Cooperative Crohn's Disease Study. *Gastroenterology.* 1976;70(3):439–444.
39. Drewes AM, Olesen AE, Farmer AD, Szigethy E, Rebours V, Olesen SS. Gastrointestinal pain. *Nat Rev Dis Primers.* 2020;6(1): Article 1. doi:10.1038/s41572-019-0135-7
40. Beyak MJ, Vanner S. Inflammation-induced hyperexcitability of nociceptive gastrointestinal DRG neurones: The role of voltage-gated ion channels. *Neurogastroenterol Motil.* 2005;17(2):175–186. doi:10.1111/j.1365-2982.2004.00596.x
41. Bielefeldt K, Davis B, Binion DG. Pain and inflammatory bowel disease. *Inflamm Bowel Dis.* 2009;15(5):778–788. doi:10.1002/ibd.20848
42. Fairbrass KM, Costantino SJ, Gracie DJ, Ford AC. Prevalence of irritable bowel syndrome-type symptoms in patients with inflammatory bowel disease in remission: A systematic review and meta-analysis. *Lancet Gastroenterol Hepatol.* 2020;5(12):1053–1062. doi:10.1016/S2468-1253(20)30300-9
43. Bao CH, Liu P, Liu HR, et al. Differences in regional homogeneity between patients with Crohn's disease with and without abdominal pain revealed by resting-state functional magnetic resonance imaging. *Pain.* 2016;157(5):1037–1044. doi:10.1097/j.pain.0000000000000479
44. Klem F, Wadhwa A, Prokop LJ, et al. Prevalence, risk factors, and outcomes of irritable bowel syndrome after infectious enteritis: A systematic review and meta-analysis. *Gastroenterology.* 2017;152(5):1042–1054. doi:10.1053/j.gastro.2016.12.039
45. Spiller R, Lam C. An update on post-infectious irritable bowel syndrome: Role of genetics, immune activation, serotonin and altered microbiome. *J Neurogastroenterol Motil.* 2012;18(3):258–268. doi:10.5056/jnm.2012.18.3.258
46. Kellow JE, Phillips SF. Altered small bowel motility in irritable bowel syndrome is correlated with symptoms. *Gastroenterology.* 1987;92(6):1885–1893. doi:10.1016/0016-5085(87)90620-2
47. Ritchie J. Pain from distension of the pelvic colon by inflating a balloon in the irritable colon syndrome. *Gut.* 1973;14(2):125–132. doi:10.1136/gut.14.2.125
48. Tillisch K, Mayer EA, Labus JS. Quantitative meta-analysis identifies brain regions activated during rectal distension in irritable bowel syndrome. *Gastroenterology.* 2011;140(1):91–100. doi:10.1053/j.gastro.2010.07.053

49. Jharap B, Sandborn WJ, Reinisch W, et al. Randomised clinical study: Discrepancies between patient-reported outcomes and endoscopic appearance in moderate to severe ulcerative colitis. *Aliment Pharmacol Ther.* 2015;42(9):1082–1092. doi:10.1111/apt.13387
50. Bisgaard TH, Allin KH, Keefer L, Ananthakrishnan AN, Jess T. Depression and anxiety in inflammatory bowel disease: Epidemiology, mechanisms and treatment. Nat Rev *Gastroenterol Hepatol.* 2022;1911):717–726. doi:10.1038/s41575-022-00634-6
51. Barberio B, Zamani M, Black CJ, Savarino EV, Ford AC. Prevalence of symptoms of anxiety and depression in patients with inflammatory bowel disease: A systematic review and meta-analysis. *Lancet Gastroenterol Hepatol.* 2021;6(5):359–370. doi:10.1016/S2468-1253(21)00014-5
52. Schirbel A, Reichert A, Roll S, et al. Impact of pain on health-related quality of life in patients with inflammatory bowel disease. *World J Gastroenterol.* 2010;16(25):3168–3177. doi:10.3748/wjg.v16.i25.3168
53. Gracie DJ, Guthrie EA, Hamlin PJ, Ford AC. Bi-directionality of brain–gut interactions in patients with inflammatory bowel disease. *Gastroenterology.* 2018;154(6):1635–1646. doi:10.1053/j.gastro.2018.01.027
54. Zhang B, Wang HE, Bai YM, et al. Bidirectional association between inflammatory bowel disease and depression among patients and their unaffected siblings. *J Gastroenterol Hepatol.* 2022;37(7):1307–1315. doi:10.1111/jgh.15855
55. Fuller-Thomson E, Sulman J. Depression and inflammatory bowel disease: Findings from two nationally representative Canadian surveys. *Inflamm Bowel Dis.* 2006;12(8):697–707. doi:10.1097/00054725-200608000-00005
56. Sweeney L, Moss-Morris R, Czuber-Dochan W, Meade L, Chumbley G, Norton C. Systematic review: Psychosocial factors associated with pain in inflammatory bowel disease. *Aliment Pharmacol Ther.* 2018;47(6):715–729. doi:10.1111/apt.14493
57. Lackner JM, Jaccard J. Specific and common mediators of gastrointestinal symptom improvement in patients undergoing education/support vs. cognitive behavioral therapy for irritable bowel syndrome. *J Consult Clin Psychol.* 2021;89(5):435–453. doi:10.1037/ccp0000648
58. Petrini L, Arendt-Nielsen L. Understanding pain catastrophizing: Putting pieces together. *Front Psychol.* 2020;11:603420. doi:10.3389/fpsyg.2020.603420
59. Petersen MW, Schroder A, Jorgensen T, et al. The unifying diagnostic construct of bodily distress syndrome (BDS) was confirmed in the general population. *J Psychosom Res.* 2020;128:109868. doi:10.1016/j.jpsychores.2019.109868
60. Lackner JM, Ma CX, Gudleski GD, et al. Type, not number, of mental–physical comorbidities increases the severity of GI symptoms in patients with more severe irritable bowel syndrome. *Gastroenterology.* 2013;144(5):S107.
61. Baccini F, Pallotta N, Calabrese E, Pezzotti P, Corazziari E. Prevalence of sexual and physical abuse and its relationship with symptom manifestations in patients with chronic organic and functional gastrointestinal disorders. *Dig Liver Dis.* 2003;35(4):256–261. doi:10.1016/s1590-8658(03)00075-6
62. Drossman DA, Talley NJ, Leserman J, Olden KW, Barreiro MA. Sexual and physical abuse and gastrointestinal illness: Review and recommendations. *Ann Intern Med.* 1995;123(10):782–794. doi:10.7326/0003-4819-123-10-199511150-00007
63. Leserman J, Drossman DA. Sexual and physical abuse history and medical practice. *Gen Hosp Psychiatry.* 1995;17(2):71–74. doi:10.1016/0163-8343(94)00069-p
64. Lackner JM, Gudleski G, Blanchard E, Katz L, Krasner S. Beyond abuse: The association among perceived parenting style, abdominal pain, and somatization in treatment-seeking IBS patients. *Gastroenterology.* 2003;124(4):A96. doi:10.1016/S0016-5085(03)80472-9
65. Lackner JM, Gudleski GD, Blanchard EB. Beyond abuse: The association among parenting style, abdominal pain, and somatization in IBS patients. *Behav Res Ther.* 2004;42(1):41–56. doi:10.1016/S0005-7967(03)00069-X
66. Lovell RM, Ford AC. Global prevalence of and risk factors for irritable bowel syndrome: A meta-analysis. *Clin Gastroenterol Hepatol.* 2012;10(7):712–721. doi:10.1016/j.cgh.2012.02.029

67. Gwee KA. Irritable bowel syndrome in developing countries: A disorder of civilization or colonization? *Neurogastroenterol Motil.* 2005;17(3):317–324. doi:10.1111/j.1365-2982.2005.00627.x
68. Gupta A, Silman AJ, Ray D, et al. The role of psychosocial factors in predicting the onset of chronic widespread pain: Results from a prospective population-based study. *Rheumatology.* 2007;46(4):666–671. doi:10.1093/rheumatology/kel363
69. Qumseya BJ, Tayem Y, Almansa C, et al. Irritable bowel syndrome in middle-aged and elderly Palestinians: Its prevalence and effect of location of residence. *Am J Gastroenterol.* 2014;109(5):723–739. doi:10.1038/ajg.2014.27
70. Sperber AD, Friger M, Shvartzman P, et al. Rates of functional bowel disorders among Israeli Bedouins in rural areas compared with those who moved to permanent towns. *Clin Gastroenterol Hepatol.* 2005;3(4):342–348. doi:10.1016/s1542-3565(04)00553-1
71. Atherton K, Wiles NJ, Lecky FE, et al. Predictors of persistent neck pain after whiplash injury. *Emerg Med J.* 2006;23(3):195–201. doi:10.1136/emj.2005.027102
72. Keefer L, Kiebles JL, Taft TH. The role of self-efficacy in inflammatory bowel disease management: Preliminary validation of a disease-specific measure. *Inflamm Bowel Dis.* 2011;17(2):614–620. doi:10.1002/ibd.21314
73. Taft TH, McGarva J, Omprakash TA, et al. Hospitalization experiences and post-traumatic stress in inflammatory bowel disease: Opportunities for change. *Inflamm Bowel Dis.* 2023;29(5):675–683. doi:10.1093/ibd/izac148
74. Emerson C, Fuller-Tyszkiewicz M, Orr R, et al. Low subjective wellbeing is associated with psychological distress in people living with inflammatory bowel disease. *Dig Dis Sci.* 2022;67(6):2059–2066. doi:10.1007/s10620-021-07065-4
75. Keefer L, Bedell A, Norton C, Hart AL. How should pain, fatigue, and emotional wellness be incorporated into treatment goals for optimal management of inflammatory bowel disease? *Gastroenterology.* 2022;162(5):1439–1451. doi:10.1053/j.gastro.2021.08.060
76. Eswaran S. Low FODMAP in 2017: Lessons learned from clinical trials and mechanistic studies. *Neurogastroenterol Motil.* 2017;29(4). doi:10.1111/nmo.13055
77. Buscail C, Sabate JM, Bouchoucha M, et al. Western dietary pattern is associated with irritable bowel syndrome in the French NutriNet Cohort. *Nutrients.* 2017;9(9):Article 986. doi:10.3390/nu9090986
78. Verdu EF, Armstrong D, Murray JA. Between celiac disease and irritable bowel syndrome: The "no man's land" of gluten sensitivity. *Am J Gastroenterol.* 2009;104(6):1587–1594. doi:10.1038/ajg.2009.188
79. Hill P, Muir JG, Gibson PR. Controversies and recent developments of the low-FODMAP diet. *Gastroenterol Hepatol.* 2017;13(1):36–45.
80. Dionne J, Ford AC, Yuan Y, et al. A systematic review and meta-analysis evaluating the efficacy of a gluten-free diet and a low FODMAPs diet in treating symptoms of irritable bowel syndrome. *Am J Gastroenterol.* Sep 2018;113(9):1290–1300. doi:10.1038/s41395-018-0195-4
81. Parker TJ, Woolner JT, Prevost AT, Tuffnell Q, Shorthouse M, Hunter JO. Irritable bowel syndrome: Is the search for lactose intolerance justified? *Eur J Gastroenterol Hepatol.* 2001;13(3):219–225. doi:10.1097/00042737-200103000-00001
82. Bernstein CN, Kraut A, Blanchard JF, Rawsthorne P, Yu N, Walld R. The relationship between inflammatory bowel disease and socioeconomic variables. *Am J Gastroenterol.* 2001;96(7):2117–2125. doi:10.1111/j.1572-0241.2001.03946.x
83. Turner D, Ricciuto A, Lewis A, et al. STRIDE-II: An update on the Selecting Therapeutic Targets in Inflammatory Bowel Disease (STRIDE) initiative of the International Organization for the Study of IBD (IOIBD): Determining therapeutic goals for treat-to-target strategies in IBD. *Gastroenterology.* 2021;160(5):1570–1583. doi:10.1053/j.gastro.2020.12.031
84. Wils P, Caron B, D'Amico F, Danese S, Peyrin-Biroulet L. Abdominal pain in inflammatory bowel diseases: A clinical challenge. *J Clin Med.* 2022;11(15):4269. doi:10.3390/jcm11154269
85. Hart AL, Lomer M, Verjee A, et al. What are the top 10 research questions in the treatment of inflammatory bowel disease? A priority setting partnership with the James Lind Alliance. *J Crohns Colitis.* 2017;11(2):204–211. doi:10.1093/ecco-jcc/jjw144

86. Ko CW, Singh S, Feuerstein JD, et al. AGA clinical practice guidelines on the management of mild-to-moderate ulcerative colitis. *Gastroenterology*. 2019;156(3):748–764. doi:10.1053/j.gastro.2018.12.009
87. Pariente B, Mary JY, Danese S, et al. Development of the Lemann Index to assess digestive tract damage in patients with Crohn's disease. *Gastroenterology*. 2015;148(1):52–63. doi:10.1053/j.gastro.2014.09.015
88. Feuerstein JD, Ho EY, Shmidt E, et al. AGA clinical practice guidelines on the medical management of moderate to severe luminal and perianal fistulizing Crohn's disease. *Gastroenterology*. 2021;160(7):2496–2508. doi:10.1053/j.gastro.2021.04.022
89. Feuerstein JD, Isaacs KL, Schneider Y, et al. AGA clinical practice guidelines on the management of moderate to severe ulcerative colitis. *Gastroenterology*. 2020;158(5):1450–1461. doi:10.1053/j.gastro.2020.01.006
90. Joris JL, Georges MJ, Medjahed K, et al. Prevalence, characteristics and risk factors of chronic postsurgical pain after laparoscopic colorectal surgery: Retrospective analysis. *Eur J Anaesthesiol*. 2015;32(10):712–717. doi:10.1097/EJA.0000000000000268
91. Long MD, Kappelman MD, Martin CF, Chen W, Anton K, Sandler RS. Role of nonsteroidal anti-inflammatory drugs in exacerbations of inflammatory bowel disease. *J Clin Gastroenterol*. 2016;50(2):152–156. doi:10.1097/MCG.0000000000000421
92. Wynne J, Kozuch P. Medical marijuana for inflammatory bowel disease: The highs and lows. *Scand J Gastroenterol*. 2022;57(2):197–205. doi:10.1080/00365521.2021.1998604
93. Coates MD, Seth N, Clarke K, et al. Opioid analgesics do not improve abdominal pain or quality of life in Crohn's disease. *Dig Dis Sci*. 2020;65(8):2379–2387. doi:10.1007/s10620-019-05968-x
94. Ford AC, Talley NJ, Spiegel BMR, et al. Effect of fibre, antispasmodics, and peppermint oil in the treatment of irritable bowel syndrome: Systematic review and meta-analysis. *BMJ*. 2008;337:a2313. doi:ARTN a2313 10.1136/bmj.a2313
95. Lambarth A, Zarate-Lopez N, Fayaz A. Oral and parenteral anti-neuropathic agents for the management of pain and discomfort in irritable bowel syndrome: A systematic review and meta-analysis. *Neurogastroent Motil*. 2022;34(1):e14289. doi:ARTN e14289 10.1111/nmo.14289
96. Black CJ, Yuan YH, Selinger CP, et al. Efficacy of soluble fibre, antispasmodic drugs, and gut-brain neuromodulators in irritable bowel syndrome: A systematic review and network meta-analysis. *Lancet Gastroenterol*. 2020;5(2):117–131. doi:10.1016/S2468-1253(19)30324-3
97. Ford AC, Lacy BE, Harris LA, Quigley EMM, Moayyedi P. Effect of antidepressants and psychological therapies in irritable bowel syndrome: An updated systematic review and meta-analysis. *Am J Gastroenterol*. 2019;114(1):21–39. doi:10.1038/s41395-018-0222-5
98. Lackner JM, Jaccard J, Keefer L, et al. Improvement in gastrointestinal symptoms after cognitive behavior therapy for refractory irritable bowel syndrome. *Gastroenterology*. 2018;155(1):47–57. doi:10.1053/j.gastro.2018.03.063
99. Laird KT, Tanner-Smith EE, Russell AC, Hollon SD, Walker LS. Comparative efficacy of psychological therapies for improving mental health and daily functioning in irritable bowel syndrome: A systematic review and meta-analysis. *Clin Psychol Rev*. 2017;51:142–152. doi:10.1016/j.cpr.2016.11.001
100. Lackner JM, Jaccard J, Radziwon CD, et al. Durability and decay of treatment benefit of cognitive behavioral therapy for irritable bowel syndrome: 12-Month follow-up. *Am J Gastroenterol*. 2019;114(2):330–338. doi:10.1038/s41395-018-0396-x
101. Lalouni M, Ljotsson B, Bonnert M, et al. Clinical and cost effectiveness of online cognitive behavioral therapy in children with functional abdominal pain disorders. *Clin Gastroenterol Hepatol*. 2019;17(11):2236–2244. doi:10.1016/j.cgh.2018.11.043

26
Pain in People Living with HIV

Mary Catherine George, Sotonye Douglas, Kaitlyn Coyle, Shanna-Kay Christa Griffiths, and Jessica Robinson-Papp

Introduction

Vulnerability has been a key concern for people living with HIV since the epidemic first started more than 40 years ago. The presence of HIV, a serious medical condition, was compounded for many people by social and economic challenges; gender, sexual, racial, and/or ethnic minority status; substance use disorders (SUDs); trauma; and the experience of pervasive stigma. These issues have not resolved, and the stigma associated with being HIV-positive continues despite HIV disease no longer being a death sentence, as highly effective antivirals (ARVs) offer individuals a near normal life span. Given the demographics of people living with HIV (PLWH), many experience the stigma of an HIV diagnosis combined with membership in other marginalized groups within the HIV population, compounding vulnerability.[1] Personal stories abound. Consider Billy Porter, a talented award-winning entertainer who finally revealed his secret of being HIV-positive after 14 years. Porter shared that he kept his status secret for fear of being marginalized in the entertainment world and shamed by his family. Consider a young woman who posted on social media that she discovered she was HIV-positive after a casual sexual encounter. The comments to her were filled with shaming statements, and she was blocked by friends (personal communication, 2022), which created hesitancy to discuss her health status with anyone again.

In this chapter, we discuss the complex vulnerabilities within the HIV population and how they might influence the experience and management of chronic pain, a common and often debilitating comorbidity experienced by PLWH. The potentially vulnerable populations within the HIV population are many, including men who have sex with men (MSM), bisexual and transgender individuals, sex workers, prisoners, immigrants and racial and ethnic minority groups, individuals with mental health and SUDs, and people experiencing poverty including homelessness. The chapter is divided into three main sections. The first section focuses on vulnerabilities experienced by some people living with HIV and how they might contribute to the experience of chronic pain. The second section reviews the types of chronic pain that are common in people living with HIV and approaches to their treatment. Finally, the third section addresses how the lens of vulnerability might be applied to a conceptual model of pain in PLWH to identify novel treatment strategies.

What Makes People with HIV More Vulnerable to Pain?

Vulnerable Groups Within the HIV Population

In the broadest sense, vulnerability can be conceptualized as susceptibility to harm, and it can encompass physical/biological as well as psychosocial vulnerability. Vulnerability in some form often predates an HIV diagnosis and contributes to the risk of HIV acquisition. Accordingly, these pre-existing factors persist at higher prevalence among the population of PLWH. This can also be understood as diverse and layered vulnerability. The layers of vulnerability that exist in the HIV population are not a new occurrence. During the early years of the epidemic, vulnerable populations were at high risk due to sexual behavior within the lesbian, gay, bisexual, transgender, and queer community, coupled with the intravenous drug use population. Over time, additional layered vulnerabilities became apparent; for example, incarcerated individuals, who are among the most complex groups at high risk for HIV infection, are typically composed of several other groups of people who are more vulnerable to HIV/AIDS, such as individuals with SUD, sex workers, and sexual or gender minorities.[2] Due to these complex and overlapping vulnerabilities, a conceptualization of vulnerability based on an individual's particular situation or circumstance may be more helpful than attempts to categorize vulnerability according to group membership. Approaching the HIV population from this perspective would facilitate acknowledgment of the layers of vulnerability that exist[3] and how they might influence how PLWH are provided health care when presenting with a chronic pain condition.

HIV has been referred to as part of a "syndemic," a co-occurrence of the disease with related conditions and health disparities. As HIV patients are aging, they are suffering from the complexities of frailty, opioid use, alcohol and substance use, coupled with mental health challenges, racial biases, and other environmental factors, all which call for a shift in the care paradigm for the HIV population.[4,5] Over time as HIV has become a manageable disease, the predominant co-occurring physical diseases have evolved from opportunistic infections to chronic noncommunicable conditions, including chronic pain. Chronic pain diagnoses exacerbate the health care needs of these marginalized groups, and often many suffer in silence, not seeking treatment until the circumstances are urgent. Vulnerabilities may represent barriers to care and should be considered in health care models for PLWH, including those with comorbid chronic pain.[6]

Gender and Sexual Minorities and Sex Workers

The largest group, representing slightly more than half of all HIV-infected individuals, is MSM. No matter whether an individual identifies as gay, straight, or bisexual, the element of having sex with men is the criterion that places individuals at risk of becoming HIV infected.[7] One in six MSM will eventually become HIV-positive,[8] despite the emphasis on pre-exposure prophylaxis (PrEP), which is available and effective.[9] Transgender people make up approximately 2% of individuals newly diagnosed with HIV in the United States, of whom 46% are Black.[10] Sex workers can be particularly vulnerable given the physical and psychological dangers of the work and the poverty that often precedes and accompanies it.[11]

Racial and Ethnic Minorities

Black people comprise a strikingly disproportionate number of new HIV infections in the United States (42%); this is especially marked for Black men, who account for 31% of all new HIV diagnoses. Given that in the vast majority of these cases the route of infection is sex with men, addressing the intersectional vulnerabilities of racial and sexual minority status is key to preventing HIV infection and, if HIV infection does occur, reducing associated comorbidities, including pain. The Hispanic/Latinx population is also significantly overrepresented at 28% of new infections. Due to historical and ongoing inequities, racial and/or ethnic minority status is often associated with additional vulnerabilities due to poverty, lower education, communication barriers, and challenges in access to medical care or preventive treatments.[12]

Women

As of 2019, out of the 1.2 million PLWH, 263,900 were women. Although women are underrepresented among PLWH, they are overrepresented among people with chronic pain and so approximately 50% of people living with both HIV and chronic pain are women.[13] Women living with HIV may be at particular risk for experiencing stigma and discrimination from both their communities and health care professionals, and also for internalizing it.[14] Women living with HIV may face being labeled as "promiscuous," "diseased," or "prostitute" due to the history of stigma associated with HIV in women specifically.

Incarcerated Individuals

Incarcerated individuals are considered a highly vulnerable group in the United States, with a higher rate of contracting infectious diseases; more diagnoses of mental illness and SUD; and a higher mortality rate after being released from prison, mostly from opioid overdoses.[15] A study by Meyer et al.[16] found that out of 151 HIV-infected incarcerated individuals who were released from prison, 56% of them ended up in the emergency department within 12 months of being released; 20.3% of those visits were due to pain. The types of pain most frequently named were "extremity pain or swelling," "abdominal pain or swelling," "back pain," and "acute or chronic pain."

There have been efforts to decrease the spread of HIV within the prison systems, such as providing incarcerated individuals with PrEP, but many facilities would rather focus on improving security.[17] Chimoyi et al.[17] identified previous research showing that incarcerated individuals living with HIV face discrimination not only for having an HIV infection but also for being incarcerated. This discrimination, coupled with internalized stigma, is a barrier to HIV care because individuals may delay seeking treatment for fear of disclosing their status. Short-term incarceration of less than 30 days has also been identified as a barrier in HIV care. Detention centers and jails, which are used for short-term stays, stays of uncertain duration, or for individuals awaiting trial, are fast-paced environments that face overcrowding and also communication deficits with health care providers, which can cause delays or errors in medication administration for HIV-infected individuals.[18]

People Who Are Homeless

A home is more than a physical structure. It is where we enjoy privacy, comfort, and protection and take care of our health and ourselves. Homelessness within the HIV population has been a long-standing issue. Research shows that homeless individuals with HIV represent a vulnerable population at increased risk for various health and social issues, such as substance abuse, mental illness, violence, poor access and adherence to HIV medical care, and high-risk sexual practices.[19] PLWH are at higher risk of becoming homeless.[20] From 2010 to 2016, the percentage of people in HIV medical care who were homeless increased from 7.7% to 8.4%.[8,21]

Adding to the challenges homelessness presents, chronic pain in homeless PLWH is associated with poor living conditions. In a study that assessed the characteristics of chronic pain in a cohort of 296 homeless PLWH, more than 90% of participants reported having chronic pain, with 34% attributing their pain to their living conditions.[22] In another study of 503 indigent PLWH in which 39.2% reported homelessness in the prior 3 months, analyses showed food and housing insecurity were greatly associated with chronic pain. This study concluded that poor living conditions might cause, worsen, and prolong pain in PLWH.[23]

Food insecurity is especially problematic among homeless PLWH. In a study done in San Francisco that consisted of 284 homeless PLWH, 54.6% of participants were food insecure, and food insecurity was associated with low antiretroviral therapy (ART) adherence, unsuppressed viral loads, and low $CD4^+$ cell counts. In addition, food insecurity may cause homeless PLWH to engage in risky sexual practices to secure meals and survive. Chronic pain and homelessness are associated with health service utilization and incomplete viral suppression in the HIV population.[24] Limited research exists on PLWH related to food insecurity, but in a study performed in Canada, food insecurity was associated with increased chronic pain perception and misuse of opioids in their community.[25]

Housing assistance programs specifically for people with HIV have been helpful with regard to addressing homelessness and improving health outcomes. Two examples are the Housing First program and the Health Resources and Services Administration's Ryan White HIV/AIDS Program (RWHAP). Housing First provides housing and supportive services to homeless PLWH immediately. A study showed a 69% undetectable viral load among homeless PLWH who participated in the Housing First program, compared with 16% undetectable viral load among participants in other housing programs.[21] RWHAP serves more than 500,000 PLWH, including more than 25,000 unstably housed people. RWHAP provides multiple services to PLWH, including medical services, mental health treatment, and support services (case management and transportation). Griffin et al.[26] reported that between 2010 and 2017, there was an increase in stable housing from 82% to 87.1%, as reported by RWHAP participants. In addition, there was an increase in the number of participants receiving medical care from 69.5% to 85.9%. As demonstrated by these housing assistance programs, stable housing can increase quality of life in PLWH and lay the foundation for better pain management and HIV outcomes.

Lower Educational Status

In a U.S. study of 103 participants with HIV-related neuropathic pain (HIV-NeP), patients with a high school education or less were more likely to experience severe pain than patients with more than a high school education ($p < .001$).[27] Mann and colleagues[27] also reported the total annual direct HIV-NeP–related medical cost for participants averaged $5,288 per patient with mild pain, $3,944 per patient with moderate pain, and $6,861 per patient with severe pain. Sabin and colleagues[28] made a similar observation regarding education in a cross-sectional analysis of a cohort study in the United Kingdom and Ireland. HIV participants with low educational attainment had regional or widespread pain that was 50% higher than that of participants with high educational attainment.[28]

People Who Use Prescription Opioids

In the past, opioids were commonly prescribed for pain, especially to people with HIV early in the epidemic who were treated in accordance with a palliative care model prior to the advent of ARVs. However, given the current U.S. opioid epidemic, which had its origins in prescription opioid misuse, physicians are now more hesitant to prescribe opioids.[29] Although this hesitation has caused the amount of opioid prescriptions to decrease throughout the past few years, the number of fatal overdoses due to opioid misuse reached a record high in 2021,[30] largely due to increases in the use of heroin and illegally manufactured fentanyl. Some data show that the most significant decrease in opioid prescribing was in new prescriptions—that is, those for patients who had not received opioids previously.[31] This is likely positive in that it reflects fewer new opioid exposures. However, it may also reflect a new vulnerability in that PLWH who have been treated with long-term opioid therapy for chronic pain may have great difficulty finding a new prescriber should they lose access to their current prescriber.

People with Mental Health Disorders

Major depressive disorder is commonly seen in patients living with HIV and pain, which likely decreases HIV patients' responses to pain treatments.[32] Pain and depressive symptoms likely have a bidirectional relationship in which each condition may cause the other to intensify; this may be due to avoidance and withdrawal of everyday activities for fear of emotional and physical pain. One study found that participants who were experiencing moderate to severe chronic pain had higher levels of depression and depressive symptoms than the participants with no chronic pain.[33] It has also been shown that depression is a strong predictor of chronic pain development, likely due to mediators such as decreased physical activity and more focus on psychological symptoms. Depression paired with chronic pain can cause more intense and prolonged depressive symptoms, as well as higher rates of suicide. For individuals living with HIV, chronic pain, and depression, there is also an increased risk of mediating nonadherence to antiretrovirals. Increasing research in behavioral methodologies to provide supportive care earlier could aid in managing pain perception, nonadherence to ARVs, and decrease suicide rates.[34]

Physical Vulnerability: Chronic Pain in HIV

Previously, we described multiple potential vulnerabilities that are prevalent among PLWH. But do these vulnerabilities also contribute to the development of pain in PLWH? Moreover, how might society's perception and response to a vulnerability impact the affected person's experience? In this section, we provide an overview of chronic pain in HIV and then focus on specific pain syndromes. In the section thereafter, we address stigma as experienced by PLWH and its potential interaction with chronic pain. Treatment modalities are addressed in the discussion.

Chronic pain is a condition found in approximately 50–85% of the HIV population.[6] The predominant individual chronic pain conditions are musculoskeletal conditions, peripheral neuropathy, and headache. However, many PLWH may experience chronic overlapping pain conditions and multisite pain of uncertain etiology, which may reflect central sensitization (also referred to as nociplastic pain).[35] Chronic pain conditions intensify management and treatment of vulnerable groups, which makes these subgroups the most vulnerable among the vulnerable. Chronic pain also significantly affects quality of life in PLWH. Two cross-sectional studies examining sleep disturbance in PLWH showed significant sleep problems in participants with pain compared to those without pain ($p < .001$). The results also showed limited ambulation distances.[36,37] Sabin et al.[28] found that pain was associated with lower employment and poor functional status in the HIV population, regardless of age. Scott et al.[37] reported that PLWH with pain were more likely to be unemployed than those without pain ($p < .001$). Moderate to severe chronic pain is also commonly associated with poor ART outcomes.[28]

Peripheral Neuropathy

Peripheral neuropathy affects 20–50% of individuals with HIV.[36] Its most common form is sometimes referred to as distal symmetric polyneuropathy (DSP). As its name describes, DSP involves the most distal part of nerves and is usually symmetric from side to side. This distribution arises from the anatomy of nerves, which originate with the cell body at the level of the spinal cord and then travel long distances to their final destinations in the hands and feet. The portions of the nerve that are farthest from the cell body are the most vulnerable to injury; thus, DSP symptoms usually begin in the feet and may include burning, shooting pain, numbness, and/or tingling. Peripheral neuropathy in PLWH may be due to the effect of HIV itself. In addition, some of the ARVs used in the past were neurotoxic, and patients may have residual effects from these.[37] Increasingly, other medical comorbidities, especially diabetes, are also likely contributory. Patients with HIV and peripheral neuropathy are more than twice as likely to have other chronic pain disorders; they are also more likely to be older, have coexisting mental health disorders, and have a history of substance use. Peripheral neuropathy is not currently reversible, and so treatment focuses on symptom management. The complex constellation of peripheral neuropathy, other pain syndromes, and comorbidities argues for a broad and holistic approach to treatment.

Chronic Widespread Pain Syndrome

Chronic widespread pain syndrome is a long-term condition with widespread muscle pain and somatic symptoms, including fatigue, psychological distress, and concentration problems. Chronic widespread pain is also the cardinal feature of fibromyalgia. Chronic widespread pain is a common problem in the general population, with an estimated prevalence of 1 in 10 adults.[38] In patients with HIV, estimates of chronic widespread pain syndrome prevalence range from 25% to 90%.[39] These estimates are substantially higher than those for the general population, and the impact is debilitating for patients with HIV, who often have limited resources.

Bone and Joint Pain

People living with HIV commonly experience chronic focal, multifocal, or diffuse joint pain due to various forms of arthritis. In the general population, the prevalence of adults with arthritis is 23.7%.[40] It is speculated that the prevalence of arthritis in HIV may be higher given that chronic treated HIV is a systemic illness with an inflammatory component; however, this is uncertain. Bone disorders are common comorbidities associated with HIV and contribute to various pain ailments, including fractures. Pramukti et al.[41] found an almost twofold greater odds of fracture for PLWH compared with the general population due to decreased bone mineral density (BMD) in patients with HIV. Low BMD has been reported in HIV as three times higher than in HIV-negative controls. The loss of BMD increases the risk of osteoporosis, osteonecrosis, and, rarely, osteomalacia.[42,43] The proposed mechanism is chronic T-cell activation resulting in increased production of proinflammatory cytokines that enhance osteoclast activity and accelerate bone loss.[44] Osteonecrosis also presents with bone or joint pain and is due to poor blood supply to the affected bone. Miller et al.[45] found a high occurrence of osteonecrosis of the hip in patients with HIV and recommended a high suspicion for the diagnosis on presentation of hip pain. The current treatment for osteonecrosis is surgical.

Chronic Low Back Pain

According to data from the National Institutes of Health, the annual prevalence of activity-limiting low back pain is estimated at 39% in the general population.[46] The causes include mechanical back pain due to muscular strain, herniated disc, or stenosis. Low bone density, which is common in PLWH, may also be contributory if it results in microfractures, which could contribute to chronic pain. Low back pain may also commonly occur as part of chronic widespread pain syndromes. One study of 137 PLWH referred to a palliative care clinic found that 76 of them experienced low back pain, the majority of which was due to degenerative spine disease.[47] Degenerative lumbar spine disease is typically a combination of degenerative disc disease, bony changes such as osteophytes, and ligamentous hypertrophy.[48] These can be painful in and of themselves, and they typically result in axial low back pain. However, they can also combine to cause narrowing of the spinal canal and neural foramina, leading to nerve root involvement (i.e., radiculopathy) and symptoms of pain radiating into the lower limbs.

Chronic Headache

The International Classification of Headache Disorders classifies chronic headaches into five subtypes: chronic migraine headache, chronic tension-type headache, medication overuse headache, hemicrania continua, and new daily persistent headache. According to some authors, headache is the most common pain complaint in PLWH.[49] In one study, 53.5% of patients (n = 200) from an internal medicine clinic/HIV outreach clinic reported symptoms consistent with a primary headache disorder, including chronic migraine, and episodic or chronic tension type headache.[50] The study also found a statistically significant association between CD4 cell count and headache severity, frequency, and disability.

Oral and Gastrointestinal Pain

People living with HIV may experience numerous painful conditions involving the oral cavity and the gastrointestinal tract, which may be due to immunocompromise and/or the effects of HIV infection and ARVs on the microbiome.[51] Starting in the oral cavity, abnormalities have been described in 30–80% of PLWH and were often found to be inadequately addressed in medical care.[52] The most common is likely herpes simplex virus lesions, which may be exacerbated by xerostomia related to polypharmacy. Odynophagia is pain during swallowing and can arise due to infections such as candida, cytomegalovirus, and herpes simplex virus or from idiopathic esophageal ulcers or pill esophagitis caused by irritative medications. Abdominal pain is also commonly reported by PLWH; however, the typical diagnoses are the same as for the general population and include gastroesophageal reflux disease, peptic ulcer disease, and gastritis.[53] There is some preliminary evidence that PLWH more commonly experience small intestinal bacterial overgrowth,[54] but it is uncertain whether this contributes to abdominal discomfort. Anorectal pathologies, such as anal and/or rectal ulcerations, anorectal fissures, perirectal abscesses, and proctitis, are often painful and can be seen with increased frequency among PLWH, particularly MSM.[55]

Psychosocial Vulnerability, Stigma, and Discrimination

Vulnerability within the context of research is typically associated with groups such as the socially and economically disadvantaged, those with diminished cognition, and children.[3] However, as we have described in the preceding sections, some PLWH might belong to more than one vulnerable group, and so conceptualizing the vulnerability as a specific constellation of conditions present in an individual may be more relevant. Stigma and discrimination are concepts closely related to vulnerability. Whereas "vulnerable" applies to the affected individual, stigma and discrimination describe negative responses of others to that individual that have the potential to exacerbate the vulnerability.

Health care discrimination, specifically toward PLWH, still widely exists today, with 26–40% of PLWH reporting that they have experienced discrimination by a health care worker since being diagnosed with HIV.[56–58] Examples of health care discrimination include overt acts, such as verbal abuse and refusal of care, and more subtle manifestations, including avoidance of eye contact and physical touch and providing different treatment options to one patient compared to another. Fear of discrimination and stigmatization from health care workers and other social contacts can be a significant barrier to proper medical care. For example, Gonzalez et al.[59] found that early HIV care was significantly decreased in women and marginalized populations due to stigma. In addition, many individuals suffer from internalized stigma.[60,61] Tian et al.[62] reported in their study of 724 PLWH that experiences of social injustice, racial biases, or judgment were internalized, intensifying the perception of stigma, deepening depression, and worsening overall health. The study found that addressing these layers of vulnerabilities related to stigma improved health and an overall sense of well-being.

All facets of stigma, including health care–based, societal, and internalized, contribute to mental health burden in PLWH, and stigma is commonly multilayered. In addition to HIV stigma, PLWH with chronic pain also experience chronic pain stigma. This is observed most commonly when chronic pain is of unknown etiology.[63] Stigma is a significant barrier to care for PLWH and can also increase pain sensitivity.[64] In addition, HIV and chronic pain stigma together could result in less medication adherence, less retention in care, and poorer patient–provider relationships.[6] Baker et al.[65] found that PLWH with chronic pain developed negative beliefs about how seeking pain management services would result in disclosure of their HIV status and HIV stigma. They concluded that negative thoughts also created barriers to pain management and observed it would be easier for PLWH to seek pain support if there were less stigma. They also observed that participants "avoided social interactions to prevent stigma and discrimination causing social isolation."[65]

Crockett et al.[61] researched pain in women living with HIV and how it related to their internalized stigma stemming from their HIV infection. They used data from the Women's Interagency HIV Study (WIHS) to assess their hypothesis that internalized HIV stigma predicts pain. The study subjects were women living with HIV enrolled in WIHS who completed questions from the HIV Stigma Scale, the Center for Epidemiological Studies Depression Scale, and the Medical Outcomes Study Short Form Health Survey (SF-36). Through this analysis, it was found that internalized HIV stigma was a direct contributor to pain in this cohort 1 year later, with the effects of the stigma strengthened by the presence of depressive symptoms acting as a mediator. Stigma, close relationships, and life stressors have also been shown, in research by Merlin et al.,[66] to be primary mediators of chronic pain. These results provide evidence of the negative effects of chronic pain and stigma on PLWH. Stigma may impact pain perception in PLWH who identify as part of a marginalized group. A recent qualitative study interviewed patients who self-reported the years of suffering from pain, their gender identity, social challenges, and barriers to care.[65] Chronic pain was described as an enmeshed experience in which these issues of self-identity are enmeshed with the chronic pain condition.[67,68]

Discussion

Layers of stigma and marginalization undoubtedly increase suffering among people living with HIV and chronic pain. However, this has been recognized for multiple decades, and this recognition has had a lasting positive impact on the manner in which PLWH receive health care in the United States. The RWHAP, which formed the basis for multidisciplinary patient-centered HIV care, was first enacted in 1990, named for a child who personally faced tremendous stigma, being barred from attending school because of an AIDS diagnosis.[69] The care supported by the RWHAP worked to co-locate HIV primary care with other key services, including social work, nursing, pharmacy, and mental health resources. This model evolved to address the medical and psychosocial complexity of PLWH, and as such, it represents a solid foundation from which to deliver pain management services within an environment that is already uniquely aware of the needs of vulnerable persons.[70]

Enhanced models of clinical care are also being studied, such as medical–legal partnerships (MLPs).[71] The concept is to incorporate legal services within the health care paradigm to improve the overarching engagement in care by providing access to legal services. These partnerships institute systems to address social and environmental legal risks that PLWH may encounter, spanning a broad range of issues from unsafe housing to domestic or elder abuse, immigration asylum, workplace discrimination, and other relevant social and justice challenges. The Williams Institute in Los Angeles conducted a study that showed approximately 98% of PLWH will encounter a legal issue within a 12-month period. In a study examining MLPs serving veterans, participants who used more of the legal services showed improved housing, mental health, and community involvement.[72] While research on the MLP model for HIV is developing, there are smaller changes that can be instituted. For example, in a primary care setting, the addition of a "navigator" may help patients who identify as belonging to a marginalized group connect with providers sensitive to these patients' unique issues.[73] Ultimately, an ideal model would comprehensively support the vulnerability of PLWH and help those who are suffering with chronic pain by keeping them engaged in care and adherent to their HIV and pain treatments.

The medical community can be challenged when treating vulnerable patients with HIV and determining what systems will best serve these groups. In the past, health care was designed around three areas: risk, fear, and moral management.[74] A transition has moved toward key goals for PLWH to maintain quality of life, stay engaged in health care, and adhere to HIV treatments. Structures designed to support these fundamental goals can also offer stability when patients have a chronic pain condition. However, HIV health care practitioners have limited time and training to address patients' multilayered vulnerability and pain management needs.[75] This is compounded by difficulty accessing appropriate specialty pain care, given that PLWH are commonly socioeconomically disadvantaged and reliant on public forms of insurance such as Medicaid.

The aging population of PLWH and increasing burden of comorbid medical illness layer on top of the need to provide care that is sensitive to multiple potential vulnerabilities. The need to provide pain management services as well may be seen as "the straw that broke the camel's back" by some HIV providers. Many HIV care providers feel ill-prepared to provide pain management services, which is likely linked to understandable discomfort with opioid prescribing.[76,77] Moreover, the bedrock of appropriate chronic pain management in HIV, similar to other chronic pain populations, is nonpharmacologic treatment (e.g., physical therapy and cognitive–behavioral therapy [CBT]), which requires additional staff not typically present in the HIV clinic.[78] In a study assessing CBT as an alternative treatment for chronic pain in PLWH, significant improvements in chronic pain were associated with program enrollment. Although more than 50% of patients did not complete all the sessions, CBT-based pain management was shown to be effective in patients who participated and completed all sessions.[79] These patients had chronic pain at multiple sites of the body. Physical therapy is acknowledged as an affordable and safe option for chronic pain management in PLWH.[80] There is also some preliminary evidence for a positive effect of mindfulness-based stress reduction.[81] Unfortunately, if such services are not co-located in the clinic, they are often difficult to obtain given that many PLWH lack the financial resources to pay out of pocket and have public forms of insurance that seek to limit costs.

The above described factors likely conspire to create an overreliance on pharmacologic therapies. There are no medications that are U.S. Food and Drug Administration–approved specifically for any pain condition related to HIV, and so in general, pharmacologic treatment does not differ significantly from that of other patient populations. Numerous studies have tested potential pharmacologic treatments for pain due to HIV-associated peripheral neuropathy. These include anticonvulsants (gabapentin, lamotrigine, and pregabalin),[82–84] topical therapies (capsaicin and lidocaine),[85–87] antidepressants (duloxetine and amitriptyline),[88,89] smoked cannabis,[90–92] and opioids.[36,93] Due to the unacceptable risk of opioid use disorder, opioids are currently not considered appropriate as a first-line treatment for chronic pain. However, earlier in the HIV/AIDS epidemic before there were effective ARVs, many patients were treated with opioids in congruence with a palliative model for what was then an untreatable and likely fatal disease.[94] This practice persisted for many years before the risks of pharmaceutical opioids were fully appreciated, and opioid prescribing rates began to decline around 2012. It is currently uncertain how best to manage PLWH who have been on long-term opioids for chronic pain. However, preliminary evidence suggests that careful adherence to the Centers for Disease Control and Prevention guidelines for opioid prescribing in chronic pain is a safe approach.[95]

Conclusion

People living with HIV can suffer from a wide variety of chronic pain conditions, and managing pain is often not within the training or expertise of their primary treating physicians. Added to this is the complexity of vulnerability that arises from belonging to one or more marginalized groups and is compounded by the associated stigma. Integrating these issues, which make PLWH the most vulnerable among the vulnerable, involves adjusting care to be inclusive of diverse identities and mindful of the impact of factors such as food insecurity, access to housing, or transportation needs. Factors such as these can contribute to the ability of PLWH to attend their follow-up clinical sessions or adhere to treatment. Furthermore, integrating nonpharmacologic pain treatments such as mindfulness, gentle yoga, self-hypnosis, and breathing practices may help PLWH view the health care environment as a safe place.[96] Future research may shed light on ways in which the currently successful models of HIV care can become even more attentive to intersectional vulnerability and evolve toward greater integration of comprehensive and patient-centered pain management for PLWH.

References

1. O'Brien KK, Brown DA, Corbett C, et al. AIDSImpact special issue: Broadening the lens: recommendations from rehabilitation in chronic disease to advance healthy ageing with HIV. *AIDS Care*. 2020;32(Suppl 2):65–73. doi:10.1080/09540121.2020.1739203
2. Milloy MJ, Montaner JS, Wood E. Incarceration of people living with HIV/AIDS: Implications for treatment-as-prevention. *Curr HIV/AIDS Rep*. 2014;11(3):308–316. doi:10.1007/s11904-014-0214-z

3. Gordon BG. Vulnerability in research: Basic ethical concepts and general approach to review. *Ochsner J*. 2020;20(1):34–38. doi:10.31486/toj.19.0079
4. Womack JA, Justice AC. The OATH syndemic: Opioids and other substances, aging, alcohol, tobacco, and HIV. *Curr Opin HIV AIDS*. 2020;15(4):218–225. doi:10.1097/coh.0000000000000635
5. Godley BA, Adimora AA. Syndemic theory, structural violence and HIV among African-Americans. Curr Opin HIV AIDS. 2020;15(4):250–255. doi:10.1097/coh.0000000000000634
6. Madden VJ, Parker R, Goodin BR. Chronic pain in people with HIV: A common comorbidity and threat to quality of life. *Pain Manag*. 2020;10(4):253–260. doi:10.2217/pmt-2020-0004
7. Kahle EM, Suarez N, Sharma A, Sullivan S, Stephenson R. Threat and impact of HIV compared to other health conditions among an online sample of gay, bisexual and other men who have sex with men in the U.S. *AIDS Care*. 2020;32(5):608–615. doi:10.1080/09540121.2019.1626341
8. Centers for Disease Control and Prevention. CDC HIV Prevention Progress Report, 2019. 2019. Accessed September 20, 2022. https://npin.cdc.gov/publication/hiv-prevention-progress-report-2019
9. Higa DH, Crepaz N, McDonald CM, et al. HIV prevention research on men who have sex with men: A scoping review of systematic reviews, 1988–2017. *AIDS Educ Prev*. 2020;32(1):1–S7. doi:10.1521/aeap.2020.32.1.1
10. Centers for Disease Control and Prevention. (2018). HIV among transgender people. 2017. https://www. cdc. gov/hiv/group/gender/transgender/index. html. Accessed 2017-10-31.
11. Paz-Bailey G, Noble M, Salo K, Tregear SJ. Prevalence of HIV among U.S. female sex workers: Systematic review and meta-analysis. *AIDS Behav*. 2016;20(10):2318–2331. doi:10.1007/s10461-016-1332-y
12. Sullivan PS, Satcher Johnson A, Pembleton ES, et al. Epidemiology of HIV in the USA: Epidemic burden, inequities, contexts, and responses. *Lancet*. 2021;397(10279):1095–1106. doi:10.1016/s0140-6736(21)00395-0
13. Jiao JM, So E, Jebakumar J, George MC, Simpson DM, Robinson-Papp J. Chronic pain disorders in HIV primary care: Clinical characteristics and association with healthcare utilization. *Pain*. 2016;157(4):931–937. doi:10.1097/j.pain.0000000000000462
14. Paudel V, Baral KP. Women living with HIV/AIDS (WLHA), battling stigma, discrimination and denial and the role of support groups as a coping strategy: A review of literature. *Reprod Health*. 2015;12: Article 53. doi:10.1186/s12978-015-0032-9
15. Sugarman OK, Bachhuber MA, Wennerstrom A, Bruno T, Springgate BF. Interventions for incarcerated adults with opioid use disorder in the United States: A systematic review with a focus on social determinants of health. *PLoS One*. 2020;15(1):e0227968. doi:10.1371/journal.pone.0227968
16. Meyer JP, Qiu J, Chen NE, Larkin GL, Altice FL. Emergency department use by released prisoners with HIV: An observational longitudinal study. *PLoS One*. 2012;7(8):e42416. doi:10.1371/journal.pone.0042416
17. Chimoyi L, Hoffmann CJ, Hausler H, et al. HIV-related stigma and uptake of antiretroviral treatment among incarcerated individuals living with HIV/AIDS in South African correctional settings: A mixed methods analysis. *PLoS One*. 2021;16(7):e0254975. doi:10.1371/journal.pone.0254975
18. Westergaard RP, Kirk GD, Richesson DR, Galai N, Mehta SH. Incarceration predicts virologic failure for HIV-infected injection drug users receiving antiretroviral therapy. *Clin Infect Dis*. 2011;53(7):725–731. doi:10.1093/cid/cir491
19. Wolitski RJ, Pals SL, Kidder DP, Courtenay-Quirk C, Holtgrave DR. The effects of HIV stigma on health, disclosure of HIV status, and risk behavior of homeless and unstably housed persons living with HIV. *AIDS Behav*. 2009;13(6):1222–12232. doi:10.1007/s10461-008-9455-4
20. Padilla M, Frazier EL, Carree T, Luke Shouse R, Fagan J. Mental health, substance use and HIV risk behaviors among HIV-positive adults who experienced homelessness in the United States: Medical Monitoring Project, 2009–2015. *AIDS Care*. 2020;32(5):594–599. doi:10.1080/09540121.2019.1683808

21. Wainwright JJ, Beer L, Tie Y, Fagan JL, Dean HD. Socioeconomic, behavioral, and clinical characteristics of persons living with HIV who experience homelessness in the United States, 2015–2016. *AIDS Behav*. 2020;24(6):1701–1708. doi:10.1007/s10461-019-02704-4
22. Miaskowski C, Penko JM, Guzman D, Mattson JE, Bangsberg DR, Kushel MB. Occurrence and characteristics of chronic pain in a community-based cohort of indigent adults living with HIV infection. *J Pain*. 2011;12(9):1004–1016. doi:10.1016/j.jpain.2011.04.002
23. Surratt HL, Kurtz SP, Levi-Minzi MA, Cicero TJ, Tsuyuki K, O'Grady CL. Pain treatment and antiretroviral medication adherence among vulnerable HIV-positive patients. *AIDS Patient Care STDS*. 2015;29(4):186–192. doi:10.1089/apc.2014.0104
24. Weiser SD, Yuan C, Guzman D, et al. Food insecurity and HIV clinical outcomes in a longitudinal study of urban homeless and marginally housed HIV-infected individuals. *AIDS*. 2013;27(18):2953–2958. doi:10.1097/01.aids.0000432538.70088.a3
25. Men F, Fischer B, Urquia ML, Tarasuk V. Food insecurity, chronic pain, and use of prescription opioids. *SSM Popul Health*. 2021;14:100768. doi:10.1016/j.ssmph.2021.100768
26. Griffin A, Dempsey A, Cousino W, et al. Addressing disparities in the health of persons with HIV attributable to unstable housing in the United States: The role of the Ryan White HIV/AIDS Program. *PLoS Med*. 2020;17(3):e1003057. doi:10.1371/journal.pmed.1003057
27. Mann R, Sadosky A, Schaefer C, et al. Burden of HIV-related neuropathic pain in the United States. *J Int Assoc Provid AIDS Care*. 2016;15(2):114–125. doi:10.1177/2325957415592474
28. Sabin CA, Harding R, Bagkeris E, et al. The predictors of pain extent in people living with HIV. *AIDS*. 2020;34(14):2071–2079. doi:10.1097/qad.0000000000002660
29. Owens B. Opioid prescriptions down but some patients fear doctors now too strict. *CMAJ*. 2019;191(19):e546–e547. doi:10.1503/cmaj.109-5748
30. Stringfellow EJ, Lim TY, Humphreys K, et al. Reducing opioid use disorder and overdose deaths in the United States: A dynamic modeling analysis. *Sci Adv*. 2022;8(25):eabm8147. doi:10.1126/sciadv.abm8147
31. Carroll JJ, Colasanti J, Lira MC, Del Rio C, Samet JH. HIV physicians and chronic opioid therapy: It's time to raise the bar. *AIDS Behav*. 2019;23(4):1057–1061. doi:10.1007/s10461-018-2356-2
32. Uebelacker LA, Weisberg RB, Herman DS, Bailey GL, Pinkston-Camp MM, Stein MD. Chronic pain in HIV-infected patients: Relationship to depression, substance use, and mental health and pain treatment. *Pain Med*. 2015;16(10):1870–1881. doi:10.1111/pme.12799
33. Uebelacker LA, Weisberg RB, Herman DS, et al. Pilot randomized trial of collaborative behavioral treatment for chronic pain and depression in persons living with HIV/AIDS. *AIDS Behav*. 2016;20(8):1675–1681. doi:10.1007/s10461-016-1397-7
34. Moitra E, Tarantino N, Garnaat SL, et al. Using behavioral psychotherapy techniques to address HIV patients' pain, depression, and well-being. *Psychotherapy*. 2020;57(1):83–89. doi:10.1037/pst0000258
35. Nijs J, Lahousse A, Kapreli E, et al. Nociplastic pain criteria or recognition of central sensitization? Pain phenotyping in the past, present and future. *J Clin Med*. J2021;10(15):2303. doi:10.3390/jcm10153203
36. Jazebi N, Evans C, Kadaru HS, et al. HIV-related neuropathy: Pathophysiology, treatment and challenges. *J Neurol Exp Neurosci*. 2021;7(1):15–24. doi:10.17756/jnen.2021-082
37. Scott W, Arkuter C, Kioskli K, et al. Psychosocial factors associated with persistent pain in people with HIV: A systematic review with meta-analysis. *Pain*. 2018;159(12):2461–2476. doi:10.1097/j.pain.0000000000001369
38. Mansfield KE, Sim J, Jordan JL, Jordan KP. A systematic review and meta-analysis of the prevalence of chronic widespread pain in the general population. *Pain*. 2016;157(1):55–64. doi:10.1097/j.pain.0000000000000314
39. Addis DR, DeBerry JJ, Aggarwal S. Chronic pain in HIV. *Mol Pain*. 2020;16:1744806920927276. doi:10.1177/1744806920927276
40. Barbour KE, Helmick CG, Boring M, Brady TJ. Vital signs: Prevalence of doctor-diagnosed arthritis and arthritis-attributable activity limitation: United States, 2013–2015. *MMWR Morb Mortal Wkly Rep*. 2017;66(9):246–253. doi:10.15585/mmwr.mm6609e1

41. Pramukti I, Lindayani L, Chen YC, et al. Bone fracture among people living with HIV: A systematic review and meta-regression of prevalence, incidence, and risk factors. *PLoS One*. 2020;15(6):e0233501. doi:10.1371/journal.pone.0233501
42. McComsey GA, Tebas P, Shane E, et al. Bone disease in HIV infection: A practical review and recommendations for HIV care providers. *Clin Infect Dis*. 2010;51(8):937–946. doi:10.1086/656412
43. Negredo E, Bonjoch A, Clotet B. Management of bone mineral density in HIV-infected patients. *Expert Opin Pharmacother*. 2016;17(6):845–852. doi:10.1517/14656566.2016.1146690
44. Manolagas SC, Jilka RL. Bone marrow, cytokines, and bone remodeling: Emerging insights into the pathophysiology of osteoporosis. *N Engl J Med*. 1995;332(5):305–311. doi:10.1056/nejm199502023320506
45. Miller KD, Masur H, Jones EC, et al. High prevalence of osteonecrosis of the femoral head in HIV-infected adults. *Ann Intern Med*. 2002;137(1):17–25. doi:10.7326/0003-4819-137-1-200207020-00008
46. Deyo RA, Dworkin SF, Amtmann D, et al. Report of the NIH Task Force on Research Standards for Chronic Low Back Pain. *Int J Ther Massage Bodywork*. 2015;8(3):16–33. doi:10.3822/ijtmb.v8i3.295
47. Molony E, Westfall AO, Perry BA, et al. Low back pain and associated imaging findings among HIV-infected patients referred to an HIV/palliative care clinic. *Pain Med*. 2014;15(3):418–424. doi:10.1111/pme.12239
48. Moodley K, Bill PLA, Patel VB. Motor lumbosacral radiculopathy in HIV-infected patients. *South Afr J HIV Med*. 2019;20(1): Article 992. doi:10.4102/sajhivmed.v20i1.992
49. Krasenbaum LJ. A review of HIV and headache: A cross-sectional study. *Headache*. 2017;57(10):1631–1632. doi:10.1111/head.13222
50. Kirkland KE, Kirkland K, Many WJ Jr, Smitherman TA. Headache among patients with HIV disease: Prevalence, characteristics, and associations. *Headache*. 2012;52(3):455–466. doi:10.1111/j.1526-4610.2011.02025.x
51. Koay WLA, Siems LV, Persaud D. The microbiome and HIV persistence: Implications for viral remission and cure. *Curr Opin HIV AIDS*. 2018;13(1):61–68. doi:10.1097/COH.0000000000000434
52. Reznik DA. Oral manifestations of HIV disease. *Top HIV Med*. 2005;13(5):143–148.
53. Panarelli NC, Yantiss RK. Inflammatory and infectious manifestations of immunodeficiency in the gastrointestinal tract. *Mod Pathol*. 2018;31(6):844–861. doi:10.1038/s41379-018-0015-9
54. Robinson-Papp J, Nmashie A, Pedowitz E, et al. The effect of pyridostigmine on small intestinal bacterial overgrowth (SIBO) and plasma inflammatory biomarkers in HIV-associated autonomic neuropathies. *J Neurovirol*. 2019;25(4):551–559. doi:10.1007/s13365-019-00756-9
55. Poynten IM, Jin F, Garland SM, et al. HIV, immune dysfunction, and the natural history of anal high-risk human papillomavirus infection in gay and bisexual men. *J Infect Dis*. 2021;224(2):246–257. doi:10.1093/infdis/jiaa723
56. Stringer KL, Turan B, McCormick L, et al. HIV-related stigma among healthcare providers in the Deep South. *AIDS Behav*. 2016;20(1):115–125. doi:10.1007/s10461-015-1256-y
57. Centers for Disease Control and Prevention. Monitoring selected national HIV prevention and care objectives by using HIV surveillance data—United States and 6 dependent areas, 2019. *HIV Surveill Suppl Rep*. 2021;26(2). https://www.cdc.gov/hiv/library/reports/hiv-surveillance.html
58. Walcott M, Kempf MC, Merlin JS, Turan JM. Structural community factors and sub-optimal engagement in HIV care among low-income women in the Deep South of the USA. *Cult Health Sex*. 2016;18(6):682–694. doi:10.1080/13691058.2015.1110255
59. Gonzalez C, Brouwer KC, Reed E, et al. Women trading sex in a U.S.–Mexico border city: A qualitative study of the barriers and facilitators to finding community and voice. *Sexes*. 2020;1(1):1–18. doi:10.3390/sexes1010001

60. Katz IT, Ryu AE, Onuegbu AG, et al. Impact of HIV-related stigma on treatment adherence: Systematic review and meta-synthesis. *J Int AIDS Soc.* 2013;16(3 Suppl 2):18640. doi:10.7448/ias.16.3.1864018640
61. Crockett KB, Esensoy TA, Johnson MO, et al. Internalized HIV stigma and pain among women with HIV in the United States: The mediating role of depressive symptoms. *AIDS Behav.* 2020;24(12):3482–3490. doi:10.1007/s10461-020-02919-w
62. Lo Hog Tian JM, Watson JR, Ibáñez-Carrasco F, et al. Impact of experienced HIV stigma on health is mediated by internalized stigma and depression: Results from the People Living with HIV Stigma Index in Ontario. *BMC Public Health.* 2021;21(1):1595. doi:10.1186/s12889-021-11596-w
63. Goodin BR, Owens MA, White DM, et al. Intersectional health-related stigma in persons living with HIV and chronic pain: Implications for depressive symptoms. *AIDS Care.* 2018;30(Suppl 2):66–73. doi:10.1080/09540121.2018.1468012
64. Mills SEE, Nicolson KP, Smith BH. Chronic pain: A review of its epidemiology and associated factors in population-based studies. *Br J Anaesth.* 2019;123(2):e273–e283. doi:10.1016/j.bja.2019.03.023
65. Baker V, Nkhoma K, Trevelion R, et al. "I have failed to separate my HIV from this pain": The challenge of managing chronic pain among people with HIV. *AIDS Care.* 2023;35(8):1164–1172. doi:10.1080/09540121.2020.1869148
66. Merlin JS, Hamm M, de Abril Cameron F, et al. The Global Task Force for Chronic Pain in People with HIV (PWH): Developing a research agenda in an emerging field). *AIDS Care.* 2023: 35(8):1215–1223. doi:10.1080/09540121.2021.1902936
67. Strath LJ, Sorge RE, Owens MA, et al. Sex and gender are not the same: Why identity is important for people living with HIV and chronic pain. *J Pain Res.* 2020;13:829–835. doi:10.2147/jpr.S248424
68. Wong CCY, Paulus DJ, Lemaire C, et al. Examining HIV-related stigma in relation to pain interference and psychological inflexibility among persons living with HIV/AIDS: The role of anxiety sensitivity. *J HIV AIDS Soc Serv.* 2018;17(1):1–15. doi:10.1080/15381501.2017.1370680
69. Health Resources & Services Administration. Ryan White HIV/AIDS program. n.d. Accessed September 20, 2022. https://ryanwhite.hrsa.gov
70. Irvine MK, Levin B, Robertson MM, et al. PROMISE (Program Refinements to Optimize Model Impact and Scalability Based on Evidence): A cluster-randomised, stepped-wedge trial assessing effectiveness of the revised versus original Ryan White Part A HIV Care Coordination Programme for patients with barriers to treatment in the USA. *BMJ Open.* 2020;10(7):e034624. doi:10.1136/bmjopen-2019-034624
71. Munoz-Laboy M, Martinez O, Davison R, Fernandez I. Examining the impact of medical legal partnerships in improving outcomes on the HIV care continuum: Rationale, design and methods. *BMC Health Serv Res.* 2019;19(1): Article 849. doi:10.1186/s12913-019-4632-x
72. Tsai J, Middleton M, Villegas J, et al. Medical–legal partnerships at Veterans Affairs medical centers improved housing and psychosocial outcomes for vets. *Health Aff.* 2017;36(12):2195–2203. doi:10.1377/hlthaff.2017.0759
73. Furness BW, Goldhammer H, Montalvo W, et al. Transforming primary care for lesbian, gay, bisexual, and transgender people: A collaborative quality improvement initiative. *Ann Fam Med.* 2020;18(4):292–302. doi:10.1370/afm.2542
74. Chambers LA, Rueda S, Baker DN, et al. Stigma, HIV and health: A qualitative synthesis. *BMC Public Health.* 2015;15: Article 848. doi:10.1186/s12889-015-2197-0
75. Navis A, George MC, Scherer M, Weiss L, Chikamoto Y, Robinson-Papp J. What physicians need to implement safer opioid prescribing: A qualitative study. *J Opioid Manag.* 2019;15(6):479–485. doi:10.5055/jom.2019.0538
76. Robinson-Papp J, George MC. Trust and the ethics of chronic pain management in HIV. *J Assoc Nurses AIDS Care.* 2015;26(5):509–513. doi:10.1016/j.jana.2015.05.007

77. Scherer M, Weiss L, Kamler A, et al. Patient recommendations for opioid prescribing in the context of HIV care: Findings from a set of public deliberations. *AIDS Care.* 2020;32(11):1471–1478. doi:10.1080/09540121.2019.1705962
78. Pantalone DW, Budge SL. Psychotherapy research is needed to improve clinical practice for clients with HIV. *Psychotherapy.* 2020;57(1):1–6. doi:10.1037/pst0000291
79. Trafton JA, Sorrell JT, Holodniy M, et al. Outcomes associated with a cognitive-behavioral chronic pain management program implemented in three public HIV primary care clinics. *J Behav Health Serv Res.* 2012;39(2):158–173. doi:10.1007/s11414-011-9254-y
80. Pullen SD, Acker C, Kim H, et al. Physical therapy for chronic pain mitigation and opioid use reduction among people living with human immunodeficiency virus in Atlanta, GA: A descriptive case series. *AIDS Res Hum Retroviruses.* 2020;36(8):670–675. doi:10.1089/aid.2020.0028
81. George MC, Wongmek A, Kaku M, Nmashie A, Robinson-Papp J. A mixed-methods pilot study of mindfulness-based stress reduction for HIV-associated chronic pain. *Behav Med.* 2017;43(2):108–119. doi:10.1080/08964289.2015.1107525
82. Titlic M, Jukic I, Tonkic A, et al. Lamotrigine in the treatment of pain syndromes and neuropathic pain. *Bratisl Lek Listy.* 2008;109(9):421–424.
83. Wiffen PJ, Derry S, Moore RA. Lamotrigine for chronic neuropathic pain and fibromyalgia in adults. *Cochrane Database Syst Rev.* 2013;2013(12):CD006044. doi:10.1002/14651858.CD006044.pub4
84. Simpson DM, Schifitto G, Clifford DB, et al. Pregabalin for painful HIV neuropathy: A randomized, double-blind, placebo-controlled trial. *Neurology.* 2010;74(5):413–420. doi:10.1212/WNL.0b013e3181ccc6ef
85. Derry S, Rice AS, Cole P, Tan T, Moore RA. Topical capsaicin (high concentration) for chronic neuropathic pain in adults. *Cochrane Database Syst Rev.* 2017;1(1):CD007393. doi:10.1002/14651858.CD007393.pub4
86. Head KA. Peripheral neuropathy: Pathogenic mechanisms and alternative therapies. *Altern Med Rev.* 2006;11(4):294–329.
87. Voute M, Morel V, Pickering G. Topical lidocaine for chronic pain treatment. *Drug Des Dev Ther.* 2021;15:4091–4103. doi:10.2147/dddt.S328228
88. Brix Finnerup N, Hein Sindrup S, Staehelin Jensen T. Management of painful neuropathies. *Handb Clin Neurol.* 2013;115:279–290. doi:10.1016/b978-0-444-52902-2.00017-5
89. Schütz SG, Robinson-Papp J. HIV-related neuropathy: Current perspectives. *HIV AIDS.* 2013;5:243–251. doi:10.2147/hiv.S36674
90. Abrams DI, Jay CA, Shade SB, et al. Cannabis in painful HIV-associated sensory neuropathy: A randomized placebo-controlled trial. *Neurology.* 2007;68(7):515–521. doi:10.1212/01.wnl.0000253187.66183.9c
91. Wallace MS, Marcotte TD, Umlauf A, Gouaux B, Atkinson JH. Efficacy of inhaled cannabis on painful diabetic neuropathy. *J Pain.* 2015;16(7):616–627. doi:10.1016/j.jpain.2015.03.008
92. Modesto-Lowe V, Bojka R, Alvarado C. Cannabis for peripheral neuropathy: The good, the bad, and the unknown. *Cleve Clin J Med.* 2018;85(12):943–949. doi:10.3949/ccjm.85a.17115
93. Attal N, Cruccu G, Baron R, et al. EFNS guidelines on the pharmacological treatment of neuropathic pain: 2010 revision. *Eur J Neurol.* 2010;17(9):1113-e88. doi:10.1111/j.1468-1331.2010.02999.x
94. Harding R, Karus D, Easterbrook P, Raveis VH, Higginson IJ, Marconi K. Does palliative care improve outcomes for patients with HIV/AIDS? A systematic review of the evidence. *Sex Transm Infect.* 2005;81(1):5–14. doi:10.1136/sti.2004.010132
95. Robinson-Papp J, Aberg J, Benn EKT, et al. Decreasing risk among HIV patients on opioid therapy for chronic pain: Development of the TOWER intervention for HIV care providers. *Contemp Clin Trials Commun.* 2019;16:100468. doi:10.1016/j.conctc.2019.100468
96. Liampas A, Rekatsina M, Vadalouca A, Paladini A, Varrassi G, Zis P. Non-pharmacological management of painful peripheral neuropathies: A systematic review. *Adv Ther.* 2020;37(10):4096–4106. doi:10.1007/s12325-020-01462-3

27

Pain Related to Thoracic Outlet Syndrome

Rebecca Freeland, Annie T. Wang, and Paul J. Christo

Evidence for Vulnerability

Thoracic outlet syndrome (TOS) was described as early as 1818 by Sir Cooper, who recounted a young woman with a palpable neck mass, upper extremity pulselessness, and gangrenous digits. He attributed the patient's constellation of symptoms to a projection of a cervical vertebrae causing compression of the subclavian artery or "cervical rib syndrome." In a publication in *The Lancet* in 1865, Coote described his successful treatment of a patient with similar symptoms by resection of "an exostosis from the transverse process of one of the cervical vertebrae."[1(p409)] Most historical reports of TOS are consistent with the arterial type.[2] In more recent years, we have come to understand TOS to encompass a group of disorders resulting in compression of the neurovascular bundle exiting the thoracic outlet. This compression leads to a constellation of symptoms most commonly including pain, numbness, tingling, weakness, and discoloration.[3]

It is important to understand the anatomy of the thoracic outlet in order to fully conceptualize the different locations where the structures of interest may be compromised, ultimately leading to symptoms. The thoracic outlet is located between the clavicle and first rib in the scalene triangle, costoclavicular space, and subcoracoid space, and it includes the brachial plexus, subclavian artery, and subclavian vein. The interscalene triangle is the most medial compartment and is bordered anteriorly by the anterior scalene, posteriorly by the middle scalene, and inferiorly by the first rib. Both the subclavian artery and the brachial plexus course through the interscalene triangle. The second compartment of the thoracic outlet is the costoclavicular space. It is bordered anteriorly by the subclavius muscle, superiorly by the clavicle, inferiorly by the first rib, and posteriorly by the anterior scalene. The brachial plexus and both the subclavian artery and vein travel through the costoclavicular space. The most lateral compartment is the retropectoralis minor (or subcoracoid) space. It is bordered anteriorly by the pectoralis minor and posteriorly by the ribs. The brachial plexus, axillary artery, and vein course through the subcoracoid space.[3]

It is important to note that a combination of both anatomic variation (predisposition) and other risk factors, such as trauma or repetitive upper extremity use, is often necessary for the development of symptomatic TOS. For example, the prevalence of cervical ribs in the general population is estimated at roughly 1% or 2%. However, most of these cases remain asymptomatic.[3]

TOS can be classified into three main types based on whether the pathophysiology involves the brachial plexus (neurogenic) or vasculature (venous or arterial).[3.] Each of the three groups of TOS may be further subdivided into congenital, traumatic, or functionally acquired cases.[4] Congenital cases are most often secondary to osseous, fibrous, or muscular anomalies.[4,5] Examples of congenital abnormalities include cervical ribs and supernumery scalene muscles.[3] Traumatic causes are usually secondary to whiplash injuries and falls. Functional acquired cases typically occur secondary to repetitive activity causing cervicoscapular muscle hypertrophies, such as in athletes involved in sports that require overhead movements (e.g., swimming, baseball, volleyball, football, and water polo).[3,4] A variety of tumors have been well documented as a cause of TOS. Superior sulcus (pancoast) tumors are a prime example of space-occupying lesions that may lead to symptoms of TOS.[3]

Neurogenic TOS (nTOS) if often subclassified as "classic" or "common." The classic form presents with objective findings such as a complete or incomplete cervical rib along with electrodiagnostic abnormalities and clear evidence of muscular atrophy. The common form of nTOS presents with symptoms suggestive of brachial plexus compromise, although objective findings are absent. The common form of nTOS represents virtually all of the neurogenic cases. The common form can present bilaterally, whereas classic nTOS is most often a unilateral condition.[3] This discussion focuses on the three primary forms of TOS: neurogenic (common), arterial, and venous.

Because there is no universal consensus regarding the diagnostic criteria for TOS, epidemiological data should be interpreted with caution. The true prevalence of TOS remains unknown secondary to a wide variety of symptoms on presentation and unreliability of many of the diagnostic measures.[6] Current data indicate an average incidence between 3 and 80 cases per 1,000 people. nTOS comprises more than 90% of these cases, followed by approximately 3–5% for venous TOS (vTOS) and less than 1% for arterial TOS (aTOS). TOS mostly affects adolescents to middle-aged adults between ages 20 and 50 years. For nTOS, the prevalence is higher in females, with a female-to-male ratio of 3.5:1.

Conditions for Vulnerability

Arterial TOS most often arises due to mechanical compression of the subclavian artery, leading to stenosis, intimal disruption, and eventual formation of thrombi.[7,8] The axillary artery may also be implicated. Of the three subtypes of TOS, aTOS is most closely associated with congenital abnormalities such as cervical ribs, abnormalities of the first thoracic rib, and soft tissue abnormalities such as fibromuscular bands.[9] The most common congenital abnormalities noted at the time of surgery are fibromuscular.[5,10] Approximately 0.5–1% of the population is thought to have cervical ribs, 70% of whom are women. Consequently, women are at highest risk for aTOS.[6] Acquired aTOS is common in athletes who undergo repetitive overhead motions, such as swimmers, weightlifters, and baseball players, due to hypertrophy of the overlying musculature.[11,12]

Although there are no pathognomonic signs or symptoms for aTOS, patients may present with pain in a nonradicular distribution, numbness, and general discomfort in the affected extremity that worsen with activity.[11] Pain may be present at rest and usually excludes the neck and shoulder.[13] aTOS should be considered in patients presenting with an acute thrombosis of the upper extremity because it remains the most common cause in people younger than age 40 years.[9] Physical exam findings may include pallor, decreased temperature, skin changes of the affected limb, and Raynaud's phenomenon.[8] A blood pressure differential of 20 mm Hg between the upper extremities may be present, although this is an uncommon finding.[8,13] Signs of microembolic events (e.g., ulcerations) are uncommon.[14] A positive elevated arm stress test (EAST), upper limb tension test (ULTT), or Adson's test may be present on physical examination.[13]

Venous TOS most often arises secondary to obstruction of the subclavian vein (with or without thrombosis) and often presents with signs of extremity congestion such as swelling, cyanosis, and pain.[8] Patients may present with dilation of the superficial veins of the neck, chest, and upper extremity.[15,16] vTOS is most often seen in populations who are subjected to repetitive overhead shoulder movements, such as competitive athletes and manual laborers.[17] It typically presents in males aged 20–30 years.[18] The dominant arm is usually affected. These patients may occasionally present with thrombosis of the subclavian vein at the costoclavicular junction, also known as Paget–Schrotter syndrome.

Neurogenic TOS is the most common of the three subtypes of TOS. Those more vulnerable to this syndrome include patients aged 20–40 years, women (female-to-male ratio of 3–4:1), people who have jobs that require substantial computer usage in non-ergonomic positions and assembly-line workers, and patients sustaining neck trauma.[16] Varying etiologies may be involved. For example, patients may have congenital abnormalities with superimposed trauma, muscle spasm, and fibrosis, all leading to a "space problem" and compression of the brachial plexus. In addition to anatomical variants, traumatic injuries of the cervicothoracic region, whiplash, shoulder injuries, or repetitive motion to the arm can cause scalene muscle spasm with resulting symptoms. The anterior scalene muscle is the structure most implicated in the symptoms related to nTOS. Hyperextension and whiplash injuries are closely associated with the development of nTOS in vulnerable populations.[6,8] Obesity has been suggested to exacerbate poor posture and potentiate symptoms.[19] Due to the chronic repetitive motion of the upper extremities, musicians and particularly violinists and violists may also be vulnerable to developing nTOS.[20] In fact, positive EAST and ULTT and abnormal ultrasound findings with vascular compression have been significantly more frequent in musicians who play bowed string instruments.[20] EAST and ULTT can aid in the diagnosis of nTOS given that both provocative tests offer relatively high sensitivity. The most common symptoms of nTOS include pain, nonradicular numbness, paresthesias, and weakness of the affected extremity. Patients may further complain of unilateral neck, trapezius, mastoid, or anterior chest wall pain and sometimes occipital headaches. The broad and sometimes nonspecific nature of symptoms contributes to the difficulty physicians encounter with making an accurate diagnosis. Moreover, the diagnosis of nTOS is one of exclusion that requires a thorough history and physical examination while ruling out suspected cervical, shoulder, and upper extremity pathological conditions that could mimic nTOS. Imaging, electrodiagnostics, and local anesthetic injection can assist in ruling out other diagnoses that may resemble nTOS. Palpation of the brachial plexus and overlying musculature may reveal tenderness, but it is not a pathognomonic finding.[16]

Treatment Strategies

Treatment of TOS is influenced by the subtype of TOS, severity, and duration of symptoms associated with TOS.[16] For nTOS, the initial management typically includes physical therapy; ergonomic and postural changes; and pharmacotherapy, including nonsteroidal anti-inflammatory drugs, antidepressants, anticonvulsants, and muscle relaxants.[3,21] The goal of conservative management is to reduce compression of the thoracic outlet by decreasing inflammation and restoring the balance in the neighboring musculature. Exercise has been associated with significant improvement in symptoms in 50–90% of patients with TOS.[21,22] For vulnerable patients, such as obese patients and females with breast hypertrophy who are at increased risk for TOS, weight reduction and postural changes are particularly important.[19,23] Other modalities, such as heat, transcutaneous electrical nerve stimulation, manual massage, phonophoresis, biofeedback techniques, and relaxation, may also be helpful.[19]

Conservative management is often adequate for pain relief, and patients are recommended to continue conservative management for approximately 4–6 months prior to considering surgical intervention.[19] However, for patients with severe, debilitating symptoms, including significant neural loss or vascular compression, interventional treatment may be needed. Anterior scalene block with local anesthetic injection, such as lidocaine or bupivacaine with or without steroids, has been used as a supportive diagnostic and prognostic indicator of surgical outcome from decompression of the thoracic outlet due to nTOS.[24] This injection is hypothesized to temporarily block or paralyze the muscle in spasm, hence permitting the first rib to descend in a manner that decompresses the thoracic outlet and simulates the results of surgery.

Botulinum toxin A (BTX) injections into various muscles, including the anterior scalene muscle, middle scalene muscle, trapezius muscle, subclavius muscle, pectoralis minor muscle, rhomboid major, and levator scapula muscles, have all been investigated, and evidence supports the value of BTX into the cervicothoracic muscles as a treatment for nTOS.[25–27] The postulated therapeutic effects of BTX include relaxation of the scalene or other muscles compressing the neurovascular structures in the thoracic outlet, and possibly reducing both pain and inflammation.[28] The efficacy of BTX injections into the scalene muscles has been debated, but the evidence suggests more durable relief than that obtained from local anesthetic blocks.[25–27] Christo et al.[27] demonstrated significant improvement in pain relief for 3 months with a single botulinum injection into the anterior scalene muscle under computed tomographic guidance. Another study used electrophysiologic and fluoroscopic guidance to perform botulinum injections into the scalene muscles, resulting in 64% of patients with significant reduction in pain for an average of 88 days.[25] A retrospective study evaluating BTX injections into the anterior scalene and pectoralis major muscles under ultrasound guidance noted that a better response to BTX injections correlated positively with a better response to scalenectomy and first rib resection.[29] Of note, the authors found both a high degree of specificity (90%) and a positive predictive value of 99% for patients responding to BTX and who subsequently responded to surgery.[29] However, a double-blind, randomized, controlled trial by Finlayson et al.[30] found no clinically or statistically significant improvement in pain or function with botulinum injections to the anterior and middle scalene muscles. The visual analog scale scores between the studied groups did show a change from baseline in favor of the BTX group at 6 weeks. Furthermore, the study was underpowered and may have been subject to allocation bias from suboptimal blinding methods.

If symptoms continue to persist despite conservative management or symptoms are debilitating, surgical decompression with scalene resection, first rib resection, and/or pectoralis minor tenotomy may alleviate symptoms and improve patients' quality of life.[28] Although there is no standard approach, resection of the first rib is often performed via the transaxillary approach or the supraclavicular approach, as the first rib is the common culprit for neural and arterial compression in the thoracic outlet.[31] The largest series of first rib resections for severe TOS found that 92% of patients had favorable outcomes with the transaxillary approach.[32] Another study demonstrated similar findings, with 95.4% of patients demonstrating improvement in symptoms after resection of the first rib via the transaxillary approach.[33] Supraclavicular decompression has also been shown to provide a success rate of 96%.[34]

However, complications can arise, including pneumothorax, winged scapula, wound infection, hematoma, thoracic duct injury, phrenic nerve injury, brachial plexus palsy, and recurrence.[33] Regarding the adolescent patient population predisposed to TOS, Caputo et al.[35] conducted a retrospective study on 189 patients, including 35 adolescent patients and 154 adults with disabling nTOS; these patients underwent primary supraclavicular decompression consisting of scalenectomy, brachial plexus neurolysis, and first rib resection, with or without pectoralis minor tenotomy. The adolescent patients were noted to have more favorable preoperative factors and significantly improved functional outcomes at 3 months and 6 months postoperatively in comparison to adults.[35] Musicians with nTOS have also undergone first rib resection, scalenectomy, and brachial plexus neurolysis, with successful return to their career after surgery.[36]

For competitive athletes with TOS, physical therapy can provide mild to moderate improvement in symptoms; however; many athletes may still require surgical intervention.[34] Chandra et al.[37] noted that 67% of nTOS athletes elected to undergo supraclavicular first rib resection and brachial plexus neurolysis, with 83% of athletes returning to high-level performance. The authors proposed that early diagnosis and standardized treatment protocols with teams consisting of sports medicine physicians, orthopedic surgeons, physical therapists, and trainers for athletes who develop nTOS or vTOS could potentially lead to better outcomes and increased likelihood of returning to competitive sports.

Anticoagulants, thrombolysis with plasminogen activator, venoplasty, and surgical decompression have been used to treat vTOS.[37,38] Timing of treatment with thrombolysis is crucial for patients with acute vTOS, and if thrombolysis is completed within 2 weeks of the onset of symptoms, success rates range from 62% to 82%.[37] However, delaying treatment for more than 2 weeks has been associated with a 29% success rate of thrombus resolution.[15] Thrombolysis and surgical decompression can provide even higher success rates of greater than 90%.[38] Complications of anticoagulation include restriction in arm movement and recurrent thrombosis, which can be minimized with venoplasty.[37,38] For chronic vTOS, in addition to thrombolysis and anticoagulation, patients may also need surgical decompression with venoplasty if subclavian vein thrombosis is present.[38] Surgical decompression is the main treatment needed in patients with symptoms of vTOS without the presence of occlusion.[38]

For aTOS, the treatment depends on the etiology and degree of ischemia.[38] Patients with compression of the subclavian artery who have an intact artery can be closely monitored with serial arterial Doppler ultrasound and may not need surgery.[38] However, for patients who are symptomatic and have arterial thrombosis, embolization, arterial damage, and aneurysm, surgery is warranted.[38] The primary treatment for aTOS is resection of the first rib and cervical rib, with possible scalenectomy.[38,39] Other treatment approaches include arterial resection for subclavian artery aneurysms and arterial stenosis with intimal damage, as well as vascular anastomosis, graft, and axillary–brachial bypass.[38] If subclavian artery thrombosis or embolization results in acute limb ischemia, thrombo-embolectomy or intra-arterial catheter-directed thrombolysis can help restore blood flow.[38,39]

Thoracic outlet syndrome in those who are vulnerable presents both diagnostic and therapeutic challenges. Factors that can contribute to these challenges include the lack of consensus for diagnosis of nTOS, different types of TOS, a variety of clinical presentations, enigmatic diagnostic testing and imaging, controversial treatment options, and lack of objective data on outcomes for nTOS. In addition, the pathophysiology and progression of the neurogenic form of the disease are still largely unknown. Vulnerable patients who are at increased risk for nTOS, such as the obese and female patient populations, may encounter significant barriers to finding the proper treatment that will improve functional outcomes. Interestingly, the occupation of patients with TOS (e.g., manual laborers compared to non-manual laborers, such as office or health care workers) was not associated with significant differences in outcomes.[40] Early diagnosis and treatment with a multidisciplinary approach incorporating pain medicine specialists, vascular and orthopedic surgeons, and physical therapists may offer a more efficacious strategy for alleviating TOS symptoms.[37] Further research is warranted to define clear diagnostic criteria for nTOS, obtain better demographic data, and further define risk factors for TOS. Larger multicenter trials are needed to investigate the most effective treatment approaches for these patients.

Conclusion

Thoracic outlet syndrome describes compression of one or several neurovascular structures that traverse the thoracic outlet. Adolescents to middle-aged adults aged 20–50 years comprise the group most at risk for developing TOS, and this includes specific athletes, women, obese individuals, and those involved in activities that require repetitive overhead shoulder movements. Among the three forms of TOS, the neurogenic (common) form affects most patients. Furthermore, woman are more than three times as likely as men to develop nTOS.

Treatments for all three forms of TOS consist of surgical and nonsurgical interventions. Surgical approaches can produce high rates of improvement in select centers. In patients with nTOS who experience insufficient relief from conservative therapies, BTX injections into the cervicothoracic muscles can provide symptomatic relief if these patients prefer to forego surgery or in advance of surgery.

References

1. Coote. St. Bartholomew's Hospital: Good recovery in the case of recent removal of an exostosis from the transverse process of one of the cervical vertebræ. *Lancet.* 1861;77(1965):409. doi:10.1016/S0140-6736(02)45595-X
2. Gharagozloo F, Atiquzzaman N, Meyer M, Tempesta B, Werden S. Robotic first rib resection for thoracic outlet syndrome. *J Thorac Dis.* 2021;13(10):6141–6154. doi:10.21037/jtd-2019-rts-04
3. Jones MR, Prabhakar A, Viswanath O, et al. Thoracic outlet syndrome: A comprehensive review of pathophysiology, diagnosis, and treatment. *Pain Ther.* 2019;8(1):5–18. doi:10.1007/s40122-019-0124-2
4. Citisli V. Assessment of diagnosis and treatment of thoracic outlet syndrome, an important reason of pain in upper extremity, based on literature. *J Pain Relief.* 2015;4(2):1–7.
5. Laulan J, Fouquet B, Rodaix C, Jauffret P, Roquelaure Y, Descatha A. Thoracic outlet syndrome: Definition, aetiological factors, diagnosis, management and occupational impact. *J Occup Rehabil.* 2011;21(3):366–373. doi:10.1007/s10926-010-9278-9
6. DiLosa KL, Humphries MD. Epidemiology of thoracic outlet syndrome. *Semin Vasc Surg.* 2021;34(1):65–70. doi:10.1053/j.semvascsurg.2021.02.008
7. Claus I, Van Bael K, Speybrouck S, Van Der Tempel G. Subclavian artery stenosis caused by a prominent first rib. *SAGE Open Med Case Rep.* 2015;3:2050313X15578319. doi:10.1177/2050313X15578319
8. Sanders RJ, Hammond SL, Rao NM. Diagnosis of thoracic outlet syndrome. *J Vasc Surg.* 2007;46(3):601–604. doi:10.1016/j.jvs.2007.04.050
9. Davidović LB, Koncar IB, Pejkić SD, Kuzmanović IB. Arterial complications of thoracic outlet syndrome. *Am Surg.* 2009;75(3):235–239.
10. Roos DB. Congenital anomalies associated with thoracic outlet syndrome: Anatomy, symptoms, diagnosis, and treatment. *Am J Surg.* 1976;132(6):771–778. doi:10.1016/0002-9610(76)90456-6
11. Daniels B, Michaud L, Sease F Jr, Cassas KJ, Gray BH. Arterial thoracic outlet syndrome. *Curr Sports Med Rep.* 2014;13(2):75–80. doi:10.1249/JSR.0000000000000034
12. Abdollahi K, Wood VE. Thoracic outlet syndrome. In: DeLee J, Drez D, Miller MD, eds. *DeLee and Drez's Orthopaedic Sports Medicine: Principles and Practice.* 3rd ed. Saunders; 2010:1128–1137.
13. Povlsen S, Povlsen B. Diagnosing thoracic outlet syndrome: Current approaches and future directions. *Diagnostics.* 2018;8(1): Article 21. doi:10.3390/diagnostics8010021
14. Kuhn JE, Lebus V GF, Bible JE. Thoracic outlet syndrome. *J Am Acad Orthop Surg.* 2015;23(4):222–232. doi:10.5435/JAAOS-D-13-00215
15. Moore R, Wei Lum Y. Venous thoracic outlet syndrome. *Vasc Med.* 2015;20(2):182–189. doi:10.1177/1358863X14568704
16. Li N, Dierks G, Vervaeke HE, et al. Thoracic outlet syndrome: A narrative review. *J Clin Med.* 2021;10(5): Article 962. doi:10.3390/jcm10050962
17. Goss SG, Alcantara SD, Todd GJ, Lantis JC 2nd. Non-operative management of Paget–Schroetter syndrome: A single-center experience. *J Invasive Cardiol.* 2015;27(9):423-428.
18. Ferrante MA, Ferrante ND. The thoracic outlet syndromes: Part 2. The arterial, venous, neurovascular, and disputed thoracic outlet syndromes. *Muscle Nerve.* 2017;56(4):663–673. doi:10.1002/mus.25535
19. Crosby CA, Wehbé MA. Conservative treatment for thoracic outlet syndrome. *Hand Clin.* 2004;20(1):43–49. doi:10.1016/s0749-0712(03)00081-7
20. Adam G, Wang K, Demaree CJ, et al. A prospective evaluation of duplex ultrasound for thoracic outlet syndrome in high-performance musicians playing bowed string instruments. *Diagnostics.* 2018;8(1): Article 11. doi:10.3390/diagnostics8010011
21. Levine NA, Rigby BR. Thoracic outlet syndrome: Biomechanical and exercise considerations. *Healthcare.* 2018;6(2): Article 68. doi:10.3390/healthcare6020068

22. Huang JH, Zager EL. Thoracic outlet syndrome. *Neurosurgery*. 2004;55:897–903. doi:10.1227/01.NEU.0000137333.04342.4D
23. Novak CB, Collins ED, Mackinnon SE. Outcome following conservative management of thoracic outlet syndrome. *J Hand Surg Am*. 1995;20(4):542–548. doi:10.1016/S0363-5023(05)80264-3
24. Jordan SE, Machleder HI. Diagnosis of thoracic outlet syndrome using electrophysiologically guided anterior scalene blocks. *Ann Vasc Surg*. 1998;12(3):260–264. doi:10.1007/s100169900150
25. Jordan SE, Ahn SS, Freischlag JA, Gelabert HA, Machleder HI. Selective botulinum chemodenervation of the scalene muscles for treatment of neurogenic thoracic outlet syndrome. *Ann Vasc Surg*. 2000;14(4):365–369. doi:10.1007/s100169910079
26. Jordan SE, Ahn SS, Gelabert HA. Combining ultrasonography and electromyography for botulinum chemodenervation treatment of thoracic outlet syndrome: Comparison with fluoroscopy and electromyography guidance. *Pain Physician*. 2007;10(4):541–6.
27. Christo PJ, Christo DK, Carinci AJ, Freischlag JA. Single CT-guided chemodenervation of the anterior scalene muscle with botulinum toxin for neurogenic thoracic outlet syndrome. *Pain Med*. 2010;11(4):504–511. doi:10.1111/j.1526-4637.2010.00814.x
28. Foley JM, Finlayson H, Travlos A. A review of thoracic outlet syndrome and the possible role of botulinum toxin in the treatment of this syndrome. *Toxins*. 2012;4(11):1223–1235. doi:10.3390/toxins4111223
29. Donahue DM, Godoy IRB, Gupta R, Donahue JA, Torriani M. Sonographically guided botulinum toxin injections in patients with neurogenic thoracic outlet syndrome: Correlation with surgical outcomes. *Skeletal Radiol*. 2020;49(5):715–722. doi:10.1007/s00256-019-03331-9
30. Finlayson HC, O'Connor RJ, Brasher PMA, Travlos A. Botulinum toxin injection for management of thoracic outlet syndrome: A double-blind, randomized, controlled trial. *Pain*. 2011;152(9):2023–2028. doi:10.1016/j.pain.2011.04.027
31. Camporese G, Bernardi E, Venturin A, et al. Diagnostic and therapeutic management of the thoracic outlet syndrome: Review of the literature and report of an Italian experience. *Front Cardiovasc Med*. 2022;9:802183. doi:10.3389/fcvm.2022.802183
32. Roos DB. The place for scalenectomy and first-rib resection in thoracic outlet syndrome. *Surgery*. 1982;92(6):1077–1085.
33. Karamustafaoglu YA, Yoruk Y, Tarladacalisir T, Kuzucuoglu M. Transaxillary approach for thoracic outlet syndrome: Results of surgery. *Thorac Cardiovasc Surg*. 2011;59(6):349–352. doi:10.1055/s-0030-1250480
34. Ciampi P, Scotti C, Gerevini S, et al. Surgical treatment of thoracic outlet syndrome in young adults: Single centre experience with minimum three-year follow-up. *Int Orthop*. 2011;35(8):1179–1186. doi:10.1007/s00264-010-1179-1
35. Caputo FJ, Wittenberg AM, Vemuri C, et al. Supraclavicular decompression for neurogenic thoracic outlet syndrome in adolescent and adult populations. *J Vasc Surg*. 2013;57(1):149–157. doi:10.1016/j.jvs.2012.07.025
36. Demaree CJ, Wang K, Lin PH. Thoracic outlet syndrome affecting high-performance musicians playing bowed string instruments. *Vascular*. 2017;25(3):329–332. doi:10.1177/1708538116671064
37. Chandra V, Little C, Lee JT. Thoracic outlet syndrome in high-performance athletes. *J Vasc Surg*. 2014;60(4):1012–1017; discussion 1017–1018. doi:10.1016/j.jvs.2014.04.013
38. Molina, JE, Hunter, DW, Dietz, CA. Paget–Schroetter syndrome treated with thrombolytics and immediate surgery. *J Vasc Surg*. 2007;45:328–334.
39. Hussain MA, Aljabri B, Al-Omran M. Vascular thoracic outlet syndrome. *Semin Thorac Cardiovasc Surg*. 2016;28(1):151–157. doi:10.1053/j.semtcvs.2015.10.008
40. Landry GJ, Moneta GL, Taylor LM Jr, Edwards JM, Porter JM. Long-term functional outcome of neurogenic thoracic outlet syndrome in surgically and conservatively treated patients. *J Vasc Surg*. 2001;33(2):312–317; discussion 317–319. doi:10.1067/mva.2001.112950

28
Pain Related to Obesity

Barbara DeLateur

Vulnerability

A useful tool for defining vulnerability is the Social Vulnerability Index (SVI), which was developed in approximately 2011 by the Centers for Disease Control and Prevention and its subagency, the Agency for Toxic Substances and Disease Registry, as a means to allocate resources. Social vulnerability

> measures the likelihood a given population or community will need certain resources following an adverse community event, like the natural disasters and public health crises. Social vulnerability can also refer to access to certain social resources including capital (average area income), natural resources like clean water and clean air, or social resources like high-quality educational opportunities.[1]

Chia-Yuan Yu and colleagues[1] studied 205 counties in the United States with respect to SVI variables and how they affect the individual-level risk of obesity, especially with regard to the built environment. They found that counties with a high index of Hispanics, African Americans, females, single-parent families, and residents without health insurance were all linked to higher percentages of fast-food restaurants and reduced access to exercise opportunities. There was a positive relationship between a higher percentage of older adults and those with special needs and obesity. In contrast, wealthier counties and those with larger Asian populations were negatively related to obesity. This suggests a relationship between the built environment (fast-food restaurants, lack of unprocessed food opportunities, lack of opportunities, and lack of opportunities to exercise) and obesity.

Prevalence of Obesity

Obesity prevalence in the United States increased from 30.5% in 2017 to 41.9% in 2020.[2] Ogden et al.[2] noted some interesting statistics from the National Health and Nutrition Examination Survey: (1) Prevalence of obesity decreased with (rising) income in women but not in men, and (2) obesity prevalence is related in a complex way to college education. For instance, it was lower in college graduates among non-Hispanic White women and men, and among non-Hispanic Black women as well as Hispanic women. It was not lower in non-Hispanic Asian women and men, or non-Hispanic Black or Hispanic women.

Relationship Between Pain and Obesity

It is well known that patients with chronic pain tend to exercise less. When I ask patients about their physical activity, they often begin their reply with something like, "I used to run every day." But pressed for the current level, they often concede that they are doing only the most basic activities of daily living.

Patients with pain often eat more. In a study by Amy and Kozak,[3] 30 adult primary care patients with an average body mass index (BMI) of 36.8 and average pain intensity of 5.6 participated in semistructured, in-depth interviews. The authors found five themes indicating that patients with comorbid chronic pain and obesity experienced depression-magnifying symptoms, hedonic hunger triggered by physical pain, and binge eating in response to pain. O'Loughlin and Newton-John[4] found that three-fourths of their sample of persons with chronic pain engaged in comfort eating and increased eating in the presence of the stress of higher pain intensity. Not surprisingly, the pain-induced comfort eating predicted increased BMI (and BMI significantly predicted greater chronic pain). Lin et al.[5] examined how eating behavior was affected in patients with low back pain before and after they transitioned to chronic pain compared to patients whose pain subsided. Using behavioral assays and structural brain imaging, they concluded that disrupted eating behavior specifically occurs after pain becomes chronic, and it is accompanied by structural changes in the nucleus accumbens.

Pain in Patients with Obesity

It is readily apparent that increased load will aggravate pain in weight-bearing joints, such as the hip and knee. Depending on pelvis width, each pound of body weight can produce 6–8 pounds of vertical compression force on the hip; each pound is calculated to produce 4 pounds of vertical compression force on the knee. A common source of this pain is osteoarthritis (OA). But load is not the only factor, and certainly would not explain OA in the hands. For instance, Bliddal et al.[6] explored the role of load (obesity) and inflammation and suggested a model for development of OA as a result of obesity. Pro-inflammatory mediators are found in joints with OA. Independently, it is known that not all white adipose tissue (WAT) is the same. With respect to inflammation, the subcutaneous WAT is harmless, but the visceral WAT constantly produces inflammatory cytokines. The article titled "Apple or Pear: Size and Shape Matter" is of interest here.[7] The development of metabolic syndrome in association with visceral fat is important for the prediction of pain. Yates et al.,[8] in their longitudinal analysis, showed that metabolic syndrome predicted the future onset of hip and knee pain over an interval of 10 years. Interestingly, subsequent weight or dietary change did not modify this risk. Loevinger et al.[9] compared 109 women with fibromyalgia to 46 control healthy women. Hemoglobin A1c was used as a substitute or marker for glucose levels. Women with fibromyalgia were 5.6 times more likely to have metabolic syndrome as the healthy controls. In support of the "apple versus pear" shape hypothesis, the waist–hip ratio was a predictor, but BMI was not.

Li et al.[10] performed a case–control study of 71 patients and found that prevalence of hypertension, obesity, dyslipidemia, and metabolic syndrome was significantly higher in patients with OA compared to the control group. Regarding the effect of load, King et al.[11] found a dose-dependent relationship between BMI on incidence of both knee and hip OA. A 5-unit increase in BMI was associated with a 35% increased risk of knee OA. They noted that early life obesity may be particularly hazardous.[11] Grotle et al.[12] found that after adjusting for age, gender, work status, and leisure time activities, a BMI greater than 30 was significantly associated with knee OA and hand OA but not with hip OA. The authors suggested different mechanisms for development of hip versus knee OA. The hip is adapted to stability with a deep socket for the ball and socket joint. The knee is far less stable crossing the joint. McVinnie[13] acknowledged the multifactorial relationship between obesity and chronic pain and stated that obese patients are known to exhibit higher levels of the inflammatory markers interleukin-6, tumor necrosis factor-α, and C-reactive protein. Furthermore, Shoelson et al.[14] noted a chronic, subacute state of inflammation that often accompanies the accumulation of excess lipid in adipose tissue and liver, evidenced by changes in both inflammatory cells and biochemical markers of inflammation.

Depression and Obesity

Luppino and colleagues[15] carried out a meta-analysis that demonstrated increased risk of depression with obesity. Also, depression was found to be predictive of developing obesity. Wurtman and Wurtman[16] summarized the reciprocal relationship in the title of their article: "Depression Can Beget Obesity Can Beget Depression." One of the studies reviewed by Blasco and colleagues[17] showed that stress and depression alter the metabolic response to rich-in-fat foods, up to 104 kcal more per meal, a possible mechanism for increasing obesity.

Obesity and Sleep Disorders

In their review, Hargens and colleagues[18] covered sleep disorders and a number of chronic conditions, including obesity. Persons with obesity were more likely to develop chronic insomnia. In a reciprocal relationship, insomnia may predispose subjects to overconsumption of energy, leading to weight gain. They cite the Wisconsin Sleep Cohort Study.[19] Grehlin is the hunger hormone. Leptin is the hormone that signals lack of hunger (not fullness of satiety, which is prompted by peptide YY3-36, heavily concentrated at the distal ileum). The following question arises: If leptin decreases hunger, and if leptin comes from the fat cells (of which obese people have many) and full fat cells, why does obesity exist? In the opinion of Robert Lustig, insulin blocks leptin's message from reaching the hypothalamus. Lustig and colleagues[20] assessed the results of experimental weight loss using the insulin-suppressive agent octreotide-LAR. Interpretation of the results suggested that hyperinsulinemia may be a proximate cause of leptin resistance and that reduction of insulin levels may promote weight loss by improving leptin sensitivity. But exercise can help. Kline and colleagues[21] reported the results of a randomized study of 6 months duration related to one of three regimens of moderate-intensity exercise (50% of peak VO_2). They found that even a low amount of exercise resulted in reduced odds of having significant sleep disturbance.

Treatment Strategies

Good Sleep Hygiene

Encourage patients to follow good sleep hygiene. This includes an 8-h sleep opportunity, establishing a firm time to go to bed plus or minus 30 min, and maintaining that sleep schedule even on weekends or other non-workdays. The best method for developing good sleep hygiene is to set a consistent time to get out of bed in the morning. If the wake-up/arise time is 6 a.m., for example the patient should be ready to go to bed by 10 p.m. Avoid television, computers, smart devices, and all other sources of blue light for at least 1 h before sleep time. For those who insist on watching television in the evening, blue-blocking glasses can be purchased. Overhead lights, especially fluorescent lighting, should be avoided. Patients particularly sensitive to the melatonin-suppression effects of light can purchase a sleep mask. The room should be cool. The bed should be reserved for sleep and sex. If sleep apnea is suspected, refer to sleep medicine and perform a monitored sleep study. Because exercise has been shown to be helpful in promoting sleep, a combination of exercise and treatment of the apnea is ideal. The time to exercise is controversial. The best time (morning vs. late afternoon) is the time when the patient will actually do it. Avoid strenuous aerobic exercise in the late evening. If the patient has already been prescribed a continuous positive airway pressure (CPAP) device, a good interviewing technique is to ask the patient how many times a week they use it rather than asking, "Do you use it?" If the patient uses it at all, the answer may well be "yes," but if one inquires about the frequency, it might be "2 or 3 times a week." Patients should be encouraged to use the CPAP device nightly and consult a technician if there are problems with the mask or other issues.[22]

Rapid Pain Relief

Patients frequently adopt a gait strategy known as antalgic gait. This is very sensitive to pain, but the term does not necessarily refer to one particular strategy. The painful hip commonly leads to an antalgic gait. It requires a brief explanation involving the difference between rotatory forces and vertical compression forces. Body weight, *W*, is typically applied 3 arbitrary distance units farther from the axis of the hip than the site of application of the hip abductors. The fulcrum is the axis of rotation of the hip joint itself. A useful analogy is a young, 30-pound child sitting on one side of a teeter totter, three times as far from the axis of rotation as an older, 90-pound child. This gives a perfect balance when the patient is in the unilateral stance phase. The vertical compression force on the hip joint is thus 4 *W* (3 *W* exerted by the hip abductors plus *W* exerted by the body weight). Patients with a painful hip usually move the trunk to the painful side in an ipsilateral stance. If the patient succeeds in getting *W* placed exactly over the center of the hip, the vertical compression force is reduced to 0, but no more than that. In contrast, if a cane is held in the contralateral hand, every pound on the cane results in a reduction of 8 pounds of vertical compression force (6 pelvic distance units plus 2 more distance units from the pelvis to the hand in which the cane is held). If more force reduction is needed (because patients are usually restricted in the amount of force they can exert on the cane), two canes or, better, two forearm crutches can be used in a three-point gait, with the crutches advanced with the painful limb, and the contralateral limb is advanced without the crutches. If both hips (or knees) are painful, an alternating two-point gait is helpful. It is optimal for a physical therapist to teach these gaits to the patient; once learned, they persist because the relief is so great. Many patients referred to me are already using a four-wheeled rolling walker with brakes and seat so that they can obtain a maximal amount of weight-bearing relief and can lock the brakes and sit down when rest is needed. If the patient has back pain resulting from lumbar spinal stenosis, relief is often obtained by bending over a shopping cart; this is known as the shopping cart sign.

Weight Reduction

Clearly, weight reduction may be indicated. But the simple "Eat less and move more" is not effective, unless the efforts are extreme. Even then, the results are generally not maintained. Scientists from the National Institutes of Health studied participants of season 8 of the television show *The Biggest Loser* at baseline, at the end of the 30-week competition, and 6 years later. After 6 years, 41.0 ± 31.3 kg of the lost weight was regained, and resting metabolic rate was 704 ± 427 kcal/day below baseline. Weight regain was not correlated with metabolic adaptation at the end of the competition, but it was correlated at 6 years. Of interest was the finding that subjects maintaining greater weight loss at 6 years also experienced greater concurrent metabolic slowing. It suggests that successful subjects were almost constantly exerting cognitive override (a term I refer to as "willpower") to struggle against the metabolic handicap.[23]

All calories are not created equal. In a calorimeter, a calorie equals a calorie. But human metabolism is far more complex than a calorimeter. In the human subject, partitioning will occur. Simple carbohydrates raise the blood sugar. In people with normal weight, obese people, and type 2 diabetics (not type 1), the body secretes insulin to maintain glucose homeostasis. Insulin stores fat. One way of communicating this to the patient is to state, "You can burn or you store, but you can't do both at the same time." The concept of the glycemic index (GI) is important. The GI is a measure of the tendency of a substance to raise the blood sugar. The standard is glucose, which is given a value of 100. Table sugar or sucrose, which consists of the two six-carbon sugars glucose and fructose, linked together has a GI of 65. Surprising to some, orange juice has a GI between 66 and 76, both higher than that of table sugar and higher than that of Coca-Cola, which has a GI of 63. It is thus important to scrutinize the actual intake of patients who say they "eat healthy." In contrast, an orange fruit has a GI of 52. So, after examining the food and drink logs, one could suggest eating an orange and drinking a glass of water. An average orange has 3 g of fiber. Fiber is an important constituent of any healthful diet, but especially for patients attempting to lose weight. The Recommended

Daily Allowance of fiber is 25 g for an adult female and 30 g for an adult male. It has been estimated that the average adult American consumes approximately 13 g of fiber per day. In contrast, our hunter–gatherer ancestors ate approximately 100 g per day. Tiger nuts (which are not nuts but, rather, small tubers) can help provide a fiber intake similar to that of our ancestors. A 1-oz. serving has 10 g of fiber. They can be made easier to chew by soaking in water overnight. Added to a salad, they are more appealing to eat.

The Clinic Process

The process of patient care that I employ involves a referral, usually by pain management physicians, but some patients are self-referred. One hour is allowed for the first visit. The program of "healthful, anti-inflammatory eating and progressive walking"[24] is explained, including the importance of the food and drink logs (I avoid the term "diet"), in which the time of consumption should be noted because science has shown that *when* one eats is as important as *what* one eats. The patient is instructed to record in logs (two per week until the next visit) the time of getting out of bed; the time, nature, and quantity of any food or drink; and when the patient retires to bed. I explain that these logs will be analyzed by me and several strategies will be suggested, from which the patient selects one strategy to execute. If the patient does not like any of the strategies—as was the case for one of my patients—they can suggest one not on the list. In the case of the one patient who did not like any of my strategies, she selected advance meal planning rather than "grabbing" whatever was available at mealtime. In my experience, when the patient responds to the question about what they eat for breakfast by saying "I just grab . . .," the words that follow "grab" are almost never "an apple," "an orange," "a hard-boiled egg," or "a handful of celery sticks with two tablespoons of hummus."

A baseline is needed for the walking logs. The patient records the minutes walked (not the distance) one time a day every day until the next visit. At that visit, I take an average, and depending on the variability from day to day, I subtract 10–50% and that becomes the quota once the patient completes the baseline and enters the quota phase. This process was originally developed for patients with chronic pain who, when they felt a bit better, overdid their housework or yard work and were subsequently incapacitated for a number of days. It is a tool to help them learn to pace themselves. It is also designed for patients who are doing very little physical activity except basic activities of daily living. The quota set is one that the physician or health care provider thinks the patient can accomplish but, more important, the patient agrees that they can do. I explain that we are going to "stack the deck in your favor." Typically, in the quota phase, a minute of walking is added each week. Nothing is said about the walking or other activity they do throughout the day. Fulfilling the quota is something that can be praised by the clinician.

These communication techniques might seem obvious, but they are not. Many patients who carry extra weight (I avoid the term "obese") have been blamed and shamed by health care providers, family and friends, and themselves. Near the end of the first visit, I tell them, "If there is one thing I want you to take away from this visit, it's that the extra weight is not your fault. It's not." Sometimes women shed tears of relief at this point. At subsequent visits, I thank patients profusely for bringing their logs (some forget or leave them on the kitchen table). I explain that the logs are the tool they give me so that I can help them. The behavioral principle of selective reinforcement is very important. I find something on the list of consumed items to like—perhaps a floret of broccoli one day. Another behavioral principle incorporates rewarding successive approximations. For example, if there is only one serving of non-starchy vegetables or fruit per day, the patient is praised, followed by a statement such as "It would be great if you could work your way up to the recommended five servings per day" Or, even more gently, "Do you think you could increase the non-starchy vegetable or fruit to two servings a day?" When pertinent to patients' concerns or a topic we have been discussing, I supply patients with graphics or videos. Processed foods, in general (as with almost anything found in the middle aisles of the supermarket), need to have a long shelf life. To accomplish this, the fat and fiber are removed or minimized. The labels on processed foods often proudly assert that they are "low in fat"; however, the fat has to be replaced with something. Refined carbohydrates, especially those low in fat and fiber, are absorbed rapidly and raise the blood sugar rapidly. Insulin, which is the fat storage hormone, rises in response. Insulin also lowers blood sugar, which can already be very low after an overnight fast.[25] Appetite increases, along with adrenaline, such that after a breakfast of most cold cereals and skim milk, or white toast and jelly, appetite is high midmorning, along with adrenaline. This leads to tremulousness in some patients that requires food consumption. Illustrating this point, Ludwig and colleagues[26] gave 12 adolescent boys three different breakfasts after three separate overnight stays. One was instant oatmeal (highly processed), one was steel-cut oats, and the third was a veggie omelet with fruit (no grains). All meals had the same caloric content. Ludwig et al. followed the blood glucose, insulin, adrenaline, and hunger for 5 h. The glucose and insulin responded in a high, medium, or gentle way, respectively. But by 4 h, the glucose level was lower than an overnight fast in the boys who ate the instant oatmeal and the hunger followed. Adrenaline surged in those boys, producing a "metabolic crisis." The boys were given the same meal at lunch, after which they were allowed, throughout the afternoon, to eat as much as they wanted from all types of tasty foods. On average, the boys who had eaten the instant oatmeal ate 650 calories more than the boys who ate the vegetable omelet with fruit.[26] Clearly, if this pattern were done consistently, overweight would likely result.

Time-Restricted Eating

Time-restricted eating (TRE) is also known as intermittent fasting (IF). However, IF can refer to so many things that I prefer to use the term TRE. This can be early (eTRE) or midday (mTRE), or in some cases, the time of day is not referenced. Instead, TRE simply refers to the total number of hours in which calories can be consumed. It is wise to inspect the content of the foods consumed before trying to restrict the time, especially eTRE. If the food and drink consumed contain processed foods, sweet desserts, and sodas and juices, the insulin and hunger will remain elevated even during fasting and the patient is unlikely to be able to fast for 14 or more hours. Two of my patients have been observed, by a spouse or grown child, to be sleepwalking and raiding the refrigerator. Depending on methodology, studies report different outcomes with

TRE. Because the burning of fat is more important than weight loss itself, the study by Ravussin et al.[27] is particularly important. In this study, 11 overweight adults practiced both eTRE, eating from 8 a.m. to 2 p.m., and a control schedule, eating from 8 a.m. to 8 p.m. They carried out each protocol for 4 days. On the fourth day of each pattern, 24-h energy expenditure (which did not change) and substrate oxidation were carried out with whole-room calorimetry as well as appropriate enzymes. In the eTRE phase, ghrelin levels decreased; fullness increased; the desire to eat decreased; and the 24-h non-protein respiratory quotient decreased, indicating a switch to fat oxidation.

Time of Eating

I show my patients a graphic which demonstrates that the later subjects eat the identical meal, the more the blood sugar escalates.[28] Therefore, that "piece of fruit" the patient thinks is "healthy" would be better eaten earlier in the day, not as a bedtime snack.

Frequent Small Meals

Some patients cannot tolerate a full meal at one time; this might be the result of a gastric sleeve procedure or other such factor. Of course, they will have to eat smaller meals and more frequently. However, this is not a good weight-reduction strategy for obese patients who are able to eat a full meal. Why? Because the insulin never returns to baseline in the daytime and only does so for a short time when the patient finally stops eating in order to sleep. I remind patients that insulin is the fat storage hormone. Insulin stores fat. You can burn or you can store, but you cannot do both simultaneously.

Medication

As part of my program, I do not prescribe medication for weight loss. The patient's primary care physician or endocrinologist can consider medication management. One recently studied medication called tirzepatide has had such striking results that it must be mentioned here.[29] In this study, 2,539 adults with a BMI of 30 or greater and at least one weight-related complication other than diabetes received once-weekly subcutaneous injections of tirzepatide 5 mg, 10 mg, 15 mg, or placebo for 72 weeks. The weight loss was dose-related, with 15%, 19.5%, and 20.9%, respectively. Placebo, in contrast, was 3%. If the results endure, this drug might well change the whole paradigm of obesity treatment.

Summary of Strategies

An environment should be established that affirms the patient and their previous efforts to lose weight in a healthful manner. A variety of strategies can be described and the patient encouraged to select the one that they find most appealing. Only one should be selected initially to prevent the patient from feeling overwhelmed and thereby failing multiple treatment suggestions. More strategies can be added if a plateau is encountered. Behavioral techniques of selective reinforcement (finding something for which the patient can be praised) and rewarding successive approximations are important. I tell patients that the day I am perfect, I will ask perfection from them, but do not expect it anytime soon.

References

1. Yu CY, Woo A, Emrich CT, Wang B. Social Vulnerability Index and obesity: An empirical study in the US, 2020. *Cities*. 2020;97:102531.
2. Ogden CL, Fakhouri TH, Carroll MD, et al. Prevalence of obesity among adults, by household income and education—United States, 2011–2014. *MMWR Morb Mortal Wkly Rep*. 2017;66(50);1369–1373.
3. Amy E, Kozak AT. "The more pain I have, the more I want to eat": Obesity in the context of chronic pain. *Obesity*. 2012;20(10):2027–2034.
4. O'Loughlin I, Newton-John TR. "Dis-comfort eating": An investigation into the use of food as a coping strategy for the management of chronic pain. *Appetite*. 2019;140:288–297.
5. Lin Y, De Araujo I, Stanley G, Small D, Geha P. Chronic pain precedes disrupted eating behavior in low-back pain patients. *PLoS One*. 2022;17(2):e0263527.
6. Bliddal H, Leeds AR, Christensen R. Osteoarthritis, obesity and weight loss: Evidence, hypotheses and horizons—A scoping review. *Obes Rev*. 2014;15(7):578–586.
7. Ju J, Hofker M, Wijmenga D. Apple or pear: Size and shape matter. *Cell Metab*. 2015;21(4):507–508.
8. Yates M, Tsigarides J, Hayat S, et al. Metabolic syndrome precedes the onset of hip and knee pain and the risk is not modified by diet or changes in BMI. *Ann Rheum Dis*. 2019;78(Suppl 2):1026.
9. Loevinger BL, Muller D, Alonso C, Coe CL. Metabolic syndrome in women with chronic pain. *Metabolism*. 2007;56(1):87–93.
10. Li H, George DM, Jaarsma RL, Mao X. Metabolic syndrome and components exacerbate osteoarthritis symptoms of pain, depression and reduced knee function. *Ann Transl Med*. 2016;4(7): Article 133.
11. King LK, March L, Anandacoomarasamy A. Obesity and osteoarthritis. *Indian J Med Res*. 2013;138(2):185–193.
12. Grotle M, Hagen KB, Natvig B, Dahl FA, Kvien TK. Obesity and osteoarthritis in knee hip and/or hand: An epidemiological study in the general population with 10 years follow-up. *BMC Musculoskelet Disord*. 2008;9: Article 132.
13. McVinnie DS. Obesity and pain. *Br J Pain*. 2013;7(40):163–170.
14. Shoelson SE, Herrero L, Naaz A. Obesity, inflammation, and insulin resistance. *Gastroenterology*. 2007;132(6):2169–2180.
15. Luppino FS, de Wit LM, Bouvy PF, et al. Overweight, obesity, and depression: A systematic review and meta-analysis of longitudinal studies. *Arch Gen Psychiatry*. 2010;67(3):220–229.
16. Wurtman JJ, Wurtman RJ. Depression can beget obesity can beget depression. *J Clin Psychiatry*. 2015;76:e1619–e1621.
17. Blasco BV, Garcia-Jimenez J, Bodoano I, Lutierrez-Rojas L. Obesity and depression: Its prevalence and influence as a prognostic factor: A systematic review. *Psychiatry Investig*. 2020;17(8):715–724.
18. Hargens TA, Kaleth AS, Edwards ES, Butner KL. Association between sleep disorders, obesity, and exercise: A review. *Nat Sci Sleep*. 2013;5:27–35.
19. Taheri S, Lin L, Austin D, Young T, Mignot E. Short sleep duration is associated with reduced leptin, elevated ghrelin and increased body mass index. *PLoS Med*. 2004;1(3):e62.

20. Lustig RH, Sen S, Soberman JE, Velasquez-Mieyer PA. Obesity, leptin resistance, and the effects of insulin reduction. *Int J Obes Relat Metab Disord.* 2004;28(10):1244–1248.
21. Kline CE, Sui X, Hall MH, et al. Dose–response effects of exercise training on the subjective sleep quality of postmenopausal women: Exploratory analyses of a randomized controlled trial. *BMJ Open.* 2012;2(4):e00144.
22. Macey PM. Is brain injury in obstructive sleep apnea reversible? *Sleep.* 2012;35(1):9–10.
23. Fothergil E, Guo J, Howard L, et al. Persistent metabolic adaptation 6 years after "The Biggest Loser" competition. *Obesity.* 2016;24(8):1612–1619.
24. Stromsnes K, Correas AG, Lehmann J, Gambini J, Olaso-Gonzalez G. Anti-inflammatory properties of diet: Role in healthy aging. *Biomedicines.* 2021;9(8): Article 922.
25. Ludwig DS: *Always Hungry?* Grand Central Life & Style; 2016.
26. Ludwig DS, Majzoub JA, Al-Zahrani A, Dallal GE, Blanco I, Roberts SB. High glycemic index foods, overeating, and obesity. *Pediatrics.* 1999;103(3):E26.
27. Ravussin E, Beyl RA, Poggiogalle E, Hsia DS, Peterson CM. Early time-restricted feeding reduces appetite and increases fat oxidation but does not affect energy expenditure in humans. *Obesity.* 2019;27(8):1244–1254.
28. Panda S. *The Circadian Code.* Rodale; 2018.
29. Jastreboff, AM, Aronne LJ, Ahmad NN, et al. Tirzepatide once weekly for the treatment of obesity. *N Engl J Med.* 2022;387(3):205–216.

29

Pain and COVID-19

Andrew Han, Taranjeet S. Jolly, and Steven P. Cohen

Introduction

An outbreak of respiratory syndrome caused by a novel coronavirus was reported in the city of Wuhan in Hubei Province of China in December 2019.[1,2] The World Health Organization (WHO) and the International Committee on Taxonomy of Viruses later named this coronavirus and the disease caused by it severe acute respiratory syndrome coronavirus 2 (SARS-CoV-2) and coronavirus disease 2019 (COVID-19), respectively. Globally, during the week of January 24–30, 2022, the number of new COVID-19 cases remained similar to that reported during the previous week, whereas the number of new deaths increased by 9%. Across the six WHO regions, more than 22 million new cases and more than 59,000 new deaths were reported. As of January 20, 2022, more than 370 million confirmed cases and 5.6 million deaths had been reported globally.[3] As of February 7, 2022, the total number of COVID-19 cases in the United States was 78,107,377, the number of deaths totaled 926,769, and the cumulative number of recovered/discharged patients was 48,112,078.[4]

The COVID-19 pandemic has affected life across all domains, with a huge impact on personal, social, financial, and health fronts. All aspects of health care have been affected since the pandemic started. The toll of the pandemic is not limited to physical illness from the virus and its aftermath; it also extends to important psychosocial stressors that include prolonged periods of limited interpersonal contact, isolation, fear of illness, future uncertainty regarding new strains and their virulence, and school and workplace closures with their ensuing financial strain. Uncertainty is often fueled by constant media coverage, often with conflicting information, different recommendations by public health authorities in different jurisdictions, and the unknown duration and likelihood of waves of resurgence.[5] The impact of the COVID-19 pandemic has touched nearly all patients dealing with both acute and chronic pain conditions. However, the impact of the pandemic has disproportionally affected more vulnerable communities, such as pediatric patients, medically complex patients, and elderly age groups.

Chronic pain is a significant health concern in the United States, affecting 13.5–47% of the general population, and it can carry a commensurate financial burden, estimated by some at more than $600 billion annually.[6] Chronic pain is accompanied by increased suffering, increased physical disability, psychosocial consequences, increased risk of illicit drug use, more time off work with increased disability, and increased financial implications from health care and disability insurance perspectives. Even controlling for higher rates of depression, opioid use, and illicit substance use, chronic pain is associated with an increased mortality rate.[7]

During the pandemic, health care providers were at a much higher risk of infection. Pain medicine physicians and anesthetists who performed interventions and anesthetic blockades were subjected to a higher risk of infection compared to many other medical specialties.[8] Physician and health care provider burnout has been noted to be a major public health crisis in the wake of the pandemic and has led to growing concerns surrounding physician mental and health issues and an increased incidence of suicide in the health care community.[9]

Epidemiology

The COVID-19 pandemic has had a global impact, yet several populations are more vulnerable to contracting COVID-19 and the experience of pain either as a direct consequence or indirectly because of the pandemic-related stress on health care resources. The likelihood of developing complications from the virus and the interplay between COVID-19 and susceptibility to severe pain are areas ripe for investigation. This section focuses on reviewing current literature on vulnerable populations: the elderly population with multiple pre-existing conditions, children, underrepresented minorities, and low socioeconomic status populations that may be at higher risk of pain manifestations in the context of COVID-19 infection.

Although many of these vulnerable populations are more susceptible to COVID-19 and at increased risk of pain, it is important to recognize that pain and its management can by themselves lead to increased risk of contracting the virus. For example, opioids are often prescribed in managing conditions such as fibromyalgia, complex regional pain syndrome, and reflex sympathetic dystrophy. However, in addition to the commonly known side effects of opioid use such as nausea, respiratory depression, and opioid-induced hyperalgesia, opioids, as well as injectable and systemic steroids, can suppress the immune system.[10] Opioids can also cause respiratory depression and act as a cough suppressant, potentially masking early signs of COVID-19.[11]

The Elderly

The elderly are more susceptible to the impact of the COVID-19 pandemic. Approximately 74% of all deaths due to COVID-19 occur in individuals older than age 65 years.[12] The elderly tend to have more comorbidities, which is an independent risk factor for both COVID-19 infection and complications, including acute and chronic pain. The prevalence of comorbid conditions such as hypertension, diabetes, heart disease, malnutrition, functional impairments, and depression increases with age.[13,14] A meta-analysis found that a constellation of symptoms (fever, dyspnea/shortness of breath, nausea, vomiting, abdominal pain, dizziness, anorexia, and pharyngula) and comorbidities (diabetes, hypertension, coronary heart disease, chronic obstructive pulmonary disease/lung disease, and acute respiratory distress syndrome) are directly correlated with the age of COVID-19–infected patients.[15]

Age-related decrease in immune functioning can be further compounded by SARS-CoV-2 infection, which increases the risk of COVID-19–related mortality and morbidity. This is consistent with other viral illnesses such as herpes zoster and HIV.[16] Significant immune system changes also occur in COVID-19 patients. Higher mortality rates occur in the elderly population due to COVID-19 and pre-existing comorbidities (hypertension, diabetes, coronary artery disease, and chronic pulmonary disease).[17]

Among the many comorbidities, diabetes is one of the most prevalent in the elderly, with 29.2% (both diagnosed and undiagnosed) of all Americans aged 65 years or older suffering from the disease.[18] Diabetes is especially relevant because it involves significant immune system dysregulation that increases the risk of lower respiratory infections and subsequently more severe outcomes from infection.[19] Hyperglycemia is linked to impaired granulocyte and macrophage function and lymphopenia, increasing the risk of contracting all types of infections.[20] Diabetes is an independent risk factor for poorer prognosis and increased mortality in COVID-19 as well.[21] Furthermore, patients with diabetes have been shown to have insufficient Treg and Th17 response, which leads to a dysregulated, sustained pro-inflammatory cytokine response that may amplify the severity of SARS-CoV-2 infection and its concomitant pain symptoms (e.g., myalgias).[22] A study examining 5,730 diabetic patients with SARS-CoV-2 infection found that 21 patients developed throbbing craniofacial pain, which suggests that diabetes may predispose patients to new-onset pain in the setting of COVID-19.[23]

In terms of acute pain exacerbation, whether it be from a COVID-19 infection or nonspecific stressors during the pandemic, the elderly fared worse than younger cohorts. Individuals aged 60 years or older were more likely to report pain during the pandemic, most likely due to reduced physical activity and decreased pain tolerance.[24] Although COVID-19 infection accounts for new-onset pain symptoms regardless of comorbidity status, exacerbation of pre-existing pain conditions is common. Numerous studies have found that patients with existing neck, back, and knee pain experienced worsening pain during the pandemic.[25–28] A cross-sectional study further showed that patients with pre-existing headache disorders and other comorbidities develop worse headaches in terms of both frequency and intensity during COVID-19 infection.[29]

Pediatric Patients

Pediatric COVID-19 disease is generally mild and often asymptomatic, with an excellent prognosis and relatively low risk of progression to severe illness.[30,31] However, recent literature has highlighted a new phenomenon called multisystem inflammatory syndrome in children (MIS-C) or pediatric multisystem inflammatory syndrome that is often observed as a complication in children with SARS-CoV-2 infection. Although children are less susceptible to severe symptoms and long COVID, they nevertheless can develop severe gastrointestinal symptoms, most notably abdominal pain, as a consequence of MIS-C. One systematic review found a higher incidence of gastrointestinal symptoms in children with MIS-C than in those without.[32] In contrast to acute COVID-19 in children, MIS-C has a more virulent course, with 68% of cases requiring critical care support.[32]

Underrepresented Minorities

Underrepresented minorities, especially African Americans and Native Americans, are at greater risk of contracting SARS-CoV-2 and developing acute and chronic pain.[33] The prevalence of COVID-19 increases by 5% for every 1% increase in African American population density, with similar rates observed for Native American communities. This means that increased African American and Native American population densities are directly associated with an increase in COVID-19 prevalence.[34] In many minority communities, people live in close proximity, resulting in a greater opportunity for spread.[35] African and Native Americans are also disproportionately affected by substance abuse, asthma, diabetes, cardiac conditions, renal dysfunction, and obesity, which are all associated with more severe COVID-19 symptoms.[34] They are more likely to experience disruption in mood and sleep quality, and ultimately experience greater exacerbation of pain compared to other ethnic groups.[33] Finally, distrust in the health care system prevents African Americans, Native Americans, and other underrepresented minorities from seeking care, whether it be for COVID-19 or associated pain, further exacerbating these conditions (Table 29.1).[36,37]

Low Socioeconomic Status

Another vulnerable population includes those of lower socioeconomic status. Individuals living in poorer conditions and more remote communities with limited access to health care have significantly higher rates of chronic pain and comorbidities.[38] Specifically in the United States, many rural communities, including those in the Appalachian region, experience health disparities primarily due to the lack of accessible health care.[39] Access to health care in rural areas cannot solely be defined by proximity to services—high health care cost, insurance availability, and health literacy are all important considerations.[40] A study examining Appalachian preparedness for the COVID-19 pandemic showed that the communities in this region were especially susceptible to poor outcomes primarily because of a lack of intensive care unit (ICU) capacity. Although 19% of the entire U.S. population live in rural counties, one study found that only 1% of the total ICU beds in the nation are located in these counties.[41]

The previously discussed outcomes are further corroborated by a study investigating the socioeconomic impact of COVID-19 in low-income countries such as Ethiopia, Malawi, Nigeria, and Uganda, where approximately 256 million people or 77% of the population lost income during the pandemic, leading to exacerbation of food insecurity and inability to access proper health care and medicines.[42]

Acute Pain

There are many types of acute pain commonly associated with COVID-19, such as myalgias/arthralgias, headaches, abdominal pain, chest pain, spinal pain, and non-headache neurological symptoms.[43–46] Various mechanisms have been proposed to explain these different types of pain in COVID-19, such as fever, deconditioning, direct

Table 29.1 Epidemiology and Risk Factors for COVID-Related Pain and Other Complications in Vulnerable Populations

Population	Prevalence	Vulnerability	Unique Circumstances
Elderly	Approximately 74% of all deaths due to COVID-19 occur in individuals older than age 65 years.[12]	Elderly patients have more comorbidities, which is an independent risk factor for COVID-19 infection, complications, and acute and chronic pain. Prevalence of comorbid conditions such as hypertension, diabetes, heart disease, malnutrition, functional impairments, and depression increases with age.[13,14] A meta-analysis found that a group of symptoms (fever, dyspnea/shortness of breath, nausea, vomiting, abdominal pain, dizziness, anorexia, and pharyngalgia) and comorbidities (diabetes, hypertension, coronary heart disease, COPD/lung disease, and ARDS) were associated with the age of COVID-19–infected patients.[15] Those aged 60 years or older were more likely to report pain during the pandemic, most likely due to reduced physical activity.[24]	Elderly individuals have decreased immune system functioning as they age. Significant immune system changes also occur in COVID-19 patients. Higher mortality rates occur in the elderly population due to COVID-19 infection and pre-existing comorbidities (hypertension, diabetes, coronary artery disease, and chronic pulmonary disease).[17]
Underrepresented minorities	The prevalence of COVID-19 increases by 5% for every 1% increase in African American density.[34] Higher rates are also reported for Hispanic and Native American populations.[91]	Distrust in the health care system. African Americans are disproportionately affected by asthma, diabetes, cardiac conditions, renal dysfunction, and obesity, all of which are associated with more severe COVID-19 symptoms and pain.[34]	African American, Hispanic, and other minorities have higher rates of chronic pain for similar medical conditions and report greater functional and quality of life limitations.[91]

Low socioeconomic status	Low-income communities are more likely to contract COVID-19 (50% more cases in September 2020 compared to wealthier communities).[92]	Access to health care: Individuals living in poorer conditions and more remote communities with limited access to health care have significantly higher rates of chronic pain and comorbidities.[38]	Lower income individuals have unique circumstances that make them more likely to be exposed to COVID-19.[92,93] Do not have the financial means to socially isolate in the case of COVID-19 infection or exposure. More likely to live in multi-occupancy housing. Often employed in occupations that do not provide opportunities to work from home. Unstable living conditions increase stress, which weakens the immune system.
Children	Only 795 total deaths were due to COVID-19 during 2020–2022.[12] Overall incidence of MIS-C per 1 million person-months was 5.1 (95% confidence interval: 4.5–5.8) people.[94]	Exposure (classrooms, with mask and vaccine mandates beyond their control and a lower rate of vaccination in people they are exposed to). Children also have less control over their environment and circumstances.	MIS-C/PMIS Although children are less susceptible to severe symptoms and consequences from COVID-19, they can develop severe gastrointestinal symptoms (including abdominal pain) with MIS-C. A higher incidence of gastrointestinal symptoms was noted in MIS-C. In contrast to acute COVID-19 infection in children, MIS-C appears to be a condition of greater severity, with 68% of cases requiring critical care support.[32]

ARDS, acute respiratory distress syndrome; COPD, chronic obstructive pulmonary disease; MIS-C, multisystem inflammatory syndrome in children; PMIS, pediatric multisystem inflammatory syndrome.

viral invasion, or a hypervigilant immune response.[45,47] Neuropathic pain in COVID-19 may be triggered by a variety of causes, such as antiviral therapy, direct viral invasion, and various immune mechanisms, and those with pre-existing risk factors are at greater risk for developing neuropathic pain.[48] Neuropathic pain in some cases can be explained by the virus binding to angiotensin-converting enzyme-2 (ACE-2) receptors in the central and peripheral nervous system, although SARS-CoV-2 is not primarily neurotropic in itself.[45,49] ACE-2 receptors are also widely distributed in other organ systems, such as the gastrointestinal system. It has been noted that 5–15% of hospitalized COVID-19 patients present with abdominal pain that can plausibly be explained by viral binding to ACE-2 receptors specifically in the gastrointestinal tract.[45] Other explanations for abdominal pain include lymphadenopathy, referred pain from the lungs, or visceral distension.[45]

In the context of COVID-19, individuals tend to have an increased perception of musculoskeletal pain and experience greater myalgia specifically in the limbs during active infection.[50,51] Although it is essential to effectively control different types of pain during an active infection, it is also important to consider both pain that persists after a COVID-19 infection subsides and new-onset pain that arises post-infection. Studies show that COVID-19 survivors are more likely to develop de novo pain and headaches.[52,53] Paradoxically, in one cohort study, individuals who did not experience acute pain during a COVID-19 infection were more likely to require intensive care and/or subsequently die. Although the exact reasons for this are still unknown, it is possible that respiratory distress and other systemic symptoms that progress to intensive care hospitalization and mortality may mask the acute symptoms or that higher catecholamines and other neuromodulator transmitters in patients with severe illness mitigate pain.[44]

Pain Etiologies

Although studies have identified associations between COVID-19 and acute pain, little is known about the relationship between COVID-19 and populations that are vulnerable to experiencing pain. In this section, we discuss risk factors for developing different types of pain associated with COVID-19 and further elaborate on how certain vulnerable populations may be at higher risk for these types of acute pain.

Myocardial Pain

Myocardial pain is a common manifestation of COVID-19, especially in the elderly population.[54,55] There have been multiple theories regarding cardiac damage and myocardial pain in COVID-19 patients, but the leading explanation remains the hypervigilant inflammatory response to the virus' entry via ACE-2 receptors, eventually leading to injury of vascular endothelium and cardiac myocytes.[56,57] Studies have also demonstrated a higher risk of myocardial infarction and other heart manifestations in ethnic minorities.[58]

Noncardiac Chest Pain

Noncardiac chest pain may result from overuse of accessory muscles during dyspnea or coughing, referred pain from the lungs and upper abdominal viscera, or fractured ribs from excessive coughing. Chest pain may persist post-infection, with one study reporting a prevalence rate exceeding 20%.[59]

Myopathy

Musculoskeletal pain is the most common manifestation in COVID-19 patients, observed in approximately 36% of all patients.[60] Musculoskeletal pain is commonly seen during both acute and long COVID and is one of the most common symptoms across adult populations, but it is less common in children.[30–32]

In a study conducted in Spain, the risk factors for developing persistent musculoskeletal pain post-COVID were investigated. Approximately 45.1% of all patients who had COVID-19 experienced post-infectious musculoskeletal pain, with female sex, history of musculoskeletal pain, the presence of myalgia and headaches during active infection, and the number of hospitalized days all being risk factors.[61]

Low socioeconomic status is associated with higher levels of inflammatory markers.[62] Given that a hypervigilant inflammatory response to COVID is a risk factor for severe myalgia, lower socioeconomic status may potentially serve as an independent risk factor for musculoskeletal pain.[62,63]

Joint Pain

Respiratory viral infections have been associated with an increased number of cases of rheumatoid arthritis, especially in the elderly population.[64]

Headache

Headache is the most common acute pain symptom of COVID, with prevalence rates ranging from less than 10% to upwards of 30%.[44,65] There are many etiologies for headache, including endogenous and exogenous pyrogens and fever, direct and indirect effects of the virus, psychological stress, and immunological mediators. Not surprisingly, the two most common types of headaches are tension-type and migraine. In one study in which headache was the most common pain complaint, older age was a significant predictor of long COVID.[66] In another study that stratified symptoms based on race and ethnicity, the percentage of African Americans with headache (27.2%) was higher than that for other races, but the difference was not statistically significant.[67]

Abdominal/Pelvic Pain

The SARS-CoV-2 virus binds to ACE-2 receptors. The clinical features of COVID-19 seem to differ in children compared to adults, with the former experiencing more severe gastrointestinal symptoms, whereas adults experience more respiratory and systemic manifestations. Many studies have described gastrointestinal symptoms, particularly abdominal pain, to be common and prominent in children with COVID. A study examining intestinal ACE-2 expression in children and adults found that intestinal ACE-2 levels were significantly higher in children. This suggests that children are at increased risk of suffering abdominal pain during a COVID infection (Figure 29.1).[68]

Chronic Pain

Chronic pain entails an understanding of a complex interaction of factors such as medical illnesses, genetic underpinnings, psychosocial vulnerabilities, cultural considerations, and access to health care and support systems that must be considered in the context of the biopsychosocial model. Predisposing factors can include genetic factors, previous pain experiences, and physical or psychological traumatic events. Chronic pain conditions can be triggered by psychosocial stressors or organ-specific biological factors, which may preferentially occur in individuals with a fragile stress response system.[69–71] Numerous contributing factors to the COVID-19 pandemic caused or exacerbated chronic pain conditions. Pain can be a consequence of COVID-19 infection leading to a post-viral syndrome, it can be due to worsening physical and mental health secondary to stress and decreased access to care, or it can result from long-lasting emotional or psychological stress related to the pandemic.

COVID-19 can lead to chronic pain in several different ways: (1) as part of a post-viral syndrome or the result of viral-associated organ damage; (2) the exacerbation of pre-existing pain due to enhanced disease progression or physical and psychological stress; and (3) new symptoms triggered in individuals not infected with COVID through amplification of risk factors (e.g., poor sleep, inactivity, fear, anxiety, and depression).[5] Chronic pain is a complex condition resulting from of a complex and dynamic interaction between biological, psychological, and social factors. Many characteristics of the COVID-19 pandemic can potentially increase the prevalence of chronic pain, especially with unpredictable stressors extending out over many years.

Infection Acting as a Trigger for Chronic Pain

Acute viral illnesses can lead to myalgia and fatigue, as well as organ-specific symptoms, as observed with influenza and noted in the H1N1 pandemics and the SARS epidemic.[72,73] In a small study of 22 subjects infected during the SARS epidemic, a chronic post-SARS syndrome consisting of fatigue, diffuse myalgia, depression, and nonrestorative sleep persisted for almost 2 years.[74] Some infections can cause specific post-infectious syndromes, with stereotypical responses to any type of infection often observed. In one study, up to 12% of patients infected with three different

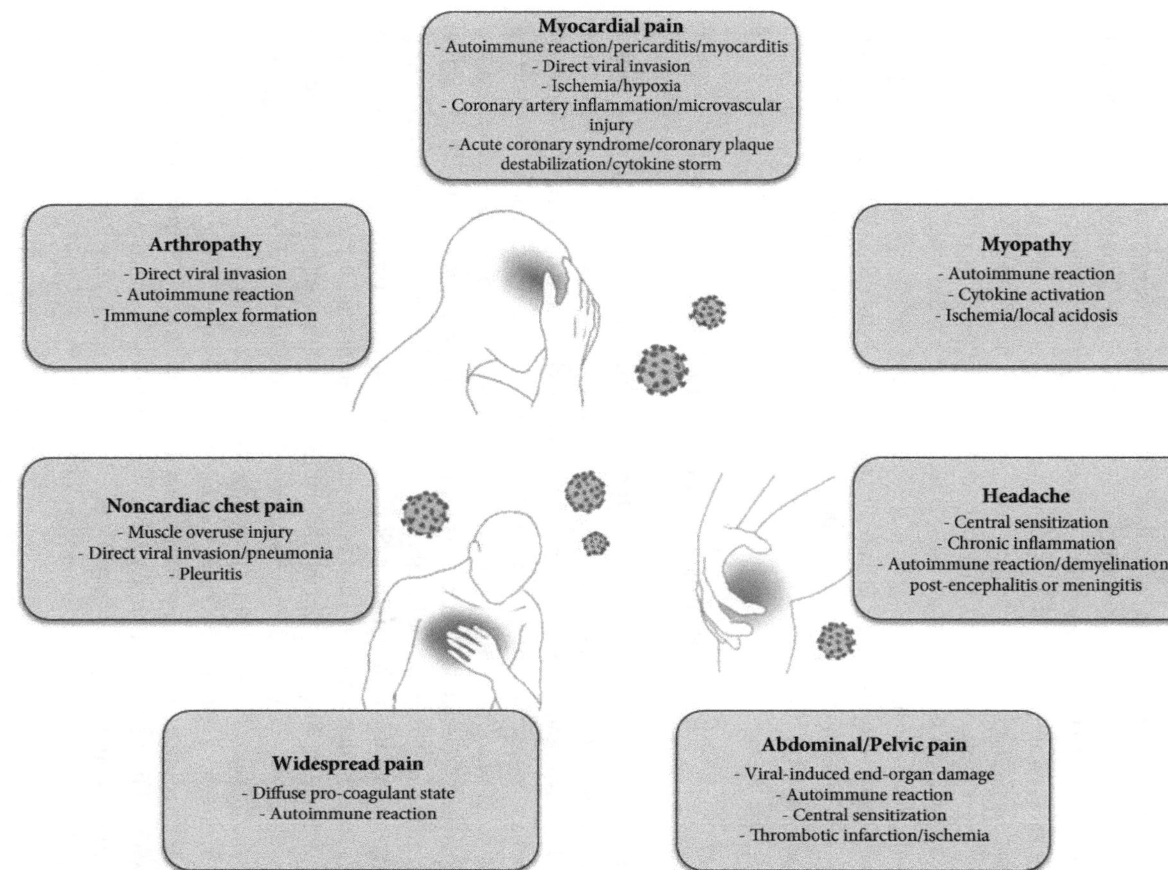

Myocardial pain
- Autoimmune reaction/pericarditis/myocarditis
- Direct viral invasion
- Ischemia/hypoxia
- Coronary artery inflammation/microvascular injury
- Acute coronary syndrome/coronary plaque destabilization/cytokine storm
Arthropathy
- Direct viral invasion
- Autoimmune reaction
- Immune complex formation
Myopathy
- Autoimmune reaction
- Cytokine activation
- Ischemia/local acidosis
Noncardiac chest pain
- Muscle overuse injury
- Direct viral invasion/pneumonia
- Pleuritis
Headache
- Central sensitization
- Chronic inflammation
- Autoimmune reaction/demyelination/post-encephalitis or meningitis
Widespread pain
- Diffuse pro-coagulant state
- Autoimmune reaction
Abdominal/Pelvic pain
- Viral-induced end-organ damage
- Autoimmune reaction
- Central sensitization
- Thrombotic infarction/ischemia

Figure 29.1 Mechanisms of chronic pain after COVID-19 infection.

Drawing by Seffrah and Zared Cohen.

pathogens—Ross River virus (the cause of epidemic polyarthritis), *Coxiella burnetii* (the cause of Q fever), and Epstein–Barr virus—experienced a post-viral syndrome of pain, fatigue, and memory difficulties for up to 12 months. Despite viral illnesses being different in their presentation, the chronic post-infectious syndromes occur at a similar rate. There was also a close correlation between somatic symptoms during the acute phase of infection and chronic fatigue and pain symptoms that occurred later on.[5,75] In a meta-analysis performed in patients with acute viral or bacterial gastroenteritis, 10% of individuals developed post-infectious irritable bowel syndrome, with psychological stressors occurring at a disproportionately high rate.[76] Similarly, an episode of acute urinary tract infection is evident in a substantial proportion of women who develop interstitial cystitis/painful bladder syndrome.[77]

Post-COVID-19 syndrome has been observed in a significant proportion of COVID survivors. According to a systematic review, 20.7% of publications on long-term COVID-19 symptoms concerned pulmonary complications, 24.1% focused on neurologic complaints and olfactory dysfunction, and 55.2% reported on widespread constitutional symptoms that included chronic fatigue and pain.[78] The most frequent long-term pain-related symptoms in post-COVID patients are myalgia, arthralgia, insomnia, and headache.[79,80]

Chronic Pain as a Result of COVID-19 Infection

Patients with COVID-19 can be asymptomatic or exhibit a broad range of symptoms, with full-blown respiratory distress syndrome being the most severe. Nonspecific constitutional symptoms can include fatigue, myalgias, chills, and headaches. A decreased immune response, which can predispose individuals to symptomatic COVID-19 infection, can be a direct result of increased mental health comorbidities, poor sleep, and opioid use.[81] Prolonged ICU stay and hospitalization secondary to COVID-19 infection can lead to worsening mental health, prolonged functional limitations, and the development or worsening of chronic pain. Studies have reported persistent pain in 38–56% of ICU survivors when evaluated 2–4 years after ICU admission.[82,83] According to a study from the United Kingdom that conducted telephone follow-ups in patients who were hospitalized for COVID-19, those who were admitted to the ICU experienced greater nonspecific pain compared to patients who were not hospitalized in the ICU.[84] This is consistent with a systematic review finding chronic pain prevalence rates between 28% and 77% lasting more than 3 months after ICU admission.[85] Numerous studies have shown significant psychiatric comorbidities in COVID survivors, including but not limited to depression, post-traumatic stress disorder, generalized anxiety, obsessive–compulsive disorder, and neurocognitive disorders.[86–88]

The Psychosocial Impact of the COVID-19 Pandemic

Some chronic pain patients may experience an exacerbation of symptoms resulting from COVID-19 due to disruption in routine medical care from lockdowns, facility closures, or fear of contracting infection. Due to the closure of ambulatory surgical centers and cancellation of elective procedures, many pain clinics throughout the world went through phases of stopping or minimizing clinical operations, including both procedural and pharmacological management appointments. Although telemedicine played a role in bridging the gap, it could not fully compensate for the reduction in the number of procedures for chronic pain, and many vulnerable patients do not have access to telemedicine.

Psychological distress related to the pandemic adds another layer to the exacerbation of existing pain due to COVID-19. Regardless of the type of pain condition, baseline pain was shown to worsen during the pandemic, which was attributed to a variety of factors, including (1) a decrease in physical activity and (2) psychological stress related to anxiety, uncertainty, lockdowns, and social distancing mandates that reduced social support structures.[25,26] Sleep problems and fear of the virus were found to be significant catalysts in worsening pain and depression.[25]

The economic impact on public health has been huge, including higher unemployment rates, job uncertainty, and the resulting lapses in health insurance. Another factor that contributed to worsening outcomes was the reduction in health-related physical activities, group therapies, and community activities such as going to gyms and pools and socializing, all of which can be crucial in managing and mitigating chronic pain.[89]

Treatment

The treatment of COVID-related pain depends on etiology, classification of pain (nociceptive, neuropathic, nociplastic, or mixed), acuity, disease burden, comorbidities, and patient preferences, in accordance with an interdisciplinary, multimodal biopsychosocial approach. Nonsteroidal anti-inflammatory drugs and opioids are more likely to be effective for acute pain, whereas muscle relaxants may be indicated in individuals with muscle spasm. Adjuvants such as gabapentinoids and antidepressants may be beneficial in patients with neuropathic and nociplastic pain, with antidepressants also having efficacy for somatic and visceral nociceptive pain. In individuals with chronic headache, preventative therapy with topiramate, antidepressants, calcitonin gene-related peptide antagonists, botulinum toxin injections, and beta and calcium channel blockers may be indicated.

The treatment of acute and chronic pain for vulnerable populations is similar to that for nonvulnerable populations, with certain caveats. Elderly patients may be more likely to experience side effects and drug–drug interactions, whereas pediatric patients and young adults are at higher risk for opioid tolerance and hyperalgesia. Physicians also tend to underestimate pain in African Americans and other minorities, which has traditionally led to them being less likely to receive opioids and other specialized interventions.[90]

Conclusion

The COVID-19 pandemic has caused major upheavals in health care, which have disproportionately affected vulnerable populations and individuals with pre-existing health problems, including chronic pain. Pain is a debilitating symptom during acute SARS-CoV-2 infection, but what is less commonly appreciated is that a substantial percentage of individuals, especially vulnerable populations, may experience long-lasting regional or diffuse chronic pain with commensurate reductions in quality of life. Reasons for this include being at increased risk for infection and having a higher rate of medical comorbidities, reduced access to health care, and greater distrust of the medical system. Future research should be devoted to identifying interventions to prevent the transition to chronic pain and developing personalized treatment pathways that can reduce disparities in treatment outcomes.

References

1. Hoffmann M, Kleine-Weber H, Schroeder S, et al. SARS-CoV-2 cell entry depends on ACE2 and TMPRSS2 and is blocked by a clinically proven protease inhibitor. *Cell.* 2020;181(2):271–280. doi:10.1016/J.CELL.2020.02.052
2. Chan JFW, Kok KH, Zhu Z, et al. Genomic characterization of the 2019 novel human-pathogenic coronavirus isolated from a patient with atypical pneumonia after visiting Wuhan. *Emerg Microbes Infect.* 2020;9(1):221–236. doi:10.1080/22221751.2020.1719902
3. World Health Organization. Weekly epidemiological update on COVID-19—1 February 2022. 2022. Accessed February 7, 2022. https://www.who.int/publications/m/item/weekly-epidemiological-update-on-covid-19---1-february-2022
4. Worldometer. United States coronavirus statistics. 2022. Accessed February 7, 2022. https://www.worldometers.info/coronavirus/country/us
5. Clauw DJ, Häuser W, Cohen SP, Fitzcharles MA. Considering the potential for an increase in chronic pain after the COVID-19 pandemic. *Pain.* 2020;161(8):1694–1697. doi:10.1097/J.PAIN.0000000000001950
6. Gaskin DJ, Richard P. The economic costs of pain in the United States. *J Pain.* 2012;13(8):715–724. doi:10.1016/J.JPAIN.2012.03.009
7. Luo Y, Liu Z, Yang L, et al. Association of body pain and chronic disease: Evidence from a 7-year population-based study in China. *Reg Anesth Pain Med.* 2021;46(9):745–751. doi:10.1136/RAPM-2021-102700
8. Song X-J, Xiong D-L, Wang Z-Y, Yang D, Zhou L, Li R-C. Pain management during the COVID-19 pandemic in China: Lessons learned. *Pain Med.* 2020;21(7):1319–1323.
9. Jain A, Gee S, Malayala SV, Laboe CW. Chronic pediatric pain and mental illness during the COVID-19 era: A case series from inpatient child psychiatry unit. *Cureus.* 2021;13(11):e20032. doi:10.7759/CUREUS.20032
10. Plein LM, Rittner HL. Opioids and the immune system—Friend or foe. *Br J Pharmacol.* 2018;175(14):2717–2725. doi:10.1111/BPH.13750
11. Widyadharma IPE, Sari NNSP, Pradnyaswari KE, et al. Pain as clinical manifestations of COVID-19 infection and its management in the pandemic era: A literature review. *Egypt J Neurol Psychiatry Neurosurg.* 2020;56(1): Article 121. doi:10.1186/S41983-020-00258-0
12. Centers for Disease Control and Prevention. COVID-19 provisional counts—Weekly updates by select demographic and geographic characteristics. n.d. Accessed February 8, 2022. https://www.cdc.gov/nchs/nvss/vsrr/covid_weekly/index.htm#SexAndAge

13. Roberts KC, Rao DP, Bennett TL, Loukine L, Jayaraman GC. Prevalence and patterns of chronic disease multimorbidity and associated determinants in Canada. *Health Promot Chronic Dis Prev Can*. 2015;35(6):87–94. doi:10.24095/HPCDP.35.6.01
14. Davis JW, Chung R, Juarez DT. Prevalence of comorbid conditions with aging among patients with diabetes and cardiovascular disease. *Hawaii Med J*. 2011;70(10):209–213.
15. Rahman MM, Bhattacharjee B, Farhana Z, et al. Age-related risk factors and severity of SARS-CoV-2 infection: A systematic review and meta-analysis. *J Prev Med Hyg*. 2021;62(2):E329. doi:10.15167/2421-4248/JPMH2021.62.2.1946
16. Cohen SP, Wang E, Doshi T, Vase L, Cawcutt K, Tontisirin N. Chronic pain and infection: Mechanisms, causes, conditions, treatments, and controversies. *BMJ Med*. 2022;1(1):e000108.
17. Wan S, Yi Q, Fan S, et al. Characteristics of lymphocyte subsets and cytokines in peripheral blood of 123 hospitalized patients with 2019 novel coronavirus pneumonia (NCP). *medRxiv*. 2020:2020.02.10.20021832.
18. American Diabetes Association. Statistics about diabetes. n.d. Accessed February 21, 2022. https://www.diabetes.org/about-us/statistics/about-diabetes
19. Muller LMAJ, Gorter KJ, Hak E, et al. Increased risk of common infections in patients with type 1 and type 2 diabetes mellitus. *Clin Infect Dis*. 2005;41(3):281–288. doi:10.1086/431587
20. Carey IM, Critchley JA, Dewilde S, Harris T, Hosking FJ, Cook DG. Risk of infection in type 1 and type 2 diabetes compared with the general population: A matched cohort study. *Diabetes Care*. 2018;41(3):513–521. doi:10.2337/DC17-2131
21. Corona G, Pizzocaro A, Vena W, et al. Diabetes is most important cause for mortality in COVID-19 hospitalized patients: Systematic review and meta-analysis. *Rev Endocr Metab Disord*. 2021;22(2):275–296. doi:10.1007/S11154-021-09630-8
22. Roberts J, Pritchard AL, Treweeke AT, et al. Why is COVID-19 more severe in patients with diabetes? The role of angiotensin-converting enzyme 2, endothelial dysfunction and the immunoinflammatory system. *Front Cardiovasc Med*. 2021;7:629933. doi:10.3389/FCVM.2020.629933
23. Badrah M, Riad A, Kassem I, Boccuzzi M, Klugar M. Craniofacial pain in COVID-19 patients with diabetes mellitus: Clinical and laboratory description of 21 cases. *J Med Virol*. 2021;93(5):2616–2619. doi:10.1002/JMV.26866
24. Hirase T, Okita M, Nakai Y, Akaida S, Shono S, Makizako H. Pain and physical activity changes during the COVID-19 state of emergency among Japanese adults aged 40 years or older: A cross-sectional study. *Medicine*. 2021;100(41):e27533. doi:10.1097/MD.0000000000027533
25. Rogers AH, Garey L, Zvolensky MJ. COVID-19 psychological factors associated with pain status, pain intensity, and pain-related interference. *Cogn Behav Ther*. 2021;50(6):466–478. doi:10.1080/16506073.2021.1874504
26. Yoshimoto T, Fujii T, Oka H, Kasahara S, Kawamata K, Matsudaira K. Pain status and its association with physical activity, psychological stress, and telework among Japanese workers with pain during the COVID-19 pandemic. *Int J Environ Res Public Health*. 2021;18(11):5595. doi:10.3390/IJERPH18115595
27. Zyznawska JM, Bartecka WM. Remote working forced by COVID-19 pandemic and its influence on neck pain and low back pain among teachers. *Med Pr*. 2021;72(6):677–684. doi:10.13075/MP.5893.01189
28. Knebel C, Ertl M, Lenze U, et al. COVID-19–related cancellation of elective orthopaedic surgery caused increased pain and psychosocial distress levels. *Knee Surg Sports Traumatol Arthrosc*. 2021;29(8):2379–2385. doi:10.1007/S00167-021-06529-4
29. Magdy R, Hussein M, Ragaie C, et al. Characteristics of headache attributed to COVID-19 infection and predictors of its frequency and intensity: A cross sectional study. *Cephalalgia*. 2020;40(13):1422–1431. doi:10.1177/0333102420965140
30. Jackson WM, Price JC, Eisler L, Sun LS, Lee JJ. COVID-19 in pediatric patients: A systematic review. *J Neurosurg Anesthesiol*. 2022;34(1):141–147. doi:10.1097/ANA.0000000000000803
31. Hoang A, Chorath K, Moreira A, et al. COVID-19 in 7780 pediatric patients: A systematic review. *EClinicalMedicine*. 2020;24:100433. doi:10.1016/j.eclinm.2020.100433

32. Radia T, Williams N, Agrawal P, et al. Multi-system inflammatory syndrome in children & adolescents (MIS-C): A systematic review of clinical features and presentation. *Paediatr Respir Rev.* 2021;38:51–57. doi:10.1016/J.PRRV.2020.08.001
33. Mun CJ, Campbell CM, McGill LS, Aaron R V. The early impact of COVID-19 on chronic pain: A cross-sectional investigation of a large online sample of individuals with chronic pain in the United States, April to May, 2020. *Pain Med.* 2021;22(2):470–480. doi:10.1093/PM/PNAA446
34. Cyrus E, Clarke R, Hadley D, et al. The impact of COVID-19 on African American communities in the United States. *medRxiv.* 2020;4(1):476–483. doi:10.1101/2020.05.15.20096552
35. KFF. Communities of color at higher risk for health and economic challenges due to COVID-19. 2020. Accessed February 9, 2022. https://www.kff.org/coronavirus-covid-19/issue-brief/communities-of-color-at-higher-risk-for-health-and-economic-challenges-due-to-covid-19
36. Nguyen TC, Gathecha E, Kauffman R, Wright S, Harris M, Harris CM. Healthcare distrust among hospitalised Black patients during the COVID-19 pandemic. *Postgrad Med J.* 2022;98(1161):539–543. doi:10.1136/postgradmedj-2021-140824
37. Best AL, Fletcher FE, Kadono M, Warren RC. Institutional distrust among African Americans and building trustworthiness in the COVID-19 response: Implications for ethical public health practice. *J Health Care Poor Underserved.* 2021;32(1):90–98. doi:10.1353/HPU.2021.0010
38. Karos K, McParland JL, Bunzli S, et al. The social threats of COVID-19 for people with chronic pain. *Pain.* 2020;161(10):2229–2235. doi:10.1097/J.PAIN.0000000000002004
39. Morrone M, Cronin CE, Schuller K, Nicks SE. Access to health care in Appalachia: Perception and reality. *J Appalach Heal.* 2021;3(4):123–136. doi:10.13023/JAH.0304.10
40. Wilson SL, Kratzke C, Hoxmeier J. Predictors of access to healthcare: What matters to rural Appalachians? *Glob J Health Sci.* 2012;4(6):23–35. doi:10.5539/GJHS.V4N6P23
41. Davoodi NM, Healy M, Goldberg EM. Rural America's hospitals are not prepared to protect older adults from a surge in COVID-19 cases. *Gerontol Geriatr Med.* 2020;6:233372142093616. doi:10.1177/2333721420936168
42. Josephson A, Kilic T, Michler JD. Socioeconomic impacts of COVID-19 in low-income countries. *Nat Hum Behav.* 2021;5(5):557–565. doi:10.1038/s41562-021-01096-7
43. Wang D, Hu B, Hu C, et al. Clinical characteristics of 138 hospitalized patients with 2019 novel coronavirus–infected pneumonia in Wuhan, China. *JAMA.* 2020;323(11):1061–1069. doi:10.1001/JAMA.2020.1585
44. Knox N, Lee CS, Moon JY, Cohen SP. Pain manifestations of COVID-19 and their association with mortality: A multicenter prospective observational study. *Mayo Clin Proc.* 2021;96(4):943–951. doi:10.1016/j.mayocp.2020.12.014
45. Weng LM, Su X, Wang XQ. Pain symptoms in patients with coronavirus disease (COVID-19): A literature review. *J Pain Res.* 2021;14:147–159. doi:10.2147/JPR.S269206
46. Zhu J, Ji P, Pang J, et al. Clinical characteristics of 3,062 COVID-19 patients: A meta-analysis. *J Med Virol.* 2020;92(10):1902–1914. doi:10.1002/jmv.25884
47. Siripanthong B, Nazarian S, Muser D, et al. Recognizing COVID-19–related myocarditis: The possible pathophysiology and proposed guideline for diagnosis and management. *Hear Rhythm.* 2020;17(9):1463–1471. doi:10.1016/J.HRTHM.2020.05.001
48. Finsterer J, Scorza FA, Scorza CA, Fiorini C. Peripheral neuropathy in COVID-19 is due to immune-mechanisms, pre-existing risk factors, anti-viral drugs, or bedding in the intensive care unit. *Arq Neuropsiquiatr.* 2021;79(10):924–928. doi:10.1590/0004-282X-ANP-2021-0030
49. Ahmad I, Rathore FA. Neurological manifestations and complications of COVID-19: A literature review. *J Clin Neurosci.* 2020;77:8–12. doi:10.1016/J.JOCN.2020.05.017
50. Carpintero-Rubio C, Torres-Chica B, Guadrón-Romero MA, Visiers-Jiménez L, Peña-Otero D. Perception of musculoskeletal pain in the state of confinement: associated factors. *Rev Lat Am Enfermagem.* 2021;29:e3454. doi:10.1590/1518-8345.4894.3454

51. Şahin T, Ayyildiz A, Gencer-Atalay K, Akgün C, Özdemir HM, Kuran B. Pain symptoms in COVID-19. *Am J Phys Med Rehabil.* 2021;100(4):307–312. doi:10.1097/PHM.0000000000001699
52. Soares FHC, Kubota GT, Fernandes AM, et al. Prevalence and characteristics of new-onset pain in COVID-19 survivours, a controlled study. *Eur J Pain.* 2021;25(6):1342–1354. doi:10.1002/EJP.1755
53. Wu L, Wu Y, Xiong H, Mei B, You T. Persistence of symptoms after discharge of patients hospitalized due to COVID-19. *Front Med.* 2021;8:761314. doi:10.3389/fmed.2021.761314
54. Basu-Ray I, Almaddah NK, Adeboye A, Soos MP. Cardiac manifestations of coronavirus (COVID-19). In: *StatPearls.* StatPearls Publishing; 2022. https://www.ncbi.nlm.nih.gov/books/NBK556152
55. Wei C, Liu Y, Liu Y, et al. Clinical characteristics and manifestations in older patients with COVID-19. *BMC Geriatr.* 2020;20(1):1–9. doi:10.1186/S12877-020-01811-5
56. Zheng YY, Ma YT, Zhang JY, Xie X. COVID-19 and the cardiovascular system. *Nat Rev Cardiol.* 2020;17(5):259–260. doi:10.1038/S41569-020-0360-5
57. Clerkin KJ, Fried JA, Raikhelkar J, et al. COVID-19 and cardiovascular disease. *Circulation.* 2020;141:1648–1655. doi:10.1161/circulationaha.120.046941
58. Rashid M, Timmis A, Kinnaird T, et al. Racial differences in management and outcomes of acute myocardial infarction during COVID-19 pandemic. *Heart.* 2021;107(9):734–740. doi:10.1136/heartjnl-2020-318356
59. Carfì A, Bernabei R, Landi F. Persistent symptoms in patients after acute COVID-19. *JAMA.* 2020;324(6):603–605. doi:10.1001/jama.2020.12603
60. Li L-Q, Huang T, Wang Y-Q, et al. COVID-19 patients' clinical characteristics, discharge rate, and fatality rate of meta-analysis. *J Med Virol.* 2020;92(6):577–583. doi:10.1002/JMV.25757
61. Fernández-de-las-Peñas C, de-la-Llave-Rincón AI, Ortega-Santiago R, et al. Prevalence and risk factors of musculoskeletal pain symptoms as long-term post-COVID sequelae in hospitalized COVID-19 survivors. *Pain.* 2022;163(9):e989–e996. doi:10.1097/j.pain.0000000000002564
62. Muscatell KA, Brosso SN, Humphreys KL. Socioeconomic status and inflammation: A meta-analysis. *Mol Psychiatry.* 2020;25(9):2189–2199. doi:10.1038/S41380-018-0259-2
63. Cascella M, Del Gaudio A, Vittori A, et al. COVID-Pain: Acute and late-onset painful clinical manifestations in COVID-19—Molecular mechanisms and research perspectives. *J Pain Res.* 2021;14:2403–2412. doi:10.2147/JPR.S313978
64. Joo Y Bin, Lim YH, Kim KJ, Park KS, Park YJ. Respiratory viral infections and the risk of rheumatoid arthritis. *Arthritis Res Ther.* 2019;21(1): Article 199. doi:10.1186/S13075-019-1977-9
65. Bobker SM, Robbins MS. COVID-19 and headache: A primer for trainees. *Headache.* 2020;60(8):1806–1811. doi:10.1111/HEAD.13884
66. Sudre CH, Murray B, Varsavsky T, et al. Attributes and predictors of long COVID. *Nat Med.* 2021;27(4):626–631. doi:10.1038/s41591-021-01292-y
67. Jones J, Sullivan PS, Sanchez TH, et al. Similarities and differences in COVID-19 awareness, concern, and symptoms by race and ethnicity in the United States: Cross-sectional survey. *J Med Internet Res.* 2020;22(7):e20001. doi:10.2196/20001
68. Berni Canani R, Comegna M, Paparo L, et al. Age-related differences in the expression of most relevant mediators of SARS-CoV-2 infection in human respiratory and gastrointestinal tract. *Front Pediatr.* 2021;9:697390. doi:10.3389/fped.2021.697390
69. Crettaz B, Marziniak M, Willeke P, et al. Stress-induced allodynia: Evidence of increased pain sensitivity in healthy humans and patients with chronic pain after experimentally induced psychosocial stress. *PLoS One.* 2013;8(8):e69460. doi:10.1371/journal.pone.0069460
70. Enck P, Mazurak N. The "biology-first" hypothesis: Functional disorders may begin and end with biology—A scoping review. *Neurogastroenterol Motil.* 2018;30(10):e13394. doi:10.1111/nmo.13394
71. McBeth J, Chiu YH, Silman AJ, et al. Hypothalamic–pituitary–adrenal stress axis function and the relationship with chronic widespread pain and its antecedents. *Arthritis Res Ther.* 2005;7(5):R992. doi:10.1186/AR1772

72. Campbell A, Rodin R, Kropp R, et al. Risk of severe outcomes among patients admitted to hospital with pandemic (H1N1) influenza. *CMAJ*. 2010;182(4):349–355. doi:10.1503/CMAJ.091823
73. Creed F. Review article: The incidence and risk factors for irritable bowel syndrome in population-based studies. *Aliment Pharmacol Ther*. 2019;50(5):507–516. doi:10.1111/apt.15396
74. Moldofsky H, Patcai J. Chronic widespread musculoskeletal pain, fatigue, depression and disordered sleep in chronic post-SARS syndrome; A case-controlled study. *BMC Neurol*. 2011;11: Article 37. doi:10.1186/1471-2377-11-37
75. Hickie I, Davenport T, Wakefield D, et al. Post-infective and chronic fatigue syndromes precipitated by viral and non-viral pathogens: Prospective cohort study. *BMJ*. 2006;333(7568):575–578. doi:10.1136/BMJ.38933.585764.AE
76. Holtmann GJ, Ford AC, Talley NJ. Pathophysiology of irritable bowel syndrome. *Lancet Gastroenterol Hepatol*. 2016;1(2):133–146. doi:10.1016/S2468-1253(16)30023-1
77. Warren JW, Brown V, Jacobs S, Horne L, Langenberg P, Greenberg P. Urinary tract infection and inflammation at onset of interstitial cystitis/painful bladder syndrome. *Urology*. 2008;71(6):1085–1090. doi:10.1016/J.UROLOGY.2007.12.091
78. Salamanna F, Veronesi F, Martini L, Landini MP, Fini M. Post-COVID-19 syndrome: The persistent symptoms at the post-viral stage of the disease: A systematic review of the current data. *Front Med*. 2021;8:653516. doi:10.3389/fmed.2021.653516/FULL
79. Gallus R, Melis A, Rizzo D, et al. Audiovestibular symptoms and sequelae in COVID-19 patients. *J Vestib Res*. 2021;31(5):381–387. doi:10.3233/VES-201505
80. Pilotto A, Cristillo V, Piccinelli SC, et al. Long-term neurological manifestations of COVID-19: Prevalence and predictive factors. *medRxiv*. 2021:2020.12.27.20248903. doi:10.1101/2020.12.27.20248903
81. Kosciuczuk U, Knapp P, Lotowska-Cwiklewsk AM. Opioid-induced immunosuppression and carcinogenesis promotion theories create the newest trend in acute and chronic pain pharmacotherapy. *Clinics*. 2020;75:e1554. doi:10.6061/clinics/2020/E1554
82. Korošec Jagodič H, Jagodič K, Podbregar M. Long-term outcome and quality of life of patients treated in surgical intensive care: A comparison between sepsis and trauma. *Crit Care*. 2006;10(5):R134. doi:10.1186/CC5047
83. Schelling G, Stoll C, Haller M, et al. Health-related quality of life and posttraumatic stress disorder in survivors of the acute respiratory distress syndrome. *Crit Care Med*. 1998;26(4):651–659. doi:10.1097/00003246-199804000-00011
84. Halpin SJ, McIvor C, Whyatt G, et al. Postdischarge symptoms and rehabilitation needs in survivors of COVID-19 infection: A cross-sectional evaluation. *J Med Virol*. 2021;93(2):1013–1022. doi:10.1002/JMV.26368
85. Mäkinen OJ, Bäcklund ME, Liisanantti J, Peltomaa M, Karlsson S, Kalliomäki ML. Persistent pain in intensive care survivors: A systematic review. *Br J Anaesth*. 2020;125(2):149–158. doi:10.1016/J.BJA.2020.04.084
86. Taquet M, Geddes JR, Husain M, Luciano S, Harrison PJ. 6-Month neurological and psychiatric outcomes in 236,379 survivors of COVID-19: A retrospective cohort study using electronic health records. *Lancet Psychiatry*. 2021;8(5):416–427. doi:10.1016/S2215-0366(21)00084-5
87. Jafri MR, Zaheer A, Fatima S, Saleem T, Sohail A. Mental health status of COVID-19 survivors: A cross sectional study. *Virol J*. 2022;19(1):1–5. doi:10.1186/S12985-021-01729-3
88. Dar S, Dar M, Sheikh S, et al. Psychiatric comorbidities among COVID-19 survivors in North India: A cross-sectional study. *J Educ Health Promot*. 2021;10(1): Article 309. doi:10.4103/jehp.jehp_119_21
89. Macfarlane GJ, Kronisch C, Dean LE, et al. EULAR revised recommendations for the management of fibromyalgia. *Ann Rheum Dis*. 2017;76(2):318–328. doi:10.1136/annrheumdis-2016-209724

90. Hoffman KM, Trawalter S, Axt JR, Oliver MN. Racial bias in pain assessment and treatment recommendations, and false beliefs about biological differences between Blacks and Whites. *Proc Natl Acad Sci USA*. 2016;113(16):4296–4301. doi:10.1073/pnas.1516047113
91. Campbell CM, Edwards RR. Ethnic differences in pain and pain management. *Pain Manag.* 2012;2(3):219–230. doi:10.2217/pmt.12.7
92. Pagel C. There is a real danger that COVID-19 will become entrenched as a disease of poverty. *BMJ*. 2021;373:n986. doi:10.1136/BMJ.N986
93. Patel JA, Nielsen FBH, Badiani AA, et al. Poverty, inequality and COVID-19: The forgotten vulnerable. *Public Health*. 2020;183:110–111. doi:10.1016/j.puhe.2020.05.006
94. Payne AB, Gilani Z, Godfred-Cato S, et al. Incidence of multisystem inflammatory syndrome in children among US persons infected with SARS-CoV-2. *JAMA Netw Open*. 2021;4(6):e2116420. doi:10.1001/jamanetworkopen.2021.16420

30
Pain and Youth Sports

Marcus Anthony, Tejas Ozarkar, Juan Andres Moncayo, and Shae Datta

Introduction

In both the medical and lay community, it is widely accepted that participation in organized sport can serve as an enjoyable and informative experience for children and adolescents that provides many potential physical and psychosocial health benefits.[1] According to several recent reports, roughly 55–60% of American youth (children and adolescents aged 6–17 years as defined by the National Youth Sports Strategy) participated in organized sport in 2019 and 2020.[2–4] These surveys defined sport participation on a spectrum ranging from regular weekly team sport activities to individual sport competitions and training sessions. Given the diverse opportunities for youth to become involved in sport, including unstructured and nonscholastic play, total youth sport participation has proven difficult to estimate and has been reported between 30 and 60 million in the United States before the COVID-19 pandemic.[5,6] Unfortunately, the pandemic had an immediate and deleterious impact on youth sport participation, most significantly in community-based sports programs. This drastic decline greatly exacerbated the steady decrease in youth sport participation that was observed in the decade before the pandemic.[7] In light of this, youth sport participation has become a growing population health concern given that many youth meet the recommended level of healthy physical activity through sport participation.[4,8,9]

What Makes Youth Athletes Vulnerable to Pain?

Numerous governmental health agencies (National Youth Sport Strategy, etc.), nongovernmental organizations (Aspen Institute, Women's Sport Foundation, etc.), and sport governing bodies (United States Olympic & Paralympic Committee, International Olympic Committee, etc.) have created public policy, consensus-based guidelines, and community programs to develop young athletes and promote public health.[4,10] These are vital to the equitable and safe development of lifelong athletes because, despite the myriad of sport's health benefits, there are also inherent risks associated with youth sport participation, namely acute and overuse musculoskeletal injuries.[11,12] As such, these efforts emphasize the prevention, diagnosis, and management of acute and overuse injuries unique to muscularly and skeletally immature athletes. Among other factors, they raise awareness of the impact of peak height velocity (PHV) on injury risk, the risk of apophyseal and physeal injuries, dilemmas cause by asynchronous skill and physical development, the importance of of training load and periodization, and the increasing levels of specialization in young athletes.[1,10,13,14]

Similar to the prevalence of sport-related injuries, pain has been shown to be common among youth athletes.[15] Although a causal relationship between sport participation and pain has not been consistently proven in the literature, many studies have revealed that pain is a common shared experience among youth athletes irrespective of injury.[16–20] Until recently, however, there has been a paucity of data describing the experience of pain not only in youth athletes but also in elite and professional athletes.[21] In addition, the limited literature available has often failed to appreciate the entire scope of pain beyond simply being a symptom of structural damage sustained during acute or chronic injury. This expression of pain is inconsistent with the reality that sport-related pain is a subjective and entirely personal experience influenced by developmental, biomechanical, and psychosocial factors (collectively referred to as biopsychosocial factors).[19,22] In the care of youth athletes, failure to recognize the many biopsychosocial factors (in addition to tissue damage) that influence the pain experience increases risk of misdiagnosis, unnecessary early withdrawal from sport, chronic pain that can extend to adulthood, and poor long-term health outcomes.[17] Furthermore, acute adolescent pain has been linked to widespread immediate harms from lower quality of life to poor academic performance.[23] The psychological burden inflicted on youth athletes by sport-related pain is also of concern because youth athletes may demonstrate greater anxiety and more persistent catastrophizing thoughts compared to adult athletes, which can greatly exacerbate the pain experience.[24]

Recognizing that pain is not synonymous with injury, the International Olympic Committee (IOC) published the first consensus-based guidelines for the diagnosis and management of pain in athletes. The guidelines advocate for a biopsychosocial approach to pain management in an attempt to overcome common cognitive biases that have historically limited sport-related pain management to analgesics, activity modification (rest), physical therapy, and surgery (i.e. typical *injury* management). To accomplish this, the consensus statement first emphasizes the importance of considering all types of pain, not just nociceptive, when encountering an athlete in pain. Management then proceeds with evaluation of the biopsychosocial factors that influence pain in order to fully address all aspects of the complex pain experience.[25] Although written for the elite athlete, the IOC recommendations can be applied to the care of youth athletes if with special considerations for the developmental, biomechanical, and psychosocial factors unique to youth athletes that both modulate the risk of injury and influence the experience of sports-related pain.[25]

Pain to Consider in Youth Athletes

Pain in youth athletes, as well as in adult athletes, is a subjective and entirely individualized personal experience. The International Association for the Study of Pain (IASP) defines pain as "an unpleasant sensory and emotional experience associated with, or resembling that associated with, actual or potential tissue damage."[26] Included in this definition is an acknowledgment that pain is a complex clinical complaint that is not predicated on the presence of tissue damage. The following review of pain types further emphasizes this point but does not minimize the influence of injury (structural damage) on the prevalence of pain. Instead, it contextualizes injury within the full spectrum of pain pathophysiology to better understand the clinical complexity of pain in youth sports.

Nociceptive Pain

Nociceptive pain is defined by IASP as "pain that arises from actual or threatened damage to non-neural tissue and is due to the activation of nociceptors."[26] Nociceptors transduce pain signals in reaction to noxious stimuli (mechanical, thermal, and/or chemical changes) in peripheral tissue that indicate potential or realized structural damage or underlying inflammation. Inflammatory pain is in fact a subset of nociceptive pain.[22,26] Nociceptive pain may be the most common cause of sports-related pain in youth athletes due to the high rates of both acute and overuse musculoskeletal injuries that result in direct tissue damage or inflammation.[27,28] Examples of acute injury leading to nociceptive pain in youth sports are plentiful and overlap with acute injuries often sustained by older athletes.[29] However, youth athletes are at risk of injury to their growth plates (physes), which close before adulthood.

Given that their developmental stage influences their risk of injury, it is critical to avoid the temptation to treat youth athletes as "little adults." Proximal humeral epiphysiolysis (Little League shoulder) is an example of nociceptive pain due to an overuse injury that only occurs in the youth athlete with an open physis.[30,31] Common among all overhead youth athletes, proximal humeral epiphysiolysis is defined as a stress fracture of the proximal humeral physis that results from excessive forces during repetitive overhead movement. During these repeated submaximal loading episodes of the physis, if there is not adequate time for recovery, tissue damage results in a physeal stress fracture. Failure to allow recovery and structural adaptation between intermittent episodes of submaximal loading is the hallmark of all overuse injuries of the musculoskeletal system and ultimately leads to structural damage.[1]

Neuropathic Pain

In contrast to nociceptive pain, which is a response to damage to non-neural peripheral tissue, neuropathic pain results from damage to the somatosensory nervous system via a direct lesion or systemic disease. Neuropathic pain requires a discrete insult to the somatosensory nervous system on diagnostic workup and is not itself a diagnosis.[26] Like nociceptive pain, neuropathic pain can result from both acute and overuse injuries.

An example of neuropathic pain that may occur in youth overhead athletes is a subscapular nerve injury, which often results in shoulder pain and posterior shoulder weakness. Injury to the subscapular nerve may be acute but is more often subacute secondary to persistent traction of the nerve through the suprascapular notch during repeated overhead movements common in tennis, volleyball, baseball, and fencing. This phenomenon is exacerbated by improper shoulder biomechanics that increase stress to the nerve.

In a theoretical case of subscapular nerve injury in a youth baseball player, a clinician may fail to consider neuropathic causes of pain if common overuse injuries of nociceptive pain more readily come to mind (availability bias). This could lead to misdiagnosis (e.g., as proximal humeral epiphysiolysis) and inappropriate treatment. Instead, if a clinician is intentionally mindful of the full spectrum of pain types during diagnostic examination, they may be more likely to assess for clinical signs of neuropathic pain (muscle weakness and atrophy) that would increase clinical suspicion of the appropriate diagnosis. Without properly diagnosing subscapular nerve injury, the clinician would further fail to consider the faulty ongoing biomechanics of the athlete's overhead movement. If the influence of the athlete's biomechanics is missed, curative treatment with focused rehabilitation to correct the overhead techniques would likely not be prescribed.[32] This injury also highlights the importance of identifying factors (in this case, biomechanical) that influence pain after appropriately defining the type of pain.

Nociplastic Pain

Unlike both nociceptive and neuropathic pain, nociplastic pain occurs from pathologically altered nociception in the absence of identifiable damage to peripheral non-neural tissue and the somatosensory nervous system.[26] In cases of nociplastic pain, the etiology is not identifiable, but individuals may present with a constellation of hypersensitivity, sympathetic nervous system dysfunction, and higher rates of chronic pain.[15] Examples of nociplastic pain in the general population that may affect youth athletes are fibromyalgia, complex regional pain syndrome, nonspecific lower back pain, and irritable bowel syndrome.[22] Rates and common causes of nociplastic pain in youth athletes have not been studied, which contributes to the difficulty of recognizing and diagnosing nociplastic pain in this population. When treating a youth athlete, pain out of proportion to physical exam and persistent pain symptoms in the setting of a negative diagnostic workup should increase clinical suspicion for nociplastic pain.

Although a clinician may be able to qualify an athlete's pain as nociceptive, neuropathic, or nociplastic, each athlete's experience of the pain is unique. Significant variability in symptomatology and symptom severity can be reported between athletes presenting with the same type of pain and also between athletes presenting with the same injury. This interpersonal variation is explained by an athlete's unique combination of biopsychosocial factors that contribute to the individualization of the pain experience.[22,27,33]

The Youth Athlete's Pain Experience: Biopsychosocial Factors

Developmental Factors

Unlike adult athletes, youth athletes face the challenges of normal physical growth and biological development in addition to the demands of training and competition. These ongoing physiologic stressors and the relative stage of muscular and skeletal maturity in the athlete influence the risk of injury and the experience of pain in unique ways.[10,34] Of particular interest are the risk of injury during skeletal growth, the influence of the immature musculoskeletal system on the risk of developing improper biomechanics, and the importance of developmentally appropriate athletic activity and expectations.[35–37]

As youth athletes mature, vertical growth and muscle mass develop asynchronously. Although wide variations can be observed, young females typically show highest vertical growth rates between ages 11 and 13 years, whereas boys achieve their highest growth rates slightly later, between ages 13 and 15 years. This time period, colloquially known as "the growth spurt," is referred to in the literature as PHV. During the entire growth process, but particularly during PHV, youth athletes are at increased risk of fracture and overuse injury of the physes.[38] One explanation of this phenomenon is that lower rates of growth in the muscle–tendon unit compared to skeletal growth rates can cause muscular imbalances and joint instability that predispose to injury.[28] Second, there is evidence that metabolic changes in growing bone may lead to less resilient growth cartilage within the articular surfaces and decreased bone mineralization that increase the risk of fracture.[1] In skeletally immature athletes, physeal fractures and stress fractures can be particularly harmful due to the risk of resultant growth disruption. Disrupted growth, especially of the femur and tibia, can result in significant limb length discrepancy and joint deformity that predispose to osteoarthritis and poor functional status as the youth athlete ages.

In addition to the risk of fracture, vertical growth in youth athletes has been identified as a risk factor for developing muscle–tendon injuries that may differ from the injuries sustained by older athletes playing the same sport.[39–41] These findings have been attributed to instability and muscular weakness (resulting from muscle mass development lagging behind the development of the axial and appendicular skeleton) that predispose to acute and overuse muscle–tendon injury.

Biomechanical Factors

An important additional factor that influences the rates of overuse injury (and therefore the pain experience) in youth athletes is the harmful biomechanics that can develop to meet performance goals when strength is still developing.[30] High-risk biomechanics can occur in all youth sports. Two such examples are a baseball pitcher's goal to maximize pitch velocity and a tennis player's goal to maximize their serve's ball speed. An understanding of the kinetic chain continuum, or how athletes generate power and force during athletic activity, helps explain how an immature musculoskeletal system can influence improper biomechanics. The kinetic chain continuum describes the system of interactive movements that lead to the transfer of forces from adjacent body segments starting from the legs (proximal) to the torso and ultimately the upper body (distal) to generate speed and power. In overhead sports, a majority of the overhead force is generated by the lower extremities and torso.[32] If the generation of force is compromised at any point in the kinetic chain continuum, distal segments experience added stress to compensate for force lost as the athlete attempts to achieve the same physiologic output that would normally be produced by an intact or fully realized system.

Like adult athletes, novice youth athletes may demonstrate improper biomechanics simply due to poor techniques that have not been corrected by coaches or training staff.[30] However, youth athletes may also develop harmful biomechanics as they attempt to push beyond the physiological limits of their muscularly immature kinetic chain to maximize performance in pursuit of lofty goals. In baseball, youth pitchers demonstrate increased torso and hip rotational velocity compared to adult pitchers to compensate for the decreased force generated in their muscularly immature legs. These changes in hip and torso biomechanics increase load on the elbow and therefore increase the risk of elbow pain and injury.[30] Biomechanics must therefore be considered within the context of the entire kinetic chain continuum in order to identify pathology that is not at the site of pain.[42] This is of particular relevance in the setting of subacute pain that is not responding to treatment. If pain is not responding to prescribed offloading, physical therapy, or if pain recurs immediately with return to sport, biomechanical assessment by a sport specialized physical therapist may reveal pathologic movements within the kinetic chain continuum away from the site of pain. In these cases, pain can only be resolved by correcting the athlete's improper biomechanics. Therefore, a clinician must be mindful of not only the kinetic chain but also the importance of collaborating with a multidisciplinary team.

Culture of Sport: Psychosocial Factors

Sports medicine organizations and sport governing bodies have attempted to decrease the risk of acute and overuse injuries in youth sport by recommending models of organized sport that emphasize skill development, rather than performance achievements, and encourage developmentally appropriate sport activities.[37,43] In the United States, national governing bodies (NGBs) that are members of the United States Olympic & Paralympic Committee (USOPC) have developed athletic development models (ADMs) that serve as guidelines for developmentally appropriate participation in youth sport. Globally, foreign national federations have created structurally similar long-term athlete development guidelines. Recommendations in each sport differ greatly due to sport-specific factors (load, estimated injury risk, etc.), but commonalities do exist. Of note is the frequent emphasis on the developmental stage of the athlete, sport-specific load considerations, and specialization.[37] USA Hockey was the first US NGB to develop an ADM in 2009. In 2014, the USOPC followed by creating a national ADM to further guide NGBs in the creation of their individualized programs. The national ADM describes five stages of youth athletic experience that are based on increasing levels of skill, progressing physiologic development, and appropriate performance expectations. This framework aims to prevent premature focus on competitive results, which has been show to be associated with higher rates of pain, injury, burnout, and early sport retirement.[44] The USOPC ADM in fact recommends postponing high performance goals until after age 15 years with 10 or more years of athletic experience in multiple sports.

Despite these national recommendations and statements made by sports medicine organizations (the American Medical Society for Sports Medicine, the American College of Sports Medicine, etc.) warning of its adverse effects, youth athletes are becoming more professionalized with increasingly intense competition occurring in increasingly younger age groups.[45] This cultural change has coincided with a trend toward youth athletes becoming more specialized as well, with an estimated 10–30% of all youth athletes focusing on only one sport by ages 12–14 years.[46] Specialization, which is defined as intense year-round training in a single sport at the expense of other sport participation, has been independently linked to pain, injury, and premature burnout in sport.[47,48] Possible explanations for the increased rate of specialization and professionalization in youth sport include increasing individual and systemic pressures to pursue scholarships; obtain name, image, and likeness opportunities; and ultimately achieve professional and/or Olympic status.[48] Despite the common perception that focusing on a single sport maximizes athletic potential, early specialization has not proven to be associated with increased likelihood of achieving professional or elite status in a number of sports.[49,50] Other harmful trends within modern youth sport that have been shown to increase the risk of pain and injury are overscheduling, decreased recovery times, and poor periodization.[5] Furthermore, these factors can contribute directly to an athlete's overall stress, which is one psychological factor that has been consistently associated with increased sport-related injury.

Defined as the result of situational demands exceeding the ability to respond to those demands, stress can increase the risk of injury through altered attention, focus, and mental fatigue. Stress also increases risk of injury through direct impact on muscular tension and coordination.[51] Other psychosocial factors can prolong and even lead to chronification of an athlete's pain resulting from injury. These factors include, but are not limited to, maladaptive behaviors (catastrophizing symptoms, fear-avoidance behaviors, etc.) and negative external influences (high performance expectation and peer and parental attitudes toward pain such as "no pain, no gain") often observed in sport culture.[15,52,53] Further research is needed to elucidate the direct impact these factors have on pain generation without identifiable injury (structure damage) in addition to their known influence of pain from nociceptive or neuropathic inputs. Advanced understanding of these factors may, in turn, improve our knowledge of nociplastic pain in youth athletes as well.

Diagnosing Pain in Youth Athletes

The following discussion on both the diagnosis and management of pain in youth athletes has been structured to demonstrate how a foundational knowledge of the aforementioned types of pain and biopsychosocial factors can be directly applied to care of the youth athlete in pain. Specific diagnostic criteria and treatment plans for common sport-related musculoskeletal and nerve injuries are not a focus of this discussion. Instead, the following sections provide a general framework for a well-intentioned diagnostic and treatment strategy that takes pain pathophysiology and important developmental, biomechanical, and psychosocial factors into consideration.[25]

History

Given the many intrinsic (peak high velocity, immediate stage of muscular and skeletal maturity, etc.) and extrinsic (biomechanics, psychosocial, etc.) factors that influence a youth athlete's pain, an appropriate diagnostic workup must begin with a comprehensive history that covers physical symptoms, developmental stage, athletic involvement, and psychosocial considerations.

When obtaining a history, common first steps include identifying the location, severity, and chronicity of pain. Pain severity and its impact on participation are important to initial risk stratification. Differentiating between acute pain (pain lasting for 6 weeks or less), subacute pain (pain lasting 6–12 weeks), and chronic pain (pain lasting more than 12 weeks) early is helpful to direct subsequent questions to identify potential factors that prolong pain. In general, the longer pain persists, the more likely it is that one or more biopsychosocial factors are influencing the pain experience.[22] In the case of acute pain, the athlete may be able to recall trauma that led to the onset of pain. Review of the mechanism of injury in acute pain cases is of particular importance and can help guide the physical exam. In subacute and chronic pain, the onset of pain may not significantly interfere with sport participation, making the immediate point in time the injury occurred more difficult to recall. In this case, loosely associating the onset of pain with changes in activity levels or type of athletic activity may be useful for identifying physical influences of pain generation.

Localization of pain provides value by informing an anatomically based differential diagnosis. However, the location of the pain must be contextualized within the youth athlete's sport-specific biomechanics and kinetic chain continuum. Considering biomechanical factors and the kinetic chain continuum can help identify causes of pain that are not localized to the site of pain, as described previously. Sport(s) of choice, sport position, experience level (skill level), and changes in training intensity (load) can also help recognize direct injury and biomechanical risk unique to the athlete.[12,54] Although a physician may be knowledgeable of sport-specific biomechanics, referral to a physical therapist or sport physiologist to perform full assessment can substitute.

Discerning the type of pain should also be an early goal during the patient interview. The type of pain can often be discerned by a thorough history with consideration of the typical characteristics that differentiate nociceptive, neuropathic, and nociplastic pain. In general, nociceptive pain is well-localized to an anatomical structure (the tissue that is damaged) and is often aggravated by mechanical load to tissue.[27,55] In contrast, neuropathic pain can be associated with patterns of motor and/or sensory deficits in the distribution of peripheral nerves or nerve roots. Both nociplastic and neuropathic pain can be described with diverse descriptors (sharp, dull, aching, etc.), but reported burning pain and numbness are among the most common complaints of a neuropathic pain input. Nociplastic pain is commonly associated with severe, sometimes widespread pain out of proportion to clinical findings, and hyperalgesia.[22]

The athlete's schedule should be evaluated for adequate time for recovery and periodization as well.[56–58] Periodization is the cyclic training schedule defined by stages of load and recovery. Without adequate recovery time, the body cannot adapt to improve performance and instead becomes at risk of overuse injury.[32] Given the aforementioned increase in the professionalization and specialization of youth athletics, training and competition burden must be established while assessing for adequate time for recovery.

Prior injuries increase the risk of reinjury and can be investigated while interviewing an athlete.[1] Historical injury at the site of pain is of obvious importance, but prior injury within the kinetic chain continuum of the athlete's activities must also be discerned. Two important details of the male and female developmental history are recent vertical growth rates and estimated PHV. Female youth athletes should additionally be asked about menarche and menstrual irregularity. If they meet criteria for the female athlete triad, which is defined by energy deprivation (possibly due to disordered eating), menstrual cycle dysfunction, and decreased bone density, female youth athletes are at even higher risk of injury.

Depression and anxiety can influence pain and recovery. Both can be identified during the athlete's mental health history.[53] More specific to sport, performance goals, coach and parent/guardian expectations, and sport specialization may impact psychosocial vulnerability and should be discussed. Poor responses to prior pain such as fear-avoidance behaviors, catastrophizing of symptoms, and unreasonable fear of recurrent pain/reinjury are important pain modulators to reveal as well.[59] The Pain Catastrophizing Scale has been clinically validated to identify and quantify the scale of pain catastrophization and can be integrated into the patient interview.[60] Similarly, youth sport specialization can be graded on a scale to better understand the degree of specialization.[61]

Physical Examination

The physical exam may vary greatly between cases but must consistently involve assessment of the site of pain and immediately surrounding structures. In many cases, a comprehensive musculoskeletal and neurologic examination is warranted. Whether focal or comprehensive, the physical exam should incorporate inspection, palpation, range of motion, strength, and reflex and sensory assessment. Special musculoskeletal exam maneuvers are performed based on the localization of pain and anatomical structures suspected to be affected. At the site of pain, well-localized point tenderness may indicate nociceptive pain and focal tissue damage. Sensory loss and decreased muscle bulk at the site of pain or at conjoining segments of the body may indicate a neuropathic pathology. Hyperalgesia and autonomic dysfunction at or near the site of pain may be a sign of nociplastic pain. Assessment of adjacent structures and even nonadjacent structures connected to the site of pain through the kinetic chain continuum may provide valuable diagnostic insights and reveal faultybiomechanics. Concern for biomechanical factors must be especially high when pain persists into the chronic phase and should be addressed by including a biomechanical assessment in the physical examination.[27] If a physician lacks the resources or experience needed to perform a particular biomechanical examination, a referral to a physical therapist or sport physiologist to perform a sport-specific biomechanical assessment is warranted when suspicion for a biomechanical influence of pain is elevated.

Further Testing

After obtaining a comprehensive history and performing an appropriate physical exam, further testing involving laboratory assays and imaging studies may be warranted on a case-by-case basis. As a general rule, advanced imaging should not replace a proper history and physical exam. Furthermore, the risks and benefits of the proposed tests should be considered. When clinical suspicion for nociceptive pain secondary to fracture or stress fracture is elevated, radiographic studies are necessary. If neuropathic pain is suspected based on history and physical exam, electromyography (EMG), nerve conduction studies (NCS), and magnetic resonance imaging (MRI) may be considered. With advances in musculoskeletal ultrasound technology and provider adoption, sonography should be considered as a first-line imaging study, especially for suspected soft tissue injury or nerve injury. Advantages of ultrasound include avoidance of radiation, point-of-care capabilities, and general tolerability compared to MRI, EMG, or NCS.[62]

Pain Management in Youth Athletes

Pain is not synonymous with injury. Even when pain is secondary to tissue damage, pain resolution does not always track with tissue recovery. Pain can even persist despite complete resolution of tissue damage.[22] As such, pain management should be informed by the biopsychosocial influences of the pain experience and account for the type of pain input and the anatomy affected.[27] Treatment strategies should take the athlete's immediate and long-term goals into consideration while attempting to maximize function and minimize harm. Explicitly partnering with the youth athlete early to help achieve their goals is one strategy to build trust and maximize the therapeutic potential of the clinician–athlete relationship.[55]

A multimodal approach including nonpharmacologic therapies and pharmacologic treatments is likely the most effective method to treating a youth athlete in pain.[63] Providing education and establishing expectations are both helpful when done early in management. Numerous studies have demonstrated the effectiveness of musculoskeletal pain education to reduce pain symptoms, decrease pain-related disability, and improve function.[55] Understanding the pathology and maintaining realistic rehabilitation expectations also protects against pain-related anxiety that interferes with recovery.[27,53] Youth athletes may in fact display numerous psychological tendencies and maladaptive behaviors that become barriers to their pain resolution. These include general and pain-related stress, catastrophization of symptoms, fear-avoidance behaviors, and pain-associated anxiety.[64] Comprehensive management should target these and similar behaviors and provide coping strategies to overcome their negative influence.[65] Mindfulness strategies that have been proven to modulate pain, reduce depressive symptoms, and enhance nonsport performance have great potential to be applied to the care of youth athletes. To date, however, their use has not been broadly validated in the youth athlete population. In some cases of severe psychological distress, athletes may require referral to mental health services to receive direct talk therapy such as cognitive–behavioral therapy.[55]

Non-mental health providers should constantly engage and counsel youth athletes on the potential negative effects of the increasingly competitive and professionalized youth sport culture. This includes correction of high-risk training and competition schedules and developmentally inappropriate activity and performance expectations. When treating the specialized youth athlete, it may be appropriate to encourage multisport participation, citing evidence contrary to the common belief that sport specialization increases likelihood of progressing to elite levels of sport and instead increases the risk of adverse outcomes.[45] Unhealthy individual, peer, coach, and parental expectations should not be normalized. Youth athletes and their guardians can be directed to sport-specific ADMs that can provide guidance on developmentally appropriate activity and goals. An additional developmental consideration is PHV. Several methods have been validated to estimate and monitor for PVH using an athlete's age, height, mass, growth rates (both height and mass), and biological parent height.[66] Clinicians can therefore monitor a youth athlete's growth and identify times during which they are at increased risk of injury. In addition to simply raising awareness of these high-risk times in an athlete's development, there is evidence that injuries may be prevented if a youth athlete's training is preemptively modified to decrease overall load, high-impact activity, and high acceleration and deceleration activity during anticipated PHV.[13]

In addition to the aforementioned psychosocial and developmental factors, the type of pain can direct treatment in youth athletes. For nociceptive pain caused by acute or overuse injuries, tissue offloading is likely the most recognized treatment strategy and is utilized frequently in the management of sprains, strains, and stress fractures. Offloading can be achieved by many mechanisms, including rest, adjustment of tissue loading through training, biomechanical retraining, and activity modification.[55] Physical therapy frequently coincides or follows offloading strategies in the treatment of amenable sports-related injuries causing nociceptive pain. When tissue damage is the definitive cause of pain, management should include heightened consideration of the anatomical structure injured given the prevalence of many high-risk injuries in youth athletes. Examples of these high-risk injuries are femoral neck injuries, medial malleolus stress fractures, fifth metatarsal proximal diaphyseal fractures (Jones fractures), osteochondritis dissecans of the capitellum, and distal radial physeal stress fractures.[1] Sport-related injuries often require specialized care, and clinicians should be wary of the limit of their clinical practice.

Similarly, neuropathic pain can be acute or subacute, depending on the mechanism of damage to the somatosensory nervous system. Treatment can also involve offloading and physical therapy, but it is important that prescribed techniques be guided by an understanding that the primary driver of neuropathic pain is a lesion to the nervous system rather than tissue damage (tissue injury).[22] An example of a physical therapy technique that targets the somatosensory nervous lesion is neurodynamic mobilization, which includes nerve glides and neural flossing. During these exercises, the affected nerve is mobilized by gentle movements, which has been shown to decrease intraneural inflammation in a number of peripheral neuropathies.[67]

Despite an overall paucity of data on pharmacologic pain management in youth athletes, recent studies show that several non-opioid and opioid medications are commonly used for the treatment of youth athletic pain.[29,68] Unsurprisingly, acetaminophen and nonsteroidal anti-inflammatory drugs (NSAIDs) are the most commonly used analgesics for treatment of youth sport-related pain. In general, NSAIDs or acetaminophen can be a practical and relatively safe first-line pharmacologic therapy for the youth athlete in pain. Still, NSAIDs and acetaminophen should only be prescribed with knowledge of their general risks and with the youth athlete's medical conditions in mind. These medications may be most utilized for the treatment of nociceptive types of pain, but they may be an effective treatment of neuropathic pain as well.[67] Analgesics commonly used for neuropathic pain in the general public, including gabapentin, pregabalin, duloxetine, and others, have not been properly studied within the youth athletes.

Although the U.S. Food and Drug Administration released a warning in 2018 that the risks of using opioids for the treatment of pain in individuals younger than age 18 years far outweigh the benefits, opioids are still commonly prescribed for the management of acute sport-related pain and postoperative pain in youth athletes.[29] If required, opioids should be used at the lowest effective dose for the shortest duration possible.[15] Even when moderate to severe pain is present, NSAIDs should be considered because several studies have shown they may be as effective at treating moderate to severe acute youth sport-related pain (including acute fracture pain) as opioids and with fewer side effects.[29] Overall, the use of all classes of pharmacologic therapies in youth athletes is understudied. Until a robust body of data from future prospective studies reveal their efficacy, safety, side effects, and impact on sport performance, these medications should be used with general caution in youth athletes. This also applies to soft-tissue and intra-articular corticosteroid injections, which are seldom used within the youth athlete population. If used, they should be performed by a specialized clinician using image guidance in order to avoid potential harms to the developing anatomical structures at the site of injection.[31,69] If pain does not respond to common nonpharmacologic interventions and a short course of acetaminophen or NSAIDs, referral to a pain specialist may be of great benefit to the youth athlete.[22] In these cases, full consideration of the many biopsychosocial factors that may be influencing the pain is paramount.

Conclusion

Pain in youth athletes is not simply defined by injury. Rather, youth athletes' pain is influenced by many developmental, biomechanical, and psychosocial factors unique to the youth athlete population. These biopsychosocial factors affect the rate of injury in youth athletes and also determine the resulting pain experience. Identification and correction of these factors are critical to optimal pain management in youth athletes, which should not be limited to diagnosing and treating structural damage at the anatomic location of pain.

References

1. DiFiori JP, Benjamin HJ, Brenner JS, et al. Overuse injuries and burnout in youth sports: A position statement from the American Medical Society for Sports Medicine. *Br J Sports Med.* 2014;48(4):287–288. doi:10.1136/bjsports-2013-093299
2. Black LI, Terlizzi EP, Vahratian A. Organized sports participation among children aged 6–17 years: United States, 2020. *NCHS Data Brief.* 2022;(441):1–8.
3. The Aspen Institute Project Play. Youth sports facts: Participation rates. n.d. Accessed January 14, 2023. https://projectplay.org/youth-sports/facts/participation-rates
4. U.S. Department of Health and Human Services. National Youth Sports Strategy. 2019. Accessed September 12, 2022. https://health.gov/sites/default/files/2019-10/National_Youth_Sports_Strategy.pdf

5. Luke A, Lazaro RM, Bergeron MF, et al. Sports-related injuries in youth athletes: Is overscheduling a risk factor? *Clin J Sport Med.* 2011;21(4):307–314. doi:10.1097/JSM.0b013e3182218f71
6. Brenner JS; Council on Sports Medicine and Fitness. Sports specialization and intensive training in young athletes. *Pediatrics.* 2016;138(3):e20162148. doi:10.1542/peds.2016-2148
7. The Aspen Institute Project Play. State of play 2022: Participation trends. 2022. Accessed January 14, 2023. https://projectplay.org/state-of-play-2022/participation-trends
8. Kliethermes SA, Marshall SW, LaBella CR, et al. Defining a research agenda for youth sport specialisation in the USA: The AMSSM Youth Early Sport Specialization Summit. *Br J Sports Med.* 2021;55(3):135–143. doi:10.1136/bjsports-2020-102699
9. Janssen I, LeBlanc AG. Systematic review of the health benefits of physical activity and fitness in school-aged children and youth. *Int J Behav Nutr Phys Act.* 2010;7(1): Article 40. doi:10.1186/1479-5868-7-40
10. Bergeron MF, Mountjoy M, Armstrong N, et al. International Olympic Committee consensus statement on youth athletic development. *Br J Sports Med.* 2015;49(13):843–851. doi:10.1136/bjsports-2015-094962
11. Emery CA. Risk factors for injury in child and adolescent sport: A systematic review of the literature. *Clin J Sport Med.* 2003;13(4):256–268. doi:10.1097/00042752-200307000-00011
12. Watkins RA, De Borja C, Ramirez F. Common upper extremity injuries in pediatric athletes. *Curr Rev Musculoskelet Med.* 2022;15(6):465–473. doi:10.1007/s12178-022-09784-1
13. Jayanthi N, Schley S, Cumming SP, et al. Developmental training model for the sport specialized youth athlete: A dynamic strategy for individualizing load-response during maturation. *Sports Health.* 2022;14(1):142–153. doi:10.1177/19417381211056088
14. Mountjoy M, Armstrong N, Bizzini L, et al. IOC consensus statement on training the elite child athlete. *Clin J Sport Med.* 2008;18(2):122–123. doi:10.1097/JSM.0b013e318168e6ea
15. Select issues in pain management for the youth and adolescent athlete. *Med Sci Sports Exerc.* 2020;52(9):2037–2046. doi:10.1249/MSS.0000000000002333
16. Maillane-Vanegas S, Fatoye F, Luiz-de-Marco R, et al. Low occurrence of musculoskeletal symptoms in swimming? Musculoskeletal symptoms and sports participation in adolescents: Cross sectional study (ABCD–Growth Study). *Int J Environ Res Public Health.* 2022;19(6):3694. doi:10.3390/ijerph19063694
17. Rathleff MS, Roos EM, Olesen JL, Rasmussen S. High prevalence of daily and multi-site pain: A cross-sectional population-based study among 3000 Danish adolescents. *BMC Pediatr.* 2013;13(1): Article 191. doi:10.1186/1471-2431-13-191
18. Hulsegge G, van Oostrom SH, Picavet HSJ, et al. Musculoskeletal complaints among 11-year-old children and associated factors: The PIAMA Birth Cohort Study. *Am J Epidemiol.* 2011;174(8):877–884.
19. Malmborg JS, Olsson MC, Bergman S, Bremander A. Musculoskeletal pain and its association with maturity and sports performance in 14-year-old sport school students. *BMJ Open Sport Exerc Med.* 2018;4(1):e000395. doi:10.1136/bmjsem-2018-000395
20. Kamada M, Abe T, Kitayuguchi J, et al. Dose–response relationship between sports activity and musculoskeletal pain in adolescents. *Pain.* 2016;157(6):1339–1345. doi:10.1097/j.pain.0000000000000529
21. Caneiro JP, Alaiti RK, Fukusawa L, Hespanhol L, Brukner P, O'Sullivan PP. There is more to pain than tissue damage: Eight principles to guide care of acute non-traumatic pain in sport. *Br J Sports Med.* 2021;55(2):75–77. doi:10.1136/bjsports-2019-101705
22. Hainline B, Turner JA, Caneiro JP, Stewart M, Lorimer Moseley G. Pain in elite athletes—Neurophysiological, biomechanical and psychosocial considerations: A narrative review. *Br J Sports Med.* 2017;51(17):1259–1264. doi:10.1136/bjsports-2017-097890
23. Rosenbloom BN, Rabbitts JA, Palermo TM. A developmental perspective on the impact of chronic pain in late adolescence and early adulthood: Implications for assessment and intervention. *Pain.* 2017;158(9):1629–1632. doi:10.1097/j.pain.0000000000000888

24. Tripp DA, Stanish WD, Reardon G, Coady C, Sullivan MJL. Comparing postoperative pain experiences of the adolescent and adult athlete after anterior cruciate ligament surgery. *J Athl Train*. 2003;38(2):154–157.
25. Hainline B, Derman W, Vernec A, et al. International Olympic Committee consensus statement on pain management in elite athletes. *Br J Sports Med*. 2017;51(17):1245–1258. doi:10.1136/bjsports-2017-097884
26. International Association for the Study of Pain. Terminology. 2021. Accessed September 5, 2022. https://www.iasp-pain.org/resources/terminology
27. Igolnikov I, Gallagher RM, Hainline B. Sport-related injury and pain classification. *Handb Clin Neurol*. 2018;158:423–430. doi:10.1016/B978-0-444-63954-7.00039-2
28. Purcell L, Micheli L. Low back pain in young athletes. *Sports Health*. 2009;1(3):212–222. doi:10.1177/1941738109334212
29. Liu DV, Lin YC. Current evidence for acute pain management of musculoskeletal injuries and postoperative pain in pediatric and adolescent athletes. *Clin J Sport Med*. 2019;29(5):430–438. doi:10.1097/JSM.0000000000000690
30. Sciascia A, Kibler WB. The pediatric overhead athlete: What is the real problem? *Clin J Sport Med*. 2006;16(6):471–477. doi:10.1097/01.jsm.0000251182.44206.3b
31. Cassas KJ, Cassettari-Wayhs A. Childhood and adolescent sports-related overuse injuries. *Am Fam Physician*. 2006;73(6):1014–1022.
32. Hainline BW. Peripheral nerve injury in sports. *Continuum*. 2014;20(6):1605–1628. doi:10.1212/01.CON.0000458971.86389.9c
33. Rajan P, Bellare B. Referring doctors' perspectives about physiotherapy management for chronic musculoskeletal pain. *Int J Ther Rehabil Res*. 2013;2(1): Article 15. doi:10.5455/ijtrr.00000018
34. Engebretsen L, Steffen K, Bahr R, et al. The International Olympic Committee consensus statement on age determination in high-level young athletes. *Br J Sports Med*. 2010;44(7):476–484. doi:10.1136/bjsm.2010.073122
35. Costa e Silva L, Teles J, Fragoso I. Sports injuries patterns in children and adolescents according to their sports participation level, age and maturation. *BMC Sports Sci Med Rehabil*. 2022;14(1): Article 35. doi:10.1186/s13102-022-00431-3
36. Gould D. The professionalization of youth sports: It's time to act! *Clin J Sport Med*. 2009;19(2):81–82. doi:10.1097/JSM.0b013e31819edaff
37. Tenforde AS, Montalvo AM, Nelson VR, et al. Current sport organization guidelines from the AMSSM 2019 Youth Early Sport Specialization Research Summit. *Sports Health*. 2022;14(1):135–141. doi:10.1177/19417381211051383
38. Bonjour JP, Chevalley T. Pubertal timing, bone acquisition, and risk of fracture throughout life. *Endocr Rev*. 2014;35(5):820–847. doi:10.1210/er.2014-1007
39. Rice RP, Roach K, Kirk-Sanchez N, et al. Age and gender differences in injuries and risk factors in elite junior and professional tennis players. *Sports Health*. 2022;14(4):466–477. doi:10.1177/19417381211062834
40. Rommers N, Rössler R, Goossens L, et al. Risk of acute and overuse injuries in youth elite soccer players: Body size and growth matter. *J Sci Med Sport*. 2020;23(3):246–251. doi:10.1016/j.jsams.2019.10.001
41. van der Sluis A, Elferink-Gemser MT, Coelho-e-Silva MJ, Nijboer JA, Brink MS, Visscher C. Sport injuries aligned to peak height velocity in talented pubertal soccer players. *Int J Sports Med*. 2014;35(4):351–355. doi:10.1055/s-0033-1349874
42. Disantis AE, Martin R. Movement system dysfunction applied to youth and young adult throwing athletes. *Int J Sports Phys Ther*. 2022;17(1):90–103. doi:10.26603/001c.30022
43. U.S. Olympic and Paralympic Committee. American development model. n.d. Accessed January 14, 2023. https://www.teamusa.org:443/About-the-USOPC/Coaching-Education/American-Development-Model
44. Bahr R. Demise of the fittest: Are we destroying our biggest talents? *Br J Sports Med*. 2014;48(17):1265–1267. doi:10.1136/bjsports-2014-093832

45. McLellan M, Allahabadi S, Pandya NK. Youth sports specialization and its effect on professional, elite, and Olympic athlete performance, career longevity, and injury rates: A systematic review. *Orthop J Sports Med.* 2022;10(11):23259671221129590. doi:10.1177/23259671221129594
46. Bell DR, Post EG, Biese K, Bay C, Valovich McLeod T. Sport specialization and risk of overuse injuries: A systematic review with meta-analysis. *Pediatrics.* 2018;142(3):e20180657. doi:10.1542/peds.2018-0657
47. Dobscha M, Peterson C, Powers WS, Goetschius J. Youth sport specialization associated with poorer lower extremity function & pain as young adults. *Phys Sportsmed.* 2023;51(3):254–259. doi:10.1080/00913847.2022.2042167
48. Jayanthi N, Kleithermes S, Dugas L, Pasulka J, Iqbal S, LaBella C. Risk of injuries associated with sport specialization and intense training patterns in young athletes: A longitudinal clinical case–control study. *Orthop J Sports Med.* 2020;8(6):2325967120922764. doi:10.1177/2325967120922764
49. LaPrade RF, Agel J, Baker J, et al. AOSSM early sport specialization consensus statement. *Orthop J Sports Med.* 2016;4(4):2325967116644241. doi:10.1177/2325967116644241
50. Kliethermes SA, Nagle K, Côté J, et al. Impact of youth sports specialisation on career and task-specific athletic performance: A systematic review following the American Medical Society for Sports Medicine (AMSSM) Collaborative Research Network's 2019 Youth Early Sport Specialisation Summit. *Br J Sports Med.* 2020;54(4):221–230. doi:10.1136/bjsports-2019-101365
51. Putukian M. The psychological response to injury in student athletes: A narrative review with a focus on mental health. *Br J Sports Med.* 2016;50(3):145–148. doi:10.1136/bjsports-2015-095586
52. Arnold JT, Franklin EV, Baker ZG, Abowd M, Santana JA. Association between fear of pain and sports-related concussion recovery in a pediatric population. *Clin J Sport Med.* 2022;32(4):369–375. doi:10.1097/JSM.0000000000000951
53. Psychological issues related to illness and injury in athletes and the team physician: A consensus statement–2016 update. *Med Sci Sports Exerc.* 2017;49(5):1043–1054. doi:10.1249/MSS.0000000000001247
54. Haus BM, Micheli LJ. Back pain in the pediatric and adolescent athlete. *Clin Sports Med.* 2012;31(3):423–440. doi:10.1016/j.csm.2012.03.011
55. Moseley GL, Baranoff J, Rio E, Stewart M, Derman W, Hainline B. Nonpharmacological management of persistent pain in elite athletes: Rationale and recommendations. *Clin J Sport Med.* 2018;28(5):472–479. doi:10.1097/JSM.0000000000000601
56. Sweeney E, Rodenberg R, MacDonald J. Overuse knee pain in the pediatric and adolescent athlete. *Curr Sports Med Rep.* 2020;19(11):479–485. doi:10.1249/JSR.0000000000000773
57. DiFiori JP. Evaluation of overuse injuries in children and adolescents. *Curr Sports Med Rep.* 2010;9(6):372–378. doi:10.1249/JSR.0b013e3181fdba58
58. Soligard T, Schwellnus M, Alonso JM, et al. How much is too much? (Part 1) International Olympic Committee consensus statement on load in sport and risk of injury. *Br J Sports Med.* 2016;50(17):1030–1041. doi:10.1136/bjsports-2016-096581
59. Alaiti RK, Reis FJJ. Pain in athletes: Current knowledge and challenges. *Int J Sports Phys Ther.* 2022;17(6):981–983. doi:10.26603/001c.37675
60. Sullivan MJL, Bishop SR, Pivik J. The Pain Catastrophizing Scale: Development and validation. *Psychol Assess.* 1995;7:524–532. doi:10.1037/1040-3590.7.4.524
61. Jayanthi NA, Post EG, Laury TC, Fabricant PD. Health consequences of youth sport specialization. *J Athl Train.* 2019;54(10):1040–1049. doi:10.4085/1062-6050-380-18
62. Chambers G, Kraft J, Kingston K. The role of ultrasound as a problem-solving tool in the assessment of paediatric musculoskeletal injuries. *Ultrasound.* 2019;27(1):6–19. doi:10.1177/1742271X18759807
63. Gai N, Naser B, Hanley J, Peliowski A, Hayes J, Aoyama K. A practical guide to acute pain management in children. *J Anesth.* 2020;34(3):421–433. doi:10.1007/s00540-020-02767-x

64. Fischerauer SF, Talaei-Khoei M, Bexkens R, Ring DC, Oh LS, Vranceanu AM. What is the relationship of fear avoidance to physical function and pain intensity in injured athletes? *Clin Orthop Relat Res*. 2018;476(4):754–763. doi:10.1007/s11999.0000000000000085
65. Ardern CL, Taylor NF, Feller JA, Webster KE. A systematic review of the psychological factors associated with returning to sport following injury. *Br J Sports Med*. 2013;47(17):1120–1126. doi:10.1136/bjsports-2012-091203
66. Malina RM, Rogol AD, Cumming SP, Coelho e Silva MJ, Figueiredo AJ. Biological maturation of youth athletes: Assessment and implications. *Br J Sports Med*. 2015;49(13):852–859. doi:10.1136/bjsports-2015-094623
67. Schmid AB, Nee RJ, Coppieters MW. Reappraising entrapment neuropathies: Mechanisms, diagnosis and management. *Man Ther*. 2013;18(6):449–457. doi:10.1016/j.math.2013.07.006
68. Pedersen JR, Andreucci A, Thorlund JB, et al. Prevalence, frequency, adverse events, and reasons for analgesic use in youth athletes: A systematic review and meta-analysis of 44,381 athletes. *J Sci Med Sport*. 2022;25(10):810–819. doi:10.1016/j.jsams.2022.08.018
69. Patel DR, Villalobos A. Evaluation and management of knee pain in young athletes: Overuse injuries of the knee. *Transl Pediatr*. 2017;6(3):190–198. doi:10.21037/tp.2017.04.05

31

Managing Pain in Patients on Long-Term Opioids

Friedhelm Sandbrink

Introduction

Opioids are considered the most potent analgesic agents clinically available, but their use is associated with potential harm, and thus a careful analysis of benefits versus risks is required taking patient factors and preference into account. Opioid therapy has been associated with serious risks, including death due to respiratory depression and sedation from overdose and development of opioid use disorder (OUD). Patients with a history of substance use disorder (SUD) and other mental health disorders are particularly vulnerable, as are younger patients, the frail or elderly, and people with medical conditions such as sleep apnea or renal disease.

Although opioids have wide efficacy and utility in the treatment of acute and cancer-related pain, they should be used only in conjunction with non-opioids, including nonpharmacological approaches. Multimodal pain care is the standard for chronic non-cancer–related pain, when the risks of long-term opioid therapy are considerable and for many patients may outweigh the potential benefit.

This chapter addresses key clinical issues related to opioids, including benefits and risks of their use in the treatment of chronic pain. It also presents clinical strategies to optimize safety and effectiveness, including risk mitigation standards.

The Role of Opioids in the Treatment of Chronic Pain

The use of opioids for pain has undergone major shifts in the past century, and the ongoing transformation in pain care away from biomedical toward a biopsychosocial model is accompanied by a shift away from opioid therapy for pain and particularly for chronic pain.

Prior to the 1980s, opioids were rarely used outside of severe acute injury or post-surgical pain, primarily due to concerns about tolerance, physical dependence, and addiction. With the hospice and palliative care movement during the 1980s, the importance of pain assessment and relief from pain was recognized and increasingly emphasized also for non-cancer pain. Subsequently, an era of aggressive pain management with pressure on providers to lower pain scores with medication including opioids emerged, whereas reimbursements for nonpharmacological interdisciplinary pain rehabilitation dwindled. Prescribing of opioids increased steadily in the

United States in the following years, with a fourfold increase from 1999 to 2010, including greater use of long-acting opioid formulations, higher dosages, and for longer durations.[1,2] With the increase in opioid prescribing, the potential risks to patients became increasingly apparent. Franklin et al.[3] reported in 2005 the association of overdose deaths with escalating opioid dosages and long-acting opioid medication for the treatment of injured workers in the Washington State workers' compensation system. In 2007, overdose deaths from prescription opioids exceeded deaths from heroin and cocaine combined, and in 2008 opioid overdose became the leading cause of accidental death in the United States ahead of car accidents.[4] In addition to the considerable risk for patients taking their prescribed opioids for pain, opioid misuse and the nonmedical use by persons without a prescription became increasingly recognized as drivers of the overdose crisis in the United States.[5,6] Reports also documented transitioning from prescription medication misuse to heroin use.[7]

The Agency for Healthcare Research and Quality published a systematic review in 2014 that not only documented the association of long-term and higher dosage prescription opioid use with greater risk of opioid overdose and misuse but also found insufficient evidence to demonstrate long-term benefits of prescription opioid treatment for chronic pain.[8] Thereafter, the U.S. Food and Drug Administration (FDA) required new safety labeling including a boxed warning on the "risks of addiction, abuse, and misuse, which can lead to overdose and death" for extended-release and long-acting opioids in 2014[9] and for immediate-release opioids in 2016.[10]

In 2016, the Centers for Disease Control and Prevention (CDC) published the "Guideline for Prescribing Opioids for Chronic Pain (CDC-CPG)."[11] The CDC noted the limited evidence of long-term effectiveness of opioids for chronic pain in the context of risks to patients and to persons using prescription opioids that were not prescribed to them and also the need for a national guideline on pain management that could improve appropriate opioid prescribing while minimizing opioid-related risks. The guideline, intended primarily for primary care providers in outpatient care settings, included recommendations regarding specific limitations for dosage and duration of opioid therapy when starting or increasing opioid therapy.[11,12] The CDC intended its recommendations to be voluntary and in support of patient–provider communication. Nevertheless, regulatory agencies, insurers, health care delivery organizations, and others reacted by imposing restrictions on opioid prescribing. For example, approximately half of all U.S. states limit initial opioid prescriptions for acute pain to a 7-day supply or less,[13] and many states require the co-prescription of naloxone, such as for high-dosage opioid therapy, or co-prescription of benzodiazepines.[12,14,15]

Other organizations and agencies issued similar guidelines. The 2017 "Canadian Guideline for Opioid Therapy and Chronic Noncancer Pain" included similar guidance regarding limits on dose escalation for patients initiating opioid therapy.[16] It made the recommendation, however, to offer a trial of opioids to select patients with chronic non-cancer pain who have not found sufficient relief with optimized non-opioid therapy. In contrast, the 2017 jointly issued clinical practice guideline (CPG) by the U.S. Department of Veterans Affairs (VA) and the U.S. Department of Defense (DoD) for opioid therapy for chronic pain specifically recommended against initiation of long-term opioid therapy due to the perceived risk of overdose and OUD and in recognition of the challenges associated with opioid tapering when long-term opioid therapy has been established.[17,18] Other notable recommendations of the VA/DoD opioid CPG included attention to suicide risk and, if tapering of opioid therapy is to be considered due to risks outweighing benefits, individualized tapering based on patient needs and preferences. In its subsequent update in 2022, the VA/DoD CPG opioid therapy for chronic pain makes a general recommendation against initiation of opioid therapy and suggests the use of buprenorphine instead of full μ-agonist opioids in patients on daily opioid therapy.[19]

Opioid prescribing has decreased in the United States from its peak in 2012, and this decline accelerated after the CDC-CPG was published in 2016. Clinicians reacted with opioid dosage reductions or discontinuations in patients with chronic pain, sometimes abruptly, and in many patients without evidence of harm or misuse and frequently unilaterally without regard to patient preferences.[20,21] Subsequently, studies documented risks related to tapering and discontinuation of long-term opioid therapy, including illicit opioid use,[22] emergency department visits and opioid-related hospitalizations,[23] mental health crises and overdose events,[24] and increased risk of death from suicide or overdose.[25] Studies also documented challenges in patient access to opioids for pain care[26,27] and patient abandonment.[23] Thus, patient advocates, professional organizations,[28] and the FDA and CDC expressed caution against the "misapplication" of the CDC-CPG based on evidence of patient harm, including undertreatment of pain, reductions in quality of life and functioning, psychological distress, overdose, and suicidal ideation and behavior.[29,30]

In 2022, the CDC updated and expanded its guideline, particularly noting the patient-centered approach to decision-making, the goal to strengthening clinician–patient communication, and strengthened the warning against abrupt reduction or discontinuation of opioid therapy (unless there are indications of a life-threatening issue, such as warning signs of impending overdose). The 2022 CDC-CPG states that opioid therapy is associated with similar or decreased effectiveness for pain and function as non-opioid analgesic across several acute pain conditions of mild to moderate severity. If used for more severe acute pain, it recommends to keep the dosage as low as possible and the duration as short as possible and as needed for the severity of the pain condition. Regarding subacute or chronic pain, there is evidence for small improvements for pain and function in the short term (1–6 months) and attenuation of any benefit for pain after 3 months. It notes no clear evidence of long-term benefit from opioids for chronic pain in general—that is, for 12 months and beyond—with studies lacking to suggest which patients, if any, may potentially benefit.

A single randomized trial evaluated outcomes at 1 year for opioid medications compared with non-opioid medications in patients with chronic musculoskeletal pain (low back and joint conditions).[31] Treatment with opioids was not superior to non-opioid medications for improving pain-related function over 12 months, pain intensity was slightly but significantly better in the non-opioid group, and adverse medication-related symptoms were more common in the opioid group. The study had significant limitations, including no blinding of patients and use of tramadol (a weak opioid agonist) in the non-opioid group).[31]

Despite the marked reduction in opioid prescribing for pain since 2012, deaths due to overdoses continue to escalate in the United States, with an annual rate of more than 100,000 overdose deaths since 2021. Opioids are the most common cause of overdose deaths, and although the percentage related to deaths from commonly prescribed opioids has been largely steady since 2010, there was an increase in overdoses from heroin after 2010, followed by a dramatic increase in overdoses from fentanyl and its derivatives since 2013 that further worsened during the COVID-19 pandemic. Provisional data from the CDC's National Center for Health Statistics indicate that there were an estimated 107,573 drug overdose deaths during the 12-month period ending in December 2021, including an estimated 80,997 overdose deaths from opioids. Of those, 71,143 were related to synthetic opioids (other than methadone)—that is, fentanyl and its derivatives; 13,674 from natural and semi-synthetic opioids—that is, prescription opioids; and 9,763 related to heroin.[32]

Vulnerable Populations and Risk Factors for Long-Term Opioid Therapy

Opioid therapy is associated with increased risk for serious harms (including overdose and OUD), in addition to other short- and long-term risks. Risk factors include patient factors and medication or prescribing factors. In addition to opioid dosage and therapy duration, other risk factors include concurrent use of sedative hypnotics, use of extended-release/long-acting opioids, and the presence of substance use and other mental health disorder comorbidities.[12,19,33]

Patient factors include the following:

- Age: younger patients (overdose, OUD)
- Age: elderly (sedation, cognitive impairment, falls)
- Medical comorbidities: sleep apnea, metabolic impairment (renal/liver)
- Mental health comorbidities: anxiety, depression, bipolar disorder, post-traumatic stress disorder, psychotic disorder
- Substance use disorder (SUD): active or history of SUD, particularly OUD; family history of SUD
- Psychological factors: negative affect, catastrophizing
- Traumatic brain injury
- Suicidal risk, history of self-directed violence
- Tobacco use (opioid misuse)

The following are prescribing factors:

- Dosage: Higher opioid dose is associated with higher risk for opioid misuse, development of OUD, and overdose death.[2,34–44] There is no safe threshold without risk. Although risk increases at 50 morphine milligram equivalents (MME)/day and higher, many patients with opioid overdose are on dosages below this level.[34] Dosage increases to greater than 50 MME/day are unlikely to substantially improve pain control for most patients, whereas overdose risk increases with dosage.
- Duration: Longer duration of opioid therapy is associated with a higher risk of being treated for OUD and a higher risk of fatal opioid overdose.[40,42,45,46] Of note, longer duration is also associated with higher risk when tapering or discontinuing

opioids, including overdose and suicide deaths, mental health crisis, and emergency department visits and hospitalizations.[22–25]

- Opioid formulations: Long-acting/extended-release (LA/ER) opioids are associated with higher risk for opioid overdose and should not be used for acute pain, when initiating opioid therapy, or as needed medication.[9,12,19] Methadone has been associated with particular high risk for respiratory depression and overdose, whereas buprenorphine has a lower risk of respiratory depression and overdose death.[19]
- Co-prescribing: Benzodiazepine, other sedative medication such as zolpidem, and possibly gabapentinoids.[12,19,35,41] In one study, the risk for opioid overdose was highest for individuals on long-term opioid therapy who also received concurrent long-term benzodiazepine therapy, with some risk, albeit lower, also noted for zolpidem.[35]

Screening Tools to Assess Risk When Initiating Opioid Therapy

Several screening tools exist to predict the risk of aberrant use behaviors (or unhealthy opioid use) for patients being considered for opioid therapy, generally based on factors assessing the patient and family history of substance use, family history of SUD, and other psychiatric comorbidities. Although these tools may indicate risk for aberrant behavior, their use has not been shown to reduce overdose or the development of SUD.[47] Commonly used tools are the Opioid Risk Tool, a five-question screen[48]; the more recently developed and slightly easier to use Opioid Risk Tool for OUD[49]; the Screener and Opioid Assessment for Patients in Pain–Revised, a 24-item self-report[50]; and the Brief Risk Interview, a clinician-administered 12-item screen.[51]

The VA has mandated risk assessment by providers when initiating opioid therapy and data-based risk reviews for patients exposed to opioid therapy, and it employs a predictive analytic tool, the Stratification Tool for Opioid Risk Mitigation, that provides estimates for death from opioid overdose or suicide.[52] The Risk Index for Overdose or Serious Opioid-Induced Respiratory Depression, which estimates the likelihood of life-threatening respiratory depression or overdose among medical users of prescription opioids, has been validated in different patient populations.[36,53,54]

Adverse Effects of Opioid Therapy and Management

Common *acute physical side effects* are sedation and cognitive dysfunction, respiratory depression, nausea and vomiting, constipation, urinary retention, and pruritus.

Cognitive dysfunction and sedation are common, especially in the elderly, and are associated with increased risk of falls and motor vehicle accidents. Sedation generally precedes respiratory depression and should always result in consideration for opioid cessation or reduction.

Respiratory depression is the usual mechanism for opioid overdose. The risk for respiratory depression is higher when opioid therapy is initiated, increased in dosage, during opioid rotation, and when administered with other medications that reduce respiratory drive. Particularly vulnerable are opioid naive patients, the elderly and frail patients, and patients with sleep-disordered breathing from obstructive or central sleep apnea. Occasionally, an improvement in the underlying pain condition may remove the stimulating effect of pain on wakefulness and contribute to respiratory depression. The opioid antagonist naloxone can rapidly reverse respiratory depression and prevent overdose death, and overdose education and issuance of naloxone are considered an important risk mitigation strategy.[55–57]

Constipation is common and is due to direct action on opioid receptors of the intestinal wall resulting in hypomotility. It usually does not resolve without specific treatment and should be treated with both a stool softener and a bowel stimulant. The best strategy is often to reduce the opioid dosage. For some patients, transdermal instead of oral opioid administration reduces the gastrointestinal side effects.

Nausea, vomiting, and pruritus are common side effects that often improve with a switch to a different opioid medication.

Side effects of *long-term opioid use* include effects on the endocrine and immune systems and hyperalgesia.

The most important hormonal effects are androgen deficiency and bone loss.[58] In men, low testosterone levels with long-term opioid use may cause low libido, erectile dysfunction, fatigue, and depressive symptoms.[59] Routine testing and treatment have been recommended.[60,61] Osteopenia and osteoporosis contribute to increased risk of fractures in the elderly, who may also be at higher risk of falls when taking opioids.[62]

Opioids have been associated with immunosuppressive effects, possibly linking opioid use and postoperative infection and carcinogenesis. Although the clinical relevance is not clear, limiting the use of opioids in acute and chronic pain treatment settings is an additional consideration.[63]

Physical dependence is a physiologic adaptation to the continuous presence of a drug that produces symptoms of withdrawal when the drug effect significantly diminishes or stops,[64] due to rapid dose reduction or discontinuation, or from administration of an antagonist. Physical dependence may develop within days (2–10 days) of opioid therapy and is an expected outcome of long-term around-the-clock opioid exposure.

Opioid withdrawal manifests with autonomic changes, diarrhea, piloerection, sweating, and mydriasis, and increases in heart rate and blood pressure. Irritability, anxiety, and sleeplessness contribute to patient discomfort. Withdrawal symptoms include hyperalgesia (increased pain sensation) and anhedonia (inability to feel pleasure). Although withdrawal symptoms comprise one of the *Diagnostic and Statistical Manual of Mental Disorders*, fifth edition (DSM-5), diagnostic criteria for OUD, they should not be considered for individuals taking opioid medication as prescribed for pain.[65] Seeking opioid medication for pain relief in patients with chronic pain may be difficult to differentiate from opioid craving in OUD.

Tolerance is indicated by the need for increasing doses of a medication to achieve the initial effects of the drug[64] and, at steady dosage, results in diminishing analgesic effect and/or reduced side effects over time, such as respiratory depression, sedation, or nausea. Tolerance to the analgesic effects of opioids administered on a continuous basis occurs over a period of several days. A progressive gradual decline of the analgesic effects from opioids, over months to years, occurs in most patients.[66] Although tolerance is one of the DSM-5 diagnostic criteria for OUD, it should not be considered for individuals taking opioids as prescribed for pain.[65]

Hyperalgesia (increased sensitivity to pain) is due to sensitization to nociceptive stimuli resulting in lowered pain threshold and/or decreased tolerance to pain, mediated by aberrant glial activation.[67] Contributing factors are the long-term presence of pain and physiological and psychological stressors such as sleep deprivation.[68] Central sensitization syndromes with hyperalgesia include fibromyalgia.[69] Opioid use may contribute to central sensitization and hyperalgesia (opioid-induced hyperalgesia [OIH]). Although the relevance of OIH for patients on opioid therapy and contributing factors are not well understood,[70] it is increasingly appreciated that opioids are generally not recommended in patients with central sensitization syndromes such as fibromyalgia.[71]

Estimates for OUD in patients taking opioids for chronic pain vary greatly. In studies of carefully assessed OUD, estimates are 8–12%.[72] Thus, the risk is likely somewhat higher than the prevalence of illicit SUDs in the U.S. population in general (6.6%).[73] Factors contributing to risk for OUD from opioids include young age, psychiatric comorbidity, and family history of SUD.[74–76] It is imperative to not abandon patients who develop OUD while on prescribed opioid therapy; rather, they should be provided urgent access to evidence-based, usually pharmacological treatment for OUD, and other therapies should be optimized for effective treatment of the pain condition. Transitioning to evidence-based medication therapy for OUD may be facilitated by using a "microdosing" approach to buprenorphine therapy for OUD.[77,78] Buprenorphine therapy for OUD, if prescribed in patients with concurring pain conditions, should be given in divided doses, usually three or four times per day, for better analgesic efficacy.[79]

Risk Mitigation Strategies When Prescribing Opioid Therapy Long Term

The "CDC Clinical Practice Guideline for Prescribing Opioids for Pain," published in 2022, provides a guiding framework for the responsible prescribing of opioids.[12] The recommendations are listed in Box 31.1. Based on this and other guidelines,[16,19] the following strategies are suggested:

- In general, nonpharmacologic therapy and non-opioid pharmacologic therapy are preferred for chronic pain. *If used, opioids are usually combined with other modalities* to reduce reliance on opioid medication and for improved outcome related to pain and function.
- Opioid therapy should only be considered *if benefits for both pain and function are anticipated to outweigh risks* to the patient. In general, any benefit from opioids for chronic pain should be expected to be only transient (not beyond 3–6 months). Thus, an endpoint in the near future supports temporary use (e.g., planned surgery; to allow someone to remain employed, while other pain measures are being instituted).
- *Risk evaluation includes assessment of medical and mental health factors* as outlined above. It is advisable to document a careful assessment of patient risk, including psychological factors, and screening tools as outlined above may facilitate this task.

Box 31.1 Centers for Disease Control and Prevention Clinical Practice Guideline for Prescribing Opioids for Pain, 2022

Recommendations for prescribing opioids for outpatients with pain, excluding pain management related to sickle cell disease, cancer-related pain treatment, palliative care, and end-of-life care.

Determining Whether or Not to Initiate Opioids for Pain

1. Nonopioid therapies are at least as effective as opioids for many common types of acute pain. Clinicians should maximize use of nonpharmacologic and nonopioid pharmacologic therapies as appropriate for the specific condition and patient and only consider opioid therapy for acute pain if benefits are anticipated to outweigh risks to the patient. Before prescribing opioid therapy for acute pain, clinicians should discuss with patients the realistic benefits and known risks of opioid therapy (B/3).
2. Nonopioid therapies are preferred for subacute and chronic pain. Clinicians should maximize use of nonpharmacologic and nonopioid pharmacologic therapies as appropriate for the specific condition and patient and only consider initiating opioid therapy if expected benefits for pain and function are anticipated to outweigh risks to the patient. Before starting opioid therapy for subacute or chronic pain, clinicians should discuss with patients the realistic benefits and known risks of opioid therapy, should work with patients to establish treatment goals for pain and function, and should consider how opioid therapy will be discontinued if benefits do not outweigh risks (A/2).

Selecting Opioids and Determining Opioid Dosages

3. When starting opioid therapy for acute, subacute, or chronic pain, clinicians should prescribe immediate-release opioids instead of extended-release and long-acting (ER/LA) opioids (A/4).
4. When opioids are initiated for opioid-naïve patients with acute, subacute, or chronic pain, clinicians should prescribe the lowest effective dosage. If opioids are continued for subacute or chronic pain, clinicians should use caution when prescribing opioids at any dosage, should carefully evaluate individual benefits and risks when considering increasing dosage, and should avoid increasing dosage above levels likely to yield diminishing returns in benefits relative to risks to patients (A/3).
5. For patients already receiving opioid therapy, clinicians should carefully weigh benefits and risks and exercise care when changing opioid dosage. If benefits outweigh risks of continued opioid therapy, clinicians should work closely with patients to optimize nonopioid therapies while continuing opioid therapy. If benefits do not outweigh risks of continued opioid therapy, clinicians should optimize other therapies and work closely with patients to gradually taper to lower dosages or, if warranted based on the individual circumstances of the patient, appropriately taper and discontinue opioids. Unless there are indications of a life-threatening issue such as warning signs of

impending overdose (e.g., confusion, sedation, or slurred speech), opioid therapy should not be discontinued abruptly, and clinicians should not rapidly reduce opioid dosages from higher dosages (B/4).

Deciding Duration of Initial Opioid Prescription and Conducting Follow-Up

6. When opioids are needed for acute pain, clinicians should prescribe no greater quantity than needed for the expected duration of pain severe enough to require opioids (A/4).
7. Clinicians should evaluate benefits and risks with patients within 1–4 weeks of starting opioid therapy for subacute or chronic pain or of dosage escalation. Clinicians should regularly reevaluate benefits and risks of continued opioid therapy with patients (A/4).

Assessing Risk and Addressing Potential Harms of Opioid Use

8. Before starting and periodically during continuation of opioid therapy, clinicians should evaluate risk for opioid-related harms and discuss risk with patients. Clinicians should work with patients to incorporate into the management plan strategies to mitigate risk, including offering naloxone (A/4).
9. When prescribing initial opioid therapy for acute, subacute, or chronic pain, and periodically during opioid therapy for chronic pain, clinicians should review the patient's history of controlled substance prescriptions using state prescription drug monitoring program (PDMP) data to determine whether the patient is receiving opioid dosages or combinations that put the patient at high risk for overdose (B/4).
10. When prescribing opioids for subacute or chronic pain, clinicians should consider the benefits and risks of toxicology testing to assess for prescribed medications as well as other prescribed and nonprescribed controlled substances (B/4).
11. Clinicians should use particular caution when prescribing opioid pain medication and benzodiazepines concurrently and consider whether benefits outweigh risks of concurrent prescribing of opioids and other central nervous system depressants (B/3).
12. Clinicians should offer or arrange treatment with evidence-based medications to treat patients with opioid use disorder. Detoxification on its own, without medications for opioid use disorder, is not recommended for opioid use disorder because of increased risks for resuming drug use, overdose, and overdose death (A/1).

Recommendation Categories

- Category A: Applies to all persons; most patients should receive the recommended course of action.
- Category B: Individual decision making needed; different choices will be appropriate for different patients. Clinicians help patients arrive at a decision consistent with patient values and preferences and specific clinical situations.

Evidence Types

- Type 1: Randomized clinical trials or overwhelming evidence from observational studies.
- Type 2: Randomized clinical trials with important limitations, or exceptionally strong evidence from observational studies.
- Type 3: Observational studies or randomized clinical trials with notable limitations.
- Type 4: Clinical experience and observations, observational studies with important limitations, or randomized clinical trials with several major limitations.

- Before starting opioid therapy for chronic pain, the clinician should *establish treatment goals* with the patients, including realistic goals for pain and function. Improvement in function is the primary goal, even if there are no changes in pain severity.
- *Initiation of opioid therapy should be considered a trial*, and it should be established with the patient that opioid therapy will be discontinued if benefits are not apparent.
- *Patient education* must include the serious adverse effects of respiratory depression and potentially fatal overdose, risk of OUD, and the expected effects of physical dependence and tolerance. The patient must be advised about the common adverse effects of constipation, nausea and vomiting, pruritus, and the risk for sedation and cognitive impairment, such as when driving or operating heavy machinery.
- Many practitioners make use of an *opioid treatment agreement* to facilitate and document the conversation about the risks and required actions by the patient, such as safeguarding the medication. In VA and DoD health care settings, a *written informed consent* is universally used for patients on long-term opioid therapy for chronic pain (with exceptions for cancer pain and in hospice settings). Informed consent, with its emphasis on patient education (including risks and benefits of opioid therapy, alternatives to opioid medication, and opioid tapering), facilitates documentation of safety considerations and risk mitigation expectations in a patient-centered format.[80] The VA/DoD patient education guide is freely available.[81]
- *Safety practices* to discuss with the patient may include opioid prescribing from a single source, taking opioids only as prescribed, refill policy, urine testing, avoidance of other psychoactive drugs or substances (including alcohol), safeguarding the medication, and not sharing with anyone.[82–84]
- *Urine drug testing* (UDT) is recommended prior to initiating of opioid therapy, at least annually for patients on long-term opioid therapy, and more often according to risk.[12,19] The testing interval should be random. UDT includes urine drug screening and confirmatory testing, if clinically indicated. Screening detects the presence of naturally occurring opioids (e.g., morphine and codeine) rather reliably, with lower sensitivity for semi-synthetic opioids (e.g., oxycodone). Drug screening for synthetic opioids such as fentanyl or buprenorphine requires specific assays for detection. UDT results should be used in a patient-centered approach,

with unexpected findings triggering a conversation with the patient, leading to enhanced safety measures if indicated, but not to patient abandonment.

- Querying the state *prescription drug monitoring program* (PDMP) database is a standard safety practice when initiating and renewing opioid therapy. State regulations vary greatly, with some states mandating PDMP queries for every controlled substance prescription event. As with UDT, an unexpected result of a PDMP query should be discussed with the patient and not result in interruption of care.
- *Opioid therapy should not be used concurrently with benzodiazepines* due to the higher risk of respiratory depression and overdose death. Similarly, concurrent use of other sedating medication such as zolpidem should be avoided.
- In addition to overdose education, the *prescribing of the opioid antagonist naloxone* is considered an important risk mitigation strategy for patients on opioid therapy, especially in higher risk situations, such as high dose (e.g., ≥50 MME/day), benzodiazepine co-prescribing, history of OUD or illicit drug use, or after recent opioid discontinuations. A family member should be educated on the signs of opioid overdose and the administration of naloxone nasal spray. Training videos are widely available. The FDA recently approved a higher dosed nasal spray formulation to be considered in patients with high risk, such as illicit opioid or stimulant use that are commonly adulterated with fentanyl.
- *Initiation of opioid therapy occurs with immediate release.* LA/ER medication should never be used for initiation of opioid therapy, for acute pain, or for as needed indications.
- *Opioid dosage should be kept at the lowest effective dose.* The update of the 2022 CDC opioid guideline does not include specific dose limits within the formal recommendations; it continues to suggest that clinicians use extra caution, including increased frequency of follow-up, for patients on opioid dosages greater than 50 mg MME/day, and generally should avoid dosage increase to greater than 90 MME/day without careful justification based on diagnosis and on individualized assessment of benefits and risks.
- *Follow-up evaluation should be timely*, usually within 1–4 weeks after dosage adjustment.
- During long-term opioid therapy, it is important to *regularly re-evaluate the opioid therapy*, usually at an interval of 3 months or less, regarding indication, risks, and benefits, including assessment of aberrant behavior and patient preference.
- For patients on long-term opioid therapy who require daily opioids, the use of *buprenorphine* as a partial agonist with lesser risk for respiratory depression than full μ-agonist opioids is an emerging practice and is suggested by recent guidelines.[19,26] It may be particularly valuable in patients with risk factors for OUD or respiratory depression due to medical comorbidities.
- If opioid therapy is not considered successful in improving function or if risks outweigh benefit for other reasons, or based on patient preference, *opioid tapering* should be considered. It is imperative that such tapering optimizes patient engagement and collaboration and that it is based on individualized assessment of risk and tolerability. In general, more gradual tapers (e.g., ≤10% per month), with

pauses as needed, are better tolerated than more rapid tapers. Sudden interruption of opioid prescribing should be avoided.

- For patients with evidence of aberrant behavior, including opioid prescription misuse or illicit drug use, clinicians should carefully assess for the presence of *OUD* and offer or arrange treatment with evidence-based medications for OUD, if indicated. Buprenorphine may be used to treat both OUD and pain in divided doses (three or four times per day). Transition to a buprenorphine product from high-dose full μ-agonist opioid therapy may be facilitated by using a "microdosing" approach, as outlined above.[77,78] For patients on long-term buprenorphine therapy for OUD and undergoing surgery, a multimodal analgesic strategy is suggested, including continuation of buprenorphine (with temporary dosage reduction if high dose) with added full μ-agonist opioid medication, if needed, in conjunction with non-opioid analgesics and regional anesthesia.[79]

References

1. Edlund MJ, Martin BC, Russo JE, DeVries A, Braden JB, Sullivan MD. The role of opioid prescription in incident opioid abuse and dependence among individuals with chronic noncancer pain: The role of opioid prescription. *Clin J Pain*. 2014;30:557–564.
2. Bohnert ASB, Valenstein M, Bair MJ, et al. Association between opioid prescribing patterns and opioid overdose-related deaths. *JAMA*. 2011;305:1315–1321.
3. Franklin GM, Mai J, Wickizer T, et al. Opioid dosing trends and mortality in Washington State workers' compensation, 1996–2002. *Am J Ind Med*. 2005;48(2):91–99
4. Paulozzi LJ, Jones C, Mack K, Rudd R. Vital signs: Overdoses of prescription opioid pain relievers—United States, 1999–2008. *MMWR Morb Mortal Wkly Rep*. 2011;60:1487–1492.
5. Centers for Disease Control and Prevention, National Center for Injury Prevention and Control. U.S. opioid dispensing rate maps. 2021. https://www.cdc.gov/drugoverdose/rxrate-maps/index.html
6. Rudd RA, Aleshire N, Zibbell JE, Gladden RM. Increases in drug and opioid overdose deaths—United States, 2000–2014. *MMWR Morb Mortal Wkly Rep*. 2016;64(50–51):1378–1382.
7. Guy GP Jr, Zhang K, Bohm MK, et al. Vital signs: Changes in opioid prescribing in the United States, 2006–2015. *MMWR Morb Mortal Wkly Rep*. 2017;66(26):697–704.
8. Chou R, Deyo R, Devine B, et al. The effectiveness and risks of long-term opioid treatment of chronic pain. Evidence report/technology assessment No. 218. AHRQ Publication No. 14-E005-EF. Agency for Healthcare Research and Quality; 2014.
9. U.S. Food and Drug Administration. Letter to application holders: ER/LA opioid analgesic class labeling changes and postmarket requirements, 2014. chrome-extension://efaidnbmnnnibpcajpcglclefindmkaj/https://www.fda.gov/media/86875/download
10. U.S. Food and Drug Administration. FDA announces enhanced warnings for immediate-release opioid pain medications related to risks of misuse, abuse, addiction, overdose and death. 2016. https://www.fda.gov/news-events/press-announcements/fda-announces-enhanced-warnings-immediate-release-opioid-pain-medications-related-risks-misuse-abuse
11. Dowell D, Haegerich TM, Chou R. CDC guideline for prescribing opioids for chronic pain—United States, 2016. *MMWR Recomm Rep*. 2016;65(RR-1):1–49.
12. Dowell D, Ragan KR, Jones CM, Baldwin GT, Chou R. CDC clinical practice guideline for prescribing opioids for pain—United States, 2022. *MMWR Recomm Rep*. 2022;71(RR-3):1–95.

13. National Conference of State Legislatures. Prescribing policies: States confront opioid overdose epidemic. 2019. https://www.ncsl.org/research/health/prescribing-policies-states-confront-opioid-overdose-epidemic.aspx
14. Bohnert ASB, Guy GP Jr, Losby JL. Opioid prescribing in the United States before and after the Centers for Disease Control and Prevention's 2016 opioid guideline. *Ann Intern Med.* 2018;169:367–375.
15. Salvatore PP, Guy GP Jr, Mikosz CA. Changes in opioid dispensing by medical specialties after the release of the 2016 CDC guideline for prescribing opioids for chronic pain. *Pain Med.* 2022;23(11):1908–1914.
16. Busse JW, Craigie S, Juurlink DN, et al. Guideline for opioid therapy and chronic noncancer pain. *CMAJ.* 2017;189(18):E659–E666.
17. U.S. Department of Defense/U.S. Department of Veterans Affairs. VA/DoD clinical practice guideline for opioid therapy for chronic pain. 2017. Accessed February 13, 2023. https://www.healthquality.va.gov/guidelines/Pain/cot/VADoDOTCPG022717.pdf
18. Rosenberg JM, Bilka BM, Wilson SM, Spevak C. Opioid therapy for chronic pain: Overview of the 2017 US Department of Veterans Affairs and US Department of Defense clinical practice guideline. *Pain Med.* 2018;19(5):928–941.
19. U.S. Department of Defense/U.S. Department of Veterans Affairs. VA/DoD clinical practice guideline for management of opioid therapy for chronic pain. 2022. Accessed February 13, 2023. https://www.healthquality.va.gov/guidelines/Pain/cot
20. Larochelle MR, Lodi S, Yan S, Clothier BA, Goldsmith ES, Bohnert ASB. Comparative effectiveness of opioid tapering or abrupt discontinuation vs no dosage change for opioid overdose or suicide for patients receiving stable long-term opioid therapy. *JAMA Netw Open.* 2022;5(8):e2226523.
21. Nataraj N, Strahan AE, Guy GP Jr, Losby JL, Dowell D. Dose tapering, increases, and discontinuity among patients on long-term high-dose opioid therapy in the United States, 2017–2019. *Drug Alcohol Depend.* 2022;234:109392.
22. Coffin PO, Rowe C, Oman N, et al. Illicit opioid use following changes in opioids prescribed for chronic non-cancer pain. *PLoS One.* 2020;15(5):e0232538.
23. Mark TL, Parish W. Opioid medication discontinuation and risk of adverse opioid-related health care events. *J Subst Abuse Treat.* 2019;103:58–63.
24. Agnoli A, Xing G, Tancredi DJ, Magnan E, Jerant A, Fenton JJ. Association of dose tapering with overdose or mental health crisis among patients prescribed long-term opioids. *JAMA.* 2021;326(5):411–419.
25. Oliva EM, Bowe T, Manhapra A, et al. Associations between stopping prescriptions for opioids, length of opioid treatment, and overdose or suicide deaths in US veterans: Observational evaluation. *BMJ.* 2020;368:m283.
26. U.S. Department of Health and Human Services. Pain management best practices interagency task force report: Updates, gaps, inconsistencies, and recommendations. 2019. https://www.hhs.gov/sites/default/files/pmtf-final-report-2019-05-23.pdf
27. Demidenko MI, Dobscha SK, Morasco BJ, Meath THA, Ilgen MA, Lovejoy TI. Suicidal ideation and suicidal self-directed violence following clinician-initiated prescription opioid discontinuation among long-term opioid users. *Gen Hosp Psychiatry.* 2017;47:29–35.
28. Kroenke K, Alford DP, Argoff C, et al. Challenges with implementing the Centers for Disease Control and Prevention opioid guideline: A consensus panel report. *Pain Med.* 2019;20:724–735.
29. McDowell D, Haegerich T, Chou R. No shortcuts to safer opioid prescribing. *N Engl J Med.* 2019;380:2285–2287.
30. U.S. Food and Drug Administration. FDA identifies harm reported from sudden discontinuation of opioid pain medicines and requires label changes to guide prescribers on gradual, individualized tapering. 2019. https://www.fda.gov/drugs/drug-safety-and-availability/fda-identifies-harm-reported-sudden-discontinuation-opioid-pain-medicines-and-requires-label-changes. Accessed February 13, 2023.

31. Krebs EE, Gravely A, Nugent S, et al. Effect of opioid vs nonopioid medications on pain-related function in patients with chronic back pain or hip or knee osteoarthritis pain: The SPACE randomized clinical trial. *JAMA*. 2018;319(9):872–882.
32. Centers for Disease Control and Prevention, National Center for Health Statistics. National Vital Statistics System: Provisional drug overdose death counts. 2023. Accessed February 13, 2023. https://www.cdc.gov/nchs/nvss/vsrr/drug-overdose-data.htm.
33. Park TW, Lin LA, Hosanagar A, Kogowski A, Paige K, Bohnert AS. Understanding risk factors for opioid overdose in clinical populations to inform treatment and policy. *J Addict Med*. 2016;10(6):369–381.
34. Bohnert AS, Logan JE, Ganoczy D, Dowell D. A detailed exploration into the association of prescribed opioid dosage and overdose deaths among patients with chronic pain. *Med Care*. 2016;54(5):435–441.
35. Turner BJ, Liang Y. Drug overdose in a retrospective cohort with non-cancer pain treated with opioids, antidepressants, and/or sedative–hypnotics: Interactions with mental health disorders. *J Gen Intern Med*. 2015;30(8):1081–1096.
36. Zedler B, Xie L, Wang L, et al. Risk factors for serious prescription opioid-related toxicity or overdose among Veterans Health Administration patients. *Pain Med*. 2014;15(11):1911–1929.
37. Dunn KM, Saunders KW, Rutter CM, et al. Opioid prescriptions for chronic pain and overdose: A cohort study. *Ann Intern Med*. 2010;152(2):85–92.
38. Ilgen MA, Bohnert AS, Ganoczy D, Bair MJ, McCarthy JF, Blow FC. Opioid dose and risk of suicide. *Pain*. 2016;157(5):1079–1084.
39. Busse JW, Wang L, Kamaleldin M, et al. Opioids for chronic noncancer pain: A systematic review and meta-analysis. *JAMA*. 2018;320(23):2448–2460.
40. Garg RK, Fulton-Kehoe D, Franklin GM. Patterns of opioid use and risk of opioid overdose death among Medicaid patients. *Med Care*. 2017;55(7):661–668.
41. Liang Y, Goros MW, Turner BJ. Drug overdose: Differing risk models for women and men among opioid users with non-cancer pain. *Pain Med*. 2016;17(12):2268–2279.
42. Papadomanolakis-Pakis N, Moore KM, Peng Y, Gomes T. Prescription opioid characteristics at initiation for non-cancer pain and risk of treated opioid use disorder: A population-based study. *Drug Alcohol Depend*. 2021;221:108601.
43. Yennurajalingam S, Arthur J, Reddy S, et al. Frequency of and factors associated with nonmedical opioid use behavior among patients with cancer receiving opioids for cancer pain. *JAMA Oncol*. 2021;7(3):404–411.
44. Hayes CJ, Krebs EE, Hudson T, Brown J, Li C, Martin BC. Impact of opioid dose escalation on the development of substance use disorders, accidents, self-inflicted injuries, opioid overdoses and alcohol and non-opioid drug-related overdoses: A retrospective cohort study. *Addiction*. 2020;115(6):1098–112.
45. Huffman KL, Shella ER, Sweis G, Griffith SD, Scheman J, Covington EC. Nonopioid substance use disorders and opioid dose predict therapeutic opioid addiction. *J Pain*. 2015;16(2):126–134.
46. Boscarino JA, Rukstalis M, Hoffman SN, et al. Risk factors for drug dependence among out-patients on opioid therapy in a large US health-care system. *Addiction*. 2010;105(10):1776–1782.
47. Keall R, Keall P, Kiani C, Luckett T, McNeill R, Lovell M. A systematic review of assessment approaches to predict opioid misuse in people with cancer. *Support Care Cancer*. 2022;30(7):5645–5658.
48. Webster LR, Webster RM. Predicting aberrant behaviors in opioid-treated patients: Preliminary validation of the Opioid Risk Tool. *Pain Med*. 2005;6(6):432–442.
49. Cheatle MD, Compton PA, Dhingra L, Wasser TE, O'Brien CP. Development of the revised Opioid Risk Tool to predict opioid use disorder in patients with chronic nonmalignant pain. *J Pain*. 2019;20(7):842–851.
50. Butler SF, Budman SH, Fernandez KC, Fanciullo GJ, Jamison RN. Cross-validation of a screener to predict opioid misuse in chronic pain patients (SOAPP-R). *J Addict Med*. 2009;3(2):66–73.

51. Jones T, Lookatch S, Grant P, McIntyre J, Moore T. Further validation of an opioid risk assessment tool: The Brief Risk Interview. *J Opioid Manag.* 2014;10:353–364.
52. Oliva EM, Bowe T, Tavakoli S, et al. Development and applications of the Veterans Health Administration's Stratification Tool for Opioid Risk Mitigation (STORM) to improve opioid safety and prevent overdose and suicide. *Psychol Serv.* 2017;14(1):34–49.
53. Zedler BK, Saunders WB, Joyce AR, Vick CC, Murrelle EL. Validation of a screening risk index for serious prescription opioid-induced respiratory depression or overdose in a US commercial health plan claims database. *Pain Med.* 2018;19(1):68–78.
54. Metcalfe L, Murrelle EL, Vu L, et al. Independent validation in a large privately insured population of the Risk Index for Serious Prescription Opioid-Induced Respiratory Depression or Overdose. *Pain Med.* 2020;21(10):2219–2228.
55. Jones CM, Compton W, Vythilingam M, Giroir B. Naloxone co-prescribing to patients receiving prescription opioids in the Medicare Part D Program, United States, 2016–2017. *JAMA.* 2019;322(5):462–464.
56. Watson A, Guay K, Ribis D. Assessing the impact of clinical pharmacists on naloxone co-prescribing in the primary care setting. *Am J Health Syst Pharm.* 2020;77(7):568–573.
57. Oliva EM, Richardson J, Harvey MA, Bellino P. Saving lives: The Veterans Health Administration (VHA) Rapid Naloxone Initiative. *Jt Comm J Qual Patient Saf.* 2021;47(8):469–480.
58. Brennan M. The effect of opioid therapy on endocrine function, *Am J Med.* 2013;126(3):S12–S18.
59. Smith HS, Elliott JA. Opioid-induced androgen deficiency (OPIAD). *Pain Physician.* 2012;15(3 Suppl):ES145–ES156.
60. De Maddalena C, Bellini M, Berra M, et al. Opioid-induced hypogonadism: Why and how to treat it. *Pain Physician.* 2012;15(Suppl 3):ES111–ES118.
61. Blick G, Khera M, Bhattacharya RK, et al. Testosterone replacement therapy outcomes among opioid users: The Testim Registry in the United States (TRiUS). *Pain Med.* 2012;13(5):688–698.
62. Miller M, Sturmer T, Azrael D, et al. Opioid analgesics and the risk of fractures in older adults with arthritis. *J Am Geriatr Soc.* 2011;59(3):430–438.
63. Kosciuczuk U, Knapp P, Lotowska-Cwiklewska AM. Opioid-induced immunosuppression and carcinogenesis promotion theories create the newest trend in acute and chronic pain pharmacotherapy. *Clinics.* 2020;75:e1554.
64. Savage SR, Joranson DE, Covington EC, et al. Definitions related to the medical use of opioids: Evolution towards universal agreement. *J Pain Symptom Manage.* 2003;26(1):655–667
65. American Psychiatric Association. About DSM-5-TR. Updated 2022. Accessed February 13, 2023. https://www.psychiatry.org/psychiatrists/practice/dsm/about-dsm
66. Roth SH, Fleischmann RM, Burch FX, et al. Around-the-clock, controlled-release oxycodone therapy for osteoarthritis-related pain: Placebo-controlled trial and long-term evaluation. *Arch Intern Med.* 2000;27(160):853–860.
67. Nijs J, Loggia ML, Polli A, et al. Sleep disturbances and severe stress as glial activators: Key targets for treating central sensitization in chronic pain patients? *Expert Opin Ther Targets.* 2017;21(8):817–826.
68. Schuh-Hofer S, Wodarski R, Pfau DB, et al. One night of total sleep deprivation promotes a state of generalized hyperalgesia: A surrogate pain model to study the relationship of insomnia and pain. *Pain.* 2013;154(9):1613–1621.
69. Sluka KA, Clauw DJ. Neurobiology of fibromyalgia and chronic widespread pain. *Neuroscience.* 2016;338:114–129.
70. Sampaio-Cunha TJ, Martins I. Knowing the enemy is halfway towards victory: A scoping review on opioid-induced hyperalgesia. J Clin Med. 2022;11(20):6161.
71. Goldenberg DL, Clauw DJ, Palmer RE, Clair AG. Opioid use in fibromyalgia: A cautionary tale. *Mayo Clin Proc.* 2016;91(5):640–648.

72. Boscarino JA, Hoffman SN, Han JJ. Opioid-use disorder among patients on long-term opioid therapy: Impact of final DSM-5 diagnostic criteria on prevalence and correlates. *Subst Abuse Rehabil.* 2015;6:83–91.
73. Substance Abuse and Mental Health Services Administration. Key substance use and mental health indicators in the United States: Results from the 2020 National Survey on Drug Use and Health. HHS Publication No. PEP21-07-01-003, NSDUH Series H-56. Center for Behavioral Health Statistics and Quality, Substance Abuse and Mental Health Services Administration; 2021. https://www.samhsa.gov/data/sites/default/files/reports/rpt35325/NSDUHFFRPDFWHTMLFiles2020/2020NSDUHFFR1PDFW102121.pdf
74. Turk D, Swanson K, Gatchel R. Predicting opioid misuse by chronic pain patients: A systematic review and literature synthesis. *Clin J Pain.* 2008;24:497–508.
75. Chou R, Fanciullo G, Fine P, et al. Opioids for chronic noncancer pain: Prediction and identification of aberrant drug-related behaviors: A review of the evidence for an American Pain Society and American Academy of Pain Medicine clinical practice guideline. *J Pain.* 2009;10:131–146.
76. Seghal N, Manchikanti L, Smith H. Prescription opioid abuse in chronic pain: A review of opioid abuse predictors and strategies to curb opioid abuse. *Pain Physician.* 2012;15:ES67–ES92.
77. Ahmed S, Bhivandkar S, Lonergan BB, Suzuki J. Microinduction of buprenorphine/naloxone: A review of the literature. *Am J Addict.* 2021;30(4):305–315.
78. Spreen LA, Dittmar EN, Quirk KC, Smith MA. Buprenorphine initiation strategies for opioid use disorder and pain management: A systematic review. *Pharmacotherapy.* 2022;42(5):411–427.
79. Hickey T, Abelleira A, Acampora G, et al. Perioperative buprenorphine management: A multidisciplinary approach. *Med Clin North Am.* 2022;106(1):169–185.
80. Sandbrink F, Oliva EM, McMullen TL, et al. Opioid prescribing and opioid risk mitigation strategies in the Veterans Health Administration. *J Gen Intern Med.* 2020;35(Suppl 3):927–934.
81. U.S. Department of Veterans Affairs. Safe and responsible use of opioids for chronic pain: A patient information guide. Updated October 2018. Accessed February 13, 2023. https://www.ethics.va.gov/docs/policy/Safe_and_Responsible_Use_of_Opioids.pdf#
82. Cheatle MD, Savage SR. Informed consent in opioid therapy: A potential obligation and opportunity. *J Pain Symptom Manage.* 2012;44(1):105–116.
83. Argoff CE, Kahan M, Sellers EM. Preventing and managing aberrant drug-related behavior in primary care: Systematic review of outcomes evidence. *J Opioid Manag.* 2014;10(2):119–134.
84. Christo PJ, Manchikanti L, Ruan X, et al. Urine drug testing in chronic pain. *Pain Physician.* 2011;14(2):123–143.

32
Pain in Critically Ill Patients

Kellie Jaremko, Brinda Krish, Katarina Nikolic, and Hassan Rayaz

Each year in the United States, more than 5 million patients are admitted to intensive care units (ICUs). In 2010, a health care cost report information system analysis showed that of 150.9 million hospital days, 25 million were ICU days.[1] Patients admitted to ICUs are in a uniquely vulnerable position in which poorly controlled acute pain may progress to chronic pain. Studies have reported that 65% of patients recalled moderate to severe pain while in the ICU.[2] Poorly controlled acute pain has been shown to be associated with increased pain, functional limitations, and lower quality of life 6–18 months later.[3,4] Because of a decreased ability to communicate due to sedation, intubation, and delirium, critically ill patients are at higher risk for poor pain control. Poor sleep, situational depression, and psychological distress can also exacerbate pain perception, leading to a negative feedback cycle. Effective multimodal adjuncts are important because they can decrease the reliance on opioids for sedation, which can lead to tolerance, iatrogenic withdrawal, and chronic opioid use.

This chapter discusses the prevalence of pain in critically ill adult patients; validated pain scales for accurate assessment; and existing research-based guidelines for management of sedation, delirium, and psychological distress. Postoperative and post-traumatic analgesia optimization, including multimodal adjuncts, is discussed to ideally balance the risks of opioids with the benefits of early aggressive pain treatment in this critically ill population.

Pain Prevalence and Consequences in the Critically Ill

Despite improved attention to assessment and management, pain at rest is present in more than half of ICU patients without an appreciable difference between medical, trauma, or surgical reasons for admission.[5] In addition to post-traumatic or postoperative pain, procedural pain with ICU interventions such as lines, tubes, dressing changes, and turns has been reported. The Thunder Project-II, a multicenter study of more than 6,000 patients, found turns in adults, and dressing changes in adolescents, to be the highest rated pain events with noticeable behavioral changes.[6] Comparable results were found in other studies, with up to 15% of patients reporting severe pain occurring more than half of their ICU stay.[7] Likewise, in a population of critically ill patients, pain at an injury site was reported 96% of the time, with a doubling of "at rest" pain on the visual analog scale during turns, and 36% reported pain related to biomedical devices.[8] Lower pain scores correlated with lower anxiety, but patients were more likely to remember the most bothersome events, such as pain, fear, anxiety, lack of sleep, inability to speak/communicate, lack of control, nightmares, and loneliness.[8,9] This is consistent with the words ICU survivors chose to describe their pain experiences, with 20% including "bad" or "awful" and 6–13% stating it was "fearful–frightening," "sickening," and "punishing–cruel."[10]

There is evidence that recall of pain, distress, and trauma during an ICU stay is associated with post-traumatic stress disorder (PTSD) symptoms and is a major contributor to post-ICU syndrome (PCIS), which encompasses mental, cognitive, and physical disorders after a serious illness. PCIS prevalence is associated with a lower 2-year survival rate and has been reported as 60% and 35% at 6 and 12 months, respectively.[11] One established tool for PTSD screening is the Impact of Events Scale (IES), which was validated in patients following acute lung injury with rates of PTSD of 13% at interview and 28% at any point since their injury.[12,13] Severe PTSD was found 25% of the time in one study of more than 250 critical care patients, with higher risk related to increased age, unemployment status, the presence of pain memories, profound feelings of loss of control, and trouble communicating needs.[14] Higher IES scores, suggestive of PTSD, correlated with higher recorded pain intensity in the ICU, and they have been associated with ongoing pain at 3- to 16-month follow-up.[15]

Taken together, there are multiple sources of pain in critically ill patients, with the prevalence of persistent post-discharge reported as 12–77%. Chronicity was particularly associated with higher intensity and longer duration of uncontrolled pain at ICU discharge and 1 week postoperatively.[16–18] Six months after ICU discharge, new chronic pain was reported in 16% of individuals, whereas 17% of those with pre-existing chronic pain had new distinct pain sites and disabling pain limiting their activities of daily living.[19] This body of work suggests that there are several contributing factors to ongoing pain, associated with both emotional and physical dysfunction after an ICU admission.

Vulnerabilities Innate to Sedation and Delirium Management

The first step in effectively treating acute pain in critically ill patients is to be cognizant of their unique vulnerabilities while utilizing validated screening tools to monitor sedation, delirium, and pain with treatment effects. Sedation and delirium are intertwined contributors to poor communication and pain screening. Sedation is often necessary in critically ill patients to improve tolerance of mechanical ventilation and decrease anxiety, discomfort, and the risk of agitation-related self-harm.[20] Suboptimal sedation level is prevalent in the literature, noted in 33–57% of cases within several cohort studies that also showed routine sedation assessments present in only 42–63% of cases.[21–24] The depth of sedation required should be assessed on a case-by-case basis. However, early and prolonged deep sedation is associated with poor outcomes, including prolonged mechanical ventilation; longer ICU/hospital stay; and increased delusional memories, PTSD, and mortality.[25,26]

Validated tools used to maintain optimal levels of sedation include the Richmond Agitation Sedation Scale (RASS), the Riker Sedation Agitation Scale (SAS), the Ramsey Sedation Scale, and the Glasgow Coma Scale (GCS).[20] Bispectral index readings (derived from electroencephalogram) correlate significantly with RASS, SAS, and GCS, offering a sedation assessment adjunct that can be used without stimulating the patient during subjective assessments.[20,27]

The Pain, Agitation/Sedation, Delirium, Immobility, and Sleep panel (PADIS), within the Society of Critical Care Medicine congress, updated its recommendations for management of critically ill patients. Lighter sedation depth, within the RASS range of −2 to 1, is recommended. In one randomized control trial (RCT), this approach led to 1 less day mechanically ventilated and 1.5 less days spent in the ICU.[20,25] Guidelines on sedative choice have shifted away from benzodiazepines due to evidence of worse short-term outcomes in RCTs.[28,29] An early multicenter ICU trial sedation with dexmedetomidine resulted in less need for additional sedatives, significantly lower morphine requirements, and less memory of pain or discomfort than their propofol sedated counterparts.[30] Major contributors to this field were the MIDEX and PRODEX trials, a collection of European, multicenter, randomized, double-blind studies that first compared midazolam with dexmedetomidine and subsequently compared propofol with dexmedetomidine.[31] Results from MIDEX/PRODEX showed non-inferiority of dexmedetomidine for maintaining light to moderate sedation and decreased duration of mechanical ventilation compared with midazolam, as well as documented improvement in patients' ability to communicate pain compared with midazolam and propofol, despite higher adverse events of hypotension and bradycardia.[31] Adequate sedation and the need for fewer analgesics were replicated in a neurosurgical population following dexmedetomidine bolus of 1 μg/kg over 15 min as a loading dose, followed by 0.4–0.7 μg/kg/h.[28] In the DEXACET trial, less breakthrough analgesia was required.[32] In addition to choice of agent, having a protocol-directed sedation was found to decrease hospital length of stay but not ICU duration or mortality.[20]

Delirium is a neuropsychiatric condition characterized by acute changes in mental status, including disordered attention and cognition, which is often seen in the ICU. Delirium in the elderly is associated with several adverse outcomes, including mortality.[33] The causative factors leading to the development of delirium are multifactorial, and prospectively validated prediction models across clinical populations show the leading risk factors are cognitive impairment, functional impairment, visual impairment, history of alcohol misuse, and advanced age.[34] Reliable diagnostic instruments validated for delirium assessment include the Confusion Assessment Method for the ICU (CAM-ICU) and the Delirium Rating Scale (DRS).[35–37]

Treating delirium should be a multicomponent intervention focused on reducing modifiable risk factors. These include strategies to reduce or shorten delirium (reorientation, cognitive stimulation, and use of clocks), improve sleep (minimizing light and noise), improve wakefulness (reduced sedation), reduce immobility (early rehabilitation/mobilization), and reduce hearing and/or visual impairment (enable use of devices such as hearing aids or eyeglasses).[20] These multicomponent bundles improve duration of ICU delirium and mortality.[38,39] Research has shown a link between higher pain levels and the development of delirium, with studies showing that moderate to severe pain is an independent risk factor equal to age.[40,41] Pain should be treated aggressively while minimizing pharmacological agents associated with delirium-worsening analgesics, posing a cyclical conundrum requiring awareness and implementation of evolving best practice guidelines. Regional analgesic techniques and indwelling perineural catheters may be helpful because they are associated with a reduced incidence of postoperative delirium and offer a method of treating pain without solely relying on systemic analgesics.[42]

Pain Assessment Tools

Once sedation and delirium management is optimized, consistent pain assessments are paramount to prevent uncontrolled pain. Based on literature and practicality, a hierarchical approach of pain assessments in the critically ill is suggested with patient self-reporting (gold standard), observed behavioral changes, and finally physiologic changes as a last resort. In verbal sighted patients, the two most used scales are the numerical rating scale (NRS) and the visual analog scale (VAS). Both scales are patients' subjective assessments of pain intensity. Using a numeric scale, the patient indicates verbally or by pointing to the number that correlates with pain intensity from 0 (none) to 10 (unbearable pain). When using a VAS, the patient is asked to mark on a 10-cm line their current pain along a continuum between "no pain" and "worst pain."[43] Many studies have shown correlation between scales, but the NRS has been reported to have better experimental compliance across studies due to its unidimensionality and ease of administration.[44] One study across 111 ICUs investigated five different self-reported pain scales and found that the visual NRS had the highest response rate, sensitivity, negative predictive value, and accuracy, whereas VAS horizontal had the lowest success rate.[45] This is consistent with findings that errors on VAS increase with age and cognitive impairment.[46] Regardless of scale, a clinically meaningful change in results is approximately 20–30%, a reduction of 2 points on the NRS.[47]

The Behavioral Pain Scale (BPS) and Critical-Care Pain Observation Tool (CPOT) are validated scales for pain assessment in uncommunicative and sedated patients in the ICU. Systematic reviews demonstrated reliability and validity for assessing pain via these tools in intubated patients admitted to ICUs from various cultures.[20,48] Both instruments were sensitive when applied during painful procedures, showing increases in various indicators: facial expression on the BPS and muscle tension/stiffness, facial tension, and ventilator tolerance/cough on the CPOT, as well as blood pressure on both scales.[49] Unlike the BPS, CPOT also has a vocalization domain, helping its application with extubated patients.[50]

Although both the BPS and CPOT are accepted assessments in ICU patients, the latter has demonstrated greater discriminant validity and sensitivity, whereas the BPS may have greater reliability and sensitivity.[48,51,52] Specificity of the CPOT was high for all assessments of intubated and conscious patients (no exposure and nociceptive exposure); thus, the risks of administering an analgesic to a patient who does not need it and the potential adverse effects that could result from the medication would be avoided.[50] The use of one or both of these scales can reduce the administration of analgesics and sedatives.

Multimodal Medications

An early and effective multimodal analgesic approach aims to minimize medications that contribute to delirium and limit prolonged high-dose opioids. Consultation with an acute pain service is beneficial in developing multidisciplinary plans and multimodal regimens, resulting in decreased pain scores at transfer; fewer adverse events; and improved quality of postoperative pain, perception of care, and patient satisfaction.[53,54] Perioperative pain medicine has evolved, adding more complementary tools for the practitioner during the past decade with evidence of enhanced recovery after surgery protocols.[55,56]

Nonsteroidal anti-inflammatory drugs (NSAIDs) are known to inhibit the cyclooxygenase (COX) enzymes, mitigating prostaglandin synthesis and inflammation-induced hyperalgesia. COX enzymes are involved in hemostasis, gastric mucosal protection, and platelet aggregation. Blocking this pathway can predispose patients to a higher risk of bleeding and should be avoided in patients with a history of gastrointestinal ulcers or bariatric surgery.[57,58] Regardless of COX selectivity, decreased prostaglandins may result in renal ischemia via reduction in peritubular blood flow and altered local afferent vasodilation.[59] Furthermore, blocking the production of prostacyclins can lead to unopposed thromboxane A2 production, which may promote coronary thrombosis, and thus caution should be exercised in patients at risk for cardiovascular events.[60] In summary, patients without cardiovascular disease, ongoing bleeding/anticoagulation, gastrointestinal sensitivity, history of gastric bypass, acute renal injury, allergic reactions, or long bone fractures may be candidates for NSAIDs. Ketorolac is an intravenous (IV) nonselective NSAID, with equivalent analgesia observed at modest doses of 15 mg compared with higher doses; it can be administered every 6 h in appropriate patients for up to 5 days.[61] Consultation with the primary surgical team prior to NSAID initiation is recommended.

Synergism of scheduled acetaminophen and NSAIDs can be more effective for decreasing morphine consumption postoperatively than the use of either agent alone.[62,63] Acetaminophen administered at higher doses of 1000 mg versus 500 mg has been observed to be superior in the treatment of pain.[64] In patients with chronic hepatic failure, some sources advocate for safe dosing at a maximum of 2 g/day, but many recommend avoiding acetaminophen altogether (especially in acute hepatic injury). Although the IV form has better bioavailability and faster onset than other formulations, it is more expensive without being significantly superior to oral dosing for the treatment of postoperative pain.[65] However, because many patients remain NPO (nothing by mouth) in the ICU with questionable gastrointestinal absorption, the increased cost of IV formulation may be offset by earlier time to pain control and discharge.[20] In addition, IV acetaminophen has been deemed safe and effective in intensive care patients following cardiac surgery, resulting in less delirium, more opioid sparing, and decreased length of ICU stay in the DEXACET trial.[32]

Ketamine is a noncompetitive *N*-methyl-D-aspartate (NMDA) receptor antagonist traditionally used as an intraoperative anesthetic. At sub-anesthetic doses, it functions on multiple additional pathways, including μ- and δ-opioid receptors, monoaminergic, and serotonin receptors.[66,67] Through these mechanisms, ketamine decreases activity within nociceptive neurons, modulates crosstalk with opioid receptors involved in tolerance, and activates descending inhibitory pain pathways. In the dorsal horn, it can attenuate NMDA receptor-mediated hyperalgesia and the wind-up phenomenon that may lead to central sensitization, pain sensitivity, and chronic pain.[68,69] These qualities make ketamine particularly effective in opioid-tolerant, neuropathic pain, and chronic pain patients.

In 2018, the American Society of Regional Anesthesia and Pain Medicine in conjunction with the American Academy of Pain Medicine and the American Society of Anesthesiologists published consensus guidelines on the use of IV ketamine for the treatment of acute pain.[70] Perioperative ketamine can be opioid-sparing while reducing postoperative nausea/vomiting and decreasing postoperative hyperalgesia.[71] Similar benefits have been reported following perioperative ketamine infusions on immediate- and long-term pain and opioid use after spine surgery.[72–74] Ketamine has also been implicated in improving acute and chronic phantom limb pain after amputations.[75,76] Inclusion of ketamine (<0.2 mg/kg/h) in a postoperative ICU regimen for pain after major abdominal surgery was shown to decrease cumulative morphine consumption.[77] Corroborative evidence has been published showing decreased opioid and sedation requirements without adverse effects on hemodynamics or delirium in ventilated critically ill patients.[78–81]

Optimal duration and dosages of ketamine for different indications have not been well defined in the current literature, but the consensus guidelines recommend boluses not exceed 0.35 mg/kg and infusion rates between 0.1 and 1 mg/kg/h.[70] Adverse effects are rare and include hallucinations, vivid nightmares, dysphoria, and nystagmus.[70] The potential risk of elevated intracranial pressure has not been seen with subanesthetic analgesic doses in neurocritical care patients.[82] Unresolved cardiac ischemia and pathological aberrant heart rhythms remain contraindications due to ketamine's activation of the sympathetic nervous system; however, ketamine has been shown to improve outcomes by decreasing opioids without complications in cardiac patients.[80] For acute pain, poorly controlled cardiovascular disease, pregnancy, and severe hepatic dysfunction are commonly agreed-upon relative contraindications, with avoidance in patients with acute psychosis.[70]

Lidocaine is a short-acting amide local anesthetic administered via transdermal patch, IV infusion, or wound infiltration. At the molecular level, it binds and inhibits sodium channels, which within neuronal membranes have been implicated in central and peripheral components of pain and hyperalgesia. Its potential anti-inflammatory role has prompted more perioperative usage,[83–85] specifically in surgical patients undergoing abdominal surgeries, regardless of open or laparoscopic approach, and major spine surgery. Intravenous lidocaine infusions in these populations led to improvements in pain scores, decreased opioid consumption, earlier return of bowel function, and decreased hospital length of stay.[86,87] In two studies, perioperative lidocaine was found to be similarly effective as thoracic epidurals with regard to pain scores and bowel function despite having less opioid sparing effect.[88,89] One study found decreased chronic postsurgical pain after mastectomy in a perioperative lidocaine cohort.[90]

An international consensus statement classifies lidocaine as a high-risk medication due to its narrow therapeutic window. It recommends initial doses less than 1.5 mg/kg/h (ideal body weight), with prolonged high-dose infusions not to exceed 24 h.[91] Clinically, the authors utilize perioperative lidocaine starting doses of 0.5–1 mg/kg/h (ideal body weight) and check a plasma level at 24 h, adjusting if necessary and terminating the infusion at 48 h. All staff should be educated on early recognition and management of local anesthetic systemic toxicity, which is a life-threatening emergency requiring intralipid infusion and hemodynamic management.[92] Lidocaine metabolism and clearance are correlated with cardiac index impacting blood flow to the hepatic circulation, intact enzymatic functions of the liver, and metabolite clearance by the kidneys. Significant acidemia or hypoalbuminemia also impacts the amount of unbound lidocaine.[85] Benefit may be more pronounced in opioid-tolerant patients, and expert consultation is advised prior to dosing.

Dexmedetomidine, an α_2-adrenergic receptor agonist, exerts analgesic properties by inhibiting descending noradrenergic pathways that modulate pain transmission, as well as directly causing presynaptic hyperpolarization within spinal cord nociceptors.[93] Dosing involves an optional bolus of 0.5–1.0 μg/kg given over 10 min followed by an infusion titrated to effect between 0.2 and 0.7 μg/kg/h.[30,94] Bolus dosing particularly poses risks of hypotension and bradycardia, which may limit usefulness within unstable ICU patients. However, intraoperative use exhibits favorable respiratory drive properties, decreased postoperative pain intensity, and decreased postoperative opioid requirements.[94]

PADIS also recommends inclusion of a neuropathic adjuvant, such as a gabapentinoid that modulates calcium channel–induced glutamate release in nociceptive neurons.[20] The enteral route is required, and pregabalin has greater bioavailability and a wider area of gastrointestinal absorption. Perioperative research findings are mixed, showing some decreased pain scores with possible prevention of chronicity, albeit with potential risk for respiratory depression when mixed with opioids in naive patients.[95,96] Muscle relaxants can also be considered as part of a multimodal approach, when applicable.

Opioids are efficacious in treating acute pain and thus inevitable in managing ICU patients; however, due to significant side effects (respiratory depression, ileus, hormonal imbalance, and immunosuppression), the lowest dose should be utilized for the shortest duration possible.[20] In patients with rapidly evolving hepatic and renal function, choosing opioids with no or few clinically relevant active metabolites is advised, such as fentanyl and hydromorphone over morphine and oxycodone.[97] Iatrogenic tolerance and withdrawal reported as 16.7% are correlated with higher opioid dose and longer duration.[98,99] Explicit plans for inpatient and ongoing outpatient opioid monitoring and tapering are required to spare patient harm.

Finally, regional anesthesia (RA) is an excellent modality for pain relief and has been shown to decrease length of ICU stay; improve patient comfort; improve clinical workflow; facilitate neurologic assessments; and significantly reduce the need for systemic analgesics, especially in trauma patients.[100] RA techniques such as epidural analgesia, paravertebral blocks, and other single-shot or continuous peripheral nerve blocks (PNBs) facilitate earlier weaning from ventilation, reduced respiratory morbidity, better postoperative analgesia than systemic opioids, as well as decreased ICU length of stay and delirium.[42,101–103] A recent study reports the effects of combined major abdominal surgery, general anesthesia, and postsurgical pain are the main contributors to inspiratory muscle dysfunction and that epidural anesthesia may partly reverse this dysfunction.[104] Polytrauma, major thoracoabdominal, and orthopedic surgery patients have substantial nociceptive input via C afferents that can be blocked by opioids;

however, Aα and Aδ afferents are also affected and are uniquely blocked in site-specific RA, conveying greater benefits in these populations.[105,106]

Coagulopathy and clotting disorders may prevent the use of neuraxial analgesia or deep PNBs, but fascial plane blocks, such as serratus or erector spinae catheters, are efficacious. Compromised immune systems and susceptibility to infection are other concerns; however, in a large study, the rate of severe RA catheter infection was only 0.07%.[107] In a hemodynamically unstable patient, neuraxial techniques such as epidural analgesia may be contraindicated because sympatholysis may worsen instability and necessitate pressor or inotrope introduction.[108] However, thoracic paravertebral blocks have been found to be as effective as thoracic epidurals in providing adequate analgesia in patients with chest wall trauma and unilateral rib fractures, and they are associated with minimal hypotension.[109,110]

In patients who are heavily sedated, there is debate regarding whether it is safe to perform RA. First, this type of patient cannot give consent, so family members should be counseled on the advantages and disadvantages of performing the procedure. Concerns include the patient's inability to report symptoms or give feedback regarding inadvertent intravascular, intraneural, and/or intrathecal injection. Of high concern to the regional anesthesiologist is the risk of nerve injury in a sedated patient. If careful consideration is made as to the risk:benefit ratio, placement of a PNB may be warranted.[111] In pediatrics, placing blocks under general anesthesia is common and has not been found to increase risk of adverse events.[112] Since the introduction of ultrasound-guided techniques, there has been more reliable identification of both vascular and neural structures, which has made the administration of local anesthetic and placement of nerve catheters much safer, even in the heavily sedated patient.[113]

Conclusion

Pain management is a critical part of caring for the ICU patient, and pain physicians are uniquely positioned to shape multimodal approaches. Acknowledgment of vulnerabilities within this population starts with communication difficulties, which can be improved with lighter sedation, aggressive delirium prevention and treatment, as well as utilization of validated pain scales (NRS, BPS, and CPOT). Multiorgan dysfunction necessitates close monitoring of pain medications and careful selection of RA procedures. Finally, awareness and support of the psychological distress and impaired sleep in this population must be a component of the holistic pain management plan. Untreated pain significantly impacts outcomes, and inadequately treated pain can lead to prolonged mechanical ventilation, longer ICU stay, morbidity, development of PTSD, and chronic post-surgical pain. Early and aggressive interventions for pain management in the ICU are essential.

References

1. Halpern NA, Goldman DA, Tan KS, Pastores SM. Trends in critical care beds and use among population groups and Medicare and Medicaid beneficiaries in the United States: 2000–2010. *Crit Care Med.* 2016;44(8):1490–1499.

2. Puntillo KA. Pain experiences of intensive care unit patients. *Heart Lung.* 1990;19(5 Pt 1):526–533.
3. Katz J, Jackson M, Kavanagh BP, Sandler AN. Acute pain after thoracic surgery predicts long-term post-thoracotomy pain. *Clin J Pain.* 1996;12(1):50–55.
4. Peters ML, Sommer M, de Rijke JM, et al. Somatic and psychologic predictors of long-term unfavorable outcome after surgical intervention. *Ann Surg.* 2007;245(3):487–494.
5. Chanques G, Sebbane M, Barbotte E, Viel E, Eledjam JJ, Jaber S. A prospective study of pain at rest: Incidence and characteristics of an unrecognized symptom in surgical and trauma versus medical intensive care unit patients. *Anesthesiology.* 2007;107(5):858–860.
6. Puntillo KA, White C, Morris AB, et al. Patients' perceptions and responses to procedural pain: Results from Thunder Project II. *Am J Crit Care.* 2001;10(4):238–251.
7. Desbiens NA, Wu AW, Broste SK, et al. Pain and satisfaction with pain control in seriously ill hospitalized adults: Findings from the SUPPORT research investigations. For the SUPPORT investigators. Study to Understand Prognoses and Preferences for Outcomes and Risks of Treatment. *Crit Care Med.* 1996;24(12):1953–1961.
8. Stanik-Hutt JA, Soeken KL, Belcher AE, Fontaine DK, Gift AG. Pain experiences of traumatically injured patients in a critical care setting. *Am J Crit Care.* 2001;10(4):252–259.
9. Rotondi AJ, Chelluri L, Sirio C, et al. Patients' recollections of stressful experiences while receiving prolonged mechanical ventilation in an intensive care unit. *Crit Care Med.* 2002;30(4):746–752.
10. Thompson CL, White C, Wild LR, et al. Translating research into practice: Implications of the Thunder Project II. *Crit Care Nurs Clin North Am.* 2001;13(4):541–546.
11. Inoue S, Nakanishi N, Sugiyama J, et al. Prevalence and long-term prognosis of post-intensive care syndrome after sepsis: A single-center prospective observational study. *J Clin Med Res.* 2022;11(18):5257. doi:10.3390/jcm11185257
12. Bienvenu OJ, Williams JB, Yang A, Hopkins RO, Needham DM. Posttraumatic stress disorder in survivors of acute lung injury: Evaluating the Impact of Event Scale–Revised. *Chest.* 2013;144(1):24–31.
13. Hosey MM, Leoutsakos JMS, Li X, et al. Screening for posttraumatic stress disorder in ARDS survivors: Validation of the Impact of Event Scale–6 (IES-6). *Crit Care.* 2019;23(1):276.
14. Fernandes A, Jaeger MS, Chudow M. Post–intensive care syndrome: A review of preventive strategies and follow-up care. *Am J Health Syst Pharm.* 2019;76(2):119–122.
15. Puntillo KA, Max A, Chaize M, Chanques G, Azoulay E. Patient recollection of ICU procedural pain and post ICU burden: The Memory Study. *Crit Care Med.* 2016;44(11):1988–1995.
16. Mäkinen OJ, Bäcklund ME, Liisanantti J, Peltomaa M, Karlsson S, Kalliomäki ML. Persistent pain in intensive care survivors: A systematic review. *Br J Anaesth.* 2020;125(2):149–158.
17. Battle CE, Lovett S, Hutchings H. Chronic pain in survivors of critical illness: A retrospective analysis of incidence and risk factors. *Crit Care.* 2013;17(3):R101.
18. Puntillo KA, Naidu R. Chronic pain disorders after critical illness and ICU-acquired opioid dependence: Two clinical conundra. *Curr Opin Crit Care.* 2016;22(5):506–512.
19. Baumbach P, Götz T, Günther A, Weiss T, Meissner W. Prevalence and characteristics of chronic intensive care–related pain: The role of severe sepsis and septic shock. *Crit Care Med.* 2016;44(6):1129–1137.
20. Devlin JW, Skrobik Y, Gélinas C, et al. Clinical practice guidelines for the prevention and management of pain, agitation/sedation, delirium, immobility, and sleep disruption in adult patients in the ICU. *Crit Care Med.* 2018;46(9):e825–e873.
21. Jackson DL, Proudfoot CW, Cann KF, Walsh TS. The incidence of sub-optimal sedation in the ICU: A systematic review. *Crit Care.* 2009;13(6):R204.
22. Elliott D, Aitken LM, Bucknall TK, et al. Patient comfort in the intensive care unit: A multicentre, binational point prevalence study of analgesia, sedation and delirium management. *Crit Care Resusc.* 2013;15(3):213–219.
23. Payen JF, Chanques G, Mantz J, et al. Current practices in sedation and analgesia for mechanically ventilated critically ill patients: A prospective multicenter patient-based study. *Anesthesiology.* 2007;106(4):687–695; quiz 891–892.

24. Weinert CR, Calvin AD. Epidemiology of sedation and sedation adequacy for mechanically ventilated patients in a medical and surgical intensive care unit. *Crit Care Med.* 2007;35(2):393–401.
25. Treggiari MM, Romand JA, Yanez ND, et al. Randomized trial of light versus deep sedation on mental health after critical illness. *Crit Care Med.* 2009;37(9):2527–2534.
26. Shehabi Y, Chan L, Kadiman S, et al. Sedation depth and long-term mortality in mechanically ventilated critically ill adults: A prospective longitudinal multicentre cohort study. *Intensive Care Med.* 2013;39(5):910–918.
27. Deogaonkar A, Gupta R, DeGeorgia M, et al. Bispectral Index monitoring correlates with sedation scales in brain-injured patients. *Crit Care Med.* 2004;32(12):2403–2406.
28. Srivastava VK, Agrawal S, Kumar S, Mishra A, Sharma S, Kumar R. Comparison of dexmedetomidine, propofol and midazolam for short-term sedation in postoperatively mechanically ventilated neurosurgical patients. *J Clin Diagn Res.* 2014;8(9):GC04–GC07.
29. Chamorro C, de Latorre FJ, Montero A, et al. Comparative study of propofol versus midazolam in the sedation of critically ill patients: Results of a prospective, randomized, multicenter trial. *Crit Care Med.* 1996;24(6):932–939.
30. Martin E, Ramsay G, Mantz J, Sum-Ping STJ. The role of the alpha2-adrenoceptor agonist dexmedetomidine in postsurgical sedation in the intensive care unit. *J Intensive Care Med.* 2003;18(1):29–41.
31. Jakob SM, Ruokonen E, Grounds RM, et al. Dexmedetomidine vs midazolam or propofol for sedation during prolonged mechanical ventilation: Two randomized controlled trials. *JAMA.* 2012;307(11):1151–1160.
32. Subramaniam B, Shankar P, Shaefi S, et al. Effect of intravenous acetaminophen vs placebo combined with propofol or dexmedetomidine on postoperative delirium among older patients following cardiac surgery: The DEXACET randomized clinical trial. *JAMA.* 2019;321(7):686–696.
33. Francis J, Kapoor WN. Prognosis after hospital discharge of older medical patients with delirium. *J Am Geriatr Soc.* 1992;40(6):601–606.
34. Inouye SK, Westendorp RGJ, Saczynski JS. Delirium in elderly people. *Lancet.* 2014;383(9920):911–922.
35. Inouye SK, van Dyck CH, Alessi CA, Balkin S, Siegal AP, Horwitz RI. Clarifying confusion: The confusion assessment method. A new method for detection of delirium. *Ann Intern Med.* 1990;113(12):941–948.
36. Trzepacz PT, Mittal D, Torres R, Kanary K, Norton J, Jimerson N. Validation of the Delirium Rating Scale–Revised-98: Comparison with the Delirium Rating Scale and the Cognitive Test for Delirium. *J Neuropsychiatry Clin Neurosci.* 2001;13(2):229–242.
37. McNicoll L, Pisani MA, Ely EW, Gifford D, Inouye SK. Detection of delirium in the intensive care unit: Comparison of confusion assessment method for the intensive care unit with confusion assessment method ratings. *J Am Geriatr Soc.* 2005;53(3):495–500.
38. Colombo R, Corona A, Praga F, et al. A reorientation strategy for reducing delirium in the critically ill: Results of an interventional study. *Minerva Anestesiol.* 2012;78(9):1026–1033.
39. Rivosecchi RM, Kane-Gill SL, Svec S, Campbell S, Smithburger PL. The implementation of a nonpharmacologic protocol to prevent intensive care delirium. *J Crit Care.* 2016;31(1):206–211.
40. Vaurio LE, Sands LP, Wang Y, Mullen EA, Leung JM. Postoperative delirium: The importance of pain and pain management. *Anesth Analg.* 2006;102(4):1267–1273.
41. Lynch EP, Lazor MA, Gellis JE, Orav J, Goldman L, Marcantonio ER. The impact of postoperative pain on the development of postoperative delirium. *Anesth Analg.* 1998;86(4):781–785.
42. Jankowski CJ, Cook DJ, Trenerry MR, Schroeder DR. Continuous peripheral nerve block analgesia and central neuraxial anesthesia are associated with reduced incidence of postoperative delirium in the elderly. *Anesthesiology.* 2005;103:A1467.
43. Price DD, McGrath PA, Rafii A, Buckingham B. The validation of visual analogue scales as ratio scale measures for chronic and experimental pain. *Pain.* 1983;17(1):45–56.

44. Hjermstad MJ, Fayers PM, Haugen DF, et al. Studies comparing numerical rating scales, verbal rating scales, and visual analogue scales for assessment of pain intensity in adults: A systematic literature review. *J Pain Symptom Manage.* 2011;41(6):1073–1093.
45. Chanques G, Viel E, Constantin JM, et al. The measurement of pain in intensive care unit: Comparison of 5 self-report intensity scales. *Pain.* 2010;151(3):711–721.
46. Briggs M, Closs JS. A descriptive study of the use of visual analogue scales and verbal rating scales for the assessment of postoperative pain in orthopedic patients. *J Pain Symptom Manage.* 1999;18(6):438–446.
47. Farrar JT, Young JP Jr, LaMoreaux L, Werth JL, Poole RM. Clinical importance of changes in chronic pain intensity measured on an 11-point numerical pain rating scale. *Pain.* 2001;94(2):149–158.
48. Birkedal HC, Larsen MH, Steindal SA, Solberg MT. Comparison of two behavioural pain scales for the assessment of procedural pain: A systematic review. *Nurs Open.* 2021;8(5):2050–2060.
49. Payen JF, Bru O, Bosson JL, et al. Assessing pain in critically ill sedated patients by using a behavioral pain scale. *Crit Care Med.* 2001;29(12):2258–2263.
50. Gélinas C, Fillion L, Puntillo KA, Viens C, Fortier M. Validation of the Critical-Care Pain Observation Tool in adult patients. *Am J Crit Care.* 2006;15(4):420–427.
51. Nazari R, Froelicher ES, Nia HS, Hajihosseini F, Mousazadeh N. Diagnostic values of the Critical Care Pain Observation Tool and the Behavioral Pain Scale for pain assessment among unconscious patients: A comparative study. *Indian J Crit Care Med.* 2022;26(4):472–476.
52. Severgnini P, Pelosi P, Contino E, Serafinelli E, Novario R, Chiaranda M. Accuracy of Critical Care Pain Observation Tool and Behavioral Pain Scale to assess pain in critically ill conscious and unconscious patients: Prospective, observational study. *J Intensive Care Med.* 2016;4(1): Article 68.
53. Story DA, Shelton AC, Poustie SJ, Colin-Thome NJ, McIntyre RE, McNicol PL. Effect of an anaesthesia department led critical care outreach and acute pain service on postoperative serious adverse events. *Anaesthesia.* 2006;61(1):24–28.
54. Sartain JB, Barry JJ. The impact of an acute pain service on postoperative pain management. *Anaesth Intensive Care.* 1999;27(4):375–380.
55. Ljungqvist O, Scott M, Fearon KC. Enhanced recovery after surgery: A review. *JAMA Surg.* 2017;152(3):292–298.
56. Gustafsson UO, Oppelstrup H, Thorell A, Nygren J, Ljungqvist O. Adherence to the ERAS protocol is associated with 5-year survival after colorectal cancer surgery: A retrospective cohort study. *World J Surg.* 2016;40(7):1741–1747.
57. Langman MJ, Weil J, Wainwright P, et al. Risks of bleeding peptic ulcer associated with individual non-steroidal anti-inflammatory drugs. *Lancet.* 1994;343(8905):1075–1078.
58. Coblijn UK, Lagarde SM, de Castro SMM, Kuiken SD, van Wagensveld BA. Symptomatic marginal ulcer disease after Roux-en-Y gastric bypass: Incidence, risk factors and management. *Obes Surg.* 2015;25(5):805–811.
59. Huerta C, Castellsague J, Varas-Lorenzo C, García Rodríguez LA. Nonsteroidal anti-inflammatory drugs and risk of ARF in the general population. *Am J Kidney Dis.* 2005;45(3):531–539.
60. Martínez-González J, Badimon L. Mechanisms underlying the cardiovascular effects of COX-inhibition: Benefits and risks. *Curr Pharm Des.* 2007;13(22):2215–2227.
61. Motov S, Yasavolian M, Likourezos A, et al. Comparison of intravenous ketorolac at three single-dose regimens for treating acute pain in the emergency department: A randomized controlled trial. *Ann Emerg Med.* 2017;70(2):177–184.
62. Miranda HF, Puig MM, Prieto JC, Pinardi G. Synergism between paracetamol and nonsteroidal anti-inflammatory drugs in experimental acute pain. *Pain.* 2006;121(1-2):22–28.
63. Alexander L, Hall E, Eriksson L, Rohlin M. The combination of non-selective NSAID 400 mg and paracetamol 1000 mg is more effective than each drug alone for treatment of acute pain: A systematic review. *Swed Dent J.* 2014;38(1):1–14.

64. McQuay HJ, Moore RA. Dose-response in direct comparisons of different doses of aspirin, ibuprofen and paracetamol (acetaminophen) in analgesic studies. *Br J Clin Pharmacol.* 2007;63(3):271–278.
65. Patel A, Pai BHP, Diskina D, Reardon B, Lai YH. Comparison of clinical outcomes of acetaminophen IV vs PO in the peri-operative setting for laparoscopic inguinal hernia repair surgeries: A triple-blinded, randomized controlled trial. *J Clin Anesth.* 2020;61:109628.
66. Bell RF, Kalso EA. Ketamine for pain management. *Pain Rep.* 2018;3(5):e674.
67. Adams HA. [Mechanisms of action of ketamine]. *Anaesthesiol Reanim.* 1998;23(3):60–63.
68. Laulin JP, Maurette P, Corcuff JB, Rivat C, Chauvin M, Simonnet G. The role of ketamine in preventing fentanyl-induced hyperalgesia and subsequent acute morphine tolerance. *Anesth Analg.* 2002;94(5):1263–1269.
69. Price DD, Mayer DJ, Mao J, Caruso FS. NMDA-receptor antagonists and opioid receptor interactions as related to analgesia and tolerance. *J Pain Symptom Manage.* 2000;19(1 Suppl):S7–S11.
70. Schwenk ES, Viscusi ER, Buvanendran A, et al. Consensus guidelines on the use of intravenous ketamine infusions for acute pain management from the American Society of Regional Anesthesia and Pain Medicine, the American Academy of Pain Medicine, and the American Society of Anesthesiologists. *Reg Anesth Pain Med.* 2018;43(5):456–466.
71. Brinck EC, Tiippana E, Heesen M, et al. Perioperative intravenous ketamine for acute postoperative pain in adults. *Cochrane Database Syst Rev.* 2018;12:CD012033.
72. Nielsen RV, Fomsgaard JS, Siegel H, et al. Intraoperative ketamine reduces immediate postoperative opioid consumption after spinal fusion surgery in chronic pain patients with opioid dependency: A randomized, blinded trial. *Pain.* 2017;158(3):463–470.
73. Pendi A, Field R, Farhan SD, Eichler M, Bederman SS. Perioperative ketamine for analgesia in spine surgery: A meta-analysis of randomized controlled trials. *Spine.* 2018;43(5):E299–E307.
74. Nielsen RV, Fomsgaard JS, Nikolajsen L, Dahl JB, Mathiesen O. Intraoperative *S*-ketamine for the reduction of opioid consumption and pain one year after spine surgery: A randomized clinical trial of opioid-dependent patients. *Eur J Pain.* 2019;23(3):455–460.
75. Nikolajsen L, Hansen CL, Nielsen J, Keller J, Arendt-Nielsen L, Jensen TS. The effect of ketamine on phantom pain: A central neuropathic disorder maintained by peripheral input. *Pain.* 1996;67(1):69–77.
76. Eichenberger U, Neff F, Sveticic G, et al. Chronic phantom limb pain: The effects of calcitonin, ketamine, and their combination on pain and sensory thresholds. *Anesth Analg.* 2008;106(4):1265–1273.
77. Guillou N, Tanguy M, Seguin P, Branger B, Campion JP, Mallédant Y. The effects of small-dose ketamine on morphine consumption in surgical intensive care unit patients after major abdominal surgery. *Anesth Analg.* 2003;97(3):843–847.
78. Eikermann M, Grosse-Sundrup M, Zaremba S, et al. Ketamine activates breathing and abolishes the coupling between loss of consciousness and upper airway dilator muscle dysfunction. *Anesthesiology.* 2012;116(1):35–46.
79. Buchheit JL, Yeh DD, Eikermann M, Lin H. Impact of low-dose ketamine on the usage of continuous opioid infusion for the treatment of pain in adult mechanically ventilated patients in surgical intensive care units. *J Intensive Care Med.* 2019;34(8):646–651.
80. Jung H, Lee J, Ahn HY, et al. Safety and feasibility of continuous ketamine infusion for analgosedation in medical and cardiac ICU patients who received mechanical ventilation support: A retrospective cohort study. *PLoS One.* 2022;17(9):e0274865.
81. Pruskowski KA, Harbourt K, Pajoumand M, Chui SHJ, Reynolds HN. Impact of ketamine use on adjunctive analgesic and sedative medications in critically ill trauma patients. *Pharmacotherapy.* 2017;37(12):1537–1544.
82. Zeiler FA, Teitelbaum J, West M, Gillman LM. The ketamine effect on ICP in traumatic brain injury. *Neurocrit Care.* 2014;21(1):163–173.
83. Yang X, Wei X, Mu Y, Li Q, Liu J. A review of the mechanism of the central analgesic effect of lidocaine. *Medicine.* 2020;99(17):e19898.

84. Koppert W, Ostermeier N, Sittl R, Weidner C, Schmelz M. Low-dose lidocaine reduces secondary hyperalgesia by a central mode of action. *Pain.* 2000;85(1–2):217–224.
85. Weinberg L. Pharmacokinetics and pharmacodynamics of lignocaine: A review. *World J Anesthesiol.* 2015;4(2):17–29.
86. Farag E, Ghobrial M, Sessler DI, et al. Effect of perioperative intravenous lidocaine administration on pain, opioid consumption, and quality of life after complex spine surgery. *Anesthesiology.* 2013;119(4):932–940.
87. Groudine SB, Fisher HA, Kaufman RP Jr, et al. Intravenous lidocaine speeds the return of bowel function, decreases postoperative pain, and shortens hospital stay in patients undergoing radical retropubic prostatectomy. *Anesth Analg.* 1998;86(2):235–239.
88. Terkawi AS, Tsang S, Kazemi A, et al. A clinical comparison of intravenous and epidural local anesthetic for major abdominal surgery. *Reg Anesth Pain Med.* 2016;41(1):28–36.
89. Swenson BR, Gottschalk A, Wells LT, et al. Intravenous lidocaine is as effective as epidural bupivacaine in reducing ileus duration, hospital stay, and pain after open colon resection: A randomized clinical trial. *Reg Anesth Pain Med.* 2010;35(4):370–376.
90. Terkawi AS, Sharma S, Durieux ME, Thammishetti S, Brenin D, Tiouririne M. Perioperative lidocaine infusion reduces the incidence of post-mastectomy chronic pain: A double-blind, placebo-controlled randomized trial. *Pain Physician.* 2015;18(2):E139–E146.
91. Foo I, Macfarlane AJR, Srivastava D, et al. The use of intravenous lidocaine for postoperative pain and recovery: International consensus statement on efficacy and safety. *Anaesthesia.* 2021;76(2):238–250.
92. Christie LE, Picard J, Weinberg GL. Local anaesthetic systemic toxicity. *Contin Educ Anaesth Crit Care Pain.* 2015;15(3):136–142.
93. Guo TZ, Jiang JY, Buttermann AE, Maze M. Dexmedetomidine injection into the locus ceruleus produces antinociception. *Anesthesiology.* 1996;84(4):873–881.
94. Wang X, Liu N, Chen J, Xu Z, Wang F, Ding C. Effect of intravenous dexmedetomidine during general anesthesia on acute postoperative pain in adults: A systematic review and meta-analysis of randomized controlled trials. *Clin J Pain.* 2018;34(12):1180–1191.
95. Schmidt PC, Ruchelli G, Mackey SC, Carroll IR. Perioperative gabapentinoids: Choice of agent, dose, timing, and effects on chronic postsurgical pain. *Anesthesiology.* 2013;119(5):1215–1221.
96. Cavalcante AN, Sprung J, Schroeder DR, Weingarten TN. Multimodal analgesic therapy with gabapentin and its association with postoperative respiratory depression. *Anesth Analg.* 2017;125(1):141–146.
97. Coller JK, Christrup LL, Somogyi AA. Role of active metabolites in the use of opioids. *Eur J Clin Pharmacol.* 2009;65(2):121–139.
98. Wang PP, Huang E, Feng X, et al. Opioid-associated iatrogenic withdrawal in critically ill adult patients: A multicenter prospective observational study. *Ann Intensive Care.* 2017;7(1): Article 88.
99. Hyun DG, Huh JW, Hong SB, Koh Y, Lim CM. Iatrogenic opioid withdrawal syndrome in critically ill patients: A retrospective cohort study. *J Korean Med Sci.* 2020;35(15):e106.
100. Gadsden J, Warlick A. Regional anesthesia for the trauma patient: Improving patient outcomes. *Local Reg Anesth.* 2015;8:45–55.
101. Guay J, Kopp S. Epidural pain relief versus systemic opioid-based pain relief for abdominal aortic surgery. *Cochrane Database Syst Rev.* 2016;2016(1):CD005059.
102. Capdevila M, Ramin S, Capdevila X. Regional anesthesia and analgesia after surgery in ICU. *Curr Opin Crit Care.* 2017;23(5):430–439.
103. Richman JM, Liu SS, Courpas G, et al. Does continuous peripheral nerve block provide superior pain control to opioids? A meta-analysis. *Anesth Analg.* 2006;102(1):248–257.
104. von Hösslin T, Imboden P, Lüthi A, Rozanski MJ, Schnider TW, Filipovic M. Adverse events of postoperative thoracic epidural analgesia. *Eur J Anaesthesiol.* 2016;33(10):708–714.
105. De Pinto M, Dagal A, O'Donnell B, Stogicza A, Chiu S, Edwards WT. Regional anesthesia for management of acute pain in the intensive care unit. *Int J Crit Illn Inj Sci.* 2015;5(3):138–143.

106. Capdevila X, Moulard S, Plasse C, et al. Effectiveness of epidural analgesia, continuous surgical site analgesia, and patient-controlled analgesic morphine for postoperative pain management and hyperalgesia, rehabilitation, and health-related quality of life after open nephrectomy: A prospective, randomized, controlled study. *Anesth Analg.* 2017;124(1):336–345.
107. Bomberg H, Bayer I, Wagenpfeil S, et al. Prolonged catheter use and infection in regional anesthesia: A retrospective registry analysis. *Anesthesiology.* 2018;128(4):764–773.
108. Carrier FM, Turgeon AF, Nicole PC, et al. Effect of epidural analgesia in patients with traumatic rib fractures: A systematic review and meta-analysis of randomized controlled trials. *Can J Anaesth.* 2009;56(3):230–242.
109. Casati A, Alessandrini P, Nuzzi M, et al. A prospective, randomized, blinded comparison between continuous thoracic paravertebral and epidural infusion of 0.2% ropivacaine after lung resection surgery. *Eur J Anaesthesiol.* 2006;23(12):999–1004.
110. Mohta M, Verma P, Saxena AK, Sethi AK, Tyagi A, Girotra G. Prospective, randomized comparison of continuous thoracic epidural and thoracic paravertebral infusion in patients with unilateral multiple fractured ribs—A pilot study. *J Trauma Acute Care Surg.* 2009;66(4):1096–1101.
111. Bernards CM, Hadzic A, Suresh S, Neal JM. Regional anesthesia in anesthetized or heavily sedated patients. *Reg Anesth Pain Med.* 2008;33(5):449–460.
112. Walker BJ, Long JB, Sathyamoorthy M, et al. Complications in pediatric regional anesthesia: An analysis of more than 100,000 blocks from the Pediatric Regional Anesthesia Network. *Anesthesiology.* 2018;129(4):721–732.
113. Wiebalck A, Grau T. Ultrasound imaging techniques for regional blocks in intensive care patients. *Crit Care Med.* 2007;35(5 Suppl):S268–S274.

33
Pain in the Emergency Room

Michael Lynch

Introduction

The emergency department (ED) presents unique sets of challenges and circumstances for patients and providers alike. The ED is the proverbial "melting pot" of patients and disease conditions. Patients from all socioeconomic classes, payer groups, and with all conceivable disease states arrive at the same triage window or through the same ambulance bay. EDs serve as a safety net for patients when they are unable to access alternative means of health care delivery. Although the circumstances of the visits and disease states that prompt patients to seek care may differ significantly, all patients share the motivating urge that medical evaluation and treatment are needed immediately. In this sense, all conditions, including pain, managed in the ED are acute even when they are parts of chronic disease. Considerations that have been explored throughout this volume relating to age, social determinants, substance use and mental health, various medical conditions, and special circumstances and their contribution to patient vulnerability are all relevant to managing patients in the ED. These factors pose significant challenges in both assessment and treatment of pain in the ED, particularly considering the continuous arrival of new patients who require evaluation and the undifferentiated nature of every new patient seen. Nevertheless, emergency medicine as a specialty has strived to recognize the unique circumstances and contributions to pain experienced by patients and has developed a body of literature to support safe and effective interventions to alleviate the suffering of people seeking emergency care.[1]

Evidence for Vulnerability

The determination of vulnerability is not clearly or consistently defined. From a population perspective, vulnerability is frequently represented in terms of communities based on characteristics of its constituents and the accessibility of resources. At the individual patient level, vulnerability is more nuanced than broadly applied population-level data. Relative vulnerability likely varies for the same individual based on a number of intrinsic and extrinsic factors. According to Sossauer et al.,[2] "Vulnerable individuals are those who are more likely to have their interests unjustly considered." Within that broad definition, their group identified five domains that influenced a patient's vulnerability: the health care system, patient characteristics, the physician caring for the patient, the treatment being considered, and communication between patient and provider. In clinical practice, a mismatch between patient needs and the care made available to the patient determines the patient's vulnerability.

The health care system creates patterns of vulnerability because individuals have unequal access to care based on insurance coverage and wealth. Socioeconomic factors are consistently cited barriers to accessing health care.[3] In 2021, 13.5% of Americans aged 18–64 years were uninsured, and another 21.7% were enrolled in a public health care coverage program.[4] Insurance status is commonly used as a surrogate for other socioeconomic factors and has historically been cited as a contributing factor to ED utilization, with the prevailing narrative being that patients without insurance are more likely to present to the ED and likely to have more advanced disease as a result of inadequate access to outpatient medical care. Interestingly, this narrative has been challenged, and published data are conflicting.[5,6] Despite having access to outpatient care, publicly insured adults and patients with Medicaid coverage have a higher rate of ED visits and serious illness requiring hospitalization compared to privately insured individuals and those who are uninsured.[6,7] These findings suggest higher vulnerability and intensity of chronic disease among publicly insured and Medicaid patients. Patients representing racial and ethnic minorities as well as those living in socioeconomically depressed neighborhoods have increased preventable ED utilization regardless of health care coverage.[5] Race is associated with increased ED utilization, which is, unfortunately, consistent with disparities encountered throughout U.S. society. The overall ED visit rate for non-Hispanic Black individuals is approximately twice the rate for non-Hispanic White individuals.[7] Many ED visits could be avoided through readily accessible outpatient care.[5] Preventable ED visits indicate a level of vulnerability because they are likely related to a real or perceived lack of alternative non-emergency care options.

In addition to patient-centered characteristics and inequities in the health care system, provider characteristics and attitudes also contribute to vulnerability experienced by patients. The presence of bias among health care providers has been demonstrated across disciplines and treatment environments.[8] Race is a common source of bias, although other factors, such as gender and gender identity, age, sexual orientation, ethnicity, religion, disability, and socioeconomic status, are also frequently reported.[9] These biases are often unrecognized or implicit. Bias has been shown in multiple studies to negatively impact patient–provider relationships, patient satisfaction, treatment decisions, and outcomes.[10] Bias is not uniform and may be variably encountered depending on the individual provider and patient.

The ED environment dictates that patient care is delivered at a rapid pace, which introduces systematic patient vulnerability because provider attention is divided and available to a given patient for only a brief assessment that is typically focused on the primary complaint rather than a holistic evaluation of the patient's entire medical history as may be accomplished in a scheduled outpatient setting. These pressures are further exacerbated during times of crowding and ED boarding of admitted patients. ED crowding can occur for a number of reasons, including increases in new arrivals or inability to move patients to other care spaces.[11] Following the peak of the COVID-19 global pandemic, staffing pressures in the ED, inpatient units, and long-term care facilities have intensified the impact of crowding and boarding. ED crowding is associated with delays in assessment and care, reduced patient satisfaction, increased staff stress, nonadherence to best practice guidelines, worsened patient outcomes, and increased mortality.[12] Physician burnout has also been increasingly recognized especially among emergency physicians, with deleterious effects on mental health and capacity for compassion. Burnout leads to medical errors, decreased physician and patient satisfaction, physician attrition from the field, provider shortages, and suicide, all of which negatively impact patient care. Burnout is the result a combination of system shortcomings.[13] ED crowding and the pressures on those providing care to patients are completely outside of patients' control yet have an enormous and unanticipated influence on the care they receive and the vulnerability they experience during an ED visit.

Communication barriers can also contribute to vulnerability. These communication barriers may arise due to differences in language or in culture. Language discordance among patients and providers can lead to frustration and increased time spent delivering care.[14] Patients with limited English proficiency are more likely to be harmed than English-proficient patients.[15] In addition to language, cultural differences between providers and patients can lead to misunderstandings, harms, and poor adherence to treatment plans.[16]

In an ideal environment, diagnostic tests and therapeutic interventions would be provided independent of social variables; however, it is well established that many treatment decisions are the result of deliberation that considers both implicit and explicit factors.[9] In some cases, decision-making may be influenced by financial and cultural concerns as well as communication barriers. Many patients avoid or delay seeking care due to concern for the costs and associated medical debt.[17] Although uninsured patients face the largest risk of medical debt, patients in all categories of coverage, including public, private, and employer-based programs, cite finances as a significant barrier.[18] Delays in seeking care can result in presentations with more advanced disease as well as a higher likelihood of seeking unplanned care in an ED with higher cost-sharing burden. Not all individuals bear that burden equitably based on coverage and wealth. Once present in an ED or other care setting, interventions may be tailored to the patient's ability to afford associated costs and co-pays. These considerations impact both the immediate treatment and the long-term plan of care. Due to concerns about impact on cost and the subsequent ED bill, patients and providers may limit diagnostic tests that would otherwise be performed. Patients for whom admission to a hospital or placement in observation status is recommended may decline. Typically, treatment delivered in the ED represents the first step in a therapeutic plan that continues beyond the visit. The nature and trajectory of that plan can be adjusted based on nonmedical factors rather than pure consideration of what would be ideal for a patient. Many patients will not have rapid access to follow-up care either due to network adequacy issues or due to a lack of insurance. Even when insurance is not a barrier, many primary and specialty providers are unavailable for weeks to months following an ED visit, particularly when there is not an established relationship. Additional social determinants must also be considered, including whether a patient has work and/or childcare responsibilities that will impede their ability to engage in ongoing care and adequate access to transportation for appointments. In the setting of pain management, optimal care frequently includes physical and other movement therapies that require regular visits, often during the day. Adhering to that plan may not be an option for many Americans. Advances in pharmacotherapeutics and interventional pain management may offer relief, but those options are not available to some patients. Similarly, alternative and complementary medicine techniques may provide benefit but are frequently not covered by insurance so they require time and personal investment, making access to those services inequitable.

Vulnerability is not static. The factors that contribute to vulnerability are not manifested by the individual alone but, rather, are an amalgamation of components related to individual patients, health care providers, the health care system, and broader social determinants of health. Many of these elements are predictable and consistent across health care and other environments, whereas others may be more or less impactful in a given situation. Due to the ED environment and the nature of illness that typically brings patients to the ED, most patients experience vulnerability and lack of control, but some patients experience that vulnerability to a much greater degree.

Vulnerability and Pain in the Emergency Department

Patients visit EDs for a variety of reasons, but the experience of pain is shared by many who decide to seek urgent care. An estimated three-fourths of patients who are evaluated in EDs are experiencing some degree of pain, with nearly half of those patients reporting a chronic pain condition.[19] Chronic pain is a common condition in the United States, with 20.4% of adults suffering from chronic pain and 7.4% indicating that the pain frequently limits life or work activities.[20] Despite its prevalence, patients living with chronic pain, particularly those receiving opioid therapy, experience stigma that creates barriers to consistent, compassionate care.[21] Due to this stigma, provider fear of oversight by regulatory and law enforcement agencies, and a shortage of pain specialty providers and services, accessing comprehensive multimodal pain care with a focus on improved quality of life and functionality is difficult for patients, particularly those living outside of metropolitan areas.[20,21] Patients living with chronic pain are more likely to visit EDs than are other patients, especially if their chronic pain condition is associated with a higher level of disability.[22] The myriad underlying disease conditions that contribute to both acute pain and acute exacerbations of chronic pain pose a challenge to emergency medicine physicians and advance practice providers. The most appropriate condition-based pain management strategies vary and require expertise. The emergency management of pain is itself a specialized area of medicine that requires understanding of pathophysiology and coordination with specialty providers.

In addition to stigma faced by patients suffering from chronic pain, other common sources of inherent bias and stigma also contribute to inadequate management of pain in EDs. Black and Hispanic patients are less likely to receive analgesic therapy for acute pain in U.S. EDs.[23] Gender differences in the experience and quantification of pain as well as response to treatments also contribute to disparities in ED pain management.[24] Factors including ethnic and cultural differences, socioeconomic status, co-occurring mental health disorders, frequent ED visits, and provider state of mind, among others, can all contribute to a patient's experience of vulnerability and the way in which their pain is managed during an ED visit. Recognizing and striving to minimize the impact of these demonstrated biases is critical to providing equitable care.

Acute pain related to traumatic injuries poses a unique set of challenges with regard to pain care and vulnerability. The nature of injuries sustained from trauma requires multiple potential modalities of pain management interventions, including procedural, pharmaceutical, psychological, and movement therapies. The selection of appropriate treatments is driven by the location and severity of injury as well as the patient's pain response. However, the response to pain is frequently more complex than the physical injury alone. The experience of pain related to injury is complicated by the patient's psychological response to the traumatic experience, which could have included violence or intentional injury. The sudden and unanticipated nature of injuries creates a situation in which patients not only endure the physical injury but also must navigate a complex set of emotions related to the circumstances of the injury, potential injury to other people, and the short- and long-term impact on their lives.[25] These nonphysical dynamics contribute to the patient's perception and experience of pain. For example, some patients may face legal ramifications from the events that led to injury. A patient who has sustained serious physical injuries or is suffering an atraumatic painful acute illness may be concerned about their ability to return to work, pay bills, or provide for their family. Those burdens can be expected to intensify the overall experience of pain and are unlikely to respond to purely pharmaceutical interventions. Regardless of the specific circumstances, a patient's fear, anxiety, and uncertainty are likely to confound and potentiate their physical experience. Although this phenomenon is common, understanding those emotions and expressing their contribution to acute pain can be difficult and may go unrecognized by treating providers, serving to further exacerbate the patient's already vulnerable state. Even when they are recognized, competing demands for provider attention while managing a busy ED can make extended discussion and supportive intervention difficult to deliver.

Traumatic injuries and the related psychological trauma can result in the development of post-traumatic stress disorder (PTSD) in a significant percentage of patients.[26] However, a physical injury is not necessarily required for patients to experience PTSD following an ED visit. Nontraumatic but acutely life-threatening events are also associated with the development of PTSD.[27] Symptoms of PTSD have been linked to chronic pain in both children and adults.[28,29] Vulnerability experienced by patients suffering acutely painful or life-threatening conditions, including traumatic injuries, persists beyond the ED visit and can contribute to ongoing quality of life and functional impairments.

Co-occurring intoxication and substance use disorders are common among ED patients.[30] Patients with changes in mental status due to intoxication or brain injury are vulnerable to their surroundings and unable to communicate, including expression of the degree of pain associated with their injuries. Pain is frequently undertreated or dismissed as part of the patient's underlying substance use disorder, which, paradoxically, can contribute to increased nonmedical substance use in order to manage pain.[31,32] Post-acute treatment of pain in patients with substance use disorders following the ED visit, whether the patient is admitted or discharged, is complex and requires coordination of care and support that is not consistently available throughout the United States.[21]

The ED environment and circumstances that mandate ED utilization complicate the experience of pain regardless of the inciting physiology. Recognizing the complex interplay of personal experiences, physical injuries, psychological confounders, and social influences on a person's perception of pain and response to treatment can inform strategies to achieve analgesia, minimize adverse effects, and optimize long-term outcomes (Figure 33.1).

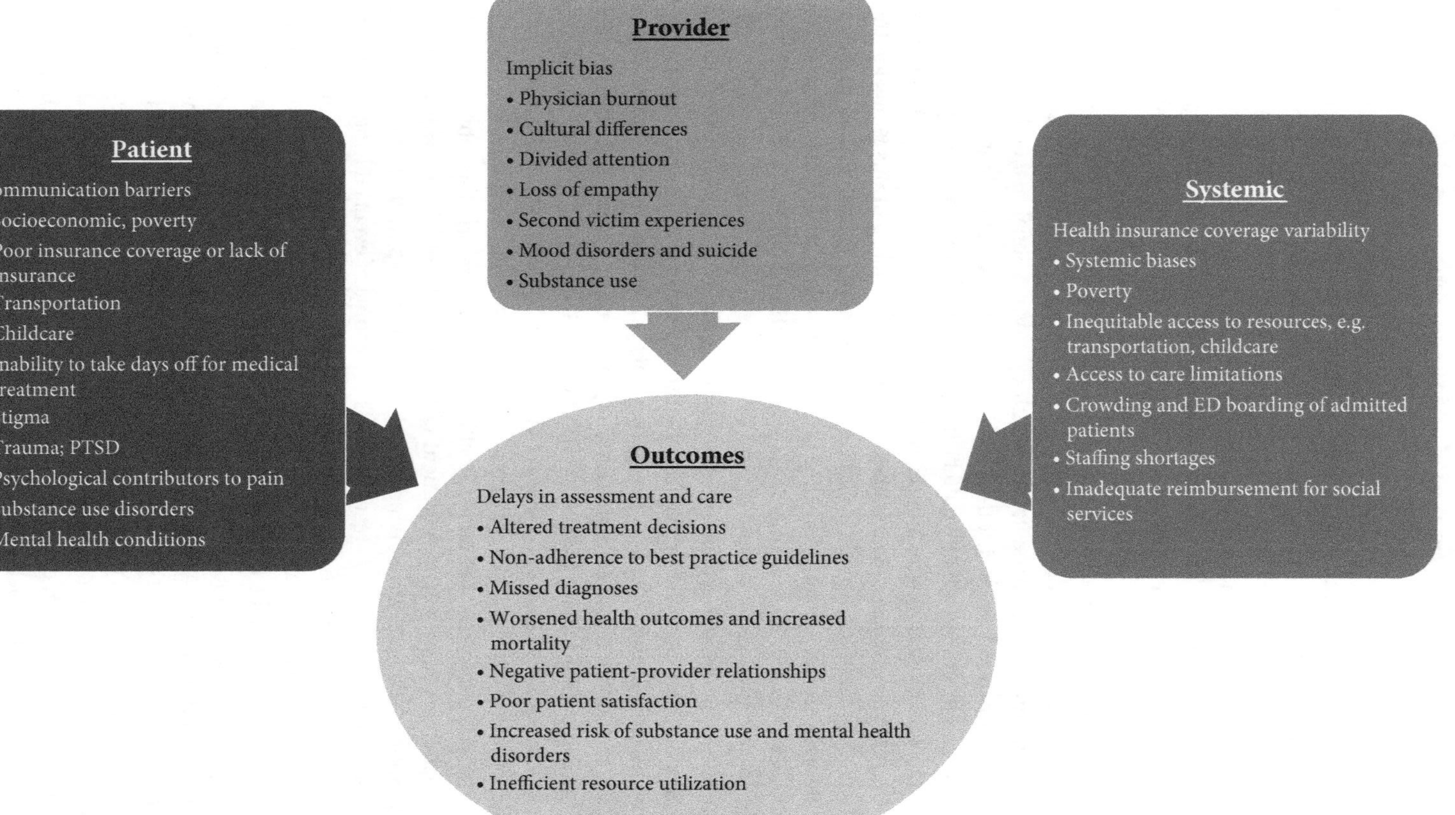

Patient
Communication barriers
• Socioeconomic, poverty
• Poor insurance coverage or lack of insurance
• Transportation
• Childcare
• Inability to take days off for medical treatment
• Stigma
• Trauma; PTSD
• Psychological contributors to pain
• Substance use disorders
• Mental health conditions
Provider
Implicit bias
• Physician burnout
• Cultural differences
• Divided attention
• Loss of empathy
• Second victim experiences
• Mood disorders and suicide
• Substance use
Systemic
Health insurance coverage variability
• Systemic biases
• Poverty
• Inequitable access to resources, e.g. transportation, childcare
• Access to care limitations
• Crowding and ED boarding of admitted patients
• Staffing shortages
• Inadequate reimbursement for social services
Outcomes
Delays in assessment and care
• Altered treatment decisions
• Non-adherence to best practice guidelines
• Missed diagnoses
• Worsened health outcomes and increased mortality
• Negative patient-provider relationships
• Poor patient satisfaction
• Increased risk of substance use and mental health disorders
• Inefficient resource utilization

Figure 33.1 Contributors to ED patient vulnerability and associated outcomes.

Mitigating the Impact of Vulnerability on Emergency Department Pain Management

Once identified, the capacity to address contributing influences of pain and vulnerability beyond the management of nociceptive pain can be challenging. As described above, many issues that result in patient vulnerability in health care and specifically in the ED are symptoms of systemic failures that are outside the control of patients and treatment providers at the time of need. For example, a system that leaves patients uninsured or underinsured, resulting in delays in seeking care or obtaining appropriate treatment due to financial considerations, will require a broad coalition of stakeholders to remediate. Potential solutions require careful thought and consideration of unintended consequences that nearly always complicate even the most well-meaning social interventions. It is critical that health care providers maintain a place in those deliberations to advocate for patients and health care professionals using data-driven, scientific expertise to inform decision-making. Any discussion of patient vulnerability and its impact on health outcomes would be incomplete without recognizing the markedly disparate economic resources and access to insurance coverage among Americans. However, a fulsome discussion of health policy and potential solutions is outside the scope of this chapter. In the current health care environment that assumes the presence of inequalities in access, there are real-time interventions that can address vulnerability and social factors that influence patients' pain and functional outcomes in and after an ED visit.

A critical step in addressing and remediating vulnerability and inequity in the ED is to recognize that they exist and understand that they require specific attention. As has been demonstrated in many fields, true equity is only achieved when interventions are tailored to the individual rather than assuming the same application of services will allow all individuals to achieve the same level of care. All boats will not rise equally, so even greater investment is needed for some patients and in some situations to achieve equity. Recognizing the dignity of each patient is a necessary starting point.

The relationship dynamic between a health care provider—whether physician, advanced practice provider, nurse, or patient care technician—and a patient is fundamentally lopsided. Patients must divulge deeply personal and potentially embarrassing information while the health care team controls the course of events during that interaction. This dynamic places patients in a position of extreme vulnerability in any health care environment, but particularly in an ED. Understanding that basic asymmetry helps guide an approach that seeks to minimize the imbalance by helping patients feel as though they have agency in the course of their evaluation and treatment. Simple actions such as sitting while talking to a patient to put yourself at the same level can improve the perception of caring and understanding. For patients who are unable to move positions, a provider can adjust their own position in order to maintain eye contact while speaking with and listening to the patient.[27] Despite the many competing priorities and demands, ED providers should try to take time to ensure that patients feel heard by asking open-ended questions as well as acknowledging and validating patients' stated concerns. Body language is also important.[33] Appearing distracted, closed off, angry, frustrated, or bored will only serve to alienate patients and contribute to a negative experience. As it relates to pain care, prioritizing assessment of pain and response to interventions is key. Utilization of care guidelines developed for specific pain complaints can minimize variability in treatment and reduce the risk of provider bias. Specific interventions will depend on multiple considerations and may not always comport with the patient's expectations. However, providing compassionate, detailed explanations of the decision-making process supports a patient's understanding of the care plan, which in turn improves outcomes.[34] A patient's perception of compassion by the treating physician reduces the risk of post-traumatic stress symptoms and associated pain independent of any other intervention.[27] Although these approaches may seem straightforward and self-evident, they are frequently neglected during the course of delivering care in a busy ED. Intentional incorporation of these basic interventions can improve care and minimize vulnerability with only a small investment of time and thought.

Emergency departments serve individuals of all backgrounds and circumstance, introducing the potential for bias to influence decision-making. In order to address stigma and bias, health care providers must first recognize and acknowledge that these are present.[35] Such recognition requires self-evaluation that can be difficult and frequently requires guidance from an external source to avoid confirmed bias stemming from unchallenged preconceived beliefs. Once recognized, education regarding the circumstances and experiences of others promotes empathy. Health care providers can then be in a better position to express understanding of the struggles patients might face both within the health care system and in society as a whole, which can inform treatment and decision-making. Moreover, advocating on behalf of patients to other team members and staff promotes a more welcoming and supportive environment, thereby minimizing adverse outcomes and experiences related to stigma.[16,36] Individual efforts to recognize and address bias are strongly encouraged, but intentional commitment by health care systems to ensure cultural competence, including diversity, equity, and inclusion training, should also be implemented.[9,37,38]

Most of a patient's vulnerability is the product of external factors applied to the individual rather than factors under the control of the patient. As such, it is important to reflect those inequities when collaborating with a patient to identify the best plan of care and to avoid a potentially paternalistic approach that further subjugates a patient to the power of the provider and the health care system as a whole.[39] Despite being well-intended, efforts to define and address perceived vulnerabilities without taking into account external variables and patient preferences risk the loss of patient autonomy, which could paradoxically potentiate the experience of vulnerability. One way to address this risk is through shared decision-making, emphasizing the patient's role in their own health care and providing some control and agency over their treatment course.[40] Shared decision-making is not always possible, but it should be used as a framework to guide provider–patient discussion of treatment in the ED when feasible.[41] In order to truly integrate the patient into the treatment and decision-making process, two-way communication must be ensured.

Failures in communication are frequently at the root of disputes and negative health care interactions. Language barriers are an obvious source of communication failure. Trained medical foreign language interpreters and individuals proficient in American Sign Language must be available and utilized. Although relying on translation by family members or potentially limited communication with a patient who has some English language skills can be tempting due to time constraints, such communication can result in errors, inefficient resource utilization, excessive testing, and missed diagnoses.[42] Beyond pure language barriers, cultural considerations regarding the meaning of words and phrases as well as variation in goals of care and anticipated outcomes can also impede the ability of both patients and health care providers to fully understand the intended message of the other. In addition to cultural competency training, taking time to ensure that all parties have the same understanding of available information and goals of care is important. In some fields, cultural brokers have been employed to bridge communication gaps.[43] The pace and patient diversity of the ED do not offer an ideal environment for the employment of cultural brokers, but the concept of educating providers and staff regarding cultural diversity in the community they serve, including anticipating potential areas for miscommunication, can help alleviate bias and improve patient experience and outcomes while potentially limiting unnecessary resource utilization.[38]

Much of the responsibility for addressing inequities and vulnerabilities in ED care delivery is placed on the health care providers themselves. As such, it is critical to optimize the environment in which they work. Loss of empathy during the course of a health care provider's career is often present.[44] Factors such as stress, burnout, and ED overcrowding also negatively impact the health and well-being of the members of the health care team, which is reflected in their interactions with patients.[12,13] There has been increased recognition of burnout, second victim experiences, mood disorders, substance use, and suicide among physicians and other health care providers.[45–47] In order to deliver compassionate care to all patients, particularly those who are most vulnerable, systematic efforts to support the professionals who provide that care must be prioritized, including peer support programs, access to confidential mental health services, adequate time away from work, and recognition of their value, among other interventions.[47]

Given the complex nature of pain and the contributions of nonphysical factors, incorporation of treatment approaches targeted to address those aspects of the pain experience would be expected to improve patient outcomes. Treating patients through a framework of trauma-informed care recognizes that many patients seeking care in the ED are suffering physical and/or emotional trauma as a part of their condition.[48] Limiting evaluation and treatment to the physical manifestations of the injury or illness, particularly when associated with the experience of pain, misses an opportunity to provide a more holistic therapeutic experience for the patient in which their concerns and fears are heard, validated, and addressed. By addressing these fears and concerns, a provider can minimize the state of vulnerability experienced by the patient and reduce the impact of post-traumatic symptoms.[27] The biopsychosocial model of health care delivery is well established as an optimal approach to address complex pathology. Psychological interventions including cognitive–behavioral therapy and acceptance and commitment therapy delivered via face-to-face, group, or asynchronous modalities have all been associated with improved pain relief and functional outcomes in the setting of chronic pain.[49,50] However, these interventions have not been evaluated in the emergency setting.[51] The compressed time frame of a typical ED encounter as well as the constant influx of patients suffering diverse illnesses and injuries are not conducive to complex, structured cognitive and psychological interventions. Nevertheless, brief interventions, motivational interviewing, and referral for comprehensive multimodal pain management services including pain psychology should be incorporated into emergency care.[21]

Screening for co-occurring mental health and substance use disorders should also be considered when formulating a treatment plan during and subsequent to the ED visit. Mental health and substance use disorders are contributing factors to vulnerability, pain, worsened medical outcomes, and increased health care utilization yet are frequently underrecognized let alone treated.[52] The ED represents the first or only contact with the health care system for many adults. Studies evaluating the prevalence of both substance use and mental health disorders in ED patients have demonstrated that the actual rates are much higher than what is reflected in documentation, making active screening to identify co-occurring substance use and mental health disorders recommended in all ED patients.[53,54] This is especially true for patients who will require pain management; untreated mental health and substance use disorders contribute to increased intensity and duration of pain as well as risk associated with treatment, particularly the maladaptive utilization of controlled substances.[55,56] The presence of these disorders should not preclude the appropriate management of pain, but recognition of the elevated risk should prompt open dialogue of potential risks and benefits with the patient; consideration of alternative pharmaceutical treatments when appropriate; assurance of close follow-up to reassess response to treatment; and, most important, initiation of treatment with rapid referral to behavioral health and/or substance use specialty treatment providers, ideally through a warm handoff process.[57,58]

The ED represents a critical focal point in the health care system where patients from all backgrounds and with all disease states receive care regardless of insurance, wealth, or cultural background. Although that episode of engagement represents a tremendous opportunity to influence the trajectory of care for patients, the demand also creates a strain on available resources. Efforts should be made to optimize health care delivery in the ED, but equally important is the need to enhance the systems of care preceding and subsequent to that emergency visit to create a more seamless continuum of care.[59] The goal of the health care system should be to minimize the need for emergency care through proactive recognition of worsening chronic disease, injury prevention, and access to primary care. In addition, patients who require emergency care will frequently need expedited follow-up to assess their response to treatment and provision of ongoing therapy to optimize return to function and reduce the likelihood of returning to the ED unnecessarily.[60] Many patients will require assistance managing social issues that influence their ability to access care. These issues may include lack of insurance, stable housing, and access to transportation; employment concerns; childcare needs; and many more. Complex social determinants of health cannot be resolved during a several-hour ED visit, but if they are not addressed at all, then it is predictable that they will continue to impede an individual's recovery and return to function. Therefore, care coordination and social work consultation are a critical part of an emergency visit to provide resources and initiate connection to support for these diverse nonmedical patient needs.[61] In ideal circumstances, all EDs would have 24/7 access to social services providers. However, many EDs do not have the resources to make those services continuously available to patients within the current reimbursement structure. Future considerations of a value-based payment approach to providing quality care, including in the ED, may offer an opportunity to more comprehensively address the medical and nonmedical needs of ED patients.[62]

Conclusion

Emergency department patients are frequently experiencing both physical and psychological pain. Complicating that experience is a condition of vulnerability. Vulnerability is complex and, for the most part, outside the control of the patients themselves. Therefore, it is incumbent upon the health care system and its constituents to recognize and ameliorate conditions that contribute to a patient's vulnerability to the greatest extent possible. These interventions should account for the inherent dignity of each patient and recognition that vulnerability is primarily a failure of the system of care rather than factors under the individual's control (Table 33.1). The role of a health care provider is to not only consider the objective data but also integrate that information with the overall condition of the person who is experiencing illness. Providing the best possible care to a patient with a goal of improving health rather than simply mitigating disease involves health care providers and the system in which they operate taking a holistic approach that includes recognition and palliation of elements that contribute to a patient's vulnerability.

Table 33.1 Summary of Interventions to Address and Mitigate Patient Vulnerability

Recognize dignity in every patient	Ensure access to health care and coverage
Sit while speaking with patients; eye contact, body language	Open-ended questions; listening and validation
Assessment of pain and response to interventions	Guideline-based therapy to minimize bias and optimize care
Shared decision-making	Detailed explanation of medical decision-making
Compassion and empathy	Bias recognition and diversity awareness
Model nonbiased, nonstigma behavior	Screening and referral for mental health and substance use disorder care
Intentional commitment by health care systems to ensure cultural competence, including diversity, equity, and inclusion training	Systematic efforts to support health care professionals—for example, peer support programs, access to confidential mental health services, adequate time away from work, and recognition of their value
Care coordination/social work to address social determinants of health, including adequate reimbursement for services	Improved transitions of care and community-based access to care

References

1. Motov S, Strayer R, Hayes BD, et al. The treatment of acute pain in the emergency department: A white paper position statement prepared for the American Academy of Emergency Medicine. *J Emerg Med.* 2018;54(5):731–736. doi:10.1016/j.jemermed.2018.01.020
2. Sossauer L, Schindler M, Hurst S. Vulnerability identified in clinical practice: A qualitative analysis. *BMC Med Ethics.* 2019;20(1): Article 87. doi:10.1186/s12910-019-0416-4
3. Daniel H, Bornstein SS, Kane GC; Health and Public Policy Committee of the American College of Physicians; Carney JK, Gantzer HE, Henry TL, et al. Addressing social determinants to improve patient care and promote health equity: An American College of Physicians position paper. *Ann Intern Med.* 2018;168(8):577–578. doi:10.7326/M17-2441
4. Cohen RA, Cha AE, Terlizzi EP, Martinez ME. Health insurance coverage: Early release of estimates from the National Health Interview Survey, 2021. National Center for Health Statistics; 2022. https://www.cdc.gov/nchs/data/nhis/earlyrelease/insur202205.pdf
5. Carlson LC, Zachrison KS, Yun BJ, et al. The association of demographic, socioeconomic, and geographic factors with potentially preventable emergency department utilization. *West J Emerg Med.* 2021;22(6):1283–1290. doi:10.5811/westjem.2021.5.50233
6. Zhou RA, Baicker K, Taubman S, Finkelstein AN. The uninsured do not use the emergency department more—They use other care less. *Health Aff.* 2017;36(12):2115–2122. doi:10.1377/hlthaff.2017.0218
7. Cairns C, Ashman JJ, Kang K. Emergency department visit rates by selected characteristics: United States, 2019. *NCHS Data Brief.* 2022;(434):1–8.
8. Hall WJ, Chapman MV, Lee KM, et al. Implicit racial/ethnic bias among health care professionals and its influence on health care outcomes: A systematic review. *Am J Public Health.* 2015;105(12):e60–e76. doi:10.2105/AJPH.2015.302903
9. Marcelin JR, Siraj DS, Victor R, Kotadia S, Maldonado YA. The impact of unconscious bias in healthcare: How to recognize and mitigate it. *J Infect Dis.* 2019;220(220 Suppl 2):S62–S73. doi:10.1093/infdis/jiz214
10. Sabin JA. Tackling implicit bias in health care. *N Engl J Med.* 2022;387(2):105–107. doi:10.1056/NEJMp2201180
11. Savioli G, Ceresa IF, Gri N, et al. Emergency department overcrowding: Understanding the factors to find corresponding solutions. *J Pers Med.* 2022;12(2): Article 279. doi:10.3390/jpm12020279
12. Morley C, Unwin M, Peterson GM, Stankovich J, Kinsman L. Emergency department crowding: A systematic review of causes, consequences and solutions. *PLoS One.* 2018;13(8):e0203316. doi:10.1371/journal.pone.0203316
13. Stehman CR, Testo Z, Gershaw RS, Kellogg AR. Burnout, drop out, suicide: Physician loss in emergency medicine, Part I. *West J Emerg Med.* 2019;20(3):485–494. doi:10.5811/westjem.2019.4.40970
14. Ngo-Metzger Q, Sorkin DH, Phillips RS, et al. Providing high-quality care for limited English proficient patients: The importance of language concordance and interpreter use. *J Gen Intern Med.* 2007;22(Suppl 2):324–330. doi:10.1007/s11606-007-0340-z
15. Divi C, Koss RG, Schmaltz SP, Loeb JM. Language proficiency and adverse events in US hospitals: A pilot study. *Int J Qual Health Care.* 2007;19(2):60–67.
16. Brach C, Fraser I. Reducing disparities through culturally competent health care: An analysis of the business case. *Qual Manag Health Care.* 2002;10(4):15–28.
17. Tipirneni R, Politi MC, Kullgren JT, Kieffer EC, Goold SD, Scherer AM. Association between health insurance literacy and avoidance of health care services owing to cost. *JAMA Netw Open.* 2018;1(7):e184796. doi:10.1001/jamanetworkopen.2018.4796
18. Wray CM, Khare M, Keyhani S. Access to care, cost of care, and satisfaction with care among adults with private and public health insurance in the US. *JAMA Netw Open.* 2021;4(6):e2110275. doi:10.1001/jamanetworkopen.2021.10275

19. Todd KH, Cowan P, Kelly N, Homel P. Chronic or recurrent pain in the emergency department: National telephone survey of patient experience. *West J Emerg Med.* 2010;11(5):408–415.
20. Zelaya CE, Dahlhamer JM, Lucas JW, Connor EM. Chronic pain and high-impact chronic pain among U.S. adults, 2019. *NCHS Data Brief.* 2020;(390):1–8.
21. U.S. Department of Health and Human Services. Pain Management Best Practices Inter-Agency Task Force Report: Updates, gaps, inconsistencies, and recommendations. 2019. https://www.hhs.gov/sites/default/files/pmtf-final-report-2019-05-23.pdf
22. Dépelteau A, Racine-Hemmings F, Lagueux É, Hudon C. Chronic pain and frequent use of emergency department: A systematic review. *Am J Emerg Med.* 2020;38(2):358–363. doi:10.1016/j.ajem.2019.158492
23. Lee P, Le Saux M, Siegel R, et al. Racial and ethnic disparities in the management of acute pain in US emergency departments: Meta-analysis and systematic review. *Am J Emerg Med.* 2019;37(9):1770–1777. doi:10.1016/j.ajem.2019.06.014
24. Musey PI Jr, Linnstaedt SD, Platts-Mills TF, et al. Gender differences in acute and chronic pain in the emergency department: Results of the 2014 Academic Emergency Medicine Consensus Conference Pain Section. *Acad Emerg Med.* 2014;21(12):1421–1430. doi:10.1111/acem.12529
25. Ahmadi A, Bazargan-Hejazi S, Heidari Zadie Z, et al. Pain management in trauma: A review study. *J Inj Violence Res.* 2016;8(2):89–98. doi:10.5249/jivr.v8i2.707
26. Joseph NM, Benedick A, Flanagan CD, Breslin MA, Vallier HA. Risk factors for posttraumatic stress disorder in acute trauma patients. *J Orthop Trauma.* 2021;35(6):e209–e215. doi:10.1097/BOT.0000000000001990
27. Moss J, Roberts MB, Shea L, et al. Healthcare provider compassion is associated with lower PTSD symptoms among patients with life-threatening medical emergencies: A prospective cohort study. *Intensive Care Med.* 2019;45(6):815–822. doi:10.1007/s00134-019-05601-5
28. Gasperi M, Afari N, Goldberg J, Suri P, Panizzon MS. Pain and trauma: The role of Criterion A trauma and stressful life events in the pain and PTSD relationship. *J Pain.* 2021;22(11):1506–1517. doi:10.1016/j.jpain.2021.04.015
29. van Meijel EPM, Gigengack MR, Verlinden E, et al. The association between acute pain and posttraumatic stress symptoms in children and adolescents 3 months after accidental injury. *J Clin Psychol Med Settings.* 2019;26(1):88–96. doi:10.1007/s10880-018-9567-6
30. London JA, Battistella FD. Testing for substance use in trauma patients: Are we doing enough? *Arch Surg.* 2007;142(7):633–638. doi:10.1001/archsurg.142.7.633
31. Speed TJ, Parekh V, Coe W, Antoine D. Comorbid chronic pain and opioid use disorder: Literature review and potential treatment innovations. *Int Rev Psychiatry.* 2018;30(5):136–146. doi:10.1080/09540261.2018.1514369
32. Coffin PO, Rowe C, Oman N, et al. Illicit opioid use following changes in opioids prescribed for chronic non-cancer pain. *PLoS One.* 2020;15(5):e0232538. doi:10.1371/journal.pone.0232538
33. Patel S, Pelletier-Bui A, Smith S, et al. Curricula for empathy and compassion training in medical education: A systematic review. *PLoS One.* 2019;14(8):e0221412. doi:10.1371/journal.pone.0221412
34. Hua J, Howell JL, Sweeny K, Andrews SE. Outcomes of physicians' communication goals during patient interactions. *Health Commun.* 2021;36(7):847–855. doi:10.1080/10410236.2020.1719321
35. Bucknor-Ferron P, Zagaja L. Five strategies to combat unconscious bias. *Nursing.* 2016;46(11):61–62. doi:10.1097/01.NURSE.0000490226.81218.6c
36. van Boekel LC, Brouwers EP, van Weeghel J, Garretsen HF. Stigma among health professionals towards patients with substance use disorders and its consequences for healthcare delivery: Systematic review. *Drug Alcohol Depend.* 2013;131(1–2):23–35. doi:10.1016/j.drugalcdep.2013.02.018

37. Truong M, Paradies Y, Priest N. Interventions to improve cultural competency in healthcare: A systematic review of reviews. *BMC Health Serv Res*. 2014;14: Article 99. doi:10.1186/1472-6963-14-99
38. Mechanic OJ, Dubosh NM, Rosen CL, Landry AM. Cultural competency training in emergency medicine. *J Emerg Med*. 2017;53(3):391–396. doi:10.1016/j.jemermed.2017.04.019
39. Clark B, Preto N. Exploring the concept of vulnerability in health care. *CMAJ*. 2018;190(11):E308–E309. doi:10.1503/cmaj.180242
40. Castaneda-Guarderas A, Glassberg J, Grudzen CR, et al. Shared decision making with vulnerable populations in the emergency department. *Acad Emerg Med*. 2016;23(12):1410–1416. doi:10.1111/acem.13134
41. Probst MA, Kanzaria HK, Schoenfeld EM, et al. Shared decisionmaking in the emergency department: A guiding framework for clinicians. *Ann Emerg Med*. 2017;70(5):688–695. doi:10.1016/j.annemergmed.2017.03.063
42. Wasserman M, Renfrew MR, Green AR, et al. Identifying and preventing medical errors in patients with limited English proficiency: Key findings and tools for the field. *J Healthc Qual*. 2014;36(3):5–16. doi:10.1111/jhq.12065
43. Alexander GK, Uz SW, Hinton I, Williams I, Jones R. Culture brokerage strategies in diabetes education. *Public Health Nurs*. 2008;25(5):461–470.
44. Kelm Z, Womer J, Walter JK, Feudtner C. Interventions to cultivate physician empathy: A systematic review. *BMC Med Educ*. 2014;14: Article 219. doi:10.1186/1472-6920-14-219
45. Seys D, Wu AW, Van Gerven E, et al. Health care professionals as second victims after adverse events: A systematic review. *Eval Health Prof*. 2013;36(2):135–162. doi:10.1177/0163278712458918
46. Dutheil F, Aubert C, Pereira B, et al. Suicide among physicians and health-care workers: A systematic review and meta-analysis. *PLoS One*. 2019;14(12):e0226361. doi:10.1371/journal.pone.0226361
47. Melnyk BM, Kelly SA, Stephens J, et al. Interventions to improve mental health, well-being, physical health, and lifestyle behaviors in physicians and nurses: A systematic review. *Am J Health Promot*. 2020;34(8):929–941. doi:10.1177/0890117120920451
48. Fischer KR, Bakes KM, Corbin TJ, et al. Trauma-informed care for violently injured patients in the emergency department. *Ann Emerg Med*. 2019;73(2):193–202. doi:10.1016/j.annemergmed.2018.10.018
49. Hoffman BM, Papas RK, Chatkoff DK, Kerns RD. Meta-analysis of psychological interventions for chronic low back pain. *Health Psychol*. 2007;26(1):1–9. doi:10.1037/0278-6133.26.1.1
50. Hughes LS, Clark J, Colclough JA, Dale E, McMillan D. Acceptance and commitment therapy (ACT) for chronic pain: A systematic review and meta-analyses. *Clin J Pain*. 2017;33(6):552–568. doi:10.1097/AJP.0000000000000425
51. Optimizing the treatment of acute pain in the emergency department. *Ann Emerg Med*. 2017;70(3):446–448. doi:10.1016/j.annemergmed.2017.06.043
52. Kamal R, Cox C, Rousseau D; Kaiser Family Foundation. Costs and outcomes of mental health and substance use disorders in the US. *JAMA*. 2017;318(5): Article 415. doi:10.1001/jama.2017.8558
53. Hawk K, D'Onofrio G. Emergency department screening and interventions for substance use disorders [Erratum in: Addict Sci Clin Pract. 2019 Jul 16;14(1):26]. *Addict Sci Clin Pract*. 2018;13(1): Article 18. doi:10.1186/s13722-018-0117-1
54. Kene M, Miller Rosales C, Wood S, Rauchwerger AS, Vinson DR, Sterling SA. Feasibility of expanded emergency department screening for behavioral health problems. *Am J Manag Care*. 2018;24(12):585–591.
55. Onwumere J, Stubbs B, Stirling M, et al. Pain management in people with severe mental illness: An agenda for progress. *Pain*. 2022;163(9):1653–1660. doi:10.1097/j.pain.0000000000002633
56. Quinlan J, Cox F. Acute pain management in patients with drug dependence syndrome. *Pain Rep*. 2017;2(4):e611. doi:10.1097/PR9.0000000000000611

57. Ellison AG, Jansen LAW, Nguyen F, et al. Specialty psychiatric services in US emergency departments and general hospitals: Results from a nationwide survey. *Mayo Clin Proc.* 2022;97(5):862–870. doi:10.1016/j.mayocp.2021.10.025
58. Hawk K, Hoppe J, Ketcham E, et al. Consensus recommendations on the treatment of opioid use disorder in the emergency department. *Ann Emerg Med.* 2021;78(3):434–442. doi:10.1016/j.annemergmed.2021.04.023
59. Biese K, Lash TA, Kennedy M. Emergency department care transition programs: Value-based care interventions that need system-level support. *JAMA Netw Open.* 2022;5(5):e2213160. doi:10.1001/jamanetworkopen.2022.13160
60. Hiti EA, Tamim H, Makki M, Geha M, Kaddoura R, Obermeyer Z. Characteristics and determinants of high-risk unscheduled return visits to the emergency department. *Emerg Med J.* 2020;37(2):79–84. doi:10.1136/emermed-2018-208343
61. Selby S, Wang D, Murray E, Lang E. Emergency departments as the health safety nets of society: A descriptive and multicenter analysis of social worker support in the emergency room. *Cureus.* 2018;10(9):e3247. doi:10.7759/cureus.32477
62. Gettel CJ, Tinloy B, Nedza SM, et al. The future of value-based emergency care: Development of an emergency medicine MIPS value pathway framework. *J Am Coll Emerg Physicians Open.* 2022;3(2):e12672. doi:10.1002/emp2.12672

34

Pain in Dental Settings and Facial Pain

Sydnee Chavis, Salvador L. Manrriquez, and Marcela Romero Reyes

Introduction: Dental Pain and Vulnerable Populations

Twelve-year-old Deamonte Driver and his younger brother DaShawn both had toothaches for which their mother attempted to seek treatment. Her work did not provide dental insurance, and she had difficulty finding a dentist who accepted Medicaid. The dental office was a bus ride away. She and her children were housing insecure and lived for a time in a homeless shelter, likely contributing to the loss of Medicaid coverage. Deamonte complained of severe headaches, so his mother took him to the local emergency department, where he was diagnosed and given medication for headache, sinusitis, and a tooth abscess. However, Deamonte's condition quickly worsened. He was diagnosed with an odontogenic brain abscess and underwent emergency brain surgery at a local children's hospital. He developed seizures and had a second brain surgery. He died several weeks later, succumbing to the medical consequences of an untreated dental infection.[1–4]

Deamonte Driver's case highlights both the dimensions of vulnerability a patient may experience and how health outcomes are undermined by multiple concomitant vulnerabilities, or risk factors, leading to poor health outcomes and health disparities. In Deamonte's case, these simultaneous vulnerabilities included race/ethnicity (Deamonte was African American), poverty, childhood, housing insecure, geography/transportation problems, lack of health insurance, multimorbidities, and low health literacy.

Deamonte Driver's case also demonstrates several important relationships and several diagnostic and treatment challenges, including how untreated dental infections can lead to pain and more serious medical conditions, including odontogenic brain abscess which led to Deamonte's death at age 12 years. Similarly, a case report describes a 56-year-old male with multimorbidities including an untreated toothache who developed headaches, neck pain, nausea, and vomiting and was diagnosed with an odontogenic brain abscess.[5] Odontogenic brain abscesses have a prevalence of 3–10% of all sources of brain abscess, and although not very common, they begin with symptoms of dental pain.[6–8]

People of vulnerable and underserved populations frequently overlap, and both groups are at risk for health disparities. Vulnerable populations at risk for health disparities include racial/ethnic minorities; children; the elderly; the poor; the uninsured/underinsured; housing insecure/homeless; immigrants; pregnant patients; LGBTQ+ patients; abuse/trauma victims; those with intellectual, developmental, or physical disabilities; and the terminally ill. Other factors contributing to vulnerability that put people at risk for health disparities are multiple comorbidities/high medical complexity; fear or distrust of health care providers, health care systems, and government programs; limited transportation; rural and geographically remote areas; and language/communication difficulties.[9,10]

Facial and dental pain are significant sources of disability and diminished quality of life across the life span in the United States and throughout the world.[11] The prevalence of orofacial pain has been found to range from 1% to 48%, with a median prevalence of 13% from all sources of orofacial pain, including odontogenic origins.[12,13] The mouth is the primary orifice for sustenance, communication, and vitality. As such, both pain deriving from the mouth and pain deriving from the face cause significant interference to daily activities, including eating, speaking, and even breathing.[11,14] Dental, oral, and facial pain have several etiologies, including inflammatory pathologies of the teeth, gums, and other oral structures, sinuses, as well as musculoskeletal, neuropathic, and neurovascular disorders, including primary and secondary headaches. Although the sources of facial and dental pain are often able to be diagnosed by comprehensive examination and evaluation, multiple innervations of oral and facial structures and patterns of referred pain may pose diagnostic challenges.[15] Diagnostic challenges are often exacerbated among vulnerable populations due to concerns with access to care, language barriers, and diagnostic overshadowing.[16] In assessing and addressing facial and dental pain, it is important to consider and address these barriers to obtain a correct diagnosis and appropriate treatment.

Odontogenic Pain

Odontogenic sources are the leading cause of orofacial pain.[13,17] Odontogenic pain is caused by inflammatory conditions such as caries, leading to pulpitis and dental abscesses, periodontal disease, and trauma. Dental caries is the most common chronic disease among children and adults in the United States, with significant disparities across racial, ethnic, and socioeconomic groups.[18] Dental caries that approach and enter the pulp, the neurovascular bundle of the tooth, can cause toothaches, infections including periapical pathology (inflammatory changes to the bone around the root of the tooth), and swelling that can cause excruciating pain (Figure 34.1). Treatment for

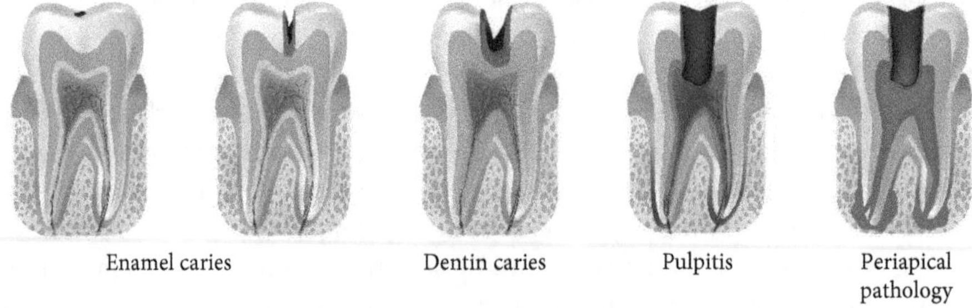

Figure 34.1 Dental caries at different stages of progression into dental tissue
Source: Royalty-free stock vector ID: 1724151628

these teeth requires removal of the instigating pulp via root canal (endodontia) or removal of the instigating tooth via extraction.

Etiologies of Dental Pain

Dental pain predominates from dental caries, but it can also result from periodontal disease and trauma. Caries is an infectious disease that results when lactobacilli and streptococci bacterium within the oral and dental biofilm produce acid and cause physical compromise to the mineral structure of teeth. The outermost enamel layer of teeth, when intact, protects the permeable inner layer of dentin from sensitivity. However, when the enamel layer is compromised by cavitation, the affected tooth can begin to feel sensitive and painful. As the cavitation gets deeper and approaches the neurovascular pulp, the inflammatory response can cause severe pain and progress to infection.

Periodontal disease is the process in which the gingiva (gums) and other supporting structures of the teeth become inflamed. The oral biofilm contains many pathogens that instigate inflammation of the gingiva. Use of substances such as tobacco and alcohol contributes to periodontal disease as well. Utilization of these substances can be higher among vulnerable population.[19] This inflammation can cause discomfort in the early stages, and it also contributes to loosening of teeth and possible infections as it progresses. As continued inflammation causes periodontal disease to worsen, there is more risk for increased pain and loss of oral and dental function.

Dental trauma contributes to approximately 5% of all bodily injuries.[20] Dental trauma can take place secondary to oral pathology, such as a tooth fracturing secondary to caries, or a tooth being lost secondary to periodontal disease. It can also stem from extraoral problems such as falling, sports injuries, or traffic accidents.[20] For people who are at risk for falling, with ambulatory instability, special needs, or diagnoses such as cerebral palsy or epilepsy, dental trauma occurs more frequently.[20–22]

Pain may also manifest in the teeth from etiologies other than dental-specific pathology. Myofascial pain, trigeminal neuropathies, orofacial pains resembling presentations of primary headaches such as neurovascular orofacial pains, and sinus infections are some of the other conditions that can cause pain within the teeth or refer to teeth independently of dental-specific pathology. Although these sources are less common etiologies for dental pain, they still contribute to diminished function and quality of life.

The Impact of Biopsychosocial Constructs in the Dental Pain Patient

The biologic etiologies of dental pain tend to stem from dietary, habits, and hygiene factors, although individual biology, including oral bacterial load, contribute as well. Caries and periodontal disease arise when pathogenic bacteria are unchecked and unmanaged. This often occurs due to a diet high in sugar and processed foods or neglecting to brush, floss, and visit a dentist. These risk factors are more prevalent among vulnerable and underserved populations due to factors such as food deserts, geographic disparities in resources, poor health literacy, poor health care access, and low socioeconomic status. Furthermore, language, insurance, and educational barriers among vulnerable populations cause a higher prevalence of dental disease, infection, and pain.

These contributors to dental pain affect vulnerable populations at a higher rate than the general population.[19] Although inherent biology does not put vulnerable populations at further risk than the general population for dental pain, psychological, social, and societal factors of vulnerable populations further instigate pain. Dental caries impact not only health but also esthetics, self-esteem, and self-efficacy. People with a higher caries rate may have poor-appearing teeth, which negatively impacts their ability to communicate, obtain and hold a job, and engage in healthy habits.[23] They may put off care for longer durations out of shame, fear, or poor access to care.[24] It usually costs more money to save a painful or infected tooth with root canal treatment (endodontics) rather than an extraction, but patients who have root canal treatments report higher quality of life than those who have an extraction.[25] Therefore, vulnerable populations may be a higher risk for losing more teeth than the general population.[24]

Limited education and health literacy can impede people from understanding the need for dental care and hygiene. Among Indigenous and immigrant populations, cultural, language, and familial tropes may not prioritize preventative or active dental care. Among patients with special needs, the reliance on others for oral care, potential intolerance to oral care and dental treatment, and potential inability to verbalize or directly communicate discomfort or pain can lead to the progression of disease and onset of severe pain.

Due to the chasm between medical and dental care, dental disease is often overlooked or undiagnosed in a medical setting. Diagnostic overshadowing, which is the attribution of maladaptive behaviors to psychiatric issues as opposed to pain or other physiologic issues, is prevalent among vulnerable and underserved populations. Dental pain can be a prominent source of behavioral changes, especially among patients with special needs and intellectual and developmental disabilities.[26] Therefore, due to the difficulty in diagnosing dental pain, whether it is because of poor access to care or the inherent intimate and invasive nature of dental diagnosis and treatment, dental pain is more readily overlooked as the source of maladaptive social or psychological signs. All of these factors contribute to the poor oral health among people from vulnerable and underserved populations, and the cycle of poor oral health status and outcomes perpetually leads to more and worse pain within these populations.

Orofacial Pain

Epidemiological studies have shown a 17–26% prevalence of orofacial pain disorders of nondental origin in the general population, of which 7–11% are chronic disorders.[13,27] These disorders include pain disorders of the mouth, jaw, face, head, and neck and comprise musculoskeletal pains such as occur in the constellation of disorders known as temporomandibular disorders (TMD), craniofacial neuropathic pains including trigeminal neuralgia, and neurovascular disorders. Orofacial pain is the specialty of dentistry involving the diagnosis and the evidence-based management of these disorders.

The most common pain experienced in the orofacial region is dental; however, the pain of these orofacial disorders is of non-odontogenic origin. A common example is that these disorders may resemble a toothache and patients may experience and report pain in their teeth, but the source is not the teeth. This pain may be due to referral from a muscle problem or as a result of a disorder of the peripheral or central nervous system. These disorders may arise from musculoskeletal problems from the temporomandibular joint or muscles of mastication; as a consequence of nerve injury; and even from a primary headache disorder but localized in the orofacial region, such as in the case of orofacial pains resembling primary headache disorders. The complexities of these disorders are supported by their diverse etiologies, pathophysiological mechanisms, and presentations, making the diagnosis a challenge and placing the sufferer at risk of unnecessary dental procedures in attempts to alleviate the pain. Therefore, it is fundamental that the care of these disorders is provided by a skilled dental professional trained and board certified in orofacial pain to provide a diagnosis and management. Moreover, even after a correct diagnosis has been provided, their management could still be challenging. Management usually includes nonpharmacological and pharmacological approaches and a multidisciplinary team approach to management, underscoring the importance of the psychosocial model of care.[28]

The orofacial pain patient possesses a vulnerability intrinsic to the nature of these disorders. Very often, these patients have visited diverse dental and medical professionals in unsuccessful attempts to relieve their pain. One of the primary barriers that this population of patients endure is the lack of recognition of the complexity of these problems, which require medical and dental management, for which advanced specialty training is necessary for diagnosis and evidence-based management. Advanced training in orofacial pain had existed in several dental schools, but it was not until March 2020 that orofacial pain was finally officially recognized by the American Dental Association as a dental specialty. This recognition may enhance the accessibility of quality care for this population of patients, decreasing the significant burden that chronic orofacial pain exerts not only for the sufferer but also within the health service utilization.[29]

Orofacial pain disorders are more prevalent in women.[30] Häggman-Henrikson et al.[31] reported that women are at higher risk of developing orofacial pain disorders, particularly TMD. It has also been reported that the prevalence of these disorders may increase over time. Chronic orofacial pain disorders dramatically affect the quality of life of the sufferer with substantial physical disability and psychological distress,[32] making it difficult to carry out daily life functions such as eating, talking, and tooth brushing; in addition, patients withdraw from social activities, lose days of work, and have poor sleep quality.[30,33,34] Moreover, the majority of patients with orofacial pain also may report pain in other parts of their body and other disorders. TMD have been shown to be comorbid with chronic fatigue, fibromyalgia, irritable bowel syndrome, post-traumatic stress disorder, other affective disorders, and headaches.[35–37] With regard to primary headaches, migraine is the most prevalent primary headache disorder in the TMD population.[38] Together, these comorbidities need to be taken into account during diagnosis and management, emphasizing even more the need for multidisciplinary management and dialogue between different health care providers.

The description of the pain experience is very subjective and personal, and as described above, the source of pain can be different from the site of pain, making the diagnosis even more challenging. These barriers intrinsic to the nature of orofacial pain disorders are more challenging when the patient presents cognitive impairment or dementia. Unfortunately, the literature lacks studies focusing on the orofacial pain diagnosis and care of this population; however, a very important review from Lobbezoo et al.[39] highlighted the imperative need of protocols and well-tested diagnostic tools to aid in the diagnosis of dental and orofacial pain in this population.

The Impact of Biopsychosocial Constructs in the Orofacial Pain Patient

In order to understand and effectively serve the chronic orofacial pain patient, a biopsychosocial framework model is necessary; this model integrates the biology of the disorder (Axis I) and the subjective psychosocial parameters of the individual (Axis II).[40,41] The Orofacial Pain: Prospective Evaluation and Risk Assessment (OPPERA) project developed a model that highlights the biopsychological framework, contributing to the development and chronicity of TMD. The OPPERA model helps clinicians integrate different factors beyond the physiological somatic parameters including psychological, genetic and environmental.[42] Moreover, a critical study by Haviv et al.[28] assessed the impact of chronic orofacial pain conditions on daily life and identified patient and pain profiles that predicted poor outcomes. From these data, they created a "vulnerable patient" profile that identifies the dramatic impact of painful post-traumatic trigeminal neuropathic pain (PTTN). This profile includes the emotional trauma history particularly associated with PTTN and the presence of medical and psychiatric comorbidities. The authors highlighted the need of a multidisciplinary approach, in accordance with the biopsychosocial model, to address patient needs to improve their outcomes.

A very thorough qualitative analysis[17] of the challenges that patients of this population suffer in their daily lives sheds light on each of the constructs of this framework, arranging them in subthemes. The biomedical subthemes included challenges in pain management that also involve perceptions of wanting to "be cured" rather than manage the pain condition; physical symptoms; medication side effects; sensory triggers; and decreased biological functions related to daily living, such as poor oral health and poor nutrition. Subthemes within the psychological construct included depression, anxiety, stress, and the uncertainty of the pain experience. Subthemes within the social construct included social relationships because pain impacts how persons relate with others, their roles and responsibilities, their experience with providers, and the impact of their socioeconomics and access to care.[43]

The careful consideration and integration of all these challenges pleads for individualized care. Unfortunately, the implementation of the biobehavioral model emphasizing the critical role of Axis II has not been optimal because the idea that the biomedical model is sufficient still prevails. Advances highlighting this necessity were implemented in the Diagnostic Criteria for Temporomandibular Disorders (DC/TMD) for Clinical and Research Applications,[44] solidifying Axis II as a core part of all TMD assessments. DC/TMD provides both the researcher and the clinician with methods

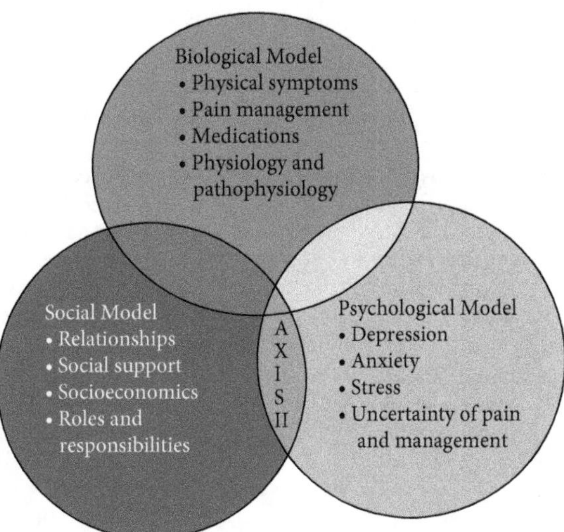

Figure 34.2. The biopsychosocial model of pain management and Axis II psychosocial components of patient assessment and management

to further assess the condition of the individual (Figure 34.2). However, their clinical implementation in the orofacial pain field has not been optimal. To help address these challenges, Sharma et al.[45] have provided a comprehensive assessment of these barriers and recommendations to improve implementation by the International RDC/TMD Consortium Network/International Network for Orofacial Pain and Related Disorders Methodology (INfORM).

The INfORM work group identified five barriers to optimize implementation, which are addressed briefly in Table 34.1.[45] This study emphasized that the stigma of mental health and pain remains pervasive and is reinforced by societal ignorance of the importance of mental health for good physical health. Although pain is recognized as a sensory and emotional experience, the psychological impact of facial and dental pain is generally overlooked in health care. The study also observed that primary care dental settings remain focused on Axis I observable and objective measurements. This focus may lead to many unnecessary and costly referrals and dental treatments such as root canals on teeth that feel painful, despite a non-odontogenic source of pain, underscoring the importance of using the simple, concise assessment tools of Axis II in patient care. These tools need to be adapted in consideration of the target population's culture.

Orofacial pain research is advancing, and orofacial pain has been recognized as a dental specialty. However, the current status of the care for this vulnerable population is in need of a revolution that can start by recognizing that (1) the orofacial pain sufferer needs specialty care and management that go beyond the training of general dentistry; (2) management requires careful individualization and may require multidisciplinary management implementing the Axis II component and addressing comorbid conditions; and (3) it is essential that the health care community in dental and medical settings, at all levels of care, has orofacial pain literacy and access to an orofacial pain specialist for the diagnosis and management of this patient population.

Table 34.1: Brief insights summary of barriers and recommendation for implementation of Axis-II*

Topics	Barriers	Recommendation
1. Society and Culture	• Most Axis-II instruments developed in English • Psychosocial interpretation considering cultural context • Stigma of Pain and mental health	• Need of cultural adaptation and translation of Axis-II instruments for a broader target population • Care giver needs to recognize social rules or cultural influences that may be affecting patient responses
2. Settings	• Integral differences between settings, levels of care and provider types	• Use of simple concise standardized screeners for Axis-II at the primary dental care provider and identify patients who need an orofacial pain referral. • Standardization of instruments and creation of uniform protocols across levels of care in healthcare systems
3. Healthcare Services	• Unclear if Axis-II is used or if its use improves behavioral health and if this is reflected in lower costs • The outcome on income disparity on access to more specialized higher level of care	• Integrate care with psychosocial modalities (Axis-II) • Clarification of costs • Assessment of infrastructure necessary in health services to accommodate Axis-II • Advocacy to support improvement in health coverage
4. Instruments and constructs	• Unknown/lack Axis-II instrument interpretation sensitive enough to capture pain phenomena in different cultures and subcultures	• INfORM workshops with broad cultural representation to assess Axis-II content and cross-cultural applicability
5. Health literacy	• Lack of standardization and education of care providers • Lack of standardization in undergraduate and graduate training • Inadequate education in pain and the biopsychosocial model	• Provide training regarding patient centered outcomes • Improving biopsychosocial model training

Table 1: Brief summary of barriers and recommendation for implementation of Axis-II. Modified from Sharma S, Breckons M, Brönnimann Lambelet B, Chung JW, List T, Lobbezoo F, Nixdorf DR, Oyarzo JF, Peck C, Tsukiyama Y, Ohrbach R. Challenges in the clinical implementation of a biopsychosocial model for assessment and management of orofacial pain. J Oral Rehabil. 2020 Jan;47(1):87-100.

Health Disparities: Underserved Populations and Vulnerable Populations

In 2003, the Institute of Medicine (IOM) released its landmark report, *Unequal Treatment: Confronting Racial and Ethnic Disparities in Health Care.*[46] It defined health care disparities as "racial or ethnic differences in the quality of healthcare that are not due to access-related factors or clinical needs, preferences, and appropriateness of intervention."[46p3] Twenty years after the report's release, racial and ethnic health disparities persist.[47] These include failure to scale the report's recommendations that mitigate structural/institutional racism as a cause of health disparities, according to the report's co-author R. J. Lavisso-Mourey, as well as the fragmentation of the U.S. health care system.[48] IOM's report stated that health care laws and regulations, health systems management, and racial discrimination were significant factors in the persistence of racial/ethnic health disparities.[46] The health disparities definition was subsequently expanded to include socioeconomic status, geography, those with disabilities, women,[49] and LGBTQ+[50] health disparities.

Health disparities are not due to random chance[51] and extend beyond the consequences of an individual's choices.[52] Health disparities result from structural inequities and social determinants of health.[52] Oral health disparities are greatest for low-income populations as well as racial/ethnic minority populations.[53] African Americans, Native Americans/American Indians, Alaskan Natives, and Latinos have greater incidence of oral cancer, orofacial pain, tooth loss, tooth decay, and periodontal disease, yet these groups have limited access to high-quality care to diagnose, treat, or manage their conditions.[53]

Trust is central to the patient–clinician encounter/relationship,[54] but it is fragile and can be eroded by both implicit and explicit biases in health care settings, contributing to poor health outcomes.[54,55] Engagement of vulnerable patients and populations is required to improve their health outcomes. That engagement relies on trust, contributing to the cyclic nature of loss of trust, lack of patient engagement, and poor health outcomes. Rebuilding and maintaining trust from vulnerable patients and populations requires sustained, concerted efforts on several levels: the patient encounter, the health system, and policy factors.

Finally, persistent racial/ethnic health disparities come at a great financial cost. In addition to the health burden caused by racial/ethnic health disparities, these disparities increased direct medical costs by more than 30% to African Americans, Asian Americans, and Latinos: From 2003 to 2006, racial/ethnic health disparities accounted for excess costs of $230 million, and racial/ethnic health disparities and premature death combined accounted for excess costs of $1.24 trillion.[56]

Vulnerable Populations: Specific Considerations

Certain vulnerable populations have specific risks when managing dental pain and/or orofacial pain. For example, during pregnancy, pain management is complex. First-line pain management is acetaminophen, considered the safest analgesic,[57] along with nonpharmacologic treatments such as ice/heat packs[58] and acupuncture/acupressure.[59] In pregnancy, the potential teratogenicity of medication is a major concern.[60] For neuropathic pain during pregnancy, gabapentin (off-label) may be used because data indicate it is not likely to be a major teratogen.[61] Nonsteroidal anti-inflammatory drugs (NSAIDs) in pregnancy must be used with caution because of kidney injury, risk of fetal ductus arteriosus constriction/premature closure (particularly after 32 weeks),[62] and risk of adverse neonatal outcomes.[63] Management of pain during pregnancy should always be done in consultation with the patient's obstetrician–gynecologist.

In pediatric patients with medical complexity such as sickle cell anemia, neurologic conditions, and sleep disorders, pain management may be part of the patient's overall management plan.[64,65] Pain management for pediatric patients in palliative care may include nonpharmacologic integrative management such as acupuncture,[66] massage, music therapy, and creative arts therapy.[67] Children who are nonverbal may show their pain by changes in their behavior, such as increased irritability. History and a thorough examination are particularly important for accurate diagnosis and proper management for nonverbal children and adults.[26]

For patients in oncology treatment, a major issue is polypharmacy and drug–drug interactions.[68] Many cancer patients are on opioids and anti-constipation and anti-nausea medications.[69] Methadone use may cause QT interval prolongation and has been better studied in adults than in pediatric patients.[70] NSAIDs are used in cancer treatment and have shown anticancer effects.[71,72] Nonpharmacologic interventions such as acupuncture, massage, music therapy, and mind–body practice have good data supporting their use in cancer treatment.[73,74]

Pain management concerns for geriatric patients include decreased renal and hepatic function as well as risk of hypotension, altered mental status, and falls.[68]

Strategies for Health Equity

There is a moral, health, and economic imperative to reduce the health disparities of people in vulnerable and underserved groups, including people with dental pain and orofacial pain. Health disparities resulting from patient vulnerabilities are complex, enduring, and vast problems. The research literature provides some strategic directions. For example, strategies for health equity should target specific interventions for health care providers and patients, as well as clinical encounter contextual factors.[75] The Commission on Social Determinants of Health recommends strategies that focus on three fundamental structural issues: "improve daily living conditions"; "tackle the inequitable distribution of power, money, and resources"; and "measure and understand the problem and assess the results of action."[76p1662] These are formidable barriers to change and therein lies the challenge.

There are strategies that can be impactful. For example, robust health literacy education programs are important strategies to reduce health outcome disparities, including for children and adolescents with chronic conditions and comorbid pain, which require health literacy for proper management.[77] Rebuilding trust in the patient–clinician relationship can be achieved through high-quality, patient-centered communication.[71] Finally, although technology can worsen or lessen health disparities based on how it is used, technology alone will not eliminate health disparities.[78]

Health care leadership and policymakers must see value in improving health outcomes for vulnerable populations and as an asset to their health systems, as well as a step in improving our nation's well-being. Health care leaders and policymakers should include in their definition of health system success the improvement of health outcomes for vulnerable people and populations. Developing health outcomes improvement measures for vulnerable populations and publishing results of their implementation strategies will grow the evidence base for improving health outcomes among vulnerable populations.

Reducing health disparities is imperative to improve health outcomes among vulnerable populations, including the management of dental pain and orofacial pain. Focusing on access to care, developing needed medical and dental infrastructure, engaging with people from vulnerable communities to ensure patient-centered care, and improving health outcomes by developing supportive policies that allow vulnerable populations to receive high-quality oral health care will help prevent, minimize, and manage dental pain and orofacial pain. Scaling these strategies to larger populations (nationally, statewide, health system-wide, etc.) will improve health equity, mitigate the disparities in dental disease and orofacial pain conditions, and reduce suffering among people of vulnerable populations.

Conclusion

Dental and facial pain are conditions that cause significant disability and diminished quality of life, more so among vulnerable populations. These conditions can be difficult to diagnose and manage, and they often require collaborative, interdisciplinary care. This care is even more challenging for patients of vulnerable populations who may have difficulties with access to care, whether geographically, financially, behaviorally, or culturally. More consideration should be given to the psychological impact of these conditions and how dental and facial pain diagnoses impact the broader physiology and psychoscial health of patients. Providers should prioritize patient-first, biopsychosocial, whole person care in order to best manage and remedy the effects of dental and facial pain.

References

1. Otto M. For want of a dentist Pr. George's boy dies after bacteria from tooth spread to brain. *The Washington Post.* February 28, 2007. Accessed August 13, 2022. https://www.washingtonpost.com/archive/local/2007/02/28/for-want-of-a-dentist-span-classbankheadpr-georges-boy-dies-after-bacteria-from-tooth-spread-to-brain-span/34055bc4-0986-4ee1-918a-fcfb0b3b541a
2. Edelman, MW. Deamonte Driver's continuing legacy. Children's Defense Fund. March 4, 2011. Accessed August 13, 2022. https://www.childrensdefense.org/child-watch-columns/health/2011/deamonte-drivers-continuing-legacy
3. Tinanoff N, Goodman H, Klein B. The legacy of Deamonte Driver. *J Public Health Dent.* 2022;82(3):251–252. doi:10.1111/jphd.12535
4. Gallagher M. Death from a toothache: The story of Deamonte Driver and where we stand today in ensuring access to dental health care for children in the District. Georgetown Law. March 9, 2018. Accessed August 13, 2022. https://oneill.law.georgetown.edu/death-from-a-toothache-the-story-of-deamonte-driver-and-where-we-stand-today-in-ensuring-access-to-dental-health-care-for-children-in-the-district
5. Clifton TC, Kalamchi S. A case of odontogenic brain abscess arising from covert dental sepsis. *Ann R Coll Surg Engl.* 2012;94(1):e41–e43. doi:10.1308/003588412X13171221499667

6. Carpenter J, Stapleton S, Holliman R. Retrospective analysis of 49 cases of brain abscess and review of the literature. *Eur J Clin Microbiol Infect Dis.* 2007;26(1):1–11. doi:10.1007/s10096-006-0236-6
7. Kao PT, Tseng HK, Liu CP, Su SC, Lee CM. Brain abscess: Clinical analysis of 53 cases. *J Microbiol Immunol Infect.* 2003;36(2):129–136.
8. Menon S, Bharadwaj R, Chowdhary A, Kaundinya DV, Palande DA. Current epidemiology of intracranial abscesses: A prospective 5 year study. *J Med Microbiol.* 2008;57(Pt 10):1259–1268. doi:10.1099/jmm.0.47814-0
9. Waisel DB. Vulnerable populations in healthcare. *Curr Opin Anaesthesiol.* 2013;26(2):186–192. doi:10.1097/ACO.0b013e32835e8c17
10. U.S. Department of Health & Human Services. Serving vulnerable and underserved populations. 2022. Accessed August 27, 2022. https://www.hhs.gov/guidance/sites/default/files/hhs-guidance-documents/vulnerable-and-underserved-populations.pdf
11. Sanders AE, Slade GD, Lim S, Reisine ST. Impact of oral disease on quality of life in the US and Australian populations. *Community Dent Oral Epidemiol.* 2009;37(2):171–181. doi:10.1111/j.1600-0528.2008.00457.x
12. Macfarlane TV, Blinkhorn AS, Davies RM, Kincey J, Worthington HV. Oro-facial pain in the community: Prevalence and associated impact. *Community Dent Oral Epidemiol.* 2002;30(1):52–60. doi:10.1034/j.1600-0528.2002.300108.x
13. Lipton JA, Ship JA, Larach-Robinson D. Estimated prevalence and distribution of reported orofacial pain in the United States. *J Am Dent Assoc.* 1993;124(10):115–121. doi:10.14219/jada.archive.1993.0200
14. Oghli I, List T, Su N, Häggman-Henrikson B. The impact of oro-facial pain conditions on oral health-related quality of life: A systematic review. *J Oral Rehabil.* 2020;47(8):1052–1064. doi:10.1111/joor.12994
15. Quail G. Facial pain: A diagnostic challenge. *Aust Fam Physician.* 2015;44(12):901–904.
16. Evans DD, Gisness C. Managing dental pain in the emergency department: Dental disparities with practice implications. *Adv Emerg Nurs J.* 2013;35(2):95–102. doi:10.1097/TME.0b013e31828f701e
17. Shetty A, James L, Nagaraj T, Abraham M. Epidemiology of orofacial pain: A retrospective study. *J Adv Clin Res Insights.* 2015;2:12–15. doi:10.15713/ins.jcri.34
18. Bagramian RA, Garcia-Godoy F, Volpe AR. The global increase in dental caries: A pending public health crisis. *Am J Dent.* 2009;22(1):3–8.
19. Northridge ME, Kumar A, Kaur R. Disparities in access to oral health care. *Annu Rev Public Health.* 2020;41:513–535. doi:10.1146/annurev-publhealth-040119-094318
20. Zaleckiene V, Peciuliene V, Brukiene V, Drukteinis S. Traumatic dental injuries: Etiology, prevalence and possible outcomes. *Stomatologija.* 2014;16(1):7–14.
21. Ferreira MCD, Guare RO, Prokopowitsch I, Santos MTBR. Prevalence of dental trauma in individuals with special needs. *Dent Traumatol.* 2011;27(2):113–116. doi:10.1111/j.1600-9657.2010.00961.x
22. Silveira ALNMS, Magno MB, Soares TRC. The relationship between special needs and dental trauma: A systematic review and meta-analysis. *Dent Traumatol.* 2020;36(3):218–236. doi:10.1111/edt.12527
23. Watt RG. Emerging theories into the social determinants of health: Implications for oral health promotion. *Community Dent Oral Epidemiol.* 2002;30(4):241–247. doi:10.1034/j.1600-0528.2002.300401.x
24. Elani HW, Batista AFM, Thomson WM, Kawachi I, Chiavegatto Filho ADP. Predictors of tooth loss: A machine learning approach. *PLoS One.* 2021;16(6):e0252873. doi:10.1371/journal.pone.0252873
25. Wigsten E, Kvist T, Jonasson P, et al. Comparing quality of life of patients undergoing root canal treatment or tooth extraction. *J Endod.* 2020;46(1):19–28.e1. doi:10.1016/j.joen.2019.10.012
26. Dubois A, Capdevila X, Bringuier S, Pry R. Pain expression in children with an intellectual disability. *Eur J Pain Lond Engl.* 2010;14(6):654–660. doi:10.1016/j.ejpain.2009.10.013

27. Benoliel R, Birman N, Eliav E, Sharav Y. The International Classification of Headache Disorders: Accurate diagnosis of orofacial pain? *Cephalalgia*. 2008;28(7):752–762. doi:10.1111/j.1468-2982.2008.0186.x
28. Haviv Y, Zini A, Etzioni Y, et al. The impact of chronic orofacial pain on daily life: The vulnerable patient and disruptive pain. *Oral Surg Oral Med Oral Pathol Oral Radiol*. 2017;123(1):58–66. doi:10.1016/j.oooo.2016.08.016
29. Shephard MK, Macgregor EA, Zakrzewska JM. Orofacial pain: A guide for the headache physician. *Headache*. 2014;54(1):22–39. doi:10.1111/head.12272
30. Sharav Y, Benoliel R. *Orofacial Pain and Headache*. Elsevier; 2008.
31. Häggman-Henrikson B, Liv P, Ilgunas A, et al. Increasing gender differences in the prevalence and chronification of orofacial pain in the population. *Pain*. 2020;161:1768–1775. doi:10.1097/j.pain.0000000000001872
32. Bäck K, Hakeberg M, Wide U, Hange D, Dahlström L. Orofacial pain and its relationship with oral health-related quality of life and psychological distress in middle-aged women. *Acta Odontol Scand*. 2020;78(1):74–80. doi:10.1080/00016357.2019.1661512
33. Almoznino G, Benoliel R, Sharav Y, Haviv Y. Sleep disorders and chronic craniofacial pain: Characteristics and management possibilities. *Sleep Med Rev*. 2017;33:39–50.
34. Almoznino G, Zini A, Zakuto A, et al. Oral health-related quality of life in patients with temporomandibular disorders. *J Oral Fac Pain Headache*. 2015;29:231–241.
35. Aaron LA, Burke MM, Buchwald D. Overlapping conditions among patients with chronic fatigue syndrome, fibromyalgia, and temporomandibular disorder. *Arch Intern Med*. 2000;160:221–227.
36. Türp JC, Kowalski CJ, Stohler CS. Temporomandibular disorders: Pain outside the head and face is rarely acknowledged in the chief complaint. *J Prosthet Dent*. 1997;78:592–595.
37. Hoffmann RG, Kotchen JM, Kotchen TA, Cowley T, Dasgupta M, Cowley AW Jr. Temporomandibular disorders and associated clinical comorbidities. *Clin J Pain*. 2011;27:268–274.
38. Franco AL, Goncalves DA, Castanharo SM, Speciali JG, Bigal ME, Camparis CM. Migraine is the most prevalent primary headache in individuals with temporomandibular disorders. *J Orofac Pain*. 2011;24:287–292.
39. Lobbezoo F, Weijenberg RA, Scherder EJ. Topical review: Orofacial pain in dementia patients: A diagnostic challenge. *J Orofac Pain*. 2011;25:6–14.
40. Durham J, Raphael KG, Benoliel R, Ceusters W, Michelotti A, Ohrbach R. Perspectives on next steps in classification of oro-facial pain: Part 2. Role of psychosocial factors. *J Oral Rehabil*. 2015;42:942–955.
41. Penlington C, Ohrbach R. Biopsychosocial assessment and management of persistent orofacial pain. *Oral Surg*. 2020;13:349–357.
42. Slade GD, Fillingim RB, Sanders AE, et al. Summary of findings from the OPPERA prospective cohort study of incidence of first-onset temporomandibular disorder: Implications and future directions. *J Pain*. 2013;14(12 Suppl):T116–T124. doi:10.1016/j.jpain.2013.09.010
43. Lovette BC, Bannon SM, Spyropoulos DC, Vranceanu AM, Greenberg J. "I still suffer every second of every day": A qualitative analysis of the challenges of living with chronic orofacial pain. *J Pain Res*. 2022;15:2139–2148.
44. Schiffman E, Ohrbach R, Truelove E, et al. Diagnostic criteria for temporomandibular disorders (DC/TMD) for clinical and research applications: Recommendations of the International RDC/TMD Consortium Network and Orofacial Pain Special Interest Group. *J Oral Fac Pain Headache*. 2014;28:6–27.
45. Sharma S, Breckons M, Brönnimann Lambelet B, et al. Challenges in the clinical implementation of a biopsychosocial model for assessment and management of orofacial pain. *J Oral Rehabil*. 2020;47:87–100.
46. Smedley BD, Stith AY, Nelson AR, eds. *Unequal Treatment: Confronting Racial and Ethnic Disparities in Health Care*. National Academies Press; 2003. doi:10.17226/12875

47. Williams DR, Cooper LA. Reducing racial inequities in health: Using what we already know to take action. *Int J Environ Res Public Health.* 2019;16(4): Article 606. doi:10.3390/ijerph16040606
48. McFarling UL. Special report: Health Equity—20 years ago, a landmark report spotlighted systemic racism in medicine. Why has so little changed? STAT. February 23.2022. Accessed August 13, 2022. https://www.statnews.com/2022/02/23/landmark-report-systemic-racism-medicine-so-little-has-changed
49. SteelFisher GK, Findling MG, Bleich SN, et al. Gender discrimination in the United States: Experiences of women. *Health Serv Res.* 2019;54(Suppl 2):1442–1453. doi:10.1111/1475-6773.13217
50. Macapagal K, Bhatia R, Greene GJ. Differences in healthcare access, use, and experiences within a community sample of racially diverse lesbian, gay, bisexual, transgender, and questioning emerging adults. *LGBT Health.* 2016;3(6):434–442. doi:10.1089/lgbt.2015.0124
51. Starfield B. Equity and health: A perspective on nonrandom distribution of health in the population. *Rev Panam Salud Publica.* 2002;12(6):384–387. doi:10.1590/s1020-49892002001200004
52. National Academies of Science, Engineering, and Medicine. *Communities in Action: Pathways to Health Equity.* National Academies Press; 2017.
53. Henshaw MM, Garcia RI, Weintraub JA. Oral health disparities across the life span. *Dent Clin North Am.* 2018;62(2):177–193. doi.org/10.10.16/j.cden.2017.12.001
54. Mack JW, Kang TI. Care experiences that foster trust between parents and physicians of children with cancer. *Pediatr Blood Cancer.* 2020;76(11):e28399. doi:10.1002/pbc.28399
55. Dovido JF, Penner LA, Albrecht TL, Norton WE, Gaertner SL, Shelton JN. Disparities and distrust: The implications of psychological processes for understanding racial disparities in health and health care. *Soc Sci Med.* 2008 Aug;67(3):478–486. doi:10.1016/j.socscimed.2008.03.019
56. LaViest TA, Gaskin D, Richard P. Estimating the economic burden of racial health inequalities in the United States. *Int J Health Serv.* 2011;41(2):231–238. doi:10.2190/HS.41.2.c
57. Toda K. Is acetaminophen safe in pregnancy? *Scand J Pain.* 2017;17:445–446. doi:10.1016/j.sjpain.2017.09.007
58. Ganji Z, Shirvani MA, Rezaei-Abhari F, Danesh M. The effect of intermittent local heat and cold on labor pain and child birth outcome. *Iran J Nurs Midwifery Res.* 2013;18(4):298–303.
59. Smith CA, Collins CT, Levett KM, et al. Acupuncture or acupressure for pain management during labour. *Cochrane Database Syst Rev.* 2020;2(2):CD009232. doi:10.1002/14651858.CD009232.pub2
60. Niederhoff H, Zahradnik HP. Analgesics during pregnancy. *Am J Med.* 1983;75(5A):117–120. doi:10.1016/0002-9343(83)90242-5
61. Black E, Khor KE, Kennedy D, et al. Medication use and pain management in pregnancy: A critical review. *Pain Pract.* 2019;19(8):875–899. doi:10.1111/papr.12814
62. Schoenfeld A, Bar Y, Merlob P, Ovadia Y. NSAIDs: Maternal and fetal considerations. *Am J Reprod Immunol.* 1992;28(3–4):141–147. doi:10.1111/j.1600-0897.1992.tb00777.x
63. Zafeiri A, Raja EA, Mitchell RT, Hay DC, Bhattacharya S, Fowler PA. Maternal over-the-counter analgesics use during pregnancy and adverse perinatal outcomes: Cohort study of 151 141 singleton pregnancies. *BMJ Open.* 2022;12(5):e048092. doi:10.1136/bmjopen-2020-048092
64. Landry BW, Fischer PR, Driscoll SW, et al. Managing chronic pain in children and adolescents: A clinical review. *PM R.* 2015;7(11 Suppl):S295–S315. doi:10.1016/j.pmrj.2015.09.006
65. Danzig JA, Katz EB. Musculoskeletal and skin considerations in children with medical complexity: Common themes and approaches to management. *Curr Probl Pediatr Adolesc Health Care.* 2021;51(9):101074. doi:10.1016/j.cppeds.2021.101074
66. Tsai SL, Reynoso E, Shin DW, Tsung JW. Acupuncture as a nonpharmacologic treatment for pain in a pediatric emergency department. *Pediatr Emerg Care.* 2021;37(7):e360–e366. doi:10.1097/PEC.0000000000001619

67. Hall M, Bifano SM, Leibel L, Golding LS, Tsai SL. The elephant in the room: The need for increased integrative therapies in conventional medical settings. *Child Basel Switz.* 2018;5(11): Article 154. doi:10.3390/children5110154
68. Blower P, de Wit R, Goodin S, Aapro M. Drug–drug interactions in oncology: Why are they important and can they be minimized? *Crit Rev Oncol Hematol.* 2005;55(2):117–142. doi:10.1016/j.critrevonc.2005.03.007
69. Amaram-Davila J, Davis M, Reddy A. Opioids and cancer mortality. *Curr Treat Options Oncol.* 2020;21(3):22. doi:10.1007/s11864-020-0713-7
70. Piccininni JA, Killinger JS, Hammad HT, Gerber LM, Dayton JD. QT interval prolongation in the pediatric oncologic population on methadone. *J Pediatr Hematol Oncol.* 2020;42(2):e121–e124. doi:10.1097/MPH.0000000000001444
71. Ramos-Inza S, Ruberte AC, Sanmartín C, Sharma AK, Plano D. NSAIDs: Old acquaintance in the pipeline for cancer treatment and prevention—Structural modulation, mechanisms of action, and bright future. *J Med Chem.* 2021;64(22):16380–16421. doi:10.1021/acs.jmedchem.1c01460
72. Zappavigna S, Cossu AM, Grimaldi A, et al. Anti-inflammatory drugs as anticancer agents. *Int J Mol Sci.* 2020;21(7):2605. doi:10.3390/ijms21072605
73. Deng G. Integrative medicine therapies for pain management in cancer patients. *Cancer J.* 2019;25(5):343–348. doi:10.1097/PPO.0000000000000399
74. Eaton LH, Brant JM, McLeod K, Yeh C. Nonpharmacologic pain interventions: A review of evidence-based practices for reducing chronic cancer pain. *Clin J Oncol Nurs.* 2017;21(3 Suppl):54–70. doi:10.1188/17.CJON.S3.54-70
75. Hirsh AT, Hollingshead NA, Ashburn-Nardo L, Kroenke K. The interaction of patient race, provider bias, and clinical ambiguity on pain management decisions. *J Pain.* 2015;16(6):558–568. doi:10.1016/j.jpain.2015.03.003
76. Marmot M, Friel S, Bell R, Houweling TA, Taylor S; Commission on Social Determinants of Health. Closing the gap in a generation: Health equity through action on the social determinants of health. *Lancet.* 2008;372(9650):1661–1669. doi:10.1016/S0140-6736(08)61690-6
77. Rieman L, Lubasch JS, Heep A, Ansmann L. The role of health literacy in health behavior, health service use, health outcomes, and empowerment in pediatric patients with chronic disease: A systematic review. *Int J Environ Res Public Health.* 2021;18(23):12464. https://doi.org/10.3390/ijerph182312464
78. National Academies of Sciences, Engineering, and Medicine. *The Promise and Perils of Digital Strategies in Achieving Health Equity: Workshop Summary.* National Academies Press; 2018. doi:10.17226/23439

Index

For the benefit of digital users, indexed terms that span two pages (e.g., 52–53) may, on occasion, appear on only one of those pages.

Tables, figures, and boxes are indicated by *t*, *f*, and *b* following the page number